Fundamentals of Operative Dentistry

A Contemporary Approach

Fundamentals of Operative Dentistry

A Contemporary Approach

Richard S. Schwartz, DDS

Associate Professor
Department of General Dentistry
The University of Texas Health Science Center at San Antonio
San Antonio, Texas

James B. Summitt, DDS, MS

Associate Professor and Head
Division of Operative Dentistry
Department of Restorative Dentistry
The University of Texas Health Science Center at San Antonio
San Antonio, Texas

J. William Robbins, DDS, MA

Associate Professor
Director, AEGD
Department of General Dentistry
The University of Texas Health Science Center at San Antonio
San Antonio, Texas

ILLUSTRATIONS BY
Jose dos Santos, Jr., DDS, PhD

Associate Professor
Department of Restorative Dentistry
The University of Texas Health Science Center at San Antonio
San Antonio, Texas

Quintessence Publishing Co, Inc

Chicago, Berlin, London, Tokyo, São Paulo, Moscow, Prague, and Warsaw

Library of Congress Cataloging-in-Publication Data

Schwartz, Richard S.
    Fundamentals of operative dentistry : a contemporary approach /
Richard S. Schwartz, James B. Summitt, J. William Robbins ;
illustrations by Jose dos Santos, Jr.
      p.   cm.
    Includes bibliographical references and index.
    ISBN 0-86715-311-3
    1. Dentistry, Operative.   I. Summitt, James B.   II. Robbins, J.
William.   III. Title.
    [DNLM: 1. Dentistry, Operative.   WU 300 S399f 1996]
RK501.S436   1996
617.6'05– –dc20
DNLM/DLC
for Library of Congress   96-20651
                                       CIP

quintessence
books

© 1996 by Quintessence Publishing Co, Inc

Quintessence Publishing Co, Inc
551 North Kimberly Drive
Carol Stream, Illinois 60188

Editor: Elizabeth M. Solaro
Production: Eric S. Przybylski and Timothy M. Robbins
Cover Design: Jennifer A. Sabella

Printed in the United States of America

To my wife, Jeannette, and my daughter, Marni,
who commented that they have spent much of the past year
looking at the back of my head as I worked on this book at the computer
RSS

To my wife, Joanne, and my two children, J.B. and Carrie,
who have supported me throughout this project and many other professional endeavors,
and to three very important teachers in my life, Drs Dave Bales, Bob Cowan, and Aaron Wilson
JBS

To those who encouraged me—my grandfather, L.E. Robbins, DDS,
my uncles, Joe N. Robbins, DDS, Bruce M. Robbins, DDS,
my most important teachers, my parents, William E. Robbins, DDS, and Ina S. Robbins,
and my best friend, my wife, Brenda M. Robbins
JWR

Contents

Preface

Dental educators and practicing dentists have, at times, been slow to respond to advances in dental materials and techniques. Operative dentistry, in particular, has often been influenced more by history and tradition than by science. Until recently, many restorative procedures taught in dental schools and practiced by dentists were based primarily on Dr G. V. Black's classic textbook, *A Work on Operative Dentistry,* published in 1908. The many advances in materials and instrumentation, linked with the development of reliable dental adhesives, have allowed us to modify many of Black's original concepts to more conservative, tooth-preserving procedures and to offer a much wider range of restorative options. Black was, indeed, one of dentistry's greatest innovators and original thinkers. Were he alive today, he would be leading the advance of new technology and innovation. We best honor his memory, not by clinging to concepts of the past, but rather by looking to scientific innovations of recent years and incorporating them in our practices and dental school curricula.

This textbook is about contemporary operative dentistry. It is a blend of traditional, time-proven methods and recent scientific developments. Whereas preparations for cast-gold restorations have changed relatively little over the years, preparations for amalgam and resin composite restorations are smaller and require removal of less sound tooth structure because of the development of adhesive technologies. While we still use many luting agents in the traditional manner, adhesive cements can provide greater retention for cast restorations and allow us to expand the use of ceramic and resin composite materials. Many concepts of caries management and pulpal protection have changed drastically in recent years. It is our hope that this textbook, which represents an ardent effort to present current concepts in restorative and preventive dentistry, will be helpful to

students, educators, and practicing dentists during this period of rapidly developing technologies.

Several themes echo throughout this textbook. The first is the attempt to provide a scientific basis for the concepts described. The authors of this book are all active clinically and engaged in clinical and laboratory research in the areas of restorative dentistry and dental materials. The diagnosis and treatment options described are based, whenever possible, on current research findings. When conclusive research is not available, we have attempted to present a consensus founded on a significant depth of experience and informed thought.

A second theme reflected in the book is our commitment to conservative dentistry. The treatment modalities described involve the maintenance of as much sound tooth structure as possible within the framework of the existing destruction and the patient's expectations for esthetic results. When disease necessitates a restoration, it should be kept as small as possible. When an extensive amount of tooth structure has been destroyed and remaining cusps are significantly weakened, occlusal coverage with a restoration may be considered the most conservative treatment. When portions of axial tooth surfaces are healthy, their preservation is desirable. In the conservative philosophy on which this book is based, a complete-coverage restoration (complete crown) is generally considered to be the least desirable treatment alternative.

The book describes techniques for the restoration of health, function, and esthetics of individual teeth and of the dentition as a whole. Included are descriptions of direct conservative and conserving restorations fabricated from dental amalgam, resin composite, and resin ionomer restorative materials. Also detailed are techniques for partial- or complete-coverage indirect restorations of gold alloy, porcelain, ceramometal, and resin composite. Current concepts of nonsurgical caries management and remineralization are discussed. Another common theme running throughout the work is the preservation of pulpal and periodontal health.

Our objective in producing this textbook is to bring to students and practitioners current and practical concepts of preventive and restorative dentistry that will allow them to serve their patients well. Our wish for all readers is that they will experience exhilaration, enjoyment, and a sense of abiding pride in bringing excellent preventive and restorative dentistry services to their patients.

Special acknowledgment goes to another of dentistry's great leaders, Dr Miles R. Markley, of Denver, Colorado, whom we regard as the father of conservative dentistry. His conservative philosophy dates from the beginning of his practice of dentistry in the early 1930s. His philosophies of prevention and conservative treatment of dental disease have affected each author of this book. In 1992, one of the authors was able to examine 20 of Dr Markley's patients who had been under his care since the 1930s and 1940s. In that time, among all of those patients, only one tooth had been lost. All the patients gave Dr Markley full credit for maintaining their healthy dentitions for those many years. All clinicians should practice dentistry with the same commitment, concern, and scientific basis as Dr Markley.

Contributors

Thomas G. Berry, DDS, MA
Professor and Chairman
Department of Restorative Dentistry
The University of Texas Health Science Center
    at San Antonio
San Antonio, Texas

John O. Burgess, DDS, MS
Associate Professor
Department of Restorative Dentistry
The University of Texas Health Science Center
    at San Antonio
San Antonio, Texas

Daniel C.N. Chan, DDS, MS
Assistant Professor
Department of Restorative Dentistry
The University of Texas Health Science Center
    at San Antonio
San Antonio, Texas

Robert L. Cooley, DMD, MS
Associate Professor
Department of General Dentistry
The University of Texas Health Science Center
    at San Antonio
San Antonio, Texas

Richard D. Davis, DDS
Colonel, U.S. Air Force Dental Corps
Keesler Air Forse Base
Biloxi, Mississippi

Dennis J. Fasbinder, DDS
Clinical Associate Professor
Director, AEGD
Department of Cariology, Restorative Sciences and
    Endodontics
The University of Michigan School of Dentistry
Ann Arbor, Michigan

Sonia Gladys, DDS
Research Associate
Department of Operative Dentistry and Dental
    Materials
School of Dentistry
Catholic University of Leuven
Leuven, Belgium

Thomas J. Hilton, DMD
Chief, Dental Investigation Service
Armstrong Laboratory
Colonel, U.S. Air Force Dental Corps
Brooks Air Force Base
San Antonio, Texas

David A. Kaiser, DDS, MSD
Associate Professor
Department of Prosthodontics
The University of Texas Health Science Center
    at San Antonio
San Antonio, Texas

Paul Lambrechts, DDS, PhD
Professor
Department of Operative Dentistry and Dental
    Materials
School of Dentistry
Catholic University of Leuven
Leuven, Belgium

Bart Van Meerbeek, DDS, PhD
Postdoctoral Researcher of the Belgian National Fund
    for Scientific Research
Department of Operative Dentistry and Dental
    Materials
School of Dentistry
Catholic University of Leuven
Leuven, Belgium

Jerry W. Nicholson, DDS, MA
Assistant Professor
Department of Restorative Dentistry
The University of Texas Health Science Center
    at San Antonio
San Antonio, Texas

Jorge Perdigão, DDS, MS, PhD
Associate Professor
Department of Operative Dentistry
School of Dentistry
Instituto Superior de Ciências da Saùde
Monte da Caparica, Portugal

Guido Vanherle, MD, DDS
Professor
Department of Operative Dentistry and Dental
    Materials
School of Dentistry
Catholic University of Leuven
Leuven, Belgium

Biologic Considerations

Jerry W. Nicholson

S uccess in clinical dentistry requires a thorough understanding of the anatomic and biologic nature of the tooth, with its components of enamel, dentin, pulp, and cementum, as well as the supporting tissues of bone and gingiva (Fig 1-1). Dentistry that violates the physical, chemical, and biologic parameters of tooth tissues can lead to premature restorative failure, compromised coronal integrity, recurrent caries, patient discomfort, or even pulpal necrosis. It is only within a biologic framework that the materials, principles, and techniques that constitute operative dentistry are validated. This chapter presents a morphologic and histologic review of tooth tissues with emphasis on the clinical significance for the practice of restorative dentistry.

▇ Enamel

Enamel provides a hard, durable shape for the functions of teeth and a protective cap for the vital tissues of dentin and pulp. Enamel defines esthetics when its pearl-like, opalescent beauty is formed in harmony with the facial features. Much of the art of restorative dentistry comes from efforts to optimize the color, texture, translucency, and form of enamel with synthetic dental materials such as resin composite or porcelain. Although capable of lifelong service, its crystallized mineral makeup and rigidity, as well as stress from occlusion, make enamel vulnerable to acid demineralization (caries), attrition (wear), and fracture (Fig 1-3). Compared to other tissues, mature enamel is unique in that, except for alterations in the dynamics of mineralization, repair or replacement is only possible through dental therapy.

Permeability

At maturity, enamel is about 90% inorganic calcium phosphorous apatite mineral by volume. Enamel also contains a small amount of organic matrix, and 4%–12% water, which is contained in the intercrystalline spaces and in a network of micropores opening to the external surface.[55,90] The micropores form a dynamic connection between the external oral cavity and the systemic, pulpal, and dentinal tubule fluids.[5,156] When teeth become dehydrated, as from nocturnal mouth breathing or rubber dam isolation for dental treatment, the empty micropores make the enamel appear chalky and lighter in color (Fig 1-2). The condition is quickly reversible with a normal "wet" oral environment. Various fluids, ions, and low–molecular weight substances, whether deleterious, physiologic, or therapeutic, can diffuse through the semipermeable enamel. Therefore, the dynamics of acid demineralization,[72,141] caries,[130] reprecipitation or remineralization,[27,30,74] fluoride uptake,[35,93] and vital bleaching therapy[36] are not limited to surface contact but are active in three dimensions.

Gradual coloration and caries resistance are two consequences of lifelong exposure of semipermeable enamel to the gradual ingress of elements from the oral environment into the mineral structure of the tooth. The yellowing of older teeth may be attributed partly to accumulation of trace elements in the enamel structure[36] and perhaps to the sclerosing effect of mature dentin. Surface enamel benefits from incorporation of salivary or toothpaste fluoride to increase the ratio or conversion of hydroxyapatite to larger, more stable crystals of fluorohydroxyapatite or fluoroapatite.[35] Therefore, with aging, color is intensified and acid solubility, pore volume, water content, and permeability of enamel are reduced.[32]

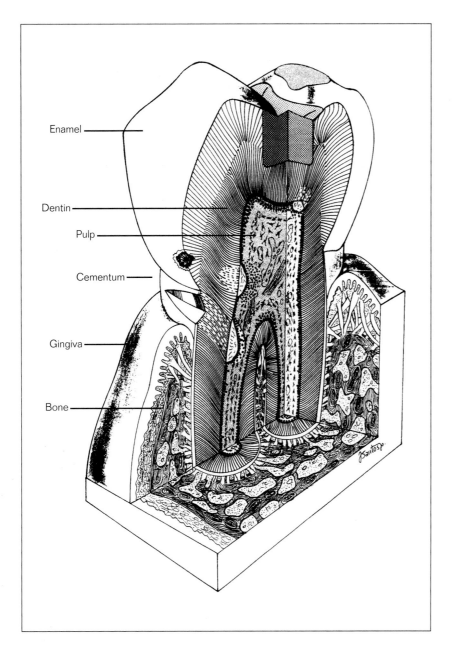

Fig 1-1 Component tissues and supporting structures of the tooth.

Enamel

Dentin

Pulp

Cementum

Gingiva

Bone

Clinical Appearance and Diagnosis

The dentist must pay close attention to the surface characteristics of enamel for evidence of pathologic or traumatic conditions. Key diagnostic signs include color changes associated with demineralization, cavitation, excessive wear, morphologic faults or fissures, and cracks (Fig 1-3).

Color

Enamel is relatively translucent; color is primarily a function of its thickness and the color of the underlying dentin. From 2.5 mm at the cusp tips and 2.0 mm at the incisal edges, enamel thickness decreases significantly below deep occlusal fissures and tapers to a negligible thickness cervically at the junction with the cementum or dentin of the root. Therefore, the young anterior tooth has a translucent gray or slightly bluish enamel tint at the thick incisal edge. A more chromatic yellow-orange shade predominates cervically, where dentin shows through thin enamel. Coincidentally, in about 10% of teeth, a gap between enamel and cementum at this juncture leaves vital, potentially sensitive dentin completely exposed.[92]

Anomalies of development and mineralization, extrinsic stains, antibiotic therapy, and excessive fluoride can

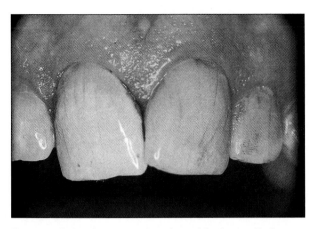

Fig 1-2 Color change resulting from dehydration. Right central incisor isolated by rubber dam for approximately 5 minutes. Color matching should be recorded with full-spectrum lighting before isolation.

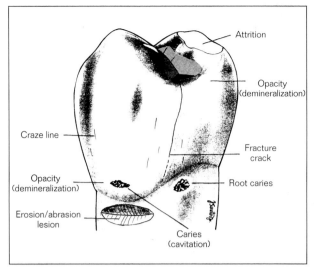

Fig 1-3 Observations of clinical importance on the enamel surface.

alter the natural color of the teeth.[36] However, because caries is the primary disease threat to the dentition, color changes related to enamel demineralization and caries are critical diagnostic observations. The translucency of enamel is directly related to the degree of mineralization. Porosity within the enamel is manifested clinically by milky white opacity. In the later stages of caries, dark subsurface cavitation imparts a blue or gray tint to the overlying enamel. Several authorities have suggested that, unless radiographic evidence of caries exists, invasive restorative procedures or replacement restorations should be initiated only if these visual changes in enamel are apparent.[18,33,98] Smooth surface enamel that is chalky white and roughened from demineralization generally indicates that the patient has inadequate oral hygiene and is at a higher risk for caries.

Cavitation

Unless prevention or remineralization can abort the carious demineralization, dentin is affected until the undermined enamel breaks away to create a "cavity"; a restoration must then be placed. Untreated, the cavitation expands to compromise the structural strength of the crown, and microorganisms infiltrate dentin in depth to jeopardize the vitality of the tooth. When caries extends below the cementoenamel junction (CEJ), or with root caries, isolation, access and gingival tissue response complicate the restorative procedure.

Wear

Enamel is as hard as steel,[25] with a Knoop Hardness Number of 343 (compared with a Knoop Hardness Number of 68 for dentin). However, enamel will wear because of attrition or frictional contact against opposing enamel or even harder restorative materials, such as porcelain. Normal physiologic contact wear for enamel is as much as 29 µm per year.[75] Restorative materials that replace or function against enamel should have compatible wear, smoothness, strength, and esthetics. Heavy occlusal wear is demonstrated when rounded cuspal contacts are ground to flat facets. Depending on factors such as bruxism, other parafunctional habits, malocclusion, age, and diet, cusps may be completely lost and enamel abraded away so that dentin is exposed and occlusal function compromised. However, the effects on vertical dimension from tooth wear may be offset by apical cementogenesis and passive eruption. Cavity outline form should be designed so that the margins of restorative materials avoid critical, high-stress areas of occlusal contact.[19]

Faults and Fissures

Various defects of the enamel surface may contribute to the accumulation and retention of acidic plaque. Perikymata (parallel ridges formed by cyclic deposition of enamel), pitting defects formed by termination of enamel rods, and other hypoplastic flaws are common, espe-

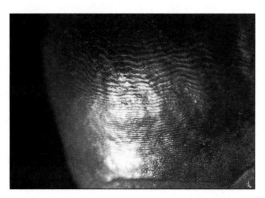

Fig 1-4 Perikymata. Magnified enamel surface morphology at cervical aspect of maxillary molar.

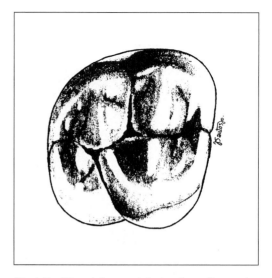

Fig 1-5 Pit and fissure defects of maxillary molar occlusal surface.

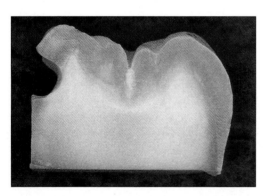

Fig 1-6a Enamel caries in deep occlusal fissure. (Note: defect on external surface is an artifact.)

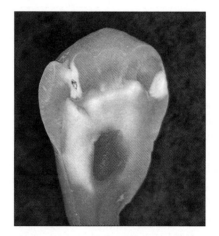

Fig 1-6b Premolar with both occlusal pit and fissure caries (Class 1) extending into the dentin and interproximal smooth-surface caries (Class 2).

cially in the cervical area[37] (Fig 1-4). Limited linear defects or craze lines result from a combination of occlusal loading and age-related loss of resiliency. Organic films of surface pellicle and dendritic cuticles extending 1 to 3 μm into the enamel may play key roles in ion exchange[133] and in adhesion and colonization of bacterial plaque on the enamel surface.[56]

Of greater concern are the fissure systems on the occlusal surfaces of posterior teeth. A deep fissure is often formed by incomplete fusion of lobes of cuspal enamel in the developing tooth.[119] The resulting narrow clefts provide a protected niche for acidogenic bacteria and the organic nutrients they require (Figs 1-5 and 1-6). Because of these fissure faults, 57.7% of total caries (decayed, missing, and filled surfaces) of US schoolchildren occurs on the occlusal surfaces; only 12.0% is found on the mesial and distal surfaces.[158] Altogether, pit and fissure defects are eight times more vulnerable to caries than are smooth surfaces.[56] Careful observation of enamel surrounding fissures for evidence of demineralization or cavitation is necessary to determine the need for restorative intervention.

Fig 1-7 Hydroxyapatite crystals of enamel and dentin. Enamel crystal length may extend the full thickness of enamel. Dentin hydroxyapatite crystals are significantly smaller and thinner, and their surface-to-volume ratio (exposure) is greater.

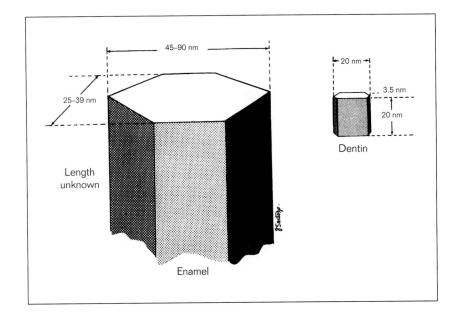

Cracks

Although craze lines in the surface enamel are of little consequence, pronounced cracks that extend from developmental grooves across marginal ridges to axial surfaces may be evidence of an incomplete or impending coronal or cuspal fracture.[1] This is especially noteworthy when the crack extends from the margin of a large restoration or when the patient has pain when chewing. An indication of a cracked tooth will dictate a restoration that provides complete cuspal coverage.[143]

Crystal Structure

Enamel is a mineralized epidermal tissue. The organic matrix gel is first formed and then later partly digested by ameloblastic cells of the developing tooth organ. Calcium and phosphorus in the form of hydroxyapatite are seeded throughout the developing matrix and immediately begin to crystallize, enlarge, and supplant the organic matrix.

The majority of hydroxyapatite crystals, $Ca_{10}(PO_4)_6(OH)_2$, exist in an impure form in which ions or molecules are missing or extrinsic substitutions occur to destabilize the crystal and make it more soluble. An important therapeutic exception is the incorporation of the fluoride ion.[93] In mature enamel, the closely packed, hexagonal crystals are 25 to 39 nm in thickness and 45 to 90 nm in width (Fig 1-7). Crystal length, whether columnar entities of full enamel thickness or segmented units, is yet to be determined.[38] The matrix proteins, enamelins, and water of hydration form a shell, or enve-

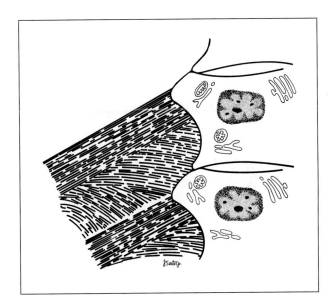

Fig 1-8 Ameloblastic formation of the enamel rod. Crystal orientation varies because crystals form perpendicular to the concave surface of the cell. (Modified from Moss-Salentijn L, Hendricks-Klyvert M. Dental and Oral Tissues, ed 2. Philadelphia: Lea & Febiger, 1985.)

lope, around each crystal. Because the crystals are oriented perpendicular to the concave contours of the secreting ameloblastic cells, the crystal orientation gradually varies by as much as 70 degrees from the center of the cell (corresponding to the core center of the enamel rod) to the periphery[84] (Fig 1-8). The crystal deposition, repeated in symmetric pattern, forms the basic structural units of enamel, the prisms or rods.

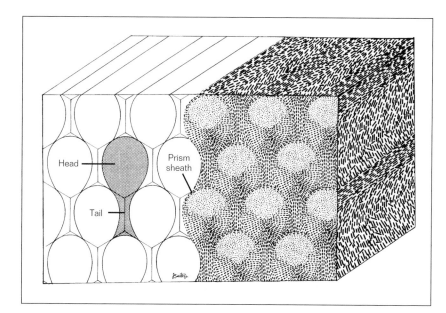

Fig 1-9 Enamel rod. Rod head (core) is formed from the center of a single ameloblast; its crystal direction is essentially parallel to the long axis. A combination of peripheries of several adjacent, hexagonal ameloblasts form the tail or interrod extension with divergent crystal orientation. A nearly perpendicular crystal interface around the rod head periphery results in greater intracrystalline space to form the prism sheath. (Modified from Moss-Salentijn L, Hendricks-Klyvert M. Dental and Oral Tissues, ed 2. Philadelphia: Lea & Febiger, 1985 and several other sources).

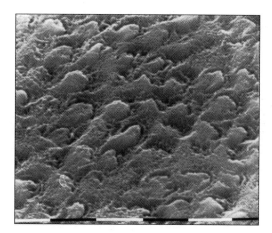

Fig 1-10 Scanning electron microscopic photomicrograph of an acid-etched enamel surface. Note the keyhole-shaped rod and uneven surface formed by the disparity in depth of rod heads and rod peripheries. (Bar = 10 μm.)

Enamel Rods

The enamel rods are described as keyhole or mushroom shaped with a circular core, or head, 4 to 5 μm in diameter in which the long axis of crystals runs approximately parallel to the rod. Cervically, the progressive disinclination of the crystals produced from the boundaries of adjacent ameloblasts forms a fan-shaped tail known as the *interprismatic* or *interrod area* (Fig 1-9). Except for a narrow, highly mineralized aprismatic zone both at the surface and at the dentinoenamel junction (DEJ), each rod runs the full thickness of the enamel. Because each row of rods is offset, the core of each rod is surrounded by the interrod substance of adjacent rods. As a result, the occlusal three fourths of each core boundary is characterized by a junction of crystals meeting at acute angles. This interface, called the *prism sheath*, is unique because of its increased intercrystalline space, location of micropores, and higher amounts of organic matrix.

The spacing and orientation of the crystals and amount of organic matrix make the enamel rod boundary and central core differentially soluble when exposed for a brief time to weak acids. Acid etchants remove about 10 μm of surface enamel and then preferentially dissolve either the prism core or periphery to form a variegated, pitted surface with microporosities greater than 20 μm in depth[53,54,131] (Fig 1-10). The acid-treated enamel surface has a high surface energy, so that resin polymer flows into and intimately adheres to the etched depressions to polymerize and form retentive resin tags.[52] Because there are 30,000 to 40,000 enamel prisms/mm² and the etch penetration increases the bondable surface area 10- to 20-fold, micromechanical bonding of resin restorative materials to enamel is achieved.[12,13] Acid-etch modification of the enamel rod to provide micromechanical retention has provided a conservative, reliable alternative to traditional surgical methods of tooth preparation and restoration.

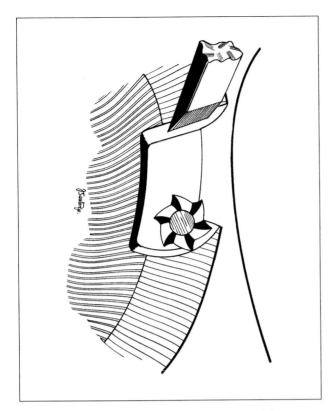

Fig 1-11a Coronal section through interproximal box cavity preparation. Use of a rotary bur, which may leave the proximal wall with an acute enamel angle and undermined enamel, requires careful planing.

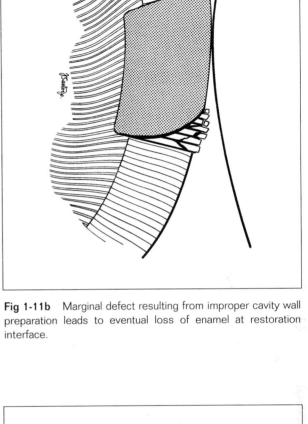

Fig 1-11b Marginal defect resulting from improper cavity wall preparation leads to eventual loss of enamel at restoration interface.

The enamel rod boundaries form natural cleavage lines through which longitudinal fracture may occur. The enamel prisms are especially weakened if the underlying dentinal support is pathologically destroyed or mechanically removed by a dental instrument (Figs 1-11a and 1-11b). Loss of enamel rods where they abut a dental restoration creates an artificial gap defect similar to an occlusal fissure. Leakage or ingress of toxic or bacterial irritants may lead to secondary caries.[67] Therefore, a basic tenet of cavity wall preparation is to bevel or parallel the direction of the enamel rods and to avoid undercutting them.[86]

However, a common precept, that cavity preparations should always be cut perpendicular to the external coronal surface, is not supported histologically. Each successive row of enamel rods runs a slightly different course in a wave pattern, both horizontally and vertically, through the inner half of the enamel thickness and then continues in a relatively straight parallel course to the surface.[32] However, on axial surfaces and cuspal slopes, the path of each row terminates at an oblique angulation rather than at a perpendicular tangent of 90 degrees (Fig 1-12).

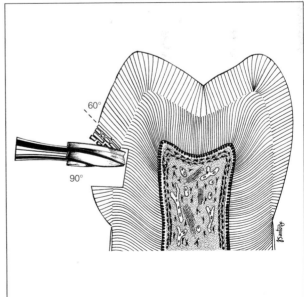

Fig 1-12 Buccal pit preparation of a molar that is cut perpendicular to the external facial, lingual, or approximal surface, would not have occlusal walls oriented with the occlusal direction of the enamel rods.[40]

Starting at 1.0 mm from the CEJ, the rods on the vertical surfaces run occlusally or incisally at a 60-degree inclination and progressively incline approaching the marginal ridges and cusp tips, where the rods are essentially parallel to the long axis of the crown. The rods beneath the occlusal fissures are also parallel to the long axis, but rods on each side of the fissure vary up to 20 degrees from the long axis.[40] Therefore, if cut perpendicular to the external surface, occlusal walls of preparations on axial surfaces might incorporate compromised enamel (Fig 1-12). An oblique enamel-cavosurface angle would more closely parallel the rod direction and preserve the integrity of the enamel margin.

Considering the wide variation in prism direction and the structural damage caused by high-speed eccentric bur rotation, a finishing step of planing the cavosurface margin with hand or low-speed rotary instruments to remove any friable or fragile enamel structure is recommended.

Resilience

Although vulnerable and incapable of self-repair, the protective and functional adaptation of enamel is noteworthy. Although the enamel is almost totally mineralized, carious demineralization, to the point of cavitation, generally takes 3 to 4 years.[115] The apatite crystals in enamel are 10 times larger than those in dentin[132] (see Fig 1-7) and therefore offer less surface-to-volume exposure, and there is very little space between the crystals. With preventive measures and exogenous or salivary renewal of calcium, phosphorus, and especially fluoride, the dynamics of demineralization can be stopped or therapeutically reversed.

Enamel thickness and degree of mineralization are greatest at the occlusal and incisal surfaces where masticatory contact occurs.[23] If enamel were uniformly crystalline, it would shatter with occlusal function. A substructure organized into discrete, parallel rods and a scalloped DEJ minimizes the transfer of occlusal stress laterally and directs it anisotropically or unidirectionally to the resilient dentinal foundation.[135] The interwoven paths and interlocked keyhole morphology of the enamel rods help control lateral cleavage. As a functional adaptation to occlusal stress, the spiraling weave is so pronounced at the cusp tips of posterior teeth that it is referred to as *gnarled enamel*. Finally, the further subdivision of enamel rods into distinct crystals separated by a thin organic matrix provides additional strain relief to help prevent fracture.[8]

Dentin

Function

The coronal (crown) dentin provides an elastic foundation for the brittle enamel. Together with the radicular (root) dentin, which is covered with cementum, dentin forms the bulk of the tooth and a protective encasement for the pulp. As a vital tissue without vascular supply or innervation, it is nevertheless able to respond to thermal, chemical, or tactile external stimuli.

Support

Tooth strength and rigidity are ensured by an intact dentinal substrate. Several investigators have reported that resistance to fracture is significantly lower with increasing depth and/or width of cavity preparation.[7,91,153] A tooth with the deepest possible Class 1 amalgam restoration, restoration of endodontic access, retains only a third of the fracture resistance of a normal tooth.[121] To appreciate the magnitude of occlusal loading, a clenching or bruxing force of 460 N[4] applied to an average tooth contact area of 4 mm^2 yields more than 17,000 psi distributed over about 20 centric contacts.[60] In vitro studies report that large mesio-occlusodistal preparations increase the strain or deflection of facial cusps by three times that of a normal tooth and decrease coronal stiffness by more than 60%.[83,122] Elastic deformation and excessive cuspal flexure are etiologic factors contributing to Class 5 abrasion/erosion lesions,[79] cervical debonding,[59] marginal breakdown,[116] fatigue failure, crack propagation, and fracture.[83] Therefore, to preserve coronal stiffness, a conservative restorative approach is recommended that combines localized removal of caries, placement of a bonded restoration, and placement of sealant. If large preparations are required, the dentist should consider placement of a crown or an onlay.

Morphology

Dentin is composed of inorganic apatite crystals embedded in a cross-linked organic matrix of collagen fibrils. The extended cytoplasmic processes of the formative cells, the odontoblasts, form channels or tubules traversing the full thickness of the tissue. Unlike enamel, which is acellular and predominantly mineralized, dentin is, by

Fig 1-13 Dentin near the DEJ (peripheral) and near the pulp (inner), compared to show relative differences in intertubular and peritubular dentin and their lumen spacing and volume.

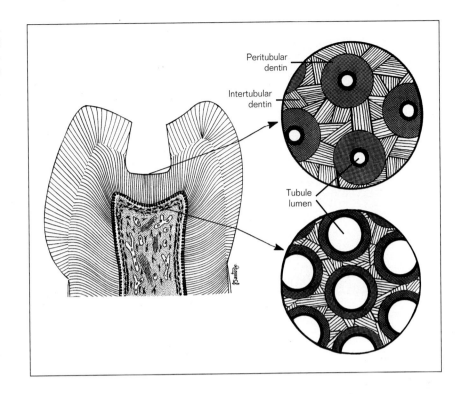

volume, 45-50% inorganic apatite crystals, about 30% organic matrix, and about 25% water. Dentin is pale yellow and slightly harder than bone. Two main types of dentin are present: *(1)* the primary structural component, *intertubular dentin*, the hydroxyapatite-embedded collagen matrix between tubules; and *(2) peritubular dentin*, the collagen-free, hypermineralized tubular wall.[149] The relative and changing proportions of mineralized solid matrix and cellular and fluid-filled tubular volume determine the clinical and biologic response of dentin. These component ratios vary according to depth of dentin, age, and traumatic history of the tooth.

Depth

Peripheral dentin. (Figs 1-13 to 1-15) During formation of dentin, the odontoblastic cells converge from the dentinoenamel junction pulpally, creating a tapered channel surrounding their extended cytoplasmic processes. By secreting precursor collagen, these cells produce and nourish the developing dentinal matrix. At the first-formed dentin near the DEJ, the tubules of the peripheral dentin are relatively far apart and the intertubular dentin makes up 96% of the surface area.[109] Although the tubules are 0.8 µm in diameter and consti-

tute about 4% of the surface area of peripheral dentin, there are as many as 20,000 tubules/mm².[47] In addition, there is extensive terminal branching of the tubules in the peripheral dentin along with regularly spaced connections, or canaliculi, between tubules, so that the cellular processes make up a highly interconnected system.[103] This structure may account for the paradox that superficial dentin, furthest from the pulpal nerve receptors, is more sensitive than is deeper dentin, even to a stimulus as localized as an explorer tip.

Inner dentin. The dentinal substrate near the pulp is quite different from that near the DEJ; these differences affect the permeability and bonding characteristics of the inner dentin. The formative odontoblast cells converge concentrically to terminate in a single, tightly packed layer at the wall of the pulp chamber. The distance between tubule centers within the inner dentin is half that of tubules at the DEJ. Thus, deep dentin may have as many as 65,000 tubules/mm² of dentin. The intertubular matrix area is only 12% of the surface area, and tubule diameters are greater, 2.5 to 3.0 µm.[42,47,149] Estimates of volume occupied by tubule lumens at the inner or predentin level vary but range up to 80%.[47,90] As a result, the dentin close to the pulp is about eight times more permeable than dentin near the DEJ.[106]

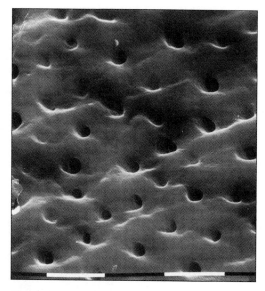

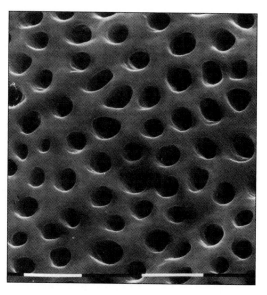

Fig 1-14a Scanning electron miscroscopic photomicrograph of tubules in peripheral dentin. All highly mineralized peritubular dentin has been removed in the specimen preparation. (Bar = 10 μm.)

Fig 1-14b Scanning electron miscroscopic photomicrograph of inner dentin. Compare to Fig 1-14a. All highly mineralized peritubular dentin has been removed in the specimen preparation. (Bar = 10 μm.)

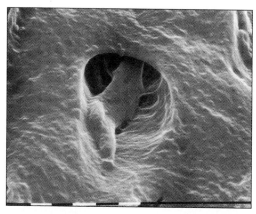

Fig 1-14c Magnified tubule orifice with collagen matrix of intertubular border and odontoblastic process. (Bar = 1.0 μm.)

Fig 1-15 Odontoblastic cell, process, and tubule system through dentinal thickness. Continual deposition of peritubular dentin and minerals, accelerated by a chronic, noxious stimulus, gradually occludes the tubules peripherally. Note terminal branching and interconnections between odontoblastic cell processes and between cellular walls. Direct neural penetration of dentin is limited to less than 20% of the tubules, and then, rarely beyond the predentin. (Modified from Avery JK. Oral Development and Histology. Baltimore: Williams & Wilkins, 1987.)

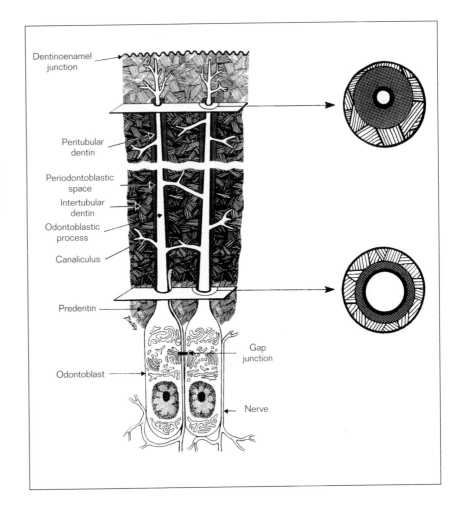

Permeability

The permeability of dentin is directly related to its protective function (Fig 1-16). When the external "cap" of enamel or cementum is lost from the periphery of the dentinal tubules through caries, preparation with burs, or abrasion and erosion, the exposed tubules become conduits between the pulp and the external oral environment. Restored teeth are also at risk of toxic seepage through the phenomenon of microleakage between the restorative material and the cavity wall. No restorative material can provide a completely hermetic seal against the cavity wall.[6] Gaps of 10 µm or more exist between newly placed amalgam and cavity walls,[16] and increased leakage at the cemental margins of resin-bonded restorations is commonly reported (Figs 1-17a and 1-17b).

Through capillary action, differential thermal expansion, and diffusion, fluids containing various acidic and bacterial products can penetrate the gap and initiate demineralization and secondary caries of the internal cavity walls.[66,67] From this base, bacterial substances can continue by diffusion through permeable dentinal tubules to reach the pulp. Conduits to the external oral environment amount to a pulpal exposure, putting the tooth at risk for pulpal inflammation and sensitivity.[10,21,110] Dentinal depth, the remaining dentinal thickness, is the key determinant of the diffusion gradient.[106,110] Restorative techniques that incorporate varnishes, liners, or dentin bonding resin adhesives are effective to the extent to which they provide reliably sealed margins and a sealed dentinal surface.

Sensitivity

Although sensitive to thermal, tactile, chemical, and osmotic stimuli across its 3.0- to 3.5-mm thickness, dentin is neither vascularized nor innervated, except for about 20% of tubules that have nerve fibers penetrating the layer of inner dentin by no more than a few microns. Therefore, attention has been focused on the odontoblast and its process as a possible stimulus receptor.

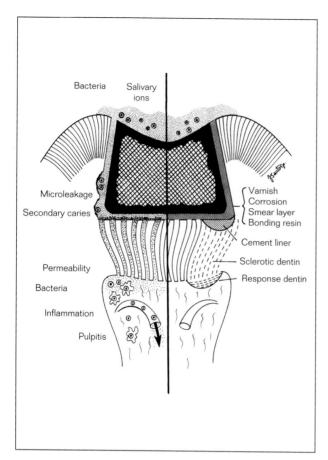

Fig 1-16 Microleakage is exacerbated by polymerization shrinkage, condensation gaps around the restorative material, and/or differences in thermal expansion. When microleakage is present, the tubule openings in dentin form a potential pathway between the oral environment and the pulp. Various restorative materials together with the tooth's defenses of tubule sclerosis and reparative dentin mitigate the noxious infiltration.

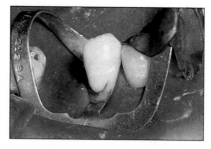

Fig 1-17a Failed resin composite restoration. Polymerization shrinkage and cervical debonding created a margin-wall gap defect, leading to microleakage and secondary caries.

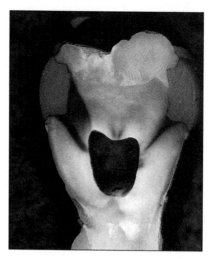

Fig 1-17b In vitro dye penetration reveals of microleakage and dentinal diffusion.

However, although the peripheral dentin is acutely sensitive, neither electron microscopy nor new research technologies have yet settled the question of whether the odontoblastic cellular process extends to the peripheral DEJ in mature dentin.[14,129,149] Nonetheless, the cell membrane of odontoblasts is nonconductive, and there is no synaptic connection between the odontoblastic cell and the adjacent terminal branches of the pulpal nerve plexus. Finally, pain sensation remains even when the odontoblastic layer is disrupted.[150]

Brännström et al[9] proposed a theory based on the capillary flow dynamics of the fluid-filled dentinal tubules (Fig 1-18). Tubular fluid flow of 4 to 6 mm/s is produced by application of stimuli, such as air evaporation, cold, or heat (ie, generated from a dental bur), osmotic stimuli such as contact with sugar-rich fluids, or tactile pressure. The "current," or hydrostatic pressure, displaces the odontoblastic cell bodies and stretches the intertwined terminal branches of the nerve plexus to allow entry of sodium and depolarization. Evidence supporting the hydrodynamic theory includes in vivo confirmation of tubule patency in hypersensitive roots.[26] Also, Ahlquist et al[3] correlated intensity of pain with rapid hydrostatic pressure changes applied to the sealed, smear-free dentinal axial wall of cavity preparations. Therefore, the knowledge that permeable dentin is sensitive dentin may help the dentist avert postoperative discomfort associated with tooth preparation.[3]

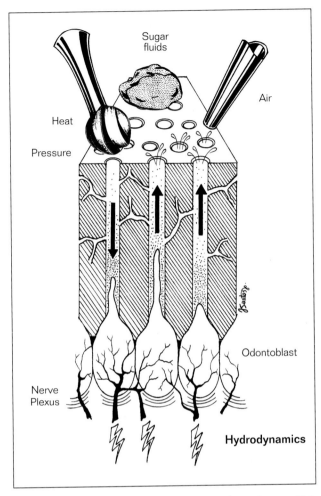

Fig 1-18 A hydrodynamic phenomenon explains the sensitivity of dentin, which is without significant innervation. Fluid dynamics of the tubules move the odontoblastic cell bodies and mechanically depolarize approximating nerve endings

Substrate for Bonding

Early attempts to bond resins to etched dentin were relatively unsuccessful because of the variability of the dentinal substrate, the hydrolytic deterioration of the bonding agents, or interference with the smear layer, a tenacious, semipermeable film of organic debris on the prepared dentinal surface. The newer dentin bonding systems remove the smear layer to penetrate the exposed collagen fibrils, etch up to a 5.0-μm depth of the intertubular dentinal surface, and demineralize the peritubular walls. Hydrophilic bonding resin then forms a limited-depth interdiffusion or hybrid zone of micromechanical bonding between the restorative resin composite and the dentin.[95,154]

Deeper levels of dentin offer an altogether different substrate for bonding that is wetter and less solid (see Figs 1-13 to 1-15). A positive pulpal pressure of 11 mm Hg creates an outward flow of dentinal tubular fluid.[112] The functional lumen of the uncut dentinal tubule, constricted by the cellular process, mineral deposits, and intertubular collagen, provides a resistance to flow. When dentin is cut at deeper levels, flow is unimpeded, and the dentinal surface becomes wet, which can interfere with the adhesion of hydrophobic resin polymers. Not all bonding systems are equally effective in both deep and peripheral dentin.[34,114,117]

Another substrate variable that reduces bond strength is excessive sclerosis or hypermineralization, indicated by a deeper yellow color and glossy surface of exposed dentin. Aging and response to external stimuli are associated with tubule occlusion through continued mineralization.[88] These conditions are typical of long-standing root surface abrasion/erosion lesions.[29,155]

Physiologic Dentin

Primary dentin is formed at a relatively fast pace until root formation is completed; then the odontoblasts become relatively quiescent. After this, the slowly formed dentin that continues to constrict the dimensions of the pulp chamber is termed *secondary dentin*. The morphology of the pulp chamber approximates the external tooth contours, but pronounced extensions, or pulp horns, into buccal cusps of premolars and mesiobuccal cusps of molars must be carefully avoided during cavity preparation in young teeth to prevent exposure. Perhaps in response to a mild occlusal stimulus, secondary dentin is preferentially deposited in the pulp horns and on the roof and floor of the pulp chamber so that, after many decades, the chamber becomes quite narrow occlusogingivally.[119] The dentist must allow for the size and location of the pulp chamber, for it may be a deciding factor in the design of the preparation and placement of retentive features, such as pins.

Another physiologic or age-related process, perhaps mediated by the odontoblastic process, is the continual mineralization of tubule walls (see Fig 1-15). As a result, the peritubular dentinal wall progressively thickens and occludes the tubule lumen. Deposition of both peritubular and secondary dentin is considered physiologic, because reduction of the pulp chamber is found in unerupted teeth, and sclerosis is reported in radicular dentin in the premolars of 18-year-olds.[149] However, with sufficient external stimulus or irritation, the rate of sclerosis or deposition of added dentin can be accelerated proportionally.

Sclerotic Dentin

Accelerated closure of the tubules protects the pulp by rendering the dentin less subject to the effects of external stimuli, such as attrition, abrasion, caries, or operative procedures. As many as one in seven adult patients suffer from hypersensitivity of exposed root surfaces,[50] which is directly correlated with open dentinal tubules. Treatment modalities close the tubules, either by sealing the tubule orifice with bonded resin or by precipitating intratubular protein or crystals with application of fluoride or potassium nitrate compounds to the root surface.[46,125] When dentin is suddenly exposed by fracture or a lost restoration, plasma proteins are transported to the exposed tubules. Within 6 to 24 hours, a fibrin-like intratubular clot forms to constrain the hydrodynamic flow and diminish sensitivity.[108]

With initial enamel caries or microleakage, the outward flow of the dentinal fluid under positive pulpal pressure counteracts pulpal diffusion of endotoxins and acids.[112] As caries progresses, immunoglobulins are transported and concentrated in tubular fluid and cellular processes within the subcarious dentin.[2,105] Withdrawal, injury, or necrosis of the cytoplasmic contents would leave the tubule open to bacterial toxins and deeper invasion. However, calcium and phosphorus released by carious acid demineralization of the peripheral hydroxyapatite crystals reprecipitate deeper within the tubules below the infected lesion. Platelike or rhomboid mineral crystals fill and barricade the open lumen[128] (Fig 1-19a and 1-19b). Also, accelerated mineralization and constriction of the peritubular walls below the level of bacterial penetration forms a protective confinement barrier, the sclerotic or translucent zone.[45,104,130]

With the added layer of response or reparative dentin formed at the dentin-pulp border, the in vitro permeability or hydraulic conductance of chronically carious dentin is reduced to only 7.6% of that recorded for normal dentin.[113] One unfortunate consequence, however, is that sclerosed, insensitive dentin blocks painful warning symptoms that might alert the patient to the presence of caries. Because of altered dentinal permeability, indications for placement of dentin bonding resin cavity sealers may differ between deep restorations due to active primary caries and replacement restorations in the presence of chronic caries.

Occasionally, with virulent bacteria and in young, permeable teeth, there is insufficient time for sclerosis. The tubules, empty and vulnerable, are described as "dead tracts."[71] Fortunately, sclerosis is a predictable, protective dentinal response observed in more than 95% of carious teeth and often in conjunction with tertiary or reparative dentin, another protective response that occurs in more than 63% of affected teeth.[139]

Reparative Dentin

Traumatic insult to the tooth, whether caused by mechanically exposed dentin, caries, or heat generated by the dental bur, may be severe enough to destroy the supporting odontoblasts (Figs 1-19a and 1-20). Within 3 weeks, fibroblasts or mesenchymal cells of the pulp are converted or differentiated to simulate the organization, matrix secretion, and mineralizing activities of the original odontoblasts. The matrix includes cellular and vascular components of the pulp and sparse, irregularly organized tubules. This reparative dentin is also called *tertiary, reactive, response,* or *secondary irregular dentin.* The pulp is further protected from diffusion or penetration of bacteria or metabolic products because there is no continuity between the affected permeable tubules of the regular dentin and those within the reparative dentin.

The rate of formation, the thickness, and the organization of the reparative dentin are commensurate with the intensity and duration of the stimulus.[149] Reparative dentin usually forms at a rate of about 1.5 μm/d, but the rate may be as high as 3.5 μm/d. At 50 days after trauma, a 70-μm thickness of reparative dentin has been reported. Thus, the tooth is able to compensate for the traumatic or carious loss of peripheral dentin with deposition of internal dentin sufficient for thermal insulation and control of permeability.[137,138]

Unless the lesion is either arrested or restored before it is about 0.5 mm from the pulp, the diffusion gradient of bacterial metabolites reaching the pulp can initiate a strong inflammatory response.[101] If the reparative dentin is breached to allow sufficient bacteria to overwhelm the vascular, inflammatory, and phagocytic defenses of the pulp, the result is pulpal necrosis.[71,123]

▇ Pulp

The dental pulp, 75% water and 25% organic,[90] is a viscous connective tissue of collagen fibers and ground substance supporting the vital cellular, vascular, and nerve structures of the tooth. It is a unique connective tissue in that its vascularization is essentially channeled through one opening, the apical foramen, and it is completely encased within relatively rigid dentinal walls. Therefore, it is without the advantage of a collateral blood supply or an expansion space for the swelling that

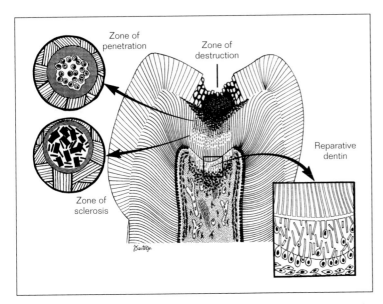

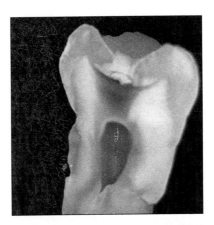

Figs 1-19a and **1-19b** Carious response. Acid demineralization and enzymatic destruction of the collagen matrix lead to irreversible cavitation.

Fig 1-19a Bacteria fill and demineralize the lumens of the tubules peripherally, but dissolved minerals reprecipitate deeper to augment sclerosis and hypermineralization of subcarious dentin. Reparative dentin with irregular and noncontinuous tubules forms a final barricade against bacterial metabolites.

Fig 1-19b Note the lateral spread of caries at the DEJ and hypermineralized sclerotic zone around the pulp.

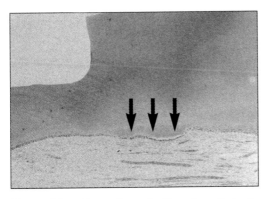

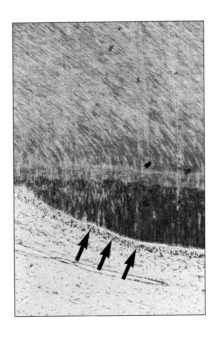

Fig 1-20a Reparative dentin deposited in response to microleakage and bacterial invasion under a dental restoration.

Fig 1-20b Reparative dentin deposited in response to infected primary and secondary dentin. (Courtesy of Dr Charles Cox, University of Alabama School of Dentistry.)

accompanies the typical inflammatory response of tissue to injurious conditions. However, the protected and isolated position of the pulp belies the fact that it is a sensitive and resilient tissue with a great potential for healing.

The dental pulp fulfills several functions[118]: *(1) formative,* creating the primary and secondary dentin as well as the protective response or reparative dentin; *(2) nutritive,* providing the vascular supply and ground substance transfer medium for metabolic functions and maintenance of cells and organic matrix; *(3) sensory,* transmitting afferent pain response (nociception) and proprioceptive response; and *(4) protective,* responding to inflammatory and antigenic stimuli and removing detrimental substances through its circulation and lymphatic systems.

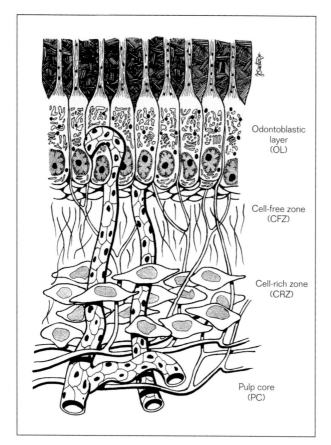

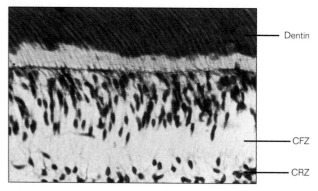

Fig 1-21a Pulpal histology. Odontoblastic layer, cell-free zone (filled with both nerve and vascular plexuses), cell-rich zone (fibroblasts), and pulp core. (Modified from Avery JK. Oral Development and Histology. Baltimore: Williams & Wilkins, 1987.)

Figs 1-21b and 1-21c Photomicrographs of the odontoblast layer. (Courtesy of Dr Charles Cox, University of Alabama School of Dentistry.)

Morphology

The pulpal tissue is traditionally described in histologically distinct, concentric zones: the innermost peripheral pulp core, the cell-rich zone, the cell-free zone, and the peripheral odontoblastic layer (Figs 1-21a, 1-21b and 1-21c).

The radicular and coronal pulp core is largely ground substance, an amorphous protein matrix gel surrounding both discrete collagen fibers and the channels of vascular and sensory supply. Neural and vascular components, which divide and multiply extensively in the subodontoblastic zones, combine into a bundled main trunk to pass through the pulp core to or from the apical foramina. Both matrix and collagen components are formed and maintained by a dispersed network of interconnected fibroblastic cells.

Fibrocytes and undifferentiated mesenchymal cells are particularly concentrated in the outer coronal pulp to form the cell-rich zone subjacent to the peripheral layer of odontoblastic cells. Functioning like troops in reserve, the mesenchymal cells and/or fibrocytes are capable of accelerated mitotic differentiation and collagen matrix production to serve as functional replacements for destroyed odontoblastic cells. They are responsible for production of additional reparative dentin when the permeable dentinal wall is breeched or a pulpal exposure occurs.[41,149,151] A dense and extensive capillary bed and nerve plexus form the cell-free zone, which separates and infiltrates the cell-rich zone internally and the cellular bodies of the odontoblastic layer peripherally.

Vascular System

The circulatory system supplies the oxygen and nutrients that dissolve in and diffuse through the viscous ground substance to reach the cells. In turn, the circulation removes waste products, such as carbon dioxide, by-products of inflammation,[71] or diffusion products that may have permeated through the dentin before they accumulate to toxic levels[107] (see Fig 1-16). The equilibrium between diffusion and clearance may be threatened by use of long-acting anesthetics that contain epinephrine or another vasoconstrictor. A ligamental injection of canine teeth with 2% lidocaine with 1:100,000 epinephrine will cause pulpal blood flow to cease for 20 minutes or more.[70] Fortunately, the respiratory requirements of mature pulp cells are low so that no permanent cellular damage ensues.

Inflammation, the normal tissue response to injury and the first stage of repair, is somewhat complicated within the noncompliant walls of the pulp chamber. Inflammation begins with increased capillary permeability and leakage of proteins, plasma fluids, and leukocytes into the confined extracellular space, causing an increase in tissue interstitial fluid pressure.[140] Theoretically, elevated extravascular tissue pressure could collapse the thin venule walls and start a destructive cycle of restricted circulation and expanding ischemia. However, the pulpal circulation is unique because it contains numerous arteriole "U-turns" or reverse flow loops, and arteriole-venule anastomoses, or shunts, to bypass the affected capillary bed.[146] Also, at the periphery of the affected area, where high tissue pressure is attenuated so that circulation may resume, capillary recapture and lymphatic adsorption of edematous fluids are expedited.[58] These processes confine the area of edema and elevated tissue pressure to the immediate inflamed area. Although tissue pressure at an area of pulpal inflammation is two to three times higher than normal, it quickly falls to nearly normal levels 1.0 mm or so from the affected area.[147]

Elevated pulpal tissue pressure resulting from inflammation or a protective neuroactive response to hydrodynamic stimuli[87] counteracts the diffusion of solutes through dentin into the pulpal space.[49] However, an inflammatory condition and higher tissue pressure may also induce hyperalgesia, a lowered threshold of sensitivity of pulpal nerves. Thus, an afflicted tooth exposed to the added stress of cavity preparation and restoration may become symptomatic as hypersensitive to cold or other stimuli.[150]

Innervation

Dental nerves are either efferent autonomic fibers to regulate blood flow or afferent sensory nerves derived from the second and third divisions of the fifth intercranial (trigeminal) nerve. Nerves are classified according to their purpose, myelin sheathing, diameter, and conduction velocity. Although a few large and very high–conduction velocity A-β (beta) nerves with a proprioceptive function have been identified, most sensory interdental nerves are either myelinated A-δ nerves or smaller, unmyelinated C fibers.[150] The innervation of a premolar, for example, consists of about 500 individual A-δ nerves that gradually lose their myelin coating and Schwann cell sheathing as they branch and form a sensory plexus of free nerve endings around and below the odontoblastic layer.[64] The A-δ nerves have conduction velocities of 13.0 m/s and low sensitization thresholds to react to hydrodynamic pressure phenomena.[96,97] Activation of the A-δ system results in a sharp, intense "jolt."

There are three to four times more of the smaller, unmyelinated C fibers, which are more uniformly distributed through the pulp. The conduction velocities of C fibers are slower, 0.5 to 1.0 m/s, and C fibers are only activated by a level of stimuli capable of creating tissue destruction, such as prolonged high temperatures or pulpitis. The C fibers are also resistant to tissue hypoxia and are not affected by reduction of blood flow or high tissue pressure. Therefore, pain may persist in anesthetized, infected, or even nonvital teeth.[31,148] The sensation resulting from activation of the C fibers is a diffuse, burning or throbbing pain, and the patient may have difficulty locating the affected tooth.

Odontoblastic Layer

The outer cellular component of the pulp, the odontoblasts, produce the primary and regular secondary dentinal matrix and control or affect peritubular mineralization and sclerosis as a defense mechanism (see Fig 1-15).[71] Postmitotic and irreplaceable, odontoblastic cell bodies line the tubule-perforated predentin wall of the pulp chamber in a single layer. Each cell has an indefinite life span but crowding from continued deposition of secondary dentin constricts the pulpal chamber, to reduce the initial number of cells by half.[119] The odontoblastic cells are packed closely together, and both permanent and variable junctions between the cellular membranes have been described. Just as the peripheral processes of the odontoblasts are physically interconnected, a third type of intercellular interface, a communicating junction, mediates transfer of chemical and electronic signals that permit coordinated response and reaction of the odontoblastic layer.[61,73,126] Thus, as an additional protective response, the integrity and spacing of the odontoblastic layer mediates the passage of tissue fluids and molecules between the pulp and the dentin. Routine operative procedures, such as cavity preparation and air drying of the cut dental surface, can temporarily disrupt the odontoblastic layer and may sometimes inflict permanent cellular damage.[11,152]

Restorative Dentistry and Pulpal Health

Surgical and restorative treatments generate considerable physical, chemical, and thermal irritation of the pulp. However, if the dentist uses an acceptable technique and achieves bacterial control, even a mechanical pulp exposure or use of acidic restorative materials poses few problems for pulpal health.[6,10,21,22,65,111,134] Although microleakage around restorations is ubiquitous, the fact that almost all pulps remain healthy is related to the pathogenicity of the bacteria, permeability of the dentin, and healing potential of the pulp.[71,94] The capacity for pulpal healing is limited by the effects of aging and by extensive and/or repeated restorative procedures. Two clinical reviews of patients who had received either a fixed prosthesis or single complete crowns reported that 6%[63] and 13%[39] of crowned teeth revealed some sign of pulpal necrosis requiring root canal treatment.

Although pressure, desiccation, and disruption of cellular processes (by cutting) accompany dental surgery, excessive heat generated by the friction of rotary instrumentation is considered the most damaging insult to the pulp. Heat may cause coagulation, extensive burn lesions, and temporary stasis of the pulpal circulation.[69,138] Studies of heat applied externally to enamel surfaces or cavity floors have produced equivocal results. Zach and Cohen[160] reported 15% irreversible pulpal necrosis after a 5.5°C increase of intrapulpal temperature and up to 60% necrosis after an 11°C rise. However, against prepared cavity walls of orthodontically condemned teeth with about 0.5 mm of remaining dentinal thickness, a 30-second heat application of 150°C (200°F) produced few symptoms, relatively minor pulpal changes, and no necrosis.[102] Interpretation of the studies indicates that the presence of a sufficient remaining dentinal thickness (0.5 mm or more) is a critical factor in limiting thermal conduction (insulation), just as it is in limiting dentinal permeability.[24,138]

Other in vitro studies have shown damaging temperature thresholds are possible if improper amalgam finishing and polishing techniques, such as continuous contact and excessive speed or pressure, are used.[51,57,142] Another study reported that 25 seconds of continuous contact of a dental bur against a tooth without water coolant could produce a critical 6°C rise in intrapulpal temperature.[159] Therefore, an important safeguard to prevent the buildup of pulpal heat is use of a water coolant combined with intermittent instrument-tooth contact, especially during high-speed enamel or dentin reduction.[144] Other steps recommended to minimize pulpal damage associated with restorative procedures include the following[20]: use of sharp burs or single-use diamonds, use of concentrically rotating instruments, avoidance of overdrying and prolonged desiccation of cut dentin, and use of accurately fitting provisional restorations with low exothermic heat on setting.

Although the aged tooth is less permeable, some biologists suggest that it has less reparative potential. Age-related changes include reduced blood supply, a smaller pulp chamber, lower ratio of cells to collagen fiber, loss and degeneration of myelinated and unmyelinated nerves, loss of water from the ground substance, and increased intrapulpal mineralizations (denticles).[127,149] Restorative procedures easily tolerated in the younger patient may pose problems for the older patient. Nevertheless, the newer concepts of treatment, including new preventive measures; restorative materials with antibacterial properties; improved bonding and seal of enamel fissures, margins, and dentinal tubules; and conservative tooth preparations should promote extended durability and compatibility of dental services.

Gingiva and Biologic Width

The gingiva is that part of the oral mucosa that covers the alveolar bone, defines the cervical contours of the clinical crown, and seals the tooth root and periodontal structures from the external environment. A normal, healthy gingiva presents a scalloped marginal outline, firm texture, coral pink or normally pigmented coloration, and, in about 40% of the population, a stippled surface. A healthy, stable gingiva without hyperplastic, swollen, bleeding, or receding tissue is essential to both esthetic and restorative success. Gingivitis, an inflammatory soft tissue response to bacterial plaque, affects up to 44% of the US adult population.[158] Gingival bacteria, associated with poor oral hygiene or defective restorations, can cause periodontal disease. Because periodontitis is a major cause of adult tooth loss, the status of the alveolar bone and soft tissues of the periodontium must be evaluated along with that of the teeth.

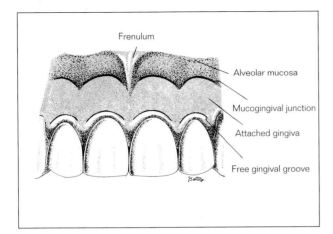

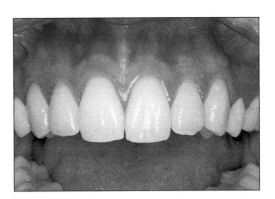

Figs 1-22a and 1-22b   Clinically healthy, normal gingiva.

External Appearance

The two primary components of the oral mucosa are masticatory gingiva and lining mucosa (Figs 1-22a and 1-22b).[80] Attached gingiva is keratinized and firmly affixed to the periosteum of the alveolar bone and hard palate and to the supra-alveolar cementum of the root. It extends coronally around the teeth to form the free marginal gingiva, a scalloped, unattached cuff that also fills the gingival embrasure between adjacent teeth with a facial and lingual papilla. Attached and marginal gingiva are separated by an external free gingival groove in about 30% to 40% of the healthy adult population. The vertical width (height) of the keratinized gingiva (attached and marginal gingiva) is clearly measured from the mucogingival junction separating it from the alveolar lining mucosa, which is mobile, darker red, and nonkeratinized. The width of keratinized gingiva varies by location, from less than 2.0 mm wide on the lingual aspect of the mandibular incisors to 9.0 mm on the lingual aspect of mandibular molars.[76]

Histologically, the surface oral epithelium and connective tissue form an irregular boundary of papillary connective tissue projecting between ridges, or rete pegs, of oral epithelium (Figs 1-23a and 1-23b). The epithelial layer is characterized by progressive zones in which the active mitotic cells of the basement membrane completely differentiate into scales of synthesized keratin protein as they migrate to the surface for desquamation.[136]

Dentogingival Junction

The complex of epithelial cell types and connective tissue forming the gingival attachment to the tooth and alveolar bone is called the *dentogingival junction* (Figs 1-23a to 1-23c).[15,43,82] Coronally, the keratinized marginal gingiva invaginates against the cervical enamel to form a partial or nonkeratinized epithelium-lined crevice with an average depth of 1.8 mm. A depth of more than 3.0 mm is generally considered pathologic and termed a *periodontal pocket.*[119]

From the base of the sulcus, which corresponds to the level of the CEJ in the young adult tooth, a layer of junctional epithelial cells forms an adhesive basement membrane seal against the cementum of the root. The thickness of the junctional epithelium narrows from 15 to 30 cells at the base of the sulcus to one to three cells apically. Over time, cumulative bacterial and mechanical irritation often result in a lower gingival level (longer clinical crown) and a corresponding increase in the width of the junctional epithelium.[48] Like other oral epithelial cells, the junctional epithelial cells exhibit high mitotic activity, and the cells migrate coronally to the base of the sulcus to be desquamated. An extensive vascular plexus underlies the junctional epithelial cells, which are widely spaced to facilitate the passage of vascular and inflammatory cells into the gingival fluid of the sulcus. Bacterial colonization within the sulcus is discouraged by the combination of a rapidly disrupted cellular base and the

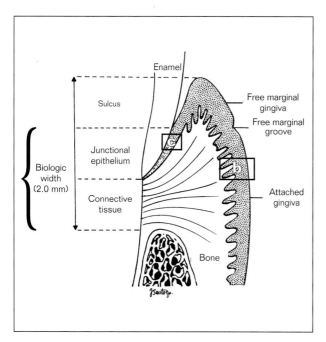

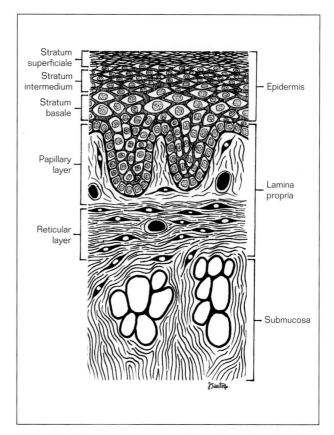

Fig 1-23a Dentogingival junction. The attachment tissues of the gingiva to the tooth and periosteum consist of superficial and deep connective tissues (see Fig 1-24) and three types of epithelium: masticatory keratinized epithelium (Fig 1-23b), a nonkeratinized inner sulcus lining epithelium, and a junctional epithelium specialized for attachment to the tooth surface (Fig 1-23c).

Fig 1-23b Masticatory keratinized epithelium. (Modified from Avery JK, Oral Development and Histology. Baltimore: Williams & Wilkins, 1987.)

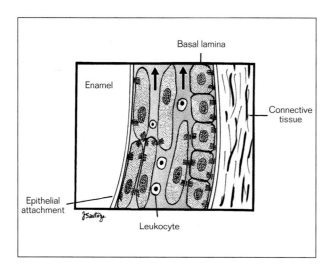

Fig 1-23c Maturing junctional epithelial cells and inflammatory cells from the connective tissue move coronally (arrows) to reach the base of the gingival sulcus and the gingival fluid.

lavage and antibacterial action of the vascular transudate of gingival fluid.[68,78]

The supra-alveolar connective tissue and lamina propria of the gingiva are made up of dense interlaced bundles of collagen fibers supporting the gingiva and affixing it to the periosteum and cementum of the hard tissues (Fig 1-24). The fibers are classified by attachment and function into the following groups: *(1)* dentogingival, attaching the gingiva to the cementum; *(2)* alveologingival, affixing gingiva to alveolar bone; *(3)* transseptal, connecting interproximal cemental surfaces; *(4)* dentoperiosteal, from alveolar crest to cementum, an extension of the periodontal ligament; and *(5)* circular, around the tooth.[44]

Biologic Width

An autopsy study of individuals of various ages and gingival levels revealed variations in depths of the sulcus and junctional epithelium, but the supra-alveolar connective tissue attachment consistently measured approximately 1.07 mm (see Fig 1-23a).[48] In health, the connective tissue and epithelial attachments occupy the space between the base of the sulcus and the alveolar crest and measure approximately 2.0 mm—this is termed the *biologic width*.[99] This dimension is assumed to be a physiologic minimum required to preserve the attachment and health of the gingiva; thus, its preservation is a prime goal of the restorative dentist.

It is generally agreed that supragingival margins are preferable in restorations, but esthetics, caries, and requirements for access and retention may dictate preparations within the biologic width. Root caries, tooth fracture, or operator error may create conditions in which the 2.0-mm dentogingival junction below the sulcus is surgically prepared or traumatized. Theoretically, irreversible or uncontrolled bone loss and inflammation may occur, as the body attempts to restore the biologic width at a more apical level. Therefore, many clinicians insist that prerestorative osseous surgery (crown lengthening) should be performed to preserve the biologic width whenever the restorative margin cannot be located at least 2.0 mm to 3.0 mm above the alveolar crest.[17,62,85]

The significance of keratinized tissue in restorative dentistry is somewhat controversial. Lang and Löe[76] concluded that a minimum width of 2.0 mm of keratinized gingiva is required to prevent chronic gingival inflammation. However, several clinical studies report that, with good oral hygiene, a healthy and stable gingival margin is possible even when the attached gingiva is

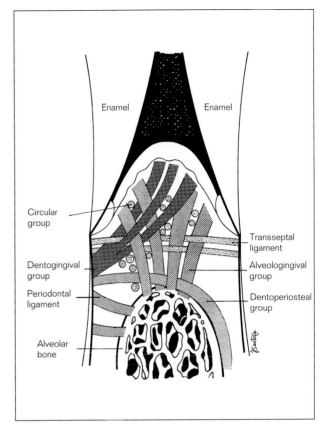

Fig 1-24 Interproximal gingival tissue the demonstrating gingival collagen fiber groups: dentogingival, alveologingival, dentoperiosteal, circular (circumferential), and transseptal. (Modified from Ten Cate AR. Oral Histology, ed 4. St Louis: Mosby, 1994.)

minimal, missing, or remodeled.[28,89,157] In a 1-year animal study in which Class 5 amalgam restorations were placed directly at the alveolar crest, the remodeled bone crest was less than 1.0 mm from the original level and the diminished junctional attachment and periodontium appeared normal.[145]

Nonetheless, placement and location of a subgingival restorative margin may preclude a healthy gingival response. Margins placed deeper than 1.0 mm into the sulcus are increasingly associated with problems of inflammation, bleeding, hyperplasia, gingival recession, and pathologic bacteria.[77,81,100] However, the quality of the restoration, marginal integrity, smoothness, and contour may be more critical to periodontal response than the location within the attachment zone.[120,124]

References

1. Abou-Rass M. Crack lines: The precursor of tooth fractures—Their diagnosis and treatment. Quintessence Int 1983;4:437-443.

2. Ackermans F, Klein JP, Frank RM. Ultrastructural localization of immunoglobulins in carious human dentine. Arch Oral Biol 1981;26:879-886.

3. Ahlquist M, Franzein O, Coffey J, Pashley D. Dental pain evoked by hydrostatic pressures applied to exposed dentin in man: A test of the hydrodynamic theory of dental sensitivity. J Endod 1994;20:130-137.

4. Anderson DJ. Measurement of stress in mastication. J Dent Res 1956;35:671-673.

5. Bartelstone HJ, Mandel ID, Oshry E, Seidlin SM. Use of radioactive iodine as a tracer in the study of the physiology of the teeth. Science 1947;106:132-133.

6. Bergenholtz G, Cox CF, Loesche WJ, Syed SA. Bacterial leakage around dental restorations: Its effect on the dental pulp. J Oral Pathol 1982;11:439-450.

7. Blaser PK, Lund MR, Cochran MA. Effects of designs of Class 2 preparations on resistance of teeth to fracture. Oper Dent 1983;8:6-10.

8. Boyde A. Enamel structure and cavity margins. Oper Dent 1976;1:13-28.

9. Brännström M, Johnson G, Linden LA. Fluid flow and pain response in the dentin produced by hydrostatic pressure. Odontol Rev 1969;20:15-16.

10. Brännström M, Vojinovic O, Nordenvall KJ. Bacteria and pulpal reactions under silicate cement restorations. J Prosthet Dent 1979;41:290-295.

11. Brännström M. Communication between the oral cavity and the dental pulp associated with restorative treatment. Oper Dent 1984;9:57-68.

12. Buonocore MG. A simple method of increasing the adhesion of acrylic filling materials to enamel surfaces. J Dent Res 1955;34:849-853.

13. Buonocore MG. The Use of Adhesives in Dentistry. Springfield, IL: Thomas, 1975:75.

14. Byers MR, Sugaya A. Odontoblast processes in dentin revealed by fluorescent Di-I. J Histochem Cytochem 1995;43:159-168.

15. Carranza FA. Clinical Periodontology, ed 7. Philadelphia: Saunders, 1990:19-69.

16. Cassin AM, Pearson GJ, Picton DCA. Fissure sealants as a means of prolonging longevity of amalgam restorations. Clin Mater 1991;7:203-207.

17. Casullo DP. Periodontal considerations in restorative dentistry. In: Genco RJ, Goldman HM, Cohen DW (eds). Contemporary Periodontics, ed 7. St Louis: Mosby, 1990:629.

18. Chan DCN. Current methods and criteria for caries diagnosis in North America. J Educ Dent 1993;57:422-427.

19. Christensen GT. Alternatives for Class 2 restorations. Clin Res Assoc Newsletter, 1994;18(5):1-3.

20. Christensen GT. Fixed prosthesis—Avoiding pulp death. Clin Res Assoc Newsletter, 1995;19(1):1.

21. Cox CF. Biocompatibility of dental materials in the absence of bacterial infection. Oper Dent 1987;12:146-152.

22. Cox CF, Keall CL, Keall HJ, Ostro E. Biocompatibility of surface-sealed dental materials against exposed pulps. J Prosthet Dent 1987;57:1-8.

23. Crabb HS, Darling AI. The gradient of mineralization in developing enamel. Arch Oral Biol 1960; 52:118-122.

24. Craig RG, Peyton FA (eds). Restorative Dental Materials, ed 5. St Louis: Mosby, 1975:47.

25. Craig RG. Restorative Dental Materials, ed 8. St Louis: Mosby, 1989:100.

26. Cuenin MF, Scheidt MJ, O'Neal RM, Strong SL, Pashley DH, Hoener DH, Van Dyke TE. An in vivo study of dentin sensitivity: The relation of dentin sensitivity and patency of dentin tubules. J Periodontol 1991;62:668-673.

27. Dijkman A, Huizinga E, Ruben J, Arends J. Remineralization of human enamel in situ after three months: The effect of not brushing versus the effect of an F dentifrice and an F-free dentifrice. Caries Res 1990;24:263-266.

28. Dorfman HS, Kennedy JE. Gingival parameters associated with varying widths of attached gingiva [abstract 301]. J Dent Res 1981;60(special issue A):386.

29. Duke ES, Lindemuth J. Variability of clinical dentin substrates. Am J Dent 1991;4:241-246.

30. Edgar WM, Geddes DAM, Jenkins GN, Rugg-Gunn AJ, Howell R. Effects of calcium gylcerophosphate and sodium fluoride on the induction in vivo of caries-like changes in human dental enamel. Arch Oral Biol 1978;66:1730-1734.

31. Edwall L, Scott D Jr. Influence of changes in microcirculation on the excitability of the sensory unit in the tooth of the cat. Acta Physiol Scand 1971;82:555.

32. Eisenmann DR. Enamel structure. In: Ten Cate AR (ed) Oral Histology—Development Structure and Function, ed 4. St Louis: Mosby, 1994:239-256.

33. Elderton RJ, Mjör IA. Changing scene in cariology and operative dentistry. Int Dent J 1992;42:165-169.

34. Elhabashy A, Swift EJ, Boyer DB, Denehy GE. Effects of dentin permeability and hydration on the bond strengths of dentin bonding systems. Am J Dent 1993;6:123-126.

35. Featherstone JDB, Ten Cate JM. Physicochemical aspects of fluoride enamel interactions. In: Ekstrand J, Fejerskov O, Silverstone LM (eds). Fluoride in Dentistry. Copenhagen: Munksgaard, 1988.

36. Feinman RA, Goldstein RE, Garber DA. Bleaching Teeth. Chicago: Quintessence, 1987.

37. Fejerskov O, Thylstrup A. Dental enamel. In: Mjör IA, Fejerskov O (eds). Human Oral Embryology and Histology. Copenhagen: Munksgaard, 1986:81-88.

38. Fejerskov O, Thylstrup A. Dental enamel. In: Mjör IA, Fejerskov O (eds). Human Oral Embryology and Histology. Copenhagen: Munksgaard, 1986:68-69.

39. Felton D. Long term effects of crown preparation on pulp vitality [abstract 1139]. J Dent Res 1989;69:1009.

40. Fernandes CP, Chevitarese O. The orientation and direction of rods in dental enamel. J Prosthet Dent 1991;65:793-800.

41. Fitzgerald M, Chiego DJ, Heys D. Autoradiographic analysis of odontoblast replacement following pulp exposure in primate teeth. Arch Oral Biol 1990;35:707.

42. Fosse G, Saele PK, Eide R. Numerical density and distributional pattern of dentin tubules. Acta Odontol Scand 1992;50:201-210.

43. Freeman E. Periodontium. In: Ten Cate AR (ed). Oral Histology—Development, Structure, and Function, ed 4. St Louis: Mosby, 1994:276-312.

44. Furseth R, Selvig KA, Mjör IA. The periodontium. In: Mjör IA, Fejerskov O (eds). Human Oral Embryology and Histology. Copenhagen: Munksgaard, 1986:136-137.

45. Fusayama T. Two layers of carious dentin; diagnosis and treatment. Oper Dent 1979;4:63-70.

46. Fusayama T. Etiology and treatment of sensitive teeth. Quintessence Int 1988;19:921-925.

47. Garberoglio R, Brännström M. Scanning electron microscopic investigation of human dentinal tubules. Arch Oral Biol 1976;21:355-362.

48. Gargiulo AW, Wentz FM, Orban B. Dimensions and relations of the dentogingival junction in humans. J Periodontol 1961;32:261-267.

49. Gerzina TMO, Hume WR. Effect of hydrostatic pressure on the diffusion of monomers through dentin in vitro. J Dent Res 1995;74:369-373.

50. Graf H, Galasse R. Morbidity, prevalence and intra-oral distribution of hypersensitive teeth [abstract 479]. J Dent Res 1977;56 (special issue A):A162.

51. Grajower R, Kaufmann E, Rajstein J. Temperature in the pulp chamber during polishing of amalgam restorations. J Dent Res 1974;53:1189-1195.

52. Gwinnett AJ, Matsui A. A study of enamel adhesives. The physical relationship between enamel and adhesive. Arch Oral Biol 1967;12:1615-1620.

53. Gwinnett AJ. Morphology of the interface between adhesive resins and treated enamel surfaces as seen by scanning electron microscopy. Arch Oral Biol 1971;16:237-238.

54. Gwinnett AJ. Histologic changes in human enamel following treatment with acidic adhesive conditioning agents. Arch Oral Biol 1971;16:731-738.

55. Gwinnett AJ. Structure and composition of enamel. Oper Dent 1992; (suppl 5):10-17.

56. Harris NO, Christen AG. Primary Preventive Dentistry, ed 3. Norwalk, CT: Appleton & Lange, 1991.

57. Hatton JG, Holtzmann DH, Ferrillo PJ, Steward GP. Effect of handpiece pressure and speed on intrapulpal temperature rise. Am J Dent 1994;7:108-110.

58. Heyeraas KJ. Interstitial fluid pressure and transmicrovascular fluid flow. In: Inoki R, Judo T, Olgart L (eds). Dynamic Aspects of Dental Pulp. London: Chapman and Hall, 1990.

59. Heymann HO, Sturdevant JR, Bayne SC, Wilder AD, Sluder TB, Brunson WD. Examining tooth flexure effects on cervical restorations: A two-year clinical study. J Am Dent Assoc 1991;122:41-47.

60. Hoffmann F, Eismann D. The total surface and number of occlusal contacts in static and dynamic occlusion. Bilt Udrux Ortodonata Jugosl. 1991;24:71-78.

61. Holland GR. Membrane junctions on cat odontoblasts. Arch Oral Biol 1975;20:551.

62. Ingber JS, Rose LF, Coslet JG. The "biologic width"—a concept in periodontics and restorative dentistry. Alpha Omegan 1977;70(3):62-65.

63. Jackson CR, Skidmore AE, Rice RT. Pulpal evaluation of teeth restored with fixed prostheses. J Prosthet Dent 1992;67:325-325.

64. Johnsen DC, Harshabarger J, Rymer HD. Quantitative assessment of neural development in human premolars. Anat Rec 1983;205:431-439.

65. Kadehashi S, Stanley HR, Fitzgerald RJ. The effects of surgical exposures of pulps in germ-free and conventional rats. Oral Surg Oral Med Oral Pathol 1965;20:340-349.

66. Kidd EAM. Microleakage: A review. J Dent 1976;4:199-206.

67. Kidd EAM, Toffenetti F, Mjör IA. Secondary caries. Int Dent J 1992;42:127-138.

68. Kidera EJ, Mackenzie IC. Surface clearance of oral mucosa and skin [abstract 939]. J Dent Res 1981;60:544.

69. Kim S, Grayson A, Kim B, Schacter W. Effects of dental procedures on pulpal blood flow in dogs [abstract 268]. J Dent Res 1983;62:199.

70. Kim S. Ligamental injection: A physiological explanation of its efficacy. J Endod 1986;12(10):486-491.

71. Kim S, Trowbridge HO. Pulpal reaction to caries and dental procedures. In: Cohen S, Burns RC (eds). Pathways of the Pulp, ed 6. St Louis:Mosby, 1994.

72. Kirkham J, Robinson C, Strong M, Shore RC. Effects of frequency of acid exposure on demineralization/remineralization behavior of human enamel in vitro. Caries Res 1994;28:9-13.

73. Koling A. Structural relationships in the human odontoblast layer, as demonstrated by freeze-fracture electron microscopy. J Endod 1988;14:239-246.

74. Lamb WJ, Corpron RE, More FG, Beltran ED, Strachan DS, Kowalski CJ. In situ remineralization of subsurface enamel lesion after the use of a fluoride chewing gum. Caries Res 1993;27:111-116.

75. Lambrechts P, Braem M, Vuylsteke-Wauters M, Vanherle G. Quantitative in vivo wear of human enamel. J Dent Res 1989;68:1752-1754.

76. Lang NP, Löe H. The relationship between the width of keratinized gingiva and gingival health. J Periodontol 1972;43:623-627.

77. Lang NP, Kiel RA, Anderhalden K. Clinical and microbiological effects of subgingival restorations with overhanging or clinically perfect margins. J Clin Periodontol 1983;10:563-578.

78. Lavelle CLB. Applied Oral Physiology, ed 2. London: Wright, 1988:86.

79. Lee WC, Eakle WS. Possible role of tensile stress in the etiology of cervical erosive lesions of teeth. J Prosthet Dent 1984;52:374-380.

80. Lindhe J, Karring T. The anatomy of the periodontium. In: Lindhe J (ed). Textbook of Clinical Periodontology, ed 2. Copenhagen: Munksgaard, 1989:19-69.

81. Löe H. Reactions of marginal periodontal tissues to restorative procedures. Int Dent J 1968;18:759-778.

82. Löe H, Listgarten M, Terranova V. Periodontal tissues in health. In: Genco R, Goldman H, Cohen D (eds). Contemporary Periodontics. St Louis: Mosby, 1990:3-55.

83. Lopes LM, Leitac JGM, Douglas WH. Effect of a new resin inlay/onlay system on cuspal reinforcement. Quintessence Int 1991;22:641-645.

84. Lyon DG, Darling AI. Orientation of the crystallites in the human dental enamel. Br Dent J 1957;102:438.

85. Malone WFP, Koth DL. Tylman's Theory and Practice of Fixed Prosthodontics, ed 8. St Louis: Ishiyaku EuroAmerica, 1989:10.

86. Marzouk MA, Simonton AL, Gross RD. Operative Dentistry—Modern Theory and Practice. St. Louis: Ishiyaku EuroAmerica, 1985:33-37.

87. Matthews B, Vongsavan N. Interactions between neural and hydrodynamic mechanisms in dentine and pulp. Arch Oral Biol 1994;39(suppl): 87s-95s.

88. Mendis BRN, Darling AI. A scanning electron microscope and microradiography study of closure of human coronal dentinal tubules related to occlusal attrition and caries. Arch Oral Biol 1979;24:725-733.

89. Miyasato M, Crigger M, Egelberg J. Gingival condition in areas of minimal and appreciable width of keratinized gingiva. J Clin Periodontol 1977;4:200-209.

90. Mjör IA, Fejerskov O (eds). Human Oral Embryology and Histology. Copenhagen: Munksgaard, 1986.

91. Mondelli JH, Steagall L, Ishikiriama A, de Lima Navaroo MF, Soares FB. Fracture strength of human teeth with cavity preparations. J Prosthet Dent 1980;43:419-422.

92. Muller CFJ, van Wyk CW. The amelo-cemental junction. J Dent Assoc South Afr 1984;39:799-803.

93. Murray JJ, Rugg-Gunn AJ, Jenkins GN. Fluorides in Caries Prevention, ed 3. Boston: Wright, 1991.

94. Nagaoka S, Miyazaki Y, Liu HJ, Iwamoto Y, Kitano M, Kawagoe M. Bacterial invasion into dentinal tubules of human vital and nonvital teeth. J Endod 1995;21:70-73.

95. Nakabayashi N, Nakamura M, Uasuda M. Hybrid layer as a dentin-bonding mechanism. J Esthet Dent 1991;3:133-138.

96. Narhi M, Hirvonen TK, Hakamura M. Responses of intradental nerve fibers to stimulation of dentin and pulp. Acta Physiol Scand 1982;115:173-178.

97. Narhi M, Virtanen A, Huopaniemi T, Hirvonen T. Conduction velocities of single pulp nerve fiber units in the cat. Acta Physiol Scand 1982;116:209-213.

98. National Institute of Dental Research. Oral Health of United States Children. Bethesda, MD: NIH, publication 89-2247, 1989.

99. Nevins M, Skurow HM. The intracrevicular restorative margin, the biologic width, and the maintenance of the gingival margin. Int J Periodont Rest Dent 1984;4(3):30-39.

100. Newcomb GM. The relationship between the location of subgingival crown margins and gingival inflammation. J Periodontol 1974;45:151-154.

101. Nissan R, Segal H, Pashley D, Stevens R, Trowbridge H. Ability of bacterial endotoxin to diffuse through human dentin. J Endod 1995;21:62-64.

102. Nyborg H, Brännström M. Pulp reaction to heat. J Prosthet Dent 1968;19:605-612.

103. Nylen MU, Scott DB. An Electron Microscopic Study of the Early Stages of Dentinogenesis. Washington, DC: US Public Health Service, publication 613, 1958.

104. Ogawa K, Yamashita Y, Ichigo T, Fusayama T. The ultrastructure and hardness of the transparent layer of human carious dentin. J Dent Res 1983;62:7-10.

105. Okamura K, Maeda M, Nishikawa T, Tsutsui M. Dentinal response against carious invasion: Localization of antibodies in odontoblastic body and process. J Dent Res 1980;59:1368-1373.

106. Outhwaite WC, Pashley DH. Effects of changes in surface area, thickness, temperature, and post-extraction time on human dentine permeability. Arch Oral Biol 1976;21:599-603.

107. Pashley DH. The influence of dentin permeability and pulpal blood flow on pulpal solute concentrations. J Endod 1979 5:355-361.

108. Pashley DH, Galloway SE, Stewart F. Effect of fibrinogen in vivo on dentin premeability in the dog. Arch Oral Biol 1984;29:725-728.

109. Pashley DH. Dentin: A dynamic substrate—a review. Scanning Microsc 1989;3:161-176.

110. Pashley DH, Pashley EL. Dentin permeability and restorative dentistry; a status report. Am J Dent 1991;4:5-9.

111. Pashley DH. The effects of acid etching on the pulpodental complex. Oper Dent 1992;17:229-242.

112. Pashley DH, Matthews WG. The effect of outward forced convective flow on inward diffusion in human dentine in vitro. Arch Oral Biol 1993;38:577-582.

113. Pashley EL, Talman R, Horner JA, Pashley DH. Permeability of normal verses carious dentin. Endod Dent Traumatol 1991;7:207-211.

114. Pashley EL, Tao L, Matthews HG, Pashley DH. Bond strengths to superficial, intermediate and deep dentin in vivo with four dentin bonding systems. Dent Mater 1993;9:19-22.

115. Pitts NG, Kidd EAM. Some of the factors to be considered in the prescription and timing of bitewing radiographs in the diagnosis and management of dental caries: Contemporary recommendations. Br Dent J 1992;172:225-227.

116. Powell GL, Nicholls JI, Shurtz DE. Deformation of human teeth under the action of an amalgam matrix band. Oper Dent 1977;2:64-69.

117. Prati C, Pashley DH, Montanari G. Hydrostatic intrapulpal pressure and bond strength of bonding systems. Dent Mater 1991; 7:54-58.

118. Provenza DV, Seibel W. Oral Histology—Inheritance and Development, ed 2. Philadelphia: Lea & Febiger, 1986:291-292.

119. Provenza DV. Fundamentals of Oral Histology and Embryology, ed 2. Philadelphia: Lea & Febiger, 1988.

120. Ramfjord SP. Periodontal considerations of operative dentistry. Oper Dent 1988;13:144-159.

121. Reeh ES, Douglas WH, Messer HH. Stiffness of endodontically-treated teeth related to restoration technique. J Dent Res 1989;68:1540-1544.

122. Reeh ES, Messer, HH, Douglas WH. Reduction in tooth stiffness as a result of endodontic and restorative procedures. J Endod 1989;15:512-516.

123. Reeves R, Stanley HR. The relationship of bacterial penetration and pulpal pathosis in carious teeth. Oral Surg Oral Med Oral Pathol 1966;22:59-65.

124. Richter WA, Ueno H. Relationship of crown margin placement to gingival inflammation. J Prosthet Dent 1973;30:156-161.

125. Scherman A, Jacobsen PL. Managing dentin hypersensitivity: What treatment to recommend to patients. J Am Dent Assoc 1992;123:57-61.

126. Seltzer S, Bender IB. The Dental Pulp, ed 3. Philadelphia: Lippincott, 1984:86.

127. Seltzer S, Bender IB. The Dental Pulp, ed 3. Philadelphia: Lippincott; 1984:324-348.

128. Shimizu C, Yamashita Y, Ichigo T, Fusayama T. Carious change of dentin observed on longspan ultrathin sections. J Dent Res 1981;60:1826-1831.

129. Sigal MJ, Aubin HE, Ten Cate AR. An immuno cytochemical study of the human odontoblast process using antibodies against tubulin, actin, and vimentin. J Dent Res 1985;64:1348-1355.

130. Silverstone LM, Mjör IA. Dental Caries. In: Hörsted-Bindslev, Mjör IA (eds). Modern Concepts in Operative Dentistry. Copenhagen: Munksgaard, 1988:46-53.

131. Silverstone LM, Saxton CA, Dogon IL, Fejerskov O. Variation in pattern of acid etching of human dental enamel examined by scanning electron microscopy. Caries Res 1975;9:373-383.

132. Simmelink JW. Histology of enamel. In: Avery JK (ed). Oral Development and Histology. Baltimore: Williams & Wilkins, 1987:143.

133. Slomiany BL, Murty VL, Zdebska E, Slomiany A, Gwozdzinski K, Mandel ID. Tooth surface-pellicle lipids and their role in the protection of dental enamel against lactic-acid diffusion in man. Arch Oral Biol 1986;31:187-191.

134. Snuggs JM, Cox CF, Powell CS, White K. Pulpal healing and dentinal bridge formation in an acidic environment. Quintessence Int 1993;24:501-510.

135. Spears IR, van Noort R, Crompton RH, Cardew GE, Howard IC. The effects of enamel anisotrophy on the distribution of stress in a tooth. J Dent Res 1993;72:1526-1531.

136. Squier CA, Hill MW. Oral mucosa. In: Ten Cate AR (ed). Oral Histology—Development, Structure and Function, ed 4. St Louis: Mosby, 1994:389-431.

137. Stanley HR, White CL, McCray L. The rate of tertiary (reparative) dentin formation in the human tooth. Oral Surg Oral Med Oral Pathol 1966;21:180-189.

138. Stanley HR. Human Pulp Response to Restorative Dental Procedures. Gainesville, FL: Storter, 1981.

139. Stanley HR, Pereira JC, Spiegel E, Broom C, Schultz M. The detection and prevalence of reactive and physiologic sclerotic dentin, reparative dentin and dead tracts beneath various types of dental lesions according to tooth surface and age. J Oral Pathol 1983;12:257-289.

140. Stenvik A, Iverson J, Mjör IA. Tissue pressure and histology of normal and inflamed tooth pulps in Macaque monkeys. Arch Oral Biol 1972;17:1501-1511.

141. Stephan RM. Changes in hydrogen-ion concentration on tooth surfaces and in carious lesions. J Am Dent Assoc 1940;27:718-723.

142. Stewart GP, Bachman TA, Hatton JF. Temperature rise due to finishing of direct restorative materials. Am J Dent 1990;4:23-28.

143. Sugars DA, Sugars DC. Patient assessment, examination and diagnosis, and treatment planning. In: Sturdevant CM, Roberson TM, Heymann HO, Sturdevant JR (eds). The Art and Science of Operative Dentistry, ed 3. St Louis: Mosby; 1995:196-197.

144. Swerdlow H, Stanley HR. Reaction of human dental pulp to cavity preparation. J Prosthet Dent 1959;9:121-131.

145. Tai J, Soldinger M, Drelangel A, Pitaru S. Periodontal response to long-term abuse of the gingival attachment by supracrestal amalgam restorations. J Clin Periodontol 1989;16:654-659.

146. Takahashi K, Kishi Y, Kim S. A scanning electron microscope study of the blood vessels of dog pulp using corrosion resin casts. J Endod 1982;8:131-135.

147. Tonder KJ, Kvinnsland I. Micropuncture measurement of interstitial tissue pressure in normal and inflamed dental pulp in cats. J Endod 1983;9:105-109.

148. Torebjork HE, Hallin RG. Perceptual changes accompanying controlled preferential blocking of A and C fibers responses in intact human skin nerves. Exp Brain Res 1973;16:321-332.

149. Torneck CD. Dentin-pulp complex. In: Ten Cate AR (ed). Oral Histology—Development, Structure, and Function, ed 4. St Louis: Mosby, 1994:169-217.

150. Trowbridge HO. Intradental sensory units: Physiological and clinical aspects. J Endod 1985;11:489-498.

151. Trowbridge HO, Kim S. Pulp Development, structure, and function. In: Cohen S, Burns RC (eds). Pathways of the Pulp, ed 6. St Louis: Mosby, 1994:296-336.

152. Turner DF, Marfurt CF, Sattleberg C. Demonstration of physiological barrier between pulpal odontoblasts and its perturbation following routine restorative procedures: Horseradish peroxidase tracing study in the rat. J Dent Res 1989;68:1262-1268.

153. Vale WA. Cavity preparations. Ir Dent Rev 1956;2:33-41.

154. Van Meerbeek B, Dhem A, Goret-Nicaise M, Braem M, Lambrechts P. Comparative SEM and TEM examination of the ultrastructure of the resin-dentin interdiffusion zone. J Dent Res 1993;72:495-501.

155. Van Meerbeek B, Braem M, Lambrechts P, Vanherle G. Morphological characterization of the interface between resin and sclerotic dentin. J Dent 1994;22:141-146.

156. Wainwright WW, Lemoine FA. Rapid diffuse penetration of intact enamel and dentin by carbon 14 labeled urea. J Am Dent Assoc 1950;41:135-145.

157. Wennström JL. Lack of association between width of attached gingiva and development of soft-tissue recession, A five-year longitudinal study. J Clin Periodontol 1987;14:181-184.

158. White A, Caplan DJ, Weintraub JA. A quarter century of changes in oral health in the United States. J Educ Dent 1995;59:19-57.

159. Zach L, Cohen G. Thermogenesis in operative techniques. J Prosthet Dent 1962;12:977-984.

160. Zach L, Cohen G. Pulp response to externally applied heat. Oral Surg Oral Med Oral Pathol 1965;19:515-530.

Patient Evaluation and Problem-Oriented Treatment Planning

Richard D. Davis

Excellence in dental care is achieved through the dentist's ability to assess the patient, determine his or her needs, design an appropriate plan of treatment, and execute the plan with proficiency. Both the comprehensive plan that is improperly executed and the well-executed treatment that is inadequately planned will result in less-than-ideal care. The process of identifying problems and designing the treatment for those problems is the essence of treatment planning and the focus of this chapter.

As an integral part of comprehensive dental care, treatment planning for the restoration of individual teeth must be done in concert with the diagnosis of problems and treatment planning for the entire masticatory system.

The objective of this chapter is to present a problem-oriented approach to treatment planning for restorative dentistry. This approach begins with a comprehensive patient evaluation and gradually narrows its focus to the restoration of individual teeth. Emphasis will be placed on the decision-making processes involved in identifying problems related to restorative dentistry, assessing the demands of the oral environment, and selecting the materials and operative modalities best suited to the treatment of these problems.

The Problem-Oriented Treatment Planning Model

Treatment planning is generally accomplished with either a treatment-oriented model or a problem-oriented model. In the treatment-oriented model, the dentist examining the patient finds certain intraoral conditions and mentally equates those problems to the need for certain forms of treatment. The examination findings are summarized in the form of a list of needed treatments, which then becomes the treatment plan. The problem-oriented model requires that the examination lead to the formulation of a list of problems. Each problem on the list is then considered in terms of treatment options, each of which has different advantages and disadvantages. The optimal solution for each problem is then chosen, and after sequencing, this list of solutions becomes the treatment plan.

For patients with only a few, uncomplicated problems, the outcomes are similar, whether the treatment plan is problem based or treatment based. In more complex cases, problems are often interrelated, and the solution to one problem may affect the treatment needed to resolve other problems. In these instances, the process of identifying and listing the individual problems enables the dentist to think through each problem and consider the treatment options without getting lost in the magnitude of the overall task.

The problem-oriented approach is designed to direct the dentist's attention to a systematic evaluation of the patient, so that no problems are overlooked, either in diagnosis or in treatment planning. It prevents tunnel vision syndrome, in which obvious pathoses are focused on at the expense of less obvious but equally important problems.

Problem List Formulation

The dentist initially evaluates the patient from a subjective standpoint, first ascertaining the chief complaint and the patient's goals of treatment. A medical history and a dental history are then elicited. The objective portion of the assessment consists of a categorical evaluation of the patient, beginning with vital signs and an extraoral head and neck examination and progressing through a thorough intraoral evaluation. The examination procedures are standardized and routinely completed in the same order and fashion to simplify the procedure and to ensure that crucial steps are not omitted. Related non-clinical portions of the evaluation include examinations of radiographs and diagnostic casts.

The objectives of the examination are to distinguish normal from abnormal findings and to determine which of the abnormal findings constitute problems requiring treatment. From the findings of the initial examination, a problem list is established. If the problems are listed under categorical headings (eg, periodontal problems, endodontic problems), the dentist is unlikely to omit problems. This list is dynamic and can be modified as new problems arise.

Problem-Oriented Planning

In the next phase of treatment planning, the dentist formulates a mental image of the optimal condition to which the patient can be rehabilitated. This visualization requires that the dentist decide which teeth are periodontally and restoratively salvageable, which teeth need to be replaced, and which form of prosthodontic replacement is most appropriate. Once this optimal condition has been visualized, the dentist proposes a treatment solution for each problem on the problem list, planning each individual solution to coincide with the final visualized optimal treatment objective.

If the treatment plan for any of the individual problems conflicts with the optimal treatment plan, either the treatment for the individual problem or the optimal treatment goal must be altered until they are coincident. When the clinician believes that, in consideration of all the problems and proposed treatments, the optimal treatment objective is feasible, this list of individual treatments becomes the unsequenced treatment plan.

Treatment Sequencing

The final step in treatment planning, sequencing the treatment, is then completed by arranging the solutions to the various problems in a set order (see box).

The proposed treatment sequencing follows the logic of the medical model, so that disease is treated in the priority of importance to the patient's overall health.

Chief complaint
Medical/systemic care
Emergency care
Treatment plan presentation
Diagnostic procedures
Disease control
Reevaluation
Definitive care
Maintenance care

This method of sequencing ignores the common technique of treating by specialty, where, for example, all the periodontal care is provided, followed by the endodontic care, which is followed by the restorative care.

The patient's *chief complaint* should be addressed at the outset of treatment, even if only via discussion, and even if definitive treatment of this problem will be deferred.

The *medical/systemic care phase* includes aspects of treatment that affect the patient's systemic health. These take precedence over the treatment of dental problems and must be considered before dental problems are addressed. This most commonly includes medically related diagnostic tests and consultations. An example is the investigation of the status and control of a patient's hypertension and diabetes.

Problems addressed in the *emergency care phase* include those involving head and neck pain or infection. They are treated before routine dental problems but after acute problems involving the patient's systemic health. Clinical judgment is exercised to determine the relative importance of systemic problems and dental emergency problems. A review of this topic is found in the text by Little and Falace.[35]

The *treatment plan presentation* (and acceptance of the treatment plan) should precede all nonemergent dental care. Presentation and discussion of the proposed treatment form the basis of informed consent and must not be overlooked. In addition to the primary or optimal treatment plan, the dentist should be prepared to present alternative plans that may be indicated based on extenuating circumstances, such as patient finances or the response to therapy of teeth crucial to the success of the plan.

Procedures needed to provide additional diagnostic information for treatment planning purposes are accomplished in the *diagnostic phase*. This includes treatment beyond the diagnostic procedures accomplished during the initial examination. It encompasses such items as the use of an occlusal appliance to assess tolerance of changes in vertical dimension of occlusion or the use of an interim removable partial denture to evaluate modifications in esthetics. Diagnostic procedures may be employed at various stages in treatment, whenever additional information is needed to determine which form of treatment is optimal.

The *disease control phase* consists of treatment designed to control active disease. Examples include endodontic treatment to control infection, periodontal treatment to control inflammation, and restorative care to control caries. Treatment in this phase is aimed at the control of active disease, so that the disease processes would be arrested even if no treatment beyond disease control were provided.

The *reevaluation phase* consists of a formal reevaluation, during which the dentist decides if all factors, including, for example, the patient's treatment goals and oral hygiene, warrant continuing with the original treatment plan. This is an important phase of treatment because it provides a predetermined point at which both patient and clinician may elect to alter or even discontinue treatment.

The *definitive care phase* is the final phase of treatment preceding maintenance. Many of the procedures accomplished within the disease-control phase, such as removal of caries and placement of direct restorations, both control the disease and constitute the definitive restoration; however, a number of procedures that go beyond the treatment of active disease are possible. These include procedures designed to enhance function and esthetics, such as orthodontics, prosthodontics, and cosmetic restorative procedures. Treatment sequencing for most of these modalities is beyond the scope of this text. A detailed and comprehensive review of treatment sequencing is provided by Barsh.[5]

Maintenance care is an ongoing phase designed to maintain the results of the previous treatment and prevent the recurrence of disease. The maintenance phase generally focuses on assessment of plaque and oral hygiene, maintenance of periodontal health, detection and treatment of caries, and the prevention of dental attrition.

Dental History and Chief Complaint

The key to successful treatment planning lies in identifying the problems present and formulating a plan that solves each problem, so that each phase of treatment is designed to lead to the final, optimal treatment goal. The dentist who follows this approach begins by listening carefully to the patient and asking relevant questions. A thorough dental history serves as a guide for the clinical examination.

The dental history is divided into three components: the history of the chief complaint, the history of past dental treatment, and the history of symptoms related to the dentition. The chief complaint is addressed first and is recorded in the dental record in the patient's own words. By discussing the patient's chief concern at the outset, the dentist accomplishes two important goals. First, the patient feels that his or her problems have been recognized and the doctor-patient relationship begins positively; second, by writing out the chief complaint, the dentist is assured that it will not be omitted from the problem list. It is not uncommon to encounter a patient who has a multitude of significant dental problems but only a minor chief complaint. If the dentist focuses too quickly on the other problems and omits a discussion of the chief complaint, the patient may question the dentist's ability and desire to resolve the patient's problems.

A brief history of past dental treatment can provide useful information. The number and frequency of past dental visits reflects the patient's dental awareness and the priority placed on oral health. The dentist should elicit information about the past treatment of specific problems, as well as the patient's tolerance for dental treatment. All of this information can be of use in fashioning the treatment plan.

Questions about previous episodes of fractured or lost restorations, trauma, infection, sensitivity, and pain can elicit information that will alert the dentist to possible problems and guide him or her in the clinical and radiographic examination. Patients may not volunteer this information; hence specific questions regarding thermal sensitivity, discomfort during chewing, gingival bleeding, and pain are warranted. When a history of symptoms indicative of pulpal damage or incomplete tooth fracture is present, specific diagnostic tests should be performed during the clinical examination.

Clinical Examination

For the purpose of restorative treatment planning, the intraoral assessment involves an examination of the periodontium, dentition, and occlusion. Specific diagnostic tests may be performed as indicated, and a radiographic examination is completed. Each portion of the evaluation should be completed before another aspect of the examination is begun. The findings from each area are placed under the appropriate heading in the problem list. Duplication is common, because some problems are noted in the evaluation of more than one system. For example, gingival bleeding and periodontal inflammation resulting from a restoration's impingement on the periodontal attachment would be noted in both the periodontal examination and the evaluation of the existing restorations. At this stage, such duplication of effort is acceptable in the interest of completeness.

The following sections describe the intraoral examination used to establish the restorative dentistry problem list (see box).

Elements of the Clinical Examination

I. Evaluation of the dentition
    A. Assessment of caries risk and plaque
    B. Evaluation of caries
    C. Assessment of the pulp
    D. Evaluation of existing restorations
    E. Evaluation of the occlusion
    F. Assessment of attrition/abrasion
    G. Assessment of tooth integrity and fractures
    H. Evaluation of esthetics

II. Evaluation of the periodontium
    A. Assessment of disease activity
    B. Evaluation of the structure and contour of bony support
    C. Mucogingival evaluation

III. Evaluation of radiographs

IV. Evaluation of diagnostic casts

Evaluation of the Dentition

Plaque and Caries Risk

The presence of plaque should be documented with a standardized plaque index. The O'Leary index, for example, is a simple, yet effective measure of plaque accumulation.[43] The use of such an index permits an objective assessment of plaque accumulation. The determination of a baseline plaque level at the time of initial examination provides a basis for communication with the patient and other dentists and permits assessments of oral hygiene over time. This is important information in

establishing a prognosis for restorative care and provides criteria for deciding whether treatment should progress beyond the disease-control phase into the definitive rehabilitation stage.

The levels and location of plaque should be established at the outset of the examination. At the conclusion of the examination appointment, the patient can be given a toothbrush and floss and instructed to clean the teeth as well as possible. Reassessment immediately after the cleaning will establish the patient's hygiene ability and reveal the nature of hygiene instructions needed. A patient who sincerely tries to remove plaque but is unsuccessful in certain areas requires instruction in technique, whereas the patient who demonstrates effective hygiene while in the office but consistently presents with high plaque levels has a problem with motivation. This information is important in designing the treatment plan. A plan requiring a great deal of patient participation and compliance would not be appropriate for a patient with inadequate motivation. Alternatively, a motivated patient who is teachable may well be suited to such a plan.

One of the most reliable indicators of future carious activity is the presence of an existing carious lesion.[18] Patients demonstrating significant carious activity may be candidates for an evaluation that entails more than simply a determination of levels and location of plaque. In addition to traditional plaque indices, both a diet survey and a specific plaque assessment are useful in determining the patient's susceptibility to caries and the prognosis for restorative treatment.

In using a diet survey, the patient itemizes all food and drink intake for a specified period (generally 1 week). From this diary, the dentist can identify the contribution of specific dietary habits to the caries and direct the patient's attention to these areas. The identification and management of episodic carbohydrate intake (snacking), as well as overall carbohydrate consumption, should be the focus of dietary intervention.[40]

Because the character of the microflora determines the cariogenicity of the plaque, an assessment of the number of cariogenic bacteria present in the plaque can give an indication of the caries susceptibility of the patient.[61] Commercial systems designed to quantify intraoral levels of *Streptococcus mutans* are available. By monitoring the levels of *S.-Mutans* at baseline and over time, the dentist can assess the effectiveness of caries-control measures.

Once plaque assessments have been completed, an examination of other areas can be accomplished. The visual examination of the dentition should be conducted in a dry field, with adequate lighting, using a mirror and

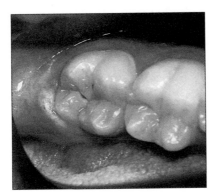

Fig 2-1a Occlusal caries. The shadowing around the stained pits in the second molar indicates the presence of caries.

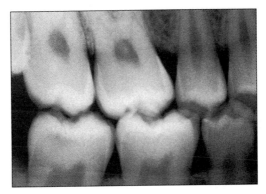

Fig 2-1b The occlusal caries shown in Fig 2-1a extends well into dentin.

explorer. If the presence of plaque and calculus partially obscures the dentition, debridement must be completed to accomplish a thorough examination.

Caries Diagnosis

Caries may be classified by location into two broad categories: smooth-surface and pit and fissure caries. Smooth-surface caries includes interproximal caries, root caries, and caries on other smooth surfaces. Diagnosis of caries involves both clinical (visual and tactile) and radiographic examinations.

Pit and fissure caries. Pit and fissure caries is generally found in areas of incomplete enamel coalescence. These areas are most commonly found on the occlusal surfaces of posterior teeth, the lingual surfaces of maxillary anterior teeth, and the buccal pits of molar teeth. Because pit and fissure caries may begin in small enamel defects that lie in close approximation to the dentino-enamel junction, this type of caries may be difficult to detect. Pit and fissure caries must be extensive to be detected radiographically, generally appearing as a crescent-shaped radiolucency immediately subjacent to the enamel[64] (Figs 2-1a to 2-1c).

Tactile examination, probing the enamel with a sharp explorer, is the clinical technique most commonly used by dentists in the United States to locate pit and fissure caries.[13] A "sticky" sensation felt on removal of the explorer is the classic sign of pit and fissure caries. Clinical studies have shown this method to be unreliable, however, producing many false-positive diagnoses.[3] In addition, an explorer can cause cavitation in a demineralized pit or fissure, precluding the possibility of remineralization.[3,7,19,21]

Visual observation, with magnification, of a clean, dry tooth has been found to be a reliable, nondestructive

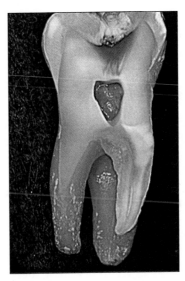

Fig 2-1c The typical pattern of occlusal caries is shown in cross section.

method of detecting pit and fissure caries.[3,19,21] Pit and fissure caries appears as a gray or gray-yellow, opaque area that shows through the enamel (Fig 2-1a). Fiber-optic transillumination may be helpful in visualizing pit and fissure and other types of caries. A variety of new imaging technologies are being evaluated for caries detection.

When the presence of pit and fissure caries is uncertain and the patient will be available for recall evaluations, sealant may be placed over the suspect area. Clinical investigations by Mertz-Fairhurst et al,[41] indicate

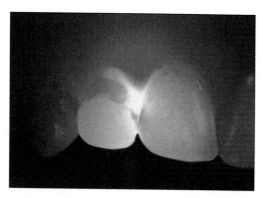

Fig 2-2 Interproximal caries is detected in an anterior tooth with the use of transillumination.

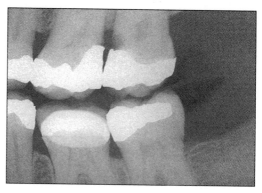

Fig 2-3 Root caries that would be difficult to detect in a routine clinical examination is revealed in a radiograph.

that sealed caries has little potential for progression. Placement of sealants over known caries cannot be recommended at present, however. The risk of sealant loss in a patient known to have caries makes this an injudicious practice.

Smooth-surface caries. Of the three types of smooth-surface caries, interproximal caries is the most difficult to detect clinically. Generally inaccessible to both visual and tactile examination, interproximal caries in posterior teeth is usually detected radiographically. Interproximal caries in anterior teeth may be diagnosed radiographically or with a visual examination using transillumination (Fig 2-2). Root caries located on the facial or lingual surface of the roots presents little diagnostic problem. When root-surface caries occurs interproximally, however, it is not readily visible during clinical examination and is generally detected through the radiographic examination (Fig 2-3). Smooth-surface caries occurring on enamel in non-interproximal areas is not difficult to detect clinically. It is most commonly found in patients with high levels of plaque and a cariogenic diet, occurring on the facial and lingual enamel surfaces. It is readily accessible to visual and tactile examination.

Pulp

Evaluation of pulpal vitality in every tooth is not warranted; however, each tooth that will receive extensive restoration, as well as all teeth that are critical to the plan of treatment and teeth with pulps of questionable vitality, should be tested.

Application of cold is a valuable method of vitality testing. A cotton pellet saturated with an aerosol skin refrigerant, such as dichlorotetrafluoroethane, is placed on the tooth to determine its vitality. A similar test can be performed by placing a "pencil of ice" (made by freezing water inside a sterilized anesthetic cartridge)

against a tooth. Skin refrigerants present minimal risk to teeth and restorations; however, carbon dioxide snow and dry ice should be avoided, because they are extremely cold (–108°F) and can damage enamel or ceramic restorations through thermal shock.[2]

An additional vitality test involves the use of an electric pulp tester. While it can provide information regarding pulp vitality, this test has limitations; it cannot be used in a wet field or on teeth with metallic interproximal restorations unless measures are taken to insulate adjacent teeth. Furthermore, the numeric scale on the instrument does not reflect the health of the pulp or its prognosis. The electronic pulp tester is merely a means of determining whether the tissue within the pulp senses electrical current. A high score may be due to the presence of a partially necrotic pulp or extensive reparative dentin or may be the result of poor contact between the tooth and the pulp tester.

When the results of the pulp tests are not congruent with the clinical impression, additional tests are indicated. When neither thermal nor electric pulp tests provide a clear picture of pulp vitality, and a restoration is indicated, the preparation can be initiated without the use of anesthetic. This is termed a test cavity. If pain or sensitivity is elicited when dentin is cut with a bur, pulpal vitality is confirmed. The restoration may then be completed after administration of local anesthetic.

When a posterior tooth receives endodontic treatment, placement of a complete–cuspal coverage restoration is generally indicated to prevent fracture.[51] The same is true for anterior teeth, except when the only significant deficiency is a conservative endodontic access.[57,58] Because endodontically treated teeth warrant this extensive restorative treatment, it is important to determine pulp vitality prior to the placement of a restoration. It is embarrassing to discover that a recently restored tooth was nonvital prior to restoration and subsequently became symptomatic, requiring endodontic treatment and a replacement restoration.

It is advantageous to ascertain the pulpal prognosis of a tooth prior to restorative treatment. At times this may be difficult, however. When pulpal prognosis is uncertain or guarded, it is often best to perform endodontic therapy prior to extensive restorative treatment. If the endodontic treatment is completed prior to restorative care, the repair or replacement of a recently completed large restoration may be avoided. An added benefit is that the endodontic prognosis can be established before the dentist commits to restorative care.

When endodontic therapy is required, the feasibility of completing the endodontic procedures should be determined early in the course of treatment. The more critical the tooth is to the overall success of the treatment, the more important it becomes to complete the necessary endodontic treatment early in the treatment schedule. It is poor planning to rely on a tooth elsewhere in the treatment plan, when that tooth cannot be successfully treated with endodontics.

Endodontic diagnosis can be a challenging task. A thorough discussion of this subject can be found in the text by Cohen and Burns.[15]

Existing Restorations

In the course of the intraoral examination, existing restorations must be evaluated to determine their serviceability. The following general criteria are used to evaluate existing restorations: *(1)* structural integrity, *(2)* marginal opening, *(3)* anatomic form, *(4)* restoration-related periodontal health, *(5)* occlusal and interproximal contacts, *(6)* caries, and *(7)* esthetics.

Structural Integrity. An evaluation of the structural integrity of a restoration involves determining whether it is intact or whether portions of the restoration are partially or completely fractured or missing. The presence of a fracture line dictates replacement of the restoration. If voids are present, the dentist must exercise clinical judgment in determining whether their size and location will weaken the restoration and predispose it to further deterioration or recurrent caries.

Marginal opening. Few restorations have perfect margins, and the point at which marginal opening dictates replacement of the restoration is difficult to determine. For amalgam restorations, it has been demonstrated that marginal ditching neither implies the presence nor necessarily portends the development of caries.[28] Therefore, the existence of marginal ditching does not dictate the replacement of amalgam restorations. Because the margins of amalgam restorations become relatively well sealed from the accumulation of corrosion products, a general guideline has been to continue to observe the restoration unless signs of recurrent caries are present. An accumulation of plaque in the marginal gap is also an indication for repair or replacement of a restoration. Recently, it has been suggested that noncarious marginal gaps in amalgam may be restored with a resin sealant to enhance the longevity of the restoration.[54] The long-term clinical efficacy of this method has yet to be documented; however, it may hold promise.

For restorations that do not seal by corrosion and do not have anticariogenic properties, a marginal gap into which the end of a sharp explorer may penetrate should be considered for repair, or the restoration should be replaced. This is especially true for resin composite restorations, because bacterial growth has been shown to progress more readily adjacent to resin composite than to amalgam or glass-ionomer cement.[55] An increased susceptibility to caries has been reported in resin composite restorations whose marginal gaps exceeded 100 to 150 µm.[44]

The presence of a marginal gap is less critical for restorations with anticariogenic properties (eg, glass-ionomer cement). Both in vitro[52] and in vivo studies[59] have shown that glass-ionomer restorations are less susceptible to caries than are resin composite restorations[59]; restorations with anticariogenic properties should be replaced when recurrent caries or some other defect indicates the need for treatment. In anterior teeth, this occurs when the marginal gap has resulted in marginal staining that is esthetically unacceptable.

Anatomic form. Anatomic form refers to the degree to which the restoration duplicates the original contour of the intact tooth. Common problems include overcontouring, undercontouring, uneven marginal ridges, inadequate facial and lingual embrasures, and lack of occlusal or gingival embrasures. Many restorations exhibit one or more of these problems yet adequately serve the needs of the patient and do not require replacement. The critical factor in determining the need for replacement is not whether the contour is ideal but whether pathoses have resulted, or are likely to result, from the poor contour.

Restoration-related periodontal health. Examination of restorations must include an assessment of the effect that existing restorations have on the health of the adjacent periodontium. Problems commonly encountered in this area are *(1)* surface roughness of the restoration, *(2)* interproximal overhangs, and *(3)* impingement on the

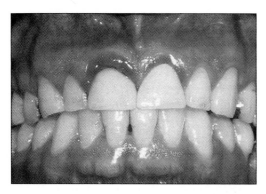

Fig 2-4a The periodontal inflammation is caused by the encroachment of the crown margins into the periodontal attachment area of the maxillary central incisors.

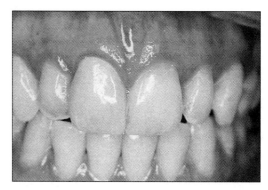

Fig 2-4b Marginal inflammation is present on the distal and facial aspects, despite supragingival margins. Encroachment on the biologic width by the mesial margin of the crown has caused a chronic inflammatory response, which has extended to the facial and distal portions of the tooth.

zone of attachment, called the *biologic width* (the area, approximately 2 mm in the apicocoronal dimension, occupied by the junctional epithelium and the connective tissue attachment) (see Fig 1-23a).

All three of these phenomena can cause inflammation of the periodontium.[39,56,62] If restorations extend vertically or horizontally beyond the cavosurface margin in the region of the periodontal attachment or impinge on the biologic width the health of the periodontal tissue should be assessed (Figs 2-4a and 2-4b). If other local etiologic factors have been removed, and periodontal inflammation persists in the presence of these conditions, treatment should be initiated. In the case of overhanging restorations, pathosis may be eliminated and the restoration may be made serviceable simply by removing the overhang. If the periodontal inflammation fails to resolve, the restoration should be replaced. In the case of biologic width impingement, space for a healthy periodontal attachment must be gained, through surgical crown lengthening or a combination of orthodontic extrusion and surgical crown lengthening.

Inflammatory changes suggestive of biologic width violations are not uncommon on the facial aspect of anterior teeth that have been restored with crowns. On occasion, however, evaluation of the marginal area reveals inflammation even when an adequate space remains between the coronal margin and the periodontal attachment apparatus, leaving the clinician puzzled as to the cause of the problem. If periodontal inflammation persists in the apparent absence of local etiologic factors, including biologic width infringement, the dentist should evaluate the entire cervical circumference of the restoration. Inflammatory changes on the facial aspect of a restoration are sometimes a manifestation of interprox-

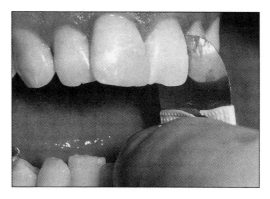

Fig 2-5 A proximal contact–smoothing device is useful for removing irregularities that impede the passage of floss.

imal inflammation. Further evaluation may reveal an interproximal violation of biologic width from which the inflammatory reaction has extended to the more visible facial area.

Even in the absence of impingement on biologic width, open or rough subgingival margins can harbor sufficient plaque to generate an inflammatory response. During assessment of existing restorations or planning of future restorations, location of margins is an important consideration. Supragingival margins result in significantly less gingival inflammation than do subgingival margins.[36] Supragingival margins should be the goal when overriding concerns (eg, esthetics or requirements for resistance and retention) do not contraindicate their use.

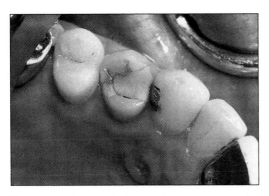

Fig 2-6a The marginal gap of a resin composite restoration is stained. Note the shadow indicating that caries extends into the dentin.

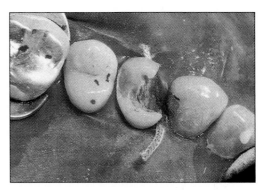

Fig 2-6b Removal of the restoration reveals that extensive caries is present.

Occlusal and interproximal contacts. All proximal contacts should be assessed with thin dental floss by the dentist. In addition, the patient should be queried regarding any problems encountered in the passing of floss through the contact during home hygiene. Contacts that do not allow the smooth passage of floss must be altered, or the restoration must be replaced, to permit the use of floss. Figure 2-5 depicts the use of a proximal contact–smoothing device that is often effective in eliminating roughness that impedes the passage of floss.

Contacts that are open or excessively light should be evaluated to determine whether pathosis, food impaction, or annoyance to the patient has resulted. When any of these features is present, steps should be taken to alleviate the problem. Generally, the placement or replacement of a restoration is required to establish an adequate proximal contact.

When an open contact is found, an attempt should be made to determine its cause. If occlusal contacts have moved a tooth, and a restoration is to be placed to close the proximal contact, the occlusal contacts must be altered to prevent the open contact from recurring after the placement of the new restoration.

The occlusal contacts of all restorations should be evaluated to determine whether they are serving their masticatory function without creating a symptomatic or pathogenic occlusion. In the absence of periodontally pathogenic bacteria, traumatic occlusion has not been found to initiate loss of periodontal attachment[63]; however, in the presence of periodontal pathogens, occlusal trauma has been found to accelerate the loss of attachment.[34] Existing restorations located on teeth exhibiting significant attachment deficits should be examined closely for the presence of hyperocclusion. Restorations whose occlusal contacts are creating primary occlusal trauma should be altered or replaced, as necessary, to resolve the problem. Restorations that are in significant infraocclusion may permit the supraeruption of opposing teeth and should be considered for replacement.

Caries. The evaluation for caries around existing restorations focuses on an examination of the margins. The dentist must use a combination of visual, tactile, and radiographic examinations to detect the presence of caries. A radiolucent area surrounding a radiopaque restoration or the presence of soft tooth structure generally indicates caries and warrants either repair or replacement of the restoration.

Discoloration in the marginal areas is a sign that is more difficult to interpret. It often indicates leakage of some degree. In non-amalgam restorations without anticariogenic properties, discoloration that penetrates the margin often indicates the need for replacement of the restoration (Figs 2-6a and 2-6b). This is not a definite indication, however, and clinical judgment is required. In restorations with anticariogenic properties, leakage and stain may be observed with less concern for caries, leaving esthetics as the primary consideration.

In the case of amalgam restorations, the decision to replace a restoration with discoloration in the adjacent tooth structure is less clear because corrosion products may discolor a tooth, even in the absence of caries, especially when little dentin is present. When there is no apparent communication between the cavosurface and the stained area and when the discoloration is primarily gray, then metal "show through" is suspected and observation is warranted (Fig 2-7). When the discolored area

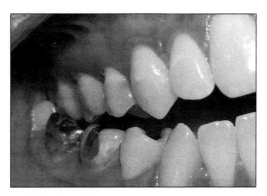

Fig 2-7 The shadow is caused by amalgam that shows through the translucent enamel. No caries is present.

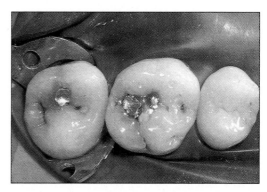

Fig 2-8 The shadow located on the mesiolingual cusp adjacent to the distal amalgam restoration on the maxillary right first molar indicates the presence of caries.

appears yellow or brown and appears to communicate with the cavosurface, replacement of the restoration is indicated (Fig 2-8).

Esthetics. The esthetic evaluation of existing restorations is highly subjective. When the functional aspects of a restoration are adequate, it is often best to simply inquire whether the patient is satisfied with the esthetic appearance of the existing restorations. If the patient expresses dissatisfaction over the appearance of a restoration, the dentist must determine whether improvement is feasible. Care should be taken to ascertain the reason that the original restoration had less-than-optimal esthetics. An underlying problem may preclude improvement of the original esthetic problem and an equally unsatisfactory result may occur in the replacement restoration.

When electively replacing a restoration for esthetic reasons, the dentist must carefully explain the risks (eg, endodontic complications) incurred in replacing the restorations.

Some of the more common esthetic problems found in existing restorations are *(1)* display of metal, *(2)* discoloration or poor shade match in tooth-colored restorations, *(3)* poor contour in tooth-colored restorations, and *(4)* poor periodontal tissue response in anterior restorations.

Occlusion and Wear

The occlusion can have significant effects on the restorative treatment plan. The following factors should be evaluated in the course of the occlusal examination: *(1)* occlusal interferences between the occlusion of centric relation (CR) and that of maximum intercuspation (MI); *(2)* the number and position of occlusal contacts, as well as the stress placed on the occlusal contacts in MI; *(3)*

the attrition of teeth and restorations resulting from occlusal function and parafunction; *(4)* the interarch space available for placement of needed restorations.

Occlusal interferences. Most people have some difference between the positions of centric relation and maximum intercuspation and have no consequent pathosis, indicating that the existence of a discrepancy between these positions is not, in itself, an indication for occlusal equilibration. Findings from the occlusal examination that should be recorded in the restorative dentistry problem list and do warrant treatment with occlusal equilibration are the following: *(1)* signs and symptoms of occlusal pathosis resulting from discrepancies between the occlusion of centric relation and maximum intercuspation (eg, mobility, excessive wear of teeth in the areas of interference between CR and MI, or periodontal ligament soreness); and *(2)* the need to restore the majority of the posterior occlusion.

This second factor does not imply the restoration of the majority of the posterior teeth but rather the restoration of the majority of the occlusal contacts. For example, insertion of a three-unit fixed partial denture in the mandibular right quadrant and several large restorations in the maxillary left quadrant results in the restoration of the majority of the occlusal contacts for the posterior teeth. There is no reason to fabricate the occlusion of the new restorations to duplicate the interferences that existed preoperatively. In such a case, occlusal equilibration should be completed prior to the restorative treatment. Through adjustment of only a very few occlusal contacts on teeth not involved in restorations and subsequent fabrication of the new restorations in centric relation, the occlusions of CR and MI become coincident.

Occlusal contacts. The number and position of occlusal contacts in the maximum intercuspation position, the force of the occlusal load, and the manner in which opposing teeth occlude in excursive function strongly influence the selection of restorative materials, as well as the design of the preparation and restoration. As the number of missing teeth increases, the proportion of the occlusal load borne by each tooth increases. As occlusal stress increases, the dentist is forced to select the strongest of the available restorative materials and to design restorations to provide the greatest strength in the areas of maximum stress. Likewise, the greater the potential for the patient to function on the restorations in lateral excursions, the greater is the need for strength in the restorative material and the greater is the imperative to select a material that will function without causing injury to the opposing dentition.

Wear. Out of concern for the opposing dentition, the clinician must consider the abrasive potential of the various restorative materials available. Clinical abrasivity is a function of a number of physical properties; no single variable is predictive of abrasivity.[45] Hardness is a useful indicator, but the best predictor of wear is the relative clinical performance of the various materials. In clinical determinations of wear behavior, the amalgam in an amalgam-enamel wear couple exhibits only slightly greater wear than does an enamel-enamel wear couple. The amalgam causes less wear to the opposing dentition than does enamel.[29] The wear rate of resin composite depends on the nature of the resin composite. Microfilled resins exhibit wear behavior similar to that of enamel, while hybrid resins exhibit more wear and generate more wear to opposing enamel than does either amalgam or enamel.[37] Polished cast gold is more wear resistant than enamel or amalgam and generates minimal wear of opposing tooth structure.

Ceramic restorations exhibit little wear themselves, but have demonstrated a consistent ability to severely abrade the enamel of the opposing dentition[42] (Fig 2-9). The castable ceramic, Dicor (Dentsply), is a notable exception among ceramic materials. The polished Dicor-enamel wear couple has been shown to perform similarly to an enamel-enamel couple.[17]

When a direct restorative material is needed, a useful guideline is to restore teeth that oppose natural teeth with amalgam or resin composite. When a crown is required, cast gold is the material of choice; it may be veneered with porcelain in nonfunctional areas. It is best to avoid occlusal coverage with porcelain in areas of excursive occlusion because of its propensity to generate wear of the natural dentition.

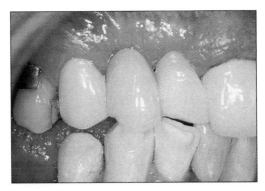

Fig 2-9 Extensive tooth structure has been lost in the mandibular teeth because of wear caused by the opposing porcelain fixed partial denture.

Wear (attrition and abrasion) of the natural dentition is a normal clinical phenomenon. Only when wear becomes excessive is it deemed a problem. The etiology of clinical wear may be varied. Excessive occlusal wear is generally caused by occlusal parafunction. In these instances, facets on opposing teeth match well, indicating the predominant path of parafunctional activity. Because altering occlusal parafunctional habits is extremely difficult, prevention of excessive occlusal wear is accomplished with the use of an occlusal acrylic resin appliance (Figs 2-10a and 2-10b). The dentist should identify patients who demonstrate signs of excessive occlusal wear (especially those patients who exhibit these signs at an early age) and include occlusal appliance therapy in the treatment plan.

Occasionally, the presence of abrasive substances in the mouth is the cause of excessive occlusal wear. When the vocation or lifestyle of a patient frequently places him or her in contact with airborne abrasives, prevention of wear is difficult. Education of the patient and use of an occlusal acrylic resin appliance will decrease the occlusal abrasion; however, decreasing the patient's exposure to the causative agent is the only reliable means of eliminating the problem.

Unlike occlusal wear, the wear found on the cervical-facial surfaces of teeth is not due to tooth-to-tooth abrasion. It is generally thought to be toothbrush related, although occlusally generated stresses may contribute to this wear in some instances. The term *abfraction* is applied to those lesions thought to have a combined etiology of abrasion and tooth flexure.[26,32] Preventive treatment for cervical abrasion is directed at altering the habit that has caused the problem. Modification of tooth-brushing habits and the use of minimally abrasive

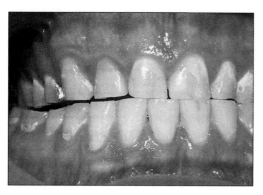

Fig 2-10a The significant occlusal attrition is caused by a habit of parafunctional grinding, in a patient less than 30 years of age.

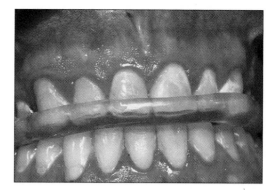

Fig 2-10b An occlusal acrylic resin appliance is used to minimize the abrasive trauma generated by the parafunctional grinding habit.

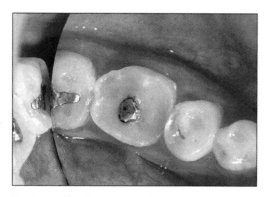

Fig 2-11 Significant loss of tooth structure in the absence of facets that would indicate occlusal wear is evidence of a chemical erosive process. Note both the amalgam restoration standing above the surrounding tooth structure and the smooth, glasslike character of the dentin.

toothpastes can reduce the rate of abrasion. If abfraction is suspected, treatment should include the nighttime wear of an occlusal acrylic resin appliance.

Another form of tooth loss, which often mimics wear, is caused by chemical erosion. Erosion can result from habits, such as lemon sucking, or from the introduction of gastric acid into the oral cavity, which can occur with repeated regurgitation (eg, with incompetent esophageal sphincter or bulimia). Chemical erosion can be distinguished from mechanical wear by the location and character of the defects. Erosion lesions have a smooth, glassy appearance. When found on the occlusal surfaces of posterior teeth, these lesions are characterized by concave defects into which abrasive agents are unlikely to penetrate. Severely "cupped out" cusp tips and teeth that have restorations standing above the surrounding

tooth structure are clinical findings commonly associated with chemical erosion (Fig 2-11). Smooth lesions appearing on the lingual surfaces are generally caused by an erosive process, while lesions on the facial surfaces might be of chemical or mechanical origin.

In instances of uncertainty, questions related to habits and tooth-brushing technique may elucidate the cause of mechanical abrasion, while a thorough history and medical evaluation may reveal the presence of acid-related erosion. When bulimia is the underlying problem, detection is often difficult. The dentist must be tactfully candid in discussing this possible etiology. Regardless of the cause of the loss of tooth structure, the primary etiology should be determined and resolved before rehabilitative therapy is undertaken.

Interarch space. When the dentist determines that significant wear of a tooth has occurred and pulpal sensitivity has arisen, or that teeth have been so weakened by abrasion or erosion as to be at risk for fracture, restorative treatment is indicated. The restoration of cervical abrasion poses little dilemma, and any of the restorative materials suited to the restoration of Class 5 lesions will serve satisfactorily. Glass-ionomer restorative materials have proven to be particularly effective in the restoration of Class 5 lesions, routinely providing longevity in excess of 5 years.[38]

When severe wear dictates the placement of a restoration covering the occlusal surface, the dentist must evaluate the occlusion of maximum intercuspation and determine whether sufficient space exists for the placement of the restoration. If inadequate space is available, the dentist must either gain space by surgical crown lengthening, shorten the opposing tooth, or select a different restorative option that requires less space. Recognition of the space's inadequacy prior to crown preparation is essential. Many a clinician has sought the advantages of a super-retentive cement to retain a short crown, when advance planning would have permitted a crown preparation of adequate height.

In those few cases where generalized wear or erosion has taken place resulting in the loss of an extensive amount of tooth structure, the dentist is faced with a significant restorative problem. In these instances, sufficient interarch space is often not available to restore the lost tooth structure, without increasing the vertical dimension of occlusion. Increasing the vertical dimension of occlusion is a complex restorative process involving more than a consideration of the mechanics of individual tooth restoration. A description of treatment of this nature is beyond the scope of this text. Dawson[16] provided an excellent review of the restoration of the severely worn dentition.

Incomplete Tooth Fracture

Incomplete tooth fracture, sometimes called *cracked-tooth syndrome*, is a fairly common clinical occurrence. Patients often report that they experience intermittent, sharp pains of short duration when they chew, sensitivity to cold, and a periodic, dull ache that is difficult to localize.[10,11,14,53]

Incomplete tooth fracture may be found in restored or unrestored teeth.[27] In restored teeth, it is usually associated with existing two- or three-surface restorations[24,30] (Fig 2-12). It has been reported to occur equally in both the maxillary and mandibular arches. In the maxillary arch, it occurs with similar frequencies in molars and premolars. In the mandibular arch, molars are the teeth most commonly found to be cracked.[12] Regardless of the location by arch, the cusps most commonly fractured are the nonfunctional cusps.[12] Often, patients with multiple cracked teeth have parafunctional habits or malocclusions that have contributed to the problem. Cracked-tooth syndrome is an age-related phenomenon; the greatest incidence is found among patients between 26 and 50 years of age.[27]

Diagnosis of incomplete tooth fracture may be difficult. The patient is often unable to identify the offending tooth, and evaluation tools, such as radiographs, clinical examination, percussion, and pulp tests, are typically nondiagnostic. Transillumination often helps identify cracks, but many teeth contain cracks and craze lines, most of which cause no symptoms. It is often possible to localize the crack responsible for the patient's pain, not only to the correct tooth but also to the specific portion of the tooth that is cracked, by having the patient bite on a wooden stick, rubber wheel, or other device, to repro-

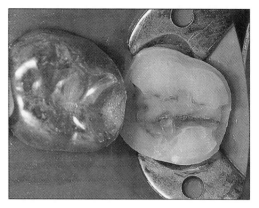

Fig 2-12 The mesiodistal crack in the pulpal floor of the mandibular right first molar causes sharp pains when the patient chews. The tooth is to be restored with an onlay to splint the tooth together during function, to relieve the patient's symptoms and prevent propagation of the crack.

duce the symptoms. Crunchy food, placed sequentially on suspect teeth, has also been suggested as a diagnostic aid.[1] Once the offending tooth has been identified, tooth preparation often allows visualization of the crack.

Where direct diagnostic methods prove unsuccessful, indirect methods may be used. An orthodontic band or sealant may be placed on suspect teeth to prevent separation of the crack during function. If the patient's symptoms subside, the diagnosis of incomplete tooth fracture has been made.

In treatment for incomplete tooth fracture, the cracked portions of the tooth are splinted together with a cuspal coverage restoration.[24] This may include amalgam restorations, crowns, or onlays of metal, ceramic, or resin composite. Because of their potential to lose bond integrity over time, bonded intracoronal restorations are presently not considered to be adequate for long-term resolution of the problem.[20,25]

Esthetic Evaluation

In addition to an esthetic evaluation of existing restorations, an assessment of the esthetics of the entire dentition should be completed. Because dental esthetics is a subjective area, patients should be questioned to discover any dissatisfaction they have regarding the esthetics of their dentition. In the absence of complaints by the patient, the impressions of the dentist regarding esthetic problems should be tactfully conveyed to determine whether the patient would like the esthetic problems addressed. When an agreement has been reached between the patient and dentist as to the existence of specific esthetic problems, the problems should be included on the restorative dentistry problem list.

Commonly encountered esthetic problems that are related to or may be addressed by restorative dentistry include *(1)* stained or discolored anterior teeth; *(2)* unesthetic contours in anterior teeth (eg, unesthetic length, width, incisal edge shape, or axial contours); *(3)* unesthetic position or spacing of anterior teeth; *(4)* carious lesions and unesthetic restorations; and *(5)* unesthetic color and/or contour of tissue adjacent to anterior restorations. The restorative treatment of esthetic problems may range from conservative therapy, such as microabrasion and bleaching, to more invasive care, such as the placement of resin veneers, ceramic veneers, or complete-coverage crowns. These restorations are discussed in subsequent chapters.

Evaluation of the Periodontium

From a restorative dentistry perspective, the periodontium must be evaluated primarily for two reasons: *(1)* to determine the effect that the periodontal health of the teeth will have on the restorative dentistry treatment plan and *(2)* to determine the effect that planned and existing restorations will have on the health of the periodontium.

Evaluation of the periodontium consists of a clinical assessment of attachment levels and bony topography, tooth mobility, a qualitative assessment of tissue health, and a radiographic evaluation of the supporting bone. The assessment of attachment levels involves periodontal probing of the entire dentition with both a straight probe for determination of vertical probing depth and a curved probe to explore furcation areas. Any bleeding induced by gentle probing should be noted. A variety of tests are available to aid in determining the presence and identity of periodontal pathogens; however, the most consistent clinical indicator of inflammation is bleeding on probing.[47] Bleeding on probing does not always indicate the presence of active periodontal disease, but periodontitis has been consistently found to be absent in the absence of bleeding on probing.[47]

The qualitative assessment of periodontal tissue health calls for a subjective assessment of the inflammatory status of the tissue; tissue color, texture, contours, edema, and sulcular exudates are noted. The presence of specific local factors, such as plaque and calculus and their relationship to tissue inflammation, should be noted. Abnormal mucogingival architecture, such as gingival dehiscences and areas of minimal attached gingiva,

should be recorded. This is especially true when these anomalies are noted in the proximity of existing or planned restorations.

During the examination of the periodontium, the dentist not only must be cognizant of periodontal inflammation adjacent to existing restorations, but also must estimate the location of margins for future restorations and their potential for impinging on the biologic width. Review of radiographs, especially correctly angulated bitewing radiographs, during the periodontal examination enables the dentist to assess the relationship of existing and planned restorations to bone levels and to correlate radiographic signs with clinical findings.

When the clinical and radiographic portion of the periodontal examination has been completed, a periodontal prognosis should be established for all teeth; special attention should be given to teeth involved in the restorative dentistry treatment plan. Teeth requiring restorative treatment that have a guarded periodontal prognosis should be noted in the restorative dentistry problem list. Until the periodontal prognosis becomes predictably positive, the restorative treatment of teeth with a guarded prognosis should be as conservative as possible, and treatment planning that relies on these teeth must remain flexible.

Evaluation of Radiographs

The radiographic examination is an essential component of the comprehensive evaluation. Problems detected during the evaluation of radiographs are listed under the appropriate heading on the problem list (eg, restorative, periodontal).

Although radiographs can provide valuable information for use in diagnosis and treatment planning, exposure of patients to ionizing radiation must be minimized; therefore, discretion is required when the dentist orders radiographs. There are no inflexible rules for radiographic evaluation; rather, clinical judgment should be exercised. The goal is to minimize unnecessary exposure and cost but to avoid underutilization, which might result in inadequate diagnosis. The use of patient-specific criteria is the key. Different patients have different requirements both in terms of the radiographic views needed and the frequency with which radiographs should be repeated.

A reasonable guideline to follow is that all dentate patients should initially have a radiographic series completed that reveals the periapical areas of the entire dentition. This will permit the detection of central lesions not visible on bitewing radiographs and will serve as a baseline, allowing the clinician to assess changes over time. Although it is not common to discover pathoses on panoramic films or complete-mouth radiograph series, it has been reported that approximately 85% of central jaw lesions are apparent in views of the apical areas of the dentition but are not visible on bitewing radiographs.[8] For patients who have periodontal disease, periapical radiographs are indicated. For patients who have no significant periodontal pathoses, a panoramic radiograph provides the necessary view. For all patients with approximating teeth, a series of films is indicated to show the interproximal areas of posterior teeth. Bitewing radiographs serve this purpose.

The frequency with which radiographs should be updated is determined by clinical judgment. The dentist should assess the etiologic factors present and determine whether new disease is likely to have occurred since the last radiographic examination. The dentist must weigh the risk of undetected disease against the cumulative risk of radiation exposure. A suggested guideline is to take new bitewing radiographs of caries-active adults on an annual basis and of caries-inactive patients every 2 to 3 years.[60] Patients may be considered minimally susceptible to caries if they have had no carious lesions in recent years, demonstrate low plaque levels, have adequate salivary flow, have a noncariogenic diet, and exhibit no clinically discernible caries. Periapical radiographs of the entire dentition should be repeated only as dictated by the specific needs of the treatment to be accomplished. For example, a patient under active treatment or maintenance for periodontal disease may require an updated radiographic series every 2 to 3 years to reevaluate bony contours, while another patient, because disease processes are controlled, may require subsequent periapical radiographic updates only every 4 to 5 years.

In evaluating radiographic findings for restorative purposes, the dentist should note open interproximal contacts, marginal openings, overhanging restorations, intrapulpal and periapical radiolucencies and radiopacities, and radiolucencies within the body of the tooth. The dentist must interpret "abnormal" radiographic findings with caution. Many phenomena that are detectable radiographically can also be detected clinically and should be verified clinically before treatment is planned. This is especially true when the clinician evaluates radiolucencies that appear to represent caries but may in fact represent nonpathologic processes. An example of this is the radiographic phenomenon commonly known as *burnout* (Fig 2-13). Burnout is a radiolucency, not caused by demineralization, that occurs when the x-ray beam traverses a portion of the tooth with less thickness than the

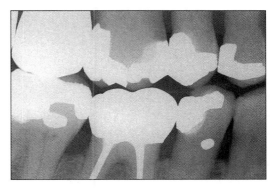

Fig 2-13 The radiolucent area beneath the restoration in the mesial surface of the maxillary first molar is radiographic burnout. No caries is present.

surrounding areas. It is most commonly found near the cervical area of a tooth and is frequently caused by concavities in the tooth or the angulation of the beam.

The dentist must be careful not to mistakenly diagnose as caries a decrease in radiopacity resulting from an abraded area. Likewise, the dentist must be cautious in diagnosing caries beneath existing restorations because certain radiolucent dental materials have a radiographic appearance similar to that of caries. A comprehensive review of dental radiology has been provided by Goaz and White.[23]

Evaluation of Diagnostic Casts

The dentist can gain valuable information through an evaluation of diagnostic casts. By examining diagnostic casts of the dentition, the dentist can see areas that are visually inaccessible during the clinical examination. Facets and marginal openings that may be difficult to discern intraorally are readily visible on the diagnostic casts. Facets on the casts of the dentition can be aligned to provide a guide to dynamic occlusal relationships. In addition, the dentist may utilize gypsum casts to complete diagnostic preparations and diagnostic waxups, simulating planned treatment. Where removable partial dentures are indicated, survey and design procedures may be completed on the diagnostic casts before restorative treatment is planned. The requirements of removable partial denture design may thus be considered during the planning of restorative care.

Although not every case requires the evaluation of casts mounted on a semiadjustable articulator, some will. Cases involving multiple missing teeth or the restoration of a significant portion of the occlusion should be evaluated with mounted diagnostic casts. If multiple teeth are missing, the articulator maintains the correct interarch relationship, permitting buccal and lingual views of interarch spaces. Using a semiadjustable articulator that provides a reasonable approximation of the patient's intercondylar distance, condylar inclination, lateral guidance, and hinge axis of rotation, the dentist can simulate the patient's mandibular movements. This enables the clinician to assess the occlusal scheme and to plan restorative care accordingly.

Treatment Plan

Having completed a comprehensive examination, the dentist lists problems related to restorative dentistry on the restorative dentistry problem list (Fig 2-14). Each of the problems on the problem list is then reevaluated. After consideration, some of the problems may be deleted from the list. For example, a tooth with a defective restoration may also have a significant loss of periodontal attachment and, therefore, a poor periodontal prognosis. In such a case, the defective restoration is initially considered a problem, but, in view of the periodontal condition, the tooth would be planned for extraction rather than restoration. The defective restoration is then omitted from the restorative problem list.

Once the final problem list is formulated, the next step is to establish a plan for the treatment of each problem on the list. A problem list worksheet is a useful tool to help organize the planning of treatment for each problem. It consists of an unsequenced list of problems and their associated solutions (Fig 2-15). Later, during the sequencing process, this list of treatments will be integrated into the comprehensive treatment plan.

Planning the restoration of individual teeth is the nuts and bolts of restorative dentistry treatment planning. It requires the consideration of four primary factors as well as a number of modifying factors. The primary considerations are *(1)* the amount and form of the remaining tooth structure; *(2)* the functional needs of each tooth; *(3)* the esthetic needs of each tooth; and *(4)* the final objective of the overall treatment plan.

Remaining Tooth Structure

The quantity and location of remaining tooth structure determine the resistance features available for the restoration and thus greatly influence the restorative design. These factors determine not only the resistance

to displacement of the restoration, but also the fracture resistance of the remaining tooth structure. The clinician should select the restoration that provides the best retention of the restoration and the optimal protection of the remaining tooth, using the least invasive design possible.

For the restoration of posterior teeth, an intracoronal restoration with amalgam or resin composite is generally the most conservative choice, and both have proven to be clinically successful. When the width of the intracoronal preparation of a posterior tooth reaches one third the intercuspal width, the tooth becomes significantly more susceptible to cuspal fracture and the concern becomes not only restoration failure but also tooth fracture.[31]

Even more significant to the fracture resistance of the tooth than restoration width is the depth of the preparation.[9] In instances of deep and/or wide preparations, the clinician must assess the need for extracoronal coverage to protect the fracture-prone portions of the tooth. Choices include cuspal coverage amalgam, partial veneer restorations (eg, onlays, three-quarters crowns, or seven-eighths crowns), and complete crowns. The clinician should resist the temptation to progress immediately to a complete crown and, instead, should select the most conservative choice that fulfils the needs of the individual tooth and the overall treatment plan.

The quantity of remaining tooth structure has an equally important effect on the choice of restorations for anterior teeth. For conservative interproximal restorations, resin composite is almost always indicated, because sufficient tooth structure is generally available for effective resin-enamel bonding. When extensive facial tooth structure has been esthetically compromised, but the facial enamel and the majority of the lingual aspect of the tooth remain intact, a resin or ceramic veneer affords a conservative alternative to a complete crown. The veneer satisfies the esthetic requirement but is considerably less invasive than complete coronal coverage. When the facial enamel has been destroyed, significant lingual tooth structure has been lost, or when occlusal stress is exceptionally heavy, veneers are not a viable option, and complete crowns are required (Fig 2-16).

Functional Needs

The choice of restorative materials and the design of restorations must accommodate the functional needs of the individual patient. This precludes the use of a cookbook approach to treatment planning and requires that the clinician assess the circumstances peculiar to each tooth prior to planning restorative procedures. The func-

PATIENT: Blank, Felina D.

PROBLEM LIST

Chief complaint: "My tooth hurts every time I chew, and lately iced tea has made it hurt, too."

Medical/systemic: Hypertension. Present blood pressure: 155/95.

Restorative (also see charting):

- Incomplete tooth fracture of mesiolingual cusp, #19
- Caries, #20, #21, #28 (high caries risk)
- Defective restorations #2, #12
- Class 5 abrasion lesions, #5, #12
- Worn incisal edges, #6–#11
- Fluorosis stain, #8
- Biologic width impingement, #3, distal
- Patient wishes to lighten maxillary anterior teeth

Periodontal:

- AAP Case Type I (see periodontal charting form)
- Generalized marginal gingivitis
- Generalized, minimal bone loss with 3- to 4-mm pockets
- Vertical defect, #3, distolingual (5 mm)
- Biologic width problem, #3, distal
- Plaque and calculus: Generalized interproximal plaque in all posterior sextants (Modified O'Leary index: 50% plaque free), subgingival calculus revealed on bitewing radiographs of #19 and #30; supragingival calculus present on lingual surfaces of mandibular anterior teeth.

Endodontic: None

Prosthodontic: Missing, #29

Orthodontic: None

Occlusion: Supraeruption, #4; Excessive wear, #6–#11

Temporomandibular dysfunction: None

Oral surgery: None

Fig 2-14 Example of a problem list.

PATIENT: Blank, Felina D.

PROBLEM LIST WORKSHEET

Problem	Treatment
Chief Complaint: cracked #19	• #19: Gold onlay
Hypertension	• Referral to physician for evaluation and treatment
Caries	• Educate patient: snacking, hygiene techniques, home fluoride use
	• Rx: stannous fluoride gel, 0.4%
	• If caries continues, complete caries risk assessment (diet survey, *Streptococcus mutans* culture)
	• #20, #21: Class 5 glass-ionomer restorations
Defective restorations	• #2 MOD amalgam
	• #4 PFM crown (shorten to level occlusal plane)
	• #12 MO resin composite
Abrasion: #5, #12	• #5, #12: Class 5 glass-ionomer restorations
Wear: #6–#11	• Protective acrylic resin occlusal splint
Fluorosis: #8	• Microabrasion #8
Biologic width: #3	• Surgical crown lengthening #3
Patient desires to lighten maxillary anterior teeth	• Home bleaching #5–#12
Periodontal inflammation associated with local factors	• Patient education and hygiene instruction; goal: 90% plaque-free index
	• Prophylaxis; scaling/root planing in mandibular sextants and any areas not responding to initial care
	• Reevaluate; goal: eliminate BOP
	• Surgical crown lengthening #3: osseous recontouring and soft tissue excision
Missing: #29	• FPD #28–#30; PFM crown #28, 3/4 crown #30
Supraeruption: #4	• Shorten #4 when PFM crown is completed

Fig 2-15 Example of a problem list worksheet to accompany the problem list in Figure 2-14.

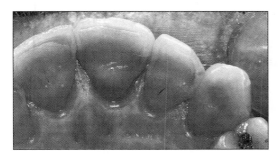

Fig 2-16 Facets and chipped incisal edges are evidence of the severe stresses placed on these anterior teeth by parafunction. Although demonstrating tetracycline staining and possessing a largely intact facial surface, these teeth would be poor candidates for veneer restorations. Complete-coverage restorations are indicated if the patient wishes to mask the tetracycline staining.

tional and parafunctional stresses of the occlusion are significant considerations in this decision process. For example, a patient with average-strength musculature, an anterior-guided disocclusion, and minimal tendency toward parafunction may require only an intracoronal amalgam or resin composite restoration to restore mesial and distal caries on a posterior tooth. In a similar circumstance, a patient with heavy musculature, signs of parafunctional activities, and no anterior-guided disocclusion may require a cast-metal restoration to minimize the chances of tooth fracture.

A useful guide in making decisions about material selection and restoration design is the evidence of functional demand provided by the existing dentition. Patients who present with a dentition exhibiting minimal destruction are good candidates for conservative, directly placed restorations. Patients whose teeth demonstrate considerable wear are often best served by materials high in strength and wear resistance, such as cast-metal restorations.

The patient's level of caries activity will influence the selection of restorative materials. Patients whose caries risk assessment indicates a high potential for caries are good candidates for treatment with anticariogenic restorative materials. Conventional glass-ionomer cements are the only restorative materials that have been found through clinical study to provide an anticariogenic effect.[59] The resin-modified glass-ionomer hybrid materials have been found to inhibit simulated caries in

vitro and may also possess anticariogenic properties in the clinical environment.[52] None of the anticariogenic restorative materials presently available is able to withstand the stresses of occlusal function.

Esthetic Needs

Establishing the patient's esthetic priorities is essential in planning restorative care. In most instances, the dentist will have the choice of a tooth-colored or a non–tooth-colored restoration for a given situation. Because non–tooth-colored materials (ie, metals) are generally superior in strength and durability, they are the materials of choice when strength and wear resistance are the overriding considerations. With the patient's input, the clinician must decide which requirement is more important, strength or esthetics.

For intracoronal, directly placed restorations in the anterior area of the mouth, resin composites are the obvious choice. They can be made to match most teeth in color and have been shown to provide an average service life of 43.5 to 72 months.[22,48] In stress-bearing areas in the posterior area of the mouth, amalgam is the material of choice for intracoronal restorations. Although resin composites have been steadily improving in terms of physical properties, clinical research indicates that they have not matched the success of amalgam for use in posterior teeth. For Class 2 restorations, amalgam restorations have an average life expectancy nearly twice that of resin composite (12.16 years for amalgam versus 6.74 years for resin composite).[46] In the posterior area of the mouth, on those occasions when esthetic concerns are paramount, however, resin composite is a viable alternative.

Large resin composite restorations do not fare as well in clinical studies as do more conservative resin composite restorations.[4] In view of this, a guideline for the use of resin composites in posterior areas of esthetic concern is to restrict their use to small or medium-sized Class 2 restorations with minimal occlusal contact.

Where cuspal coverage is required, amalgam has been found to yield favorable results, routinely providing service in excess of 10 years[49,50]; cast-metal restorations offer even greater longevity.[6,33] When cuspal coverage is required in an area of esthetic concern, the clinician must choose between an all-ceramic and a metal-ceramic restoration. All-ceramic restorations generally provide a superior cosmetic result, while metal-ceramic restorations offer greater strength. Resin composite has not yet proven to be of sufficient durability to serve in cuspal coverage restorations when occlusal stress is a factor.

Final Treatment Objective

The anticipated ultimate plan of restorative and prosthodontic rehabilitation is the final factor to consider when the design of a restoration is planned and the restorative material is selected. Teeth that may require one type of restoration to restore their function may require a different treatment to meet the needs of the final treatment plan. For example, if no prosthodontic replacement is planned for teeth that are missing, the teeth adjacent to the edentulous area may require only conservative restorative care for the treatment of small carious lesions. In a different treatment plan, one calling for replacement of the missing teeth with a removable partial denture, surveyed castings may be required on the teeth adjacent to the edentulous area. In a third variation of the same case, missing teeth may be replaced with a fixed partial denture and the teeth in question may be needed as fixed partial denture abutments.

When the final treatment objective has been visualized, it is often possible to identify certain teeth as key teeth, whose retention and restoration are crucial to the success of the treatment plan. These teeth are often potential prosthodontic abutments and/or canine teeth. Because the success of the total treatment plan often hinges on these teeth, it is crucial to ascertain their periodontal and endodontic prognosis and to plan the restorative treatment that provides the best long-term prognosis. This may dictate an aggressive restorative design to achieve the most predictable success for these key teeth.

The following example serves to illustrate this principle. A hypothetical patient has a free-standing second molar that contains a defective mesio-occlusodistal amalgam restoration. Although the facial wall of the tooth is slightly undermined, a replacement mesio-occlusodistal amalgam restoration appears likely to serve adequately. In the comprehensive treatment plan, the tooth will serve as a distal abutment for a removable partial denture. With mere replacement of the defective amalgam restoration, the tooth is at some degree of risk for cuspal fracture in the future. Fracture of the tooth would necessitate fabrication of a crown beneath the recently placed removable partial denture. By planning for a casting from the outset, a treatment plan somewhat more aggressive than would be dictated by the needs of the individual tooth, the prognosis for the ultimate treatment objective becomes more predictable and the risk of compromising the final result is reduced. This is not to be interpreted to mean that each and every removable partial denture abutment should receive a cast restoration, but is intended to convey the importance of planning for predictable longevity in key teeth.

Treatment Sequence

When the completed treatment is visualized and the design of the restorations required to address each problem on the restorative dentistry problem list is established, the final step in establishing the restorative dentistry treatment plan is sequencing the treatment. Most restorative treatment will fall into the categories, discussed at the outset of the chapter, of disease control or definitive rehabilitative treatment.

Restorative treatment aimed at the control of active disease generally consists of direct restorative procedures using amalgam, resin composite, or glass-ionomer materials. The sequence of treatment within the disease-control phase is dictated by three considerations: *(1)* severity of the disease process (ie, the deepest caries or most debilitated tooth is restored first); *(2)* esthetic needs; and *(3)* effective use of time. At each appointment, treatment is rendered in the area in most acute need of restorative treatment. When possible, the restorations should be completed quadrant by quadrant to optimize the use of time.

Treatment provided in the definitive rehabilitative phase goes beyond that needed for the stabilization of active disease and includes restorative treatment designed primarily to enhance esthetics (eg, ceramic veneers) and provide optimum function (eg, replacement of missing teeth using fixed partial dentures) and resistance to oral stresses (eg, cast restorations).

The primary benefit of segregating the restorative treatment into these categories is that a formal reevaluation is completed at the end of the disease-control phase and before the definitive treatment phase. This approach incorporates into the plan the opportunity to modify or curtail restorative treatment after the control of caries and the replacement of defective restorations. There can be many reasons for altering the original treatment plan, including the patient's desires, oral hygiene, finances, or the doctor-patient relationship.

The patient's financial situation or third-party payment guidelines often dictate that treatment be divided into stages and completed over a period of time. Organization of treatment in phases serves the patient's most urgent needs first, directing resources into the management of active disease and allowing less acute problems to be addressed as finances permit.

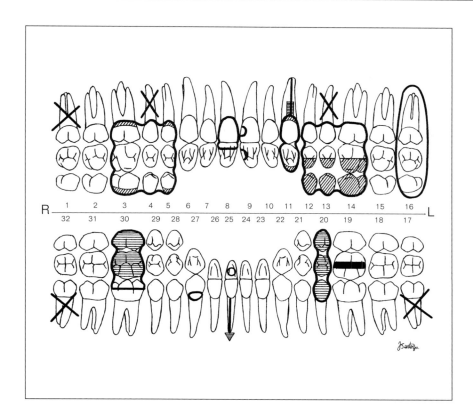

Fig 2-17 Example of a pictorial charting system used to record dental restorations. Any system that distinguishes among the various restorations is acceptable. In this example, tooth #1 is missing; tooth #4 is missing, replaced with a metal-ceramic fixed partial denture that extends from tooth #3 to tooth #5 with ceramic occlusal coverage; tooth #8 has a facial veneer; tooth #9 has a mesial resin composite restoration; tooth #11 has been endodontically treated and has a post and metal-ceramic crown; tooth #13 is missing, replaced by a metal-ceramic fixed partial denture that extends from tooth #12 to tooth #14 with metal occlusal coverage; tooth #16 is impacted; tooth #17 is missing; tooth #19 has a mesioocclusodistal amalgam restoration; tooth #20 has been restored with a metal crown; tooth #25 has been endodontically treated and received a retrograde restoration and has a resin composite restoration in the lingual access opening; tooth #27 has a facial tooth-colored restoration; tooth #30 has a metal three-quarters crown; tooth #32 is missing.

The Dental Record

Accurate and descriptive record keeping is essential to quality dental care. The dental chart should include findings from the history and examination, the problem list, the treatment plan, and a description of the treatment accomplished. This record serves several purposes:

1. Organization and documentation of the examination findings, the problem list, the treatment plan, and the treatment rendered
2. Documentation for third-party payment
3. Legal purposes
4. Forensic purposes

Organizing and documenting the examination findings and the problem list enable the dentist to evaluate the patient's dental problems and plan the treatment when the patient is no longer present. Once treatment has begun, documentation of the sequenced treatment plan also permits the dentist to review the anticipated treatment without the need to reconsider the entire treatment-planning process.

Dental records should include the following information:

1. Charting of examination findings, including existing restorations and dental relationships (eg, diastemas, supraeruptions, tilted teeth); existing periodontal and endodontic conditions; occlusal relationships; and carious lesions and defective restorations
2. Medical consultations
3. Problem list
4. Treatment plan
5. Description of treatment rendered

In addition to the usual typed or handwritten entries in a dental record, pictorial charting is an efficient means of recording a great deal of information in a small area (Figs 2-17 and 2-18). Intraoral imaging devices, either conventional cameras or videographic recording devices, provide an extremely effective means of recording findings and documenting treatment and are an ideal complement to a pictorial charting system. These offer the added advantage of simplifying communication with the patient and third-party funding agencies.

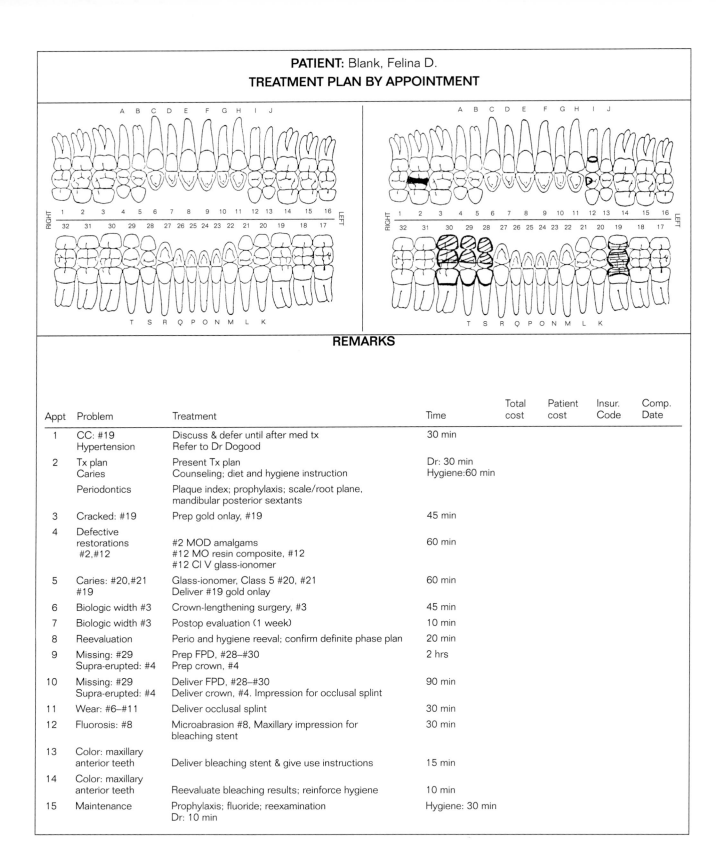

PATIENT: Blank, Felina D.
TREATMENT PLAN BY APPOINTMENT

REMARKS

Appt	Problem	Treatment	Time	Total cost	Patient cost	Insur. Code	Comp. Date
1	CC: #19 Hypertension	Discuss & defer until after med tx Refer to Dr Dogood	30 min				
2	Tx plan Caries	Present Tx plan Counseling; diet and hygiene instruction	Dr: 30 min Hygiene:60 min				
	Periodontics	Plaque index; prophylaxis; scale/root plane, mandibular posterior sextants					
3	Cracked: #19	Prep gold onlay, #19	45 min				
4	Defective restorations #2,#12	#2 MOD amalgams #12 MO resin composite, #12 #12 Cl V glass-ionomer	60 min				
5	Caries: #20,#21 #19	Glass-ionomer, Class 5 #20, #21 Deliver #19 gold onlay	60 min				
6	Biologic width #3	Crown-lengthening surgery, #3	45 min				
7	Biologic width #3	Postop evaluation (1 week)	10 min				
8	Reevaluation	Perio and hygiene reeval; confirm definite phase plan	20 min				
9	Missing: #29 Supra-erupted: #4	Prep FPD, #28–#30 Prep crown, #4	2 hrs				
10	Missing: #29 Supra-erupted: #4	Deliver FPD, #28–#30 Deliver crown, #4. Impression for occlusal splint	90 min				
11	Wear: #6–#11	Deliver occlusal splint	30 min				
12	Fluorosis: #8	Microabrasion #8, Maxillary impression for bleaching stent	30 min				
13	Color: maxillary anterior teeth	Deliver bleaching stent & give use instructions	15 min				
14	Color: maxillary anterior teeth	Reevaluate bleaching results; reinforce hygiene	10 min				
15	Maintenance	Prophylaxis; fluoride; reexamination Dr: 10 min	Hygiene: 30 min				

Fig 2-18 Example of a combined written and pictorial treatment planning sheet. The pictorial charts are for use in recording both completed treatment (left) and treatment yet to be accomplished (right). Once completed, the treatment charted in pencil on the right may be erased. The remarks section is for making comments, generally made in pencil (erased and updated as needed). The area below the remarks section is for the sequenced treatment plan. A treatment planning sheet such as this allows quick review of the overall treatment plan and provides a profile of the current status of treatment.

There are times when the identification of a deceased individual must be accomplished through the use of dental records. A complete record of the dentition and restorations, a radiographic survey, and photographic records are useful for identification purposes.

The dental record is a legal document. The nature and clarity of the entries made should reflect the knowledge that it may be needed in a court of law to document examination findings, informed consent, and treatment completed. The records should be accurate and should contain the elements listed above. They should not contain erasures or text that has been obliterated by any means. If errors are made, a single line should be drawn through the mistake and then the change should be initialed and dated. In the retrospective review of a legal investigation, the descriptiveness and clarity of the record is often held to be an indication of the quality of care provided.

Summary

Treatment planning for restorative dentistry can be a complex undertaking. Use of a logical and orderly problem-oriented approach can simplify the process. The following principles have been offered as guidelines:

1. Be aware of pathoses that may be encountered and be able to distinguish the normal from the abnormal and stable from risk-prone situations.
2. Organize findings into a problem list. It is from the list of abnormal or unhealthy findings that the problem list is developed.
3. Envision an overall restorative goal for the patient. This is the anticipated final state of rehabilitation. Not every patient can be restored to the ideal, but each patient has an optimum state of health that can be obtained, given the circumstances of that patient.
4. Determine a plan of treatment for each specific problem, so that each treatment contributes to the achievement of the anticipated ultimate treatment goal. This is the essence of restorative treatment planning; it requires that the dentist consider a number of factors before selecting the optimum restorative option. Chief among these considerations are the overall goal of treatment; the functional and esthetic needs of each restorative situation (use the existing dentition and restorations as an indicator of the performance of future restorations); the strengths and weaknesses of the various restora-

tive materials available; and the amount and location of remaining tooth structure.
5. Sequence the treatment based on a logical model. Control active disease processes first, beginning treatment with teeth in the most acute need of care. Complete as much care as feasible in each sextant at the same appointment. Establish a restorative prognosis for key teeth early in the treatment schedule. Consider nondental factors (especially third-party payment guidelines and time-related limits) when planning the treatment schedule.

References

1. Albers HF. Treating cracked teeth. ADEPT Report 1994;4:17-24.
2. Andreason JO. Traumatic Injuries of the Teeth, ed 2. Philadelphia: Saunders, 1981.
3. Bader JD, Brown JP. Dilemmas in caries diagnosis. J Am Dent Assoc 1993;124:48-50.
4. Barnes DM, Blank LW, Thompson VP, Holston AM, Gingell JC. A five-and eight-year clinical evaluation of a posterior resin composite. Quintessence Int 1991;22:143-154.
5. Barsh LI. Dental Treatment Planning for the Adult Patient. Philadelphia: Saunders, 1981.
6. Bentley C, Drake CW. Longevity of restorations in a dental school clinic. J Dent Educ 1986;50:594-600.
7. Bergman G, Linden LA. The action of the explorer on incipient caries. Sven Tandlak 1969;62:629-634.
8. Bhaskar SN. Radiographic Interpretation for the Dentist. St Louis: Mosby, 1986.
9. Blaser PK, Lund MR, Cochran MA, Potter RH. Effect of designs of class II preparations on the resistance of teeth to fracture. Oper Dent 1983;8:6-10.
10. Cameron CE. Cracked tooth syndrome. J Am Dent Assoc 1964;68:405-411.
11. Cameron CE. The cracked tooth syndrome: Additional findings. J Am Dent Assoc 1976;971-975.
12. Cavel WT, Kelsey WP, Blankenau RJ. An in vivo study of cuspal fracture. J Prosthet Dent 1985;53:38-42.
13. Chan DCN. Current methods and criteria for caries diagnosis in North America. J Dent Educ 1993;57:422-427.
14. Cohen SN, Silvestri AR. Complete and incomplete fractures of posterior teeth. Compend Contin Educ Dent 1984;5:652-663.
15. Cohen S, Burns RC. Pathways of the Pulp, ed 6. St Louis: Mosby-Year Book, 1994.
16. Dawson PE. Evaluation, Diagnosis, and Treatment of Occlusal Problems. St Louis: Mosby, 1989.
17. DeLong R, Sasik C, Pintado MR, Douglas WH. The wear of enamel when opposed by ceramic systems. Dent Mater 1989;5:266-271.
18. Disney JA, Graves RC, Stamm JW, Bohannan HM, Abernathy JR, Zack DD. The University of North Carolina Caries Risk Assessment Study: Future developments in caries predictors. Community Dent Oral Epidemiol 1992;20:64-75.
19. Dodds MWJ. Dilemmas in caries diagnosis—Applications to current practice and need for research. J Dent Educ 1993;57:433-438.

20. Eakle WS. Effect of thermocycling on fracture strength and microleakage in teeth restored with a bonded composite resin. Dent Mater 1986;2:114-117.

21. Ekstrand K, Qvist V, Thylstrup A. Light microscope study of the effect of probing in occlusal surfaces. Caries Res 1987;21:368-374.

22. Friedl K-H, Hiller K-A, Schmalz G. Placement and replacement of composite restorations in Germany. Oper Dent 1995;20:34-38.

23. Goaz PW, White SC eds. Oral Radiology: Principles and Interpretation. St Louis: Mosby, 1982.

24. Guthrie RC, Difiore PM. Treating the cracked tooth with a full crown. J Am Dent Assoc 1991;122:71-73.

25. Hansen EK. In vivo cusp fracture of endodontically treated premolars restored with MOD amalgam or MOD resin fillings. Dent Mater 1988;4:169-173.

26. Heymann HO, Sturdevant JR, Bayne S, Wilder AD, Sluder TB, Brunson WD. Examining tooth flexure effects. J Am Dent Assoc 1991; 122:41-47.

27. Hiatt WH. Incomplete crown-root fracture in pulpal-periodontal disease. J Periodontol 1973;49:369-379.

28. Kidd EAM, O'Hara JW. The caries status of occlusal amalgam restorations with marginal defects. J Dent Res 1990;69:1275-1277.

29. Lambrechts P, Braem M, Vanherle G. Evaluation of clinical performance for posterior composites and dentin adhesives. Oper Dent 1987;2:53-78.

30. Langouvardos P, Sourai P, Douvitsas G. Coronal fractures in posterior teeth. Oper Dent 1989;14:28-32.

31. Larson TO, Douglas WH, Geistfeld RE. Effects of prepared cavities on the strength of prepared teeth. Oper Dent 1981;6:2-5.

32. Lee WC, Eakle WS. Possible role of tensile stress in the etiology of cervical lesions of teeth. J Prosthet Dent 1984;52:374-380.

33. Leempoel PJB, Eschen S, DeHaan AFJ, Van't Hof MA. An evaluation of crowns and bridges in a general dental practice. J Oral Rehabil 1985;12:515-518.

34. Lindhe JA. Influence of trauma from occlusion on the progression of experimental periodontitis in beagle dogs. J Clin Periodontol 1974;1:3-14.

35. Little JW, Falace DA. Dental Management of the Medically Compromised Patient, ed 4. St Louis: Mosby-Year Book, 1993.

36. Löe H. Reaction of marginal periodontal tissue to restorative procedures. Int Dent J 1968;18:759-778.

37. Lutz F, Kreci I, Barbakow F. Chewing pressure versus wear of composites and opposing enamel cusps. J Dent Res 1992;71:1525-1529.

38. Matis BA, Carlson T, Cochran M, Phillips RW. How finishing affects glass ionomers: Results of a five-year evaluation. J Am Dent Assoc 1991;122:43-46.

39. Maynard JG, Wilson RD. Physiologic dimensions of the periodontium fundamental to successful restorative dentistry. J Periodontol 1979;50:170-174.

40. Mendoza M, Mobley CL, Hattaway K. Caries risk management and the role of dietary assessment[abstract 33]. J Dent Res 1995;74:16.

41. Mertz-Fairhurst E, Smith C, Williams J, Sherrer J, Mackert J, Richards E, et al. Cariostatic and ultraconservative sealed restorations: Six-year results. Quintessence Int 1992;23:828-838.

42. Monasky DE, Taylor DF. Studies on the wear of porcelain, enamel and gold. J Prosthet Dent 1971;25:299-306.

43. O'Leary TJ, Drake RB, Naylor JB. The plaque control record. J Periodontol 1972;43:38.

44. O'Neal SJ, Miracle RL, Leinfelder KF. Evaluating interfacial gaps for esthetic inlays. J Am Dent Assoc 1993;124:48-54.

45. Phillips RW. The Science of Dental Materials, ed 9. Philadelphia: Saunders, 1991.

46. Pink FE, Minder NJ, Simmonds S. Decisions of practitioners regarding placement of amalgam and composite restorations in a general practice setting. Oper Dent 1994;19:127-132.

47. Polson AM, Caton JG. Current status of bleeding in the diagnosis of periodontal disease. J Periodontol 1985;56(suppl):1.

48. Qvist V, Qvist J, Mjör IA. Placement and longevity of tooth-colored restorations in Denmark. Acta Odontol Scand 1990;48:305-311.

49. Robbins JW, Summitt JB. Longevity of complex amalgam restorations. Oper Dent 1988;13:54-57.

50. Smales R. Longevity of cusp-covered amalgams: Survival after 15 years. Oper Dent 1991;16:17-20.

51. Sorenson JA, Martinoff MD. Intracoronal reinforcement and coronal coverage: A study of endodontically treated teeth. J Prosthet Dent 1984;51:780-784.

52. Souto M, Donley KJ. Caries inhibition of glass ionomers. Am J Dent 1994;7:122-124.

53. Stanley HR. The cracked tooth syndrome. J Am Acad Gold Foil Oper 1968;11:36-47.

54. Summitt JB, Osborne JM. Initial preparations for amalgam restorations: Extending the longevity of the tooth-restoration unit. J Am Dent Assoc 1993;123:67-73.

55. Svanberg M, Mjör IA, Orstavik D. Mutans streptococci in plaque from margins of amalgam, composite and glass ionomer restorations. J Dent Res 1990;69:861-864.

56. Than A, Duguid R, McKendrick AJW. Relationship between restorations and the level of periodontal attachment. J Clin Periodontol 1982;9:193-202.

57. Trabert KC, Caputo AA, Abou-Rass M. Tooth fracture: A comparison of endodontic and restorative treatments. J Endod 1978;4:341-345.

58. Trope M, Maltz DO, Tronstad L. Resistance to fracture of restored endodontically treated teeth. Endod Dent Traumatol 1985;1:108-111.

59. Tyas M. Cariostatic effect of glass ionomer cement: A five year clinical study. Aust Dent J 1991;36:236-239.

60. US Department of Health and Human Services, The Selection of Patients for X-ray Examination: Dental Radiographic Examination. US Dept of Health and Human Services Publication (FDA), 1987;88-827.

61. Van Houte JH. Bacterial specificity in the etiology of dental caries. Int Dent J 1980;30:305-326.

62. Waerhaug J. Effect of rough surfaces upon the gingival tissues. J Dent Res 1956;35:323-327.

63. Waerhaug J, Hansen ER. Periodontal changes incident to prolonged occlusal overload in monkeys. Acta Odontol Scand 1966; 24:91-105.

64. Wenzel A, Larsen MJ, Fejerskov O. Detection of occlusal caries without cavitation by visual inspection, film radiographs, xeroradiographs and digitized radiographs. Caries Res 1991;25:365-371.

Caries Management and Pulpal Considerations

Richard S. Schwartz / Thomas J. Hilton

Caries is often the factor that initiates restorative treatment. Extensive research on caries over the past 30 years has greatly broadened the understanding of the carious process. Early researchers identified bacterial plaque and a dietary source of sugar as ingredients essential to formation of caries[65] (Fig 3-1). Today we have a better understanding of the carious process, including which bacteria are most important, which sugars are cariogenic, and how saliva and other factors influence caries. This chapter will discuss caries from the clinical and scientific perspectives, as well as pulpal considerations affecting the treatment of caries.

Initiation of Caries

Caries is the progressive dissolution of the mineral component of enamel, dentin, or cementum. It is essentially a bacterial disease[79] but has a multifactorial etiology. Acids produced from bacterial plaque cause demineralization of the tooth surface, which may be followed by bacterial invasion and further demineralization. If the pH of the oral environment remains below 5.5 for repeated or extended periods, the demineralization may progress to caries.[144]

Tooth surfaces are constantly undergoing demineralization and remineralization. Plaque and saliva have buffering capacities that neutralize bacterial acids, up to a point. When the pH falls below 5.5, demineralization is initiated and continues until a more neutral pH is established.[60] When the pH is neutral at the tooth surface, sufficient calcium and phosphate are present in the saliva to cause remineralization.[43] The composition and thickness of plaque, frequency and character of sugar

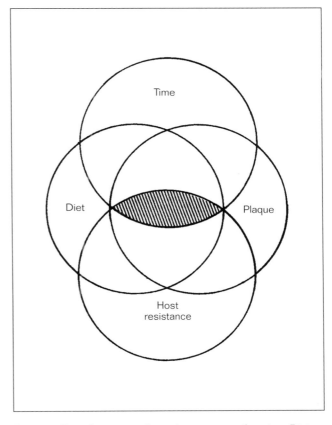

Fig 3-1 Four factors mediate the initiation of caries: Dietary intake of sugars; the presence of cariogenic plaque; the level of host resistance; and time.

intake, and composition and flow rate of saliva determine the time balance between demineralization and remineralization.[94] Fluoride also influences the equilibrium.[94]

Bacterial Etiology

Bacterial plaque is known to be essential to caries formation, but more than 300 bacterial species have been identified in plaque. Loesche[79] showed that most of the bacteria present in plaque are not etiologic factors for caries and that general removal of plaque will not necessarily prevent caries. Rather, it is necessary to eliminate specific cariogenic organisms. These principles make up the specific plaque hypothesis.[79]

A group of bacterial species collectively called mutans streptococcus (which includes *Streptococcus mutans, S sobrinus,* and others) and the Lactobacillus species have been associated with dental caries.[16,21,31,64,69,77-79] Mutans streptococci are thought to be the primary etiologic factor in formation of caries.[16,21,32,64,69,77-79] Lactobacilli are thought to be secondary organisms that flourish in the carious environment and contribute to caries progression but do not initiate it.[16,69,77,79] Mutans streptococci can be cultured at high levels in patients with caries, but are present in low levels or are undetectable in caries-free patients.[17,67,114] High levels of mutans streptococci and Lactobacilli have not proven to be predictive of new caries formation, but low levels of mutans streptococci are good predictors of low caries activity.[1,33,77-79,109]

The minimum level of mutans streptococci necessary to cause caries varies by location. Pit and fissure caries may be initiated by as few as 3,000 colony-forming units (CFU)/mL of saliva, while smooth-surface caries requires about 43,000 CFU/mL.[133]

Patients who are free of mutans streptococci may be "infected" or "reinfected." Mutans streptococci are commonly transmitted, for example, between a mother and her children.[8,16,17,133]

For many years, *Actinomyces* was thought to be the primary microbial factor in root-surface caries. However, mutans streptococci are now believed to be the most important microbes in root caries,[94] although other bacteria may be of importance because dentin has a higher critical pH and higher organic content than enamel.

Dietary Factors

A source of dietary carbohydrates is necessary for bacteria to produce the acids that initiate demineralization.[94] Simple carbohydrates are used by bacteria in the plaque as an energy source; acid is the metabolic result of glycolysis.[79,94,144] The frequency of carbohydrate consumption is more important than quantity, because repeated intake results in prolonged periods of acid production and low pH at the tooth surface.[43] Adherence (stickiness) is also an important factor in the cariogenicity of foods. The sucrose intake of individuals and populations correlates well with caries rates.[82]

Diet modification can be an effective strategy to prevent caries, although obtaining the compliance of the patient is often a problem. Small changes, such as from natural sugar to artificial sweeteners, are the strategies that are most likely to be successful.

Salivary Factors

Salivary composition and flow rate also affect initiation and progression of caries. Saliva has a buffering capacity that helps to neutralize the acids produced by bacteria. Saliva also contains calcium and phosphates that aid in the remineralization process. Thick plaque on a tooth surface may enhance the carious process by shielding the bacteria from the buffering effects of the saliva at the tooth-plaque interface and by preventing remineralization. For this reason, general plaque removal may be beneficial in preventing caries.

High levels of salivary flow have a cariostatic effect, because buffering and remineralization are enhanced, whereas xerostomia provides a favorable environment for caries development.[93] Several methods to stimulate salivary flow, for example the daily use of sugar-free chewing gum, have been advocated. Xylotol-containing gum has been shown to stimulate remineralization.[112]

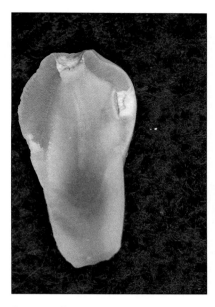

Fig 3-2a Demineralized white-spot lesions are shown at various stages of progression.

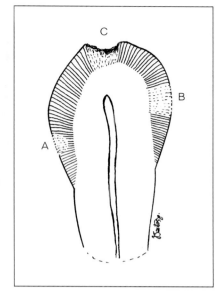

Fig 3-2b Lesion A is an example of decalcification confined to enamel. Lesion B has progressed to dentin, but no cavitation is present. Lesion C extends into dentin, and cavitation is present.

Development and Progression of Caries

Caries is usually identified by location: pit and fissure caries on the occlusal surfaces or in buccal or lingual pits, smooth-surface caries below the interproximal contacts, and root-surface caries. Pit and fissure caries tend to develop earliest in life, followed by smooth-surface caries. Root-surface caries is most common in older patients with gingival recession and in patients with low salivary flow. Each type of caries offers unique challenges in diagnosis and treatment.

Enamel caries develops initially as a subsurface phenomenon. The initial demineralization appears clinically as a white or chalky spot with an intact surface[30] (Figs 3-2a and 3-2b). As the demineralization progresses, the fragile surface breaks down and a cavitated lesion develops. Complete remineralization is possible until cavitation occurs. Even when cavitation is present, partial remineralization may occur and the carious process can be arrested. It is thought that some basic change in the etiologic factors must occur to arrest the carious process.[43] Arrested carious lesions in both enamel and dentin are becoming increasingly common,[7] and progression of caries has been shown to be slower now than it was in the past.[7]

As caries progresses through the enamel, it forms a characteristic cone-shaped lesion extending to the dentinoenamel junction. At the dentinoenamel junction, the lesion spreads laterally and penetrates the dentin (Figs 3-3a to 3-3c).

The initiation of caries in cementum and dentin is a surface phenomenon, as opposed to the subsurface demineralization of enamel. Otherwise, the process is essentially the same: Demineralization precedes bacterial invasion. Remineralization of dentin and cementum may also occur[92,95] (Figs 3-4a and 3-4b).

Diagnosis of Caries

Caries is most commonly diagnosed clinically through visual and tactile examinations and radiographs. Diagnosis of caries is discussed in chapter 2.

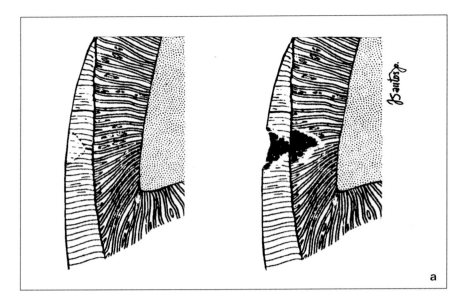

Fig 3-3a to 3-3c Smooth surface caries makes an initial cone-shaped entry through the enamel and spreads when it reaches the dentinoenamel junction. Fig 3-3a shows incipient caries confined to enamel and caries that has progressed into dentin. Figs 3-3b and 3-3c show clinical examples of this in sectioned teeth.

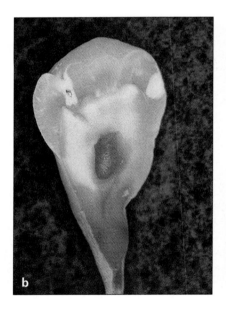

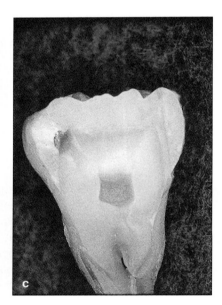

Identification and Removal of Caries

Once caries has been accessed during clinical procedures, the primary methods of identification for its removal are visual and tactile. Caries is softer and darker than the surrounding tooth structure and is usually removed mechanically with a round bur or spoon excavator. However, studies have shown that the tactile and visual methods are often inadequate for evaluating whether removal of caries is complete.[2,46,63,76,128,132]

Dyes that stain only those areas of the preparation that contain caries have been developed. These dyes are often referred to as *caries detectors*. Their mechanism of action is reported to be staining of denatured collagen,[71] but demineralized enamel also stains, so the mechanism is not totally clear. In most clinical studies, use of a caries detector has proven to be more effective than the tactile and visual methods for detecting caries.[2,46,63,76,128,132] There has not been complete agreement about the efficacy of caries detectors, however.[66] Some clinicians believe caries detectors stain some unaffected dentin (Figs 3-5a and 3-5b).

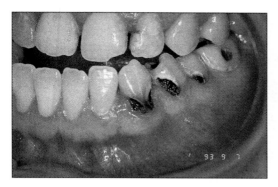

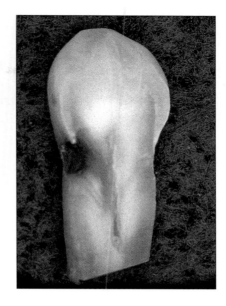

Fig 3-4a Root caries is often initiated at the cemento-enamel junction. This is a particularly severe case.

Fig 3-4b Root caries is shown in cross section.

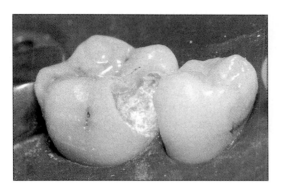

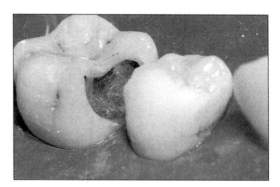

Fig 3-5a Studies have shown that practitioners often have difficulty in identifying and removing all of the caries in a lesion. To aid in removal of caries, caries detector is painted on.

Fig 3-5b When it is rinsed off, the caries detector stains any caries that is present.

Inhibition of Caries

The Role of Fluoride

Fluoridation of water has been among the most successful public health projects in the United States. Fluoride dentifrices have been credited with the dramatic worldwide drop in caries rates.[68] Fluoride provides cariostatic effects, which are somewhat cumulative with time,[96] and it aids in remineralization.[43,84] Fluoride inhibits caries in three ways:

1. It has direct antimicrobial effects on mutans streptococci and other organisms, probably by inhibition of glycolysis and glucose uptake.[94]
2. Although it is not a direct participant in remineralization, fluoride acts as a catalyst to enhance the remineralization process.[84,94]
3. Fluoride is incorporated into the mineral structure of hydroxyapatite, making it more acid resistant.[94]

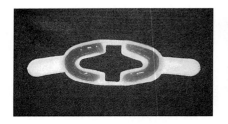

Fig 3-6a

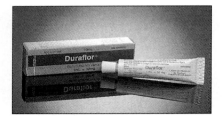

Fig 3-6b

Fig 3-6a In-office fluoride treatments are an effective preventative measure. A styrofoam carrier is often used to apply acidulated phosphate fluoride.

Fig 3-6b Fluoride varnishes, relatively new in the United States, are painted on the tooth surfaces. They hold the fluoride in intimate contact with the tooth surface for several hours.

Professional Application of Topical Fluoride

Application of topical fluoride has long been a standard procedure in dental offices with a successful track record. Acidulated phosphate fluoride in a gel form (1.23%), the most commonly used type, has been shown to reduce caries 25% to 40%.[95] Fluoride treatments are typically provided after the teeth are cleaned. A carrier or tray is commonly used to hold the gel in contact with the teeth (Fig 3-6a).

Fluoride varnishes have been used in Europe for a number of years and have shown promise for in-office application.[3] Fluoride is incorporated into an adherent varnish, which is painted onto the teeth. The varnish holds the fluoride in intimate contact with the tooth surface for several hours. Periodic applications of fluoride varnish have proven to be an effective anticaries measure that requires no compliance from the patient (Fig 3-6b).

Self-application of Fluoride

Daily self-application of topical fluoride is sometimes recommended for patients with high risk of caries. Stannous fluoride (0.40%) is often used. Fluoride may be applied to the teeth by the patient with a swab or toothbrush at bedtime. The patient is told not to rinse after the application. A more effective home method is self-application with fluoride trays for 5 minutes daily.[95] The fluoride trays keep the gel in intimate contact with the teeth and minimize dilution by saliva.

Daily application of stannous fluoride leaves brown stains on the teeth with prolonged use. Although sometimes objectionable to the patient, the stains are a good indicator of a patient's compliance or lack of compliance. The stains are easily removed with prophylaxis paste.

Fluoride mouthrinses have proven to be effective in reducing caries levels in public health settings.[95] Mouthrinse programs have been established in the public schools in a number of European countries. Low levels of sodium fluoride (0.05% to 0.20%) are typically used twice a week.

Placement of Sealants

Sealants have been used successfully for many years for the prevention of pit and fissure caries.[117] The clinical technique is quite simple and can be performed by auxiliaries. The teeth are isolated and debris is cleaned out of the pits and fissures. (A sharp explorer works well.) Air abrasion with alumina powder has also been used to clean fissures and prepare enamel for sealants. The occlusal fissures are etched with 37% phosphoric acid. A 60-second etch has been recommended for maximum penetration into the pits and fissures.[3] A lightly filled resin is then flowed into the etched fissures and polymerized (Fig 3-7).

Ideally, sealants are applied to posterior teeth shortly after their eruption. They seal pits and fissures from bacterial ingress and prevent nutrients from reaching the sealed-in bacteria. Concern has been expressed about placement of sealant over undiagnosed caries. However, there is ample evidence that caries does not progress as long as the fissure remains sealed.[53,54,86,87,93] Sealed, radiographically evident caries has been shown not to progress over a 10-year period.[14]

Sealants are now commonly used in conjunction with restorations. Simonsen[116] introduced the concept of the *preventive resin restoration,* in which small carious lesions are excavated, the tooth is restored with resin composite, and the remaining occlusal fissures are sealed. The same concept may be used with glass-ionomer cement, sometimes called *preventive glass-ionomer restorations.* Preventative glass-ionomer restorations have the added benefit of fluoride release from the restorative material. Preventive amalgam restorations, in which the remaining fissures are sealed with resin, have also been clinically successful.[87]

Management with Antimicrobial Agents

Traditional management of caries has consisted of mechanical removal of caries and replacement of lost tooth structure with a restorative material. This method

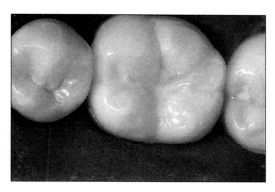

Fig 3-7 Sealants are an effective method of preventing pit and fissure caries. The sealant denies bacteria access to the pit or fissure, and prevents nutrients from reaching bacteria that are already present.

has been the basis of restorative dentistry since the founding of the dental profession. A new approach attempts to eliminate the source of the caries infection. This approach combines traditional restorative procedures and sealants with antimicrobial treatment and bacterial monitoring. The goal of treatment is to eliminate caries, suppress the cariogenic bacterial populations, encourage remineralization, and prevent reinfection. This approach has been recommended primarily for patients with high rates of caries and a history of recurrent caries.[3]

Treatment in the antimicrobial approach begins with diagnosis and removal of existing caries (that are into dentin) and placement of restorations with the usual clinical methods. Next, the most caries-susceptible areas, such as pits, fissures, and ditched margins of restorations, are eliminated or sealed. These areas require only low levels of mutans streptococci (3,000 CFU/mL of saliva) for initiation of caries. They provide a protective microenvironment for mutans streptococci that cannot be effectively treated by removal of plaque or antimicrobial therapy. Elimination of protected, caries-susceptible areas is accomplished with placement of pit and fissure sealants, sealing of the margins of existing restorations, and replacement of defective restorations.

Once active caries has been eliminated and the protected areas have been sealed, the bacterial populations are suppressed with a short, intense period of antimicrobial therapy. This is accomplished with a 2-week regimen of chlorhexidine rinses, once a day at bedtime.[3] Chlorhexidine adheres to the oral surfaces[51] and is very effective against mutans streptococci.[135,145] The 2-week regimen will suppress the oral population of mutans streptococci to low levels. Because caries and the protec-

tive environments have been eliminated, the cariogenic population will remain low unless reinfection occurs.[20,146]

The first recall examination is performed at 3 months, to check for reinfection with mutans streptococci and to check the sealants. Three months was chosen as the interval because chlorhexidine rinses have been shown to suppress mutans streptococcus populations for at least 12 weeks,[39] and because, when sealant failure occurs, it is usually in the first 3 months.[45]

At the recall appointment, the saliva is cultured to determine levels of *S. mutans*. Commercial tests available for culturing salivary *S. mutans* are inexpensive, simple, and can be administered in the office in a few minutes.[61] If a patient becomes reinfected (exhibits mutans streptococci levels of greater than 100,000 CFU/mL), the patient undergoes another 2-week regimen of chlorhexidine rinses. Three-month recalls are continued until the patient has several consecutive cultures of fewer than 100,000 CFU/mL. Recall intervals can then be extended to 6 months.

Based on the information available in the literature, a strong case can be made for this approach to caries management in patients with high rates of caries. Four randomized clinical trials have tested the effectiveness of chlorhexidine in preventing caries in limited populations.[6,50,74,145] They showed caries reduction ranging from 26% to 68%.[40] Chlorhexidine varnishes, a promising route of administration, have also been developed.[40] They are applied in the dental office, eliminating the potential problem of patient noncompliance.

Pulpal Considerations in Restorative Dentistry

Because caries is a bacterial infection, it has a deleterious effect on the pulp, ranging from mild inflammation to pulpal death. In addition, virtually all of the restorative procedures that a dentist performs cause pulpal irritation. As discussed in chapter 1, the pulp has certain inherent defense mechanisms to limit the damage from irritants. There are also a number of dental procedures with the aim of preserving pulpal health. Most of these procedures attempt to provide a barrier to external irritants by placing a protective sealer or liner on the cavity walls. The purpose of this section is to define the various protective materials, discuss how they interact with and provide protection for the pulp, review the properties of current materials, and discuss the changes that have arisen in this area of operative dentistry in recent years.

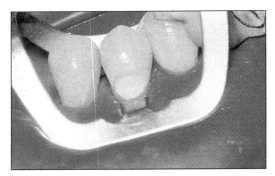

Fig 3-8a The role of liners and bases has changed in recent years, from the extensive coverage of dentin shown, to minimal or no coverage.

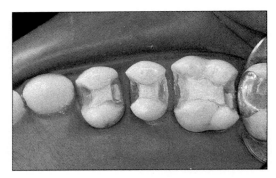

Fig 3-8b The primary use for bases is to block out undercuts in divergent preparations. Glass-ionomer bases are used here to block out undercuts in inlay preparations.

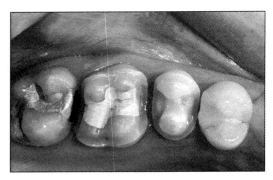

Fig 3-8c Glass-ionomer bases are used in this case to block out undercuts in porcelain onlay preparations.

Classification and Definitions

In the dental literature, terms such as *base* and *liner* are often used inconsistently. We propose the adoption of the following system of classification for intermediate materials placed under restorative materials.[129]

Cavity Sealers

Cavity sealers provide a protective coating for freshly cut tooth structure of the prepared cavity. They take two forms.

Varnish is a natural gum, such as copal or rosin, or a synthetic resin dissolved in an organic solvent, such as acetone, chloroform, or ether, that evaporates and leaves a protective film behind. It is used as a barrier against the passage of bacteria or irritants from restorative materials down dentinal tubules and to reduce the penetration of oral fluid at the restoration-tooth interface. This film is very thin (usually 2 to 5 μm) and provides no thermal insulation.[29,105,129]

The term *resin bonding agents* includes the primers and adhesives of dentin bonding systems and all-purpose bonding systems. These are used to seal dentinal tubules from bacterial ingress and reduce penetration of oral fluids at the restoration-tooth interface. They provide no thermal insulation.

Liners

Liners provide a barrier against the passage of irritants, similar to a varnish, but also provide some therapeutic effect, such as fluoride release, adhesion to tooth structure, or antibacterial action, that benefits the health of the pulp.[129] Liners are normally placed with minimal thickness (less than 0.5 mm).

Bases

In the past, a *base* was utilized to protect the pulp from thermal insult. It was placed in sufficient bulk (greater than 0.5 mm) to reduce thermal diffusion. More recently, bases have been designated as dentinal replacement materials, allowing less bulk of restorative material or blocking out undercuts for indirect restorations[129] (Figs 3-8a to 3-8c). Because bases are applied in greater thicknesses, they must possess adequate strength to support the overlying restoration.[26,105,129]

Remaining Dentinal Thickness

No artificial material that can be placed in a tooth provides better protection for the pulp than dentin, which has excellent buffering capability to neutralize the effects of cariogenic acids.[123] The remaining dentinal thickness from the depth of the cavity preparation to the pulp is the single-most important factor in protecting the pulp from insult.[125] In vitro studies have shown that a 0.5-mm thickness of dentin reduces the effect of toxic substances on the pulp by 75%; a 1.0-mm thickness of dentin reduces the effect of toxins by 90%.[89] Little if any pulpal reaction occurs with 2.0 mm of remaining dentinal thickness.[125] Conservation of remaining tooth structure is more important to pulpal health than is replacement of lost tooth structure with a cavity liner or base.

Causes of Pulpal Inflammation

As in other soft tissues of the body, the pulp reacts to an irritant with an inflammatory response.[139] It was believed for a number of years that pulpal inflammation was the result of toxic effects from dental materials.[120,127] More recent evidence, however, has demonstrated that pulpal inflammatory reactions to dental materials are mild and transitory; adverse pulpal reactions only occur as the result of pulpal invasion by bacteria or their toxins (Fig 3-9a).[13,23,138] When this does occur, severe inflammation or necrosis of the pulp is frequently observed.[138] The outward flow of fluid through dentinal tubules does not prevent bacteria or their toxins from reaching the pulp and initiating pulpal inflammation.[134]

When bacterial contamination is prevented, favorable pulpal responses have been found with amalgam, zinc phosphate cement, light-activated resin composite, silicate cement,[23] glass-ionomer cement, autocured resin composite,[97] and acrylic resin.[11] Acid etching of dentin has long been considered detrimental to the pulp, but the pulp can readily tolerate the effects of low pH if bacterial invasion is prevented.[12,72,97]

Causes of Pulpal Pain

Although not fully explained, the causes of pulpal pain and sensitivity are becoming better understood. Increased intrapulpal pressure on nerve endings secondary to an inflammatory response is one mechanism that may explain pain as a result of bacterial invasion.[121] However, this interpretation fails to explain sensitivity that occurs in the absence of inflammation.

Although alternative theories have been proposed, the one that is most accepted is the hydrodynamic theory.[13] In a vital tooth with exposed dentin, there is a constant slow movement of fluid outward through dentinal tubules. The hydrodynamic theory proposes that when a stimulus causes the slow fluid movement to become more rapid, nerve endings in the pulp are deformed, and this is interpreted as pain. Stimuli such as tooth preparation, drying with an air syringe, and application of cold have been suggested as causes of this sudden, rapid movement of fluid.[13]

Causes of Thermal Sensitivity

Prevention of postoperative thermal sensitivity has long been a rationale for placement of bases underneath metallic restorations. In vivo research documenting the alleged problem is sparse and poorly controlled. Although one study showed reduced postoperative sensitivity in patients with thick cement bases,[90] another demonstrated that, by 6 months postoperatively, few patients still have thermal sensitivity regardless of whether or not a base has been utilized.[107] In one survey fifty percent of patients questioned 24 hours after restoration placement reported some discomfort, but 78% of these patients described the discomfort as mild and fleeting.[115] Any discussion of the need for protection against postoperative thermal sensitivity must be tempered by the prospect that the prevalence and magnitude of this problem may be overestimated.

Theory of Thermal Shock

There are two theories as to the cause of thermal sensitivity (usually to cold) following restoration placement and consequently two philosophies as to how to best address the problem. The first theory states that sensitivity is the result of direct thermal shock to the pulp via temperature changes transferred from the oral cavity through the restorative material,[52,104] especially when remaining dentin is thin. Protection from this insult would then be provided by an adequate thickness of an insulating material with low thermal diffusivity.[56,104] It has been noted that resin composite exhibits such low thermal diffusivity that a thermal insulating base is unnecessary in conjunction with these restorations.[34,56] Utilization of an insulating base for thermal protection is therefore limited to metallic restorative materials that exhibit higher rates of temperature transfer.

When a base is used to provide insulation to counter thermal sensitivity in amalgam restorations, the thickness of the basing material must be minimized. Research has clearly shown that as the thickness of the base increases the fracture resistance of the overlying amalgam decreases.[42,58] Because temperature diffusion through amalgam to the floor of the cavity preparation is effectively reduced by 0.50 to 0.75 mm of basing material, thickness should be restricted to this dimension.[56] Modulus of elasticity (high modulus of elasticity indicates stiffness; low modulus of elasticity indicates flexi-

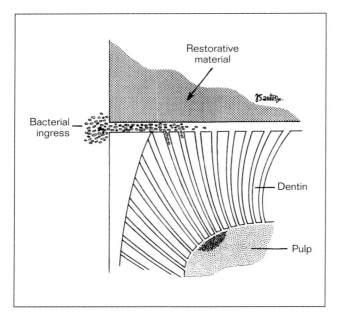

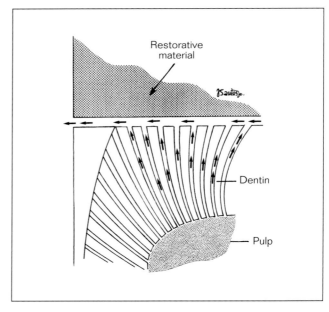

Fig 3-9a Bacteria will penetrate the marginal gap and dentinal tubules from the saliva, which may cause pulpal irritation, pulpal necrosis, or recurrent caries.

Fig 3-9b If a restoration is not well sealed, fluid flows out of the dentinal tubules and into the space between the restorative material and the tooth surface (arrows). A stimulus such as hot or cold causes a change in the flow rate, which is interpreted by mechanoreceptors as painful.

bility) is the key property that determines how effectively a base or liner will support an amalgam restoration. As the modulus of elasticity of a material decreases, the resistance to fracture of amalgam decreases.[42,58,106]

Theory of Pulpal Hydrodynamics

The more widely accepted theory holds that temperature sensitivity is based on pulpal hydrodynamics. Most restorations have a gap between the wall of the preparation and the restorative material that allows the slow outward movement of dentinal fluid (Fig 3-9b). Cold causes a sudden contraction of this fluid, resulting in a rapid increase in the flow, which is perceived by the patient as pain.[13] As dentin nears the pulp, tubule density and diameter increase,[122] as does permeability,[101] thus increasing both the volume and flow of pulpal fluid susceptible to the hydrodynamic effects of cold. This might explain why deeper restorations are associated with more problems of sensitivity.

According to this theory, if the tubules can be occluded, fluid flow is prevented and cold does not induce pain. The operative factor in reducing sensitivity to temperature thus becomes not a certain thickness of insulat-

ing material but effective sealing of dentinal tubules.[13] Credence is lent to this theory by scanning electron microscopic observations that have revealed significantly higher numbers of open tubule orifices in hypersensitive dentin.[35,143]

This theory has gained general acceptance within the dental profession in recent years and has changed the direction of restorative procedures toward dentinal sealing and away from thermal insulation. Varnish has traditionally been used to seal the interface under amalgam restorations, but numerous studies have revealed that varnishes reduce, but do not eliminate microleakage around amalgam restorations,[44,100,119,142] and others have found increased microleakage or no benefit.[83,141]

Dentin bonding systems[110] and a primer/liner[99] have demonstrated superior sealing of dentinal tubules compared to varnish. Animal research has demonstrated that dentinal primers used alone or in conjunction with dentinal adhesives can significantly reduce dentinal sensitivity.[137] Early results of research on use of dentinal primers alone or in conjunction with dentinal adhesives under amalgam restorations are promising, but long-term clinical studies are needed to confirm their efficacy.

Minimum Basing Concept

Regardless of the clinician's rationale for utilizing a base or liner under a restoration, the limitations of currently available lining materials must be considered. The best possible base for any restoration is sound tooth structure. The following are guidelines for placement of bases:

1. The need for insulating bases under amalgam is questionable. If used the minimum thickness necessary to achieve the desired result should be used, and should not exceed 0.50 to 0.75 mm.
2. The extent of the base should be minimized.
3. Sound tooth structure must not be removed to provide space for a base. Basing a preparation to "ideal" depth and outline form is contraindicated.
4. Although early results have been promising, the long-term risks or benefits of placing dentinal primers and/or adhesives under metallic restorations are unknown.

Categories of Cavity Sealers, Bases, and Liners

Varnish

Copal varnish has been utilized for many years to partially seal the amalgam-tooth interface until corrosion products form to eliminate the gap.[4,74] Two applications have been shown to be most advantageous.[99] Because the layer of varnish is so thin,[27] little or no thermal insulation is provided.

Zinc Oxide–Eugenol and Zinc Phosphate Cements

Zinc oxide–eugenol and zinc phosphate cements have been used for a number of years as bases under a variety of restorative materials. Although both provide excellent thermal insulation,[23,56] and zinc phosphate cement exhibits superior physical properties,[25] their use has diminished in recent years with the advent of materials that are adhesive to dentin and release fluoride.[81]

Calcium Hydroxide [Ca(OH)₂]

Calcium hydroxide has long been used as a liner for its pulpal compatability and purported ability to stimulate formation of reparative dentin with direct pulpal contact.[123] There is a growing belief that reparative dentin is not stimulated, but forms because $Ca(OH)_2$ has antibacterial activity that prevents bacteria from entering the pulp and inducing inflammation.[13,23,138] The antimicrobial activity is not permanent, however.[24] Conventional formulations of $Ca(OH)_2$ demonstrate poor physical properties.[27,42] High solubility may result in contamination of bonding agents and increased marginal leakage[70] as well as softening or loss of material under poorly sealed restorations.[13,103] Visible light–activated $Ca(OH)_2$ exhibits improved physical properties and significantly reduced solubility.[27] However, its modulus of elasticity[130] and subsequent ability to support amalgam restorations[106] is reduced relative to that of conventional $Ca(OH)_2$.

These unfavorable properties restrict use of $Ca(OH)_2$ to application over the smallest possible area needed to aid in the formation of reparative dentin. Two such indications may be direct and indirect pulp caps, which will be discussed later in this chapter.

Glass-Ionomer Cement

Glass-ionomer cement has been utilized as a base and liner in an attempt to take advantage of two highly desirable properties: chemical bond to tooth structure and fluoride release.[28] Although release of fluoride from glass-ionomer cement decreases with time,[98] sustained release has been demonstrated,[91] as has corresponding uptake into adjacent tooth structure.[49] This is thought to aid in anticariogenic activity.[48] Similar to zinc phosphate cement, glass-ionomer cement is acidic on initial mixing, but has a relatively neutral pH within 24 hours.[18] Pulpal response to both resin-reinforced and conventional glass-ionomer formulations is quite favorable,[47,57,59,97] probably because of glass-ionomer cement's ability to decrease bacterial penetration.[57] The exact mechanism by which glass-ionomer cement reduces bacterial invasion is uncertain, but it may be due to one or more of the following properties: fluoride release, initial low pH,[31] chemical bond to tooth structure that physically excludes bacteria,[57] or release of a metal cation.[88,113]

Both resin-reinforced and conventional glass-ionomer cements exhibit good physical properties; the conventional version exhibits a higher modulus of elasticity[15] and consequently improved support for amalgam restorations.[106] In addition, glass-ionomer cement has been shown to reduce microleakage when placed under amalgam restorations.[5] Conventional glass-ionomer cement has relatively high solubility in an acidic environment and is subject to rapid surface deterioration from acid etching.[118] Resin-reinforced glass-ionomer cements exhibit improved resistance to acid solubility,[130] while they maintain fluoride release and bond to tooth structure.[15] Therefore, this formulation is more desirable for use with resin composite restorations.

Adhesive Liners

The most recent materials to be utilized as cavity sealers have a demonstrated multisubstrate bonding ability that allows the restorative material to adhere to tooth structure. Examples include resin cements, glass-ionomer cements, and dentin bonding systems. The benefits of utilizing any one of these materials to bond resin composite restorations to tooth structure is well documented and accepted.[37,38,80,108]

Their use in conjunction with amalgam restorations is more controversial, however. The use of adhesive liners to decrease microleakage and temperature sensitivity was previously discussed. The other proposed benefits are improved retention and strengthening of adjacent tooth structure. Research results are equivocal; some studies have demonstrated these advantages,[10,38,131] and others have not.[62,111] In addition, loss of the bond between the adhesive agent and amalgam with aging has been demonstrated,[110] as has the bond of adhesive to dentin.[136] A clinical study showed that bonded resin composite restorations provide only short-term reinforcement of tooth structure.[55] Consideration of the possible effects on the physical properties of amalgam is also warranted, because incorporation of adhesive agents may have detrimental consequences.[19]

▪ Direct and Indirect Pulp Caps

Several favorable conditions must be present before considering a direct or indirect pulp cap:

1. The tooth must be vital and have no history of spontaneous pain.
2. Pain elicited during pulp testing with a hot or cold stimulus should not linger once the stimulus is removed.

3. A periapical radiograph should show no evidence of a periradicular lesion of endodontic origin.
4. Bacteria must be excluded from the site by the permanent restoration.

Given these conditions, placement of an indirect pulp cap is preferable to use of a direct pulp cap. Because of the uncertainty for success with either procedure, pulpal health should be monitored for several months in teeth that are to receive castings or serve as abutments for fixed or removable partial dentures.

Indirect Pulp Cap

In an indirect pulp cap, all caries is removed except the last portion of firm, leathery dentin immediately overlying the pulp; pulpal exposure might result if this dentin were excavated. Placement of $Ca(OH)_2$ over this layer of infected dentin has been shown to eliminate virtually all remaining bacteria and render the residual carious dentin operationally sterile.[36,41,73] A well-sealed restoration will deny remaining bacteria the nutrients for further acid production, arrest the carious lesion,[85] and provide a sound dentinal base.[127] These facts argue against a two-step procedure in which the tooth is reentered after several months for the purpose of excavating the previously carious dentin to confirm formation of reparative dentin. This procedure risks creation of a pulpal exposure and further traumatic insult to the pulp[36] (Fig 3-10).

Direct Pulp Cap

Animal studies have demonstrated that direct pulpal exposures can heal normally, but a bacteria-free environment is required.[102] The adverse consequences of bacterial contamination of the pulp have been well documented.[11,13,23,97,138] Therefore, the best chance that a direct pulp cap will form a dentinal bridge and maintain vitality is under the most ideal conditions. If the pulp has been contaminated by caries or exposure to the oral flora, the likelihood of success is diminished. In addition, aged pulps have increased fibrosis and a decreased blood supply,[9] and thus a decreased ability to mount an effective response to invading microorganisms.

Calcium hydroxide has traditionally been recommended for direct pulp caps because of its documented success,[140] although other materials with good sealing properties have also been recommended.[13,23,138] It must also be possible to restore the tooth with a well-sealed restoration that will prevent future bacterial contamina-

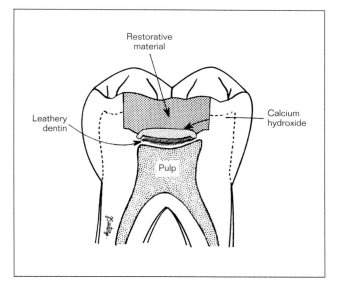

Fig 3-10 In an indirect pulp cap caries is removed until it is believed that an exposure is imminent. Calcium hydroxide is placed and the tooth is restored. If treatment is successful, the calcium hydroxide kills any remaining viable bacteria, reparative dentin forms under the caries, and the pulp remains healthy.

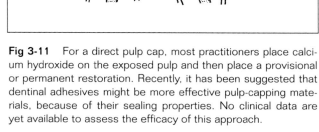

Fig 3-11 For a direct pulp cap, most practitioners place calcium hydroxide on the exposed pulp and then place a provisional or permanent restoration. Recently, it has been suggested that dentinal adhesives might be more effective pulp-capping materials, because of their sealing properties. No clinical data are yet available to assess the efficacy of this approach.

tion. Because of the uncertainty of success with this procedure, some clinicians recommend root canal therapy any time a pulpal exposure occurs. Each situation should be assessed individually and a decision to place a direct pulp cap should be based on pulpal health and the potential for a desired response from the pulp.

The use of adhesive resins for direct pulp caps is a fairly new concept that has been gaining support. Maintenance of pulpal health after an exposure is dependent on long-term exclusion of bacteria from the exposure site. Some argue that calcium hydroxide is not the best material for direct pulp caps because its antimicrobial effects are short term and microleakage under a restoration can result in bacterial invasion under the calcium hydroxide.[24] Adhesive resins are reported to be compatible with direct pulpal contact[22] and formation of a dentinal bridge has been shown to occur.[24] In addition, adhesive resins reportedly form a more effective barrier to bacterial invasion than does calcium hydroxide.[24] However, hemorrhage control is crucial to obtaining a good seal with an adhesive; this can be difficult to achieve with an inflamed pulp. There have been clinical reports of success with this technique, but long-term effectiveness is not known. Until there is more substantial evidence of the effectiveness of dentin bonding agents, calcium hydroxide may continue to be used (Fig 3-11).

References

1. Alaluusua S, Kleemola-Kujala E, Groonroos L, Evalchti M. Salivary caries-related tests as predictors of future caries increments in teenagers. A three year longitudinal study. Oral Microbiol Immunol 1990;5:77-81.

2. Anderson MH, Charbeneau GT. A comparison of digital and optical criteria for detecting carious dentine. J Prosthet Dent 1985;53:643-646.

3. Anderson MH, Bales DJ, Omnell KA. Modern management of dental caries: The cutting edge is not the dental bur. J Am Dent Assoc 1993;124:36-44.

4. Andrews JT, Hembree JH. Marginal leakage of amalgam alloys with high content of copper: A laboratory study. Oper Dent 1980;5:7-10.

5. Arcoria CJ, Fisher MA, Wagner MJ. Microleakage in alloy-glass ionomer lined amalgam restorations after thermocycling. J Oral Rehabil 1991;18:9-14.

6. Axelsson P, Kristoffersson K, Karlsson R, Bratthall D. A 30-month longitudinal study of the effects of some oral hygiene measures on *Streptococcus mutans* and approximal dental caries. J Dent Res 1987;66:761-765.

7. Bader JD, Brown JP. Dilemmas in caries diagnosis. J Am Dent Assoc 1993; 124:48-50.

8. Berkowitz R, Jordan H. Similarity of bacteriocins of *Streptococcus mutans* from mother and infant. Arch Oral Biol 1975;20:725-730.

9. Bernick S, Nedelman C. Effect of aging on the human pulp. J Endod 1975;1:88-91.

10. Boyer DB, Roth L. Fracture resistance of teeth with bonded amalgams. Am J Dent 1994;7:91-97.

11. Brännström M, Vojinovic O. Response of the dental pulp to invasion of bacteria around three filling materials. J Dent Child 1976;43:83-89.

12. Brännström M, Nordenvall KJ. Bacterial penetration, pulpal reaction and the inner surface of concise enamel bond. Composite fillings in etched and unetched cavities. J Dent Res 1978;57:3-9.

13. Brännström M. Communication between the oral cavity and the dental pulp associated with restorative treatment. Oper Dent 1984;9:57-68.

14. Briley JB, Dove SB, Mertz-Fairhurst EJ. Radiographic analysis of previously sealed carious teeth [abstract 2514]. J Dent Res 1994;73:416.

15. Burgess JO, Barghi N, Chan D, Hummert T. A comparative study of three glass ionomer base materials. Am J Dent 1993;6:137-141.

16. Carlsson J, Grahnen H, Jonsson G. Lactobacilli and Streptococci in the mouth of children. Caries Res 1975;9:333-339.

17. Caufield P, Cutter G, Dasanayake A. Initial acquisition of mutans streptococci by infants: Evidence for a discrete window of infectivity. J Dent Res 1993;72:37-45.

18. Charlton DG, Moore BK, Swartz ML. Direct surface pH determinations of setting cements. Oper Dent 1991;16:231-238.

19. Charlton DG, Murchison DF, Moore BK. Incorporation of adhesive liners in amalgam: Effect on compressive strength and creep. Am J Dent 1991;4:184-188.

20. Clark D, Stamm J, Robert G, Tessier C. Results of a 32-month fluoride varnish study in Sherbrook and Lac-Megantic, Canada. J Am Dent Assoc 1985;111:949-953.

21. Clark J. On the bacterial factor in the aetiology of dental caries. J Exp Pathol 1924;5:141.

22. Cox CF. Biocompatibility of dental materials in the absence of bacterial infection. Oper Dent 1987;12:146-152.

23. Cox CF, Keall CL, Keall HJ, Ostro E, Bergenholtz G. Biocompatibility of surface-sealed dental materials against exposed pulps. J Prosthet Dent 1987;57:1-8.

24. Cox CF, Suzuki S. Re-evaluating pulp protection: Calcium hydroxide liners vs. cohesive hybridization. J Am Dent Assoc 1994;125:823-831.

25. Craig RG (ed). Restorative Dental Materials, 8. St Louis: Mosby, 1989:200.

26. Craig RG (ed). Restorative Dental Materials, 8. St Louis: Mosby, 1989:216.

27. Craig RG (ed). Restorative Dental Materials, 8. St Louis: Mosby, 1989:218.

28. Craig RG (ed). Restorative Dental Materials, 8. St Louis: Mosby, 1989:284.

29. Craig RG (ed). Restorative Dental Materials, 9. St Louis: Mosby-Year Book, 1993:203-207.

30. Darling A. Studies of the early lesion of enamel caries with transmitted light, polarized light and microradiography. Br Dent J 1956;101:289-297.

31. De Schepper E, Thrasher M, Thurmond B. Antibacterial effects of light-cured liners. Am J Dent 1989;2:74-76.

32. de Stoppelaar J, van Houte J, Backer-Dirks O. The relationship between extracellular polysaccharide-producing streptococci and smooth surface caries in 13 year old children. Caries Res 1969;3:190-199.

33. Disney J, Graves R, Stamm J, Bohannan H, Abernathy J, Zack D. The University of North Carolina caries risk assessment study: Further developments in caries risk prediction. Community Dent Oral Epidemiol 1992;20:64-75.

34. Drummond JL, Robledo J, Garcia L, Toepke TRS. Thermal conductivity of cement base materials. Dent Mater 1993;9:68-71.

35. Duke ES, Lindemuth J. Variability of clinical dentin substrates. Am J Dent 1991;4:241-246.

36. Dumsha T, Hovland E. Considerations and treatment of direct and indirect pulp-capping. Dent Clin North Am 1985;29:251-259.

37. Eakle WS. Fracture resistance of teeth restored with class II bonded composite resin. J Dent Res 1986;65:149-153.

38. Eakle WS, Staninec M, Lacy AM. Effect of bonded amalgam on the fracture resistance of teeth. J Prosthet Dent 1992;68:257-260.

39. Emilson C, Lindquist B, Wennerholm K. Recolonization of human tooth surfaces by Streptococcus mutans after suppression by chlorhexidine treatment. J Dent Res 1987;66:1503-1508.

40. Emilson CG. Potential efficacy of chlorhexidine against mutans streptococci and human dental caries. J Dent Res 1994;73:682-691.

41. Fairbourn DR, Charbeneau GT, Loesche WJ. Effect of improved Dycal and IRM on bacteria in deep carious lesions. J Am Dent Assoc 1980;100:547-552.

42. Farah JW, Clark AE, Mohsein M, Thomas PA. Effect of cement base thicknesses on MOD amalgam restorations. J Dent Res 1983;62:109-111.

43. Featherstone J, McIntyre J, Fu J. Dentine and Dentine Reactions in the Oral Cavity. Oxford, England: IRL Press, 1987.

44. Fitchie J, Reeves G, Scarbrough A, Hembree J. Microleakage of a new cavity varnish with a high-copper spherical amalgam alloy. Oper Dent 1990;15:136-140.

45. Foreman F, Matis B. Retention of sealants placed by dental technicians without assistance. Pediatr Dent 1991;13:59-61.

46. Franco SJ, Kelsey WP. Caries removal with and without a disclosing solution of basic fuchsin. Oper Dent 1991;6:46-49.

47. Gaintantzopoulou MD, Willis GP, Kafrawy AH. Pulp reactions to light-cured glass ionomer cements. Am J Dent 1994;7:39-42.

48. Garcia-Godoy F, Jensen ME. Artificial recurrent caries in glass ionomer-lined amalgam restorations. Am J Dent 1990;3:89-93.

49. Geiger SB, Weiner S. Fluoridated carbonatoapatite in the intermediate layer between glass ionomer and dentin. Dent Mater 1993;9:33-36.

50. Gisselsson H, Birkhed D, Bjorn AL. Effect of professional flossing with chlorhexidine gel on approximal caries in 12- to 15-year old schoolchildren. Caries Res 1988;22:187-192.

51. Gjermo P, Bonesvoll P, Rolla G. Relationship between plaque-inhibiting effect and retention of chlorhexidine in the human oral cavity. Arch Oral Biol 1974;19:1031-1034.

52. Going RE. Cavity liners and dentin treatment. J Am Dent Assoc 1964;69:415-422.

53. Handelman S, Washburn F, Wopperer P. Two-year report of sealant effect on bacteria in dental caries. J Am Dent Assoc 1976;93:967-970.

54. Handelman S. Effect of sealant placement on occlusal caries progression. Clin Prevent Dent 1982;4:11-16.

55. Hansen EK. In vivo cusp fracture of endodontically treated premolars restored with MOD amalgam or MOD resin fillings. Dent Mater 1988;4:169-173.

56. Harper RH, Schnell RJ, Swartz ML, Phillips RW. In vivo measurements of thermal diffusion through restorations of various materials. J Prosthet Dent 1980;43:180-185.

57. Heys RJ, Fitzgerald M. Microleakage of three cement bases. J Dent Res 1991;70:55-58.

58. Hormati AA, Fuller JL. The fracture strength of amalgam overlying base materials. J Prosthet Dent 1980;43:52-57.

59. Hosoda H, Inokoshi S, Shimada Y, Harnirattisai C, Otsuki M. Pulpal response to a new light-cured composite placed in etched glass-ionomer lined cavities. Oper Dent 1991;16:122-129.

60. Hume W. Need for change in standards of caries diagnosis—perspective based on the structure and behavior of caries lesion. J Dent Educ 1993;57:439-443.

61. Jensen B, Bratthall D. A new method for the estimation of mutans streptococci in human saliva. J Dent Res 1989;68:468-471.

62. Joynt RB, Davis EL, Wieczkowski G, Williams DA. Fracture resistance of posterior teeth restored with glass ionomer-composite resin systems. J Prosthet Dent 1989;62:28-31.

63. Joyston-Bechal S, Kidd EA, Allan R, Smith MM. Use of a caries detector dye in cavity preparation, in vivo. Caries Res 1989;23:109.

64. Keene H, Shklair I. Relationship of Streptococcus mutans carrier status to the development of caries lesions in initially caries free recruits. J Dent Res 1974;53:1295-1299.

65. Keyes P. Present and future measures for caries control. J Am Dent Assoc 1969;79:1395-1404.

66. Kidd EA, Joyston-Bechal S, Beighton K. The use of caries detector dye during cavity preparation: A microbiological assessment. Br Dent J 1993;174:245-248.

67. Kohler B, Bratthall D. Intrafamilial levels of mutans and some aspects of the bacterial transmission. J Dent Res 1991;5:50-55.

68. Konig K. Role of fluoride toothpastes in a caries-preventative strategy. Caries Res 1993;27:23-28.

69. Krasse B. Biological factors as indicators of future caries. Int Dent J 1988;38:219-225.

70. Krejci I, Lutz F. Mixed class V restorations: The potential of a dentine bonding agent. J Dent 1990;18:263-270.

71. Kuboki Y, Lin CF, Fusayama T. Mechanism of differential staining in carious dentine. J Dent Res 1983;62:713-715.

72. Kuroske N, Kubota M, Yamamoto Y, Fusayama T. The effect of etching dentin of the clinical cavity floor. Quintessence Int 1990;21:87-92.

73. Leung RL, Loesche WJ, Charbeneau GT. Effect of Dycal on bacteria in deep carious lesions. J Am Dent Assoc 1980;100:193-197.

74. Lin JHC, Marshall GW, Marshall SJ. Microstructures of Cu-rich amalgams after corrosion. J Dent Res 1983;62:112-115.

75. Lindquist B, Edward S, Torell P, Krasse B. Effect of different caries preventive measures in children highly infected with mutans streptococci. Scand J Dent Res 1989;97:330-337.

76. List G, Lommel TJ, Tilk MA. Use of a dye in caries identification. Quintessence Int 1987;18:343-345.

77. Loesche W. Chemotherapy of dental plaque infections. Oral Sci Rev 1976;9:63-107.

78. Loesche W. Longitudinal investigation of the role of mutans in human fissure decay. Infect Immun 1979;26:498-507.

79. Loesche W. Dental caries: A Treatable Infection. Springfield, IL: Thomas, 1982.

80. Lundin SA. Studies on posterior composite resins with special reference to class II restorations. Swed Dent J 1990;73(suppl):6-33.

81. Manders CA, Garcia-Godoy F, Barnwell GM. Effect of copal varnish, ZOE, or glass ionomer cement bases on microleakage of amalgam restorations. Am J Dent 1990;3:63-66.

82. Marthaler T. Health and Sugar Substitutes. Basel: Karger, 1979.

83. Mazer RB, Rehfeld R, Leinfelder KF. Effect of cavity varnishes on microleakage of amalgam restorations. Am J Dent 1988;1:205-208.

84. Mellberg JR. Remineralization. A status report for the *American Journal of Dentistry*. Am J Dent 1988;1:39-43.

85. Mertz-Fairhurst EJ, Schuster GS, Williams JE, Fairhurst CW. Clinical progress of sealed and unsealed caries. Part I. Depth changes and bacterial counts. J Prosthet Dent 1979;42:521-526.

86. Mertz-Fairhurst E, Schuster G, Fairhurst C. Arresting caries by sealants: Results of a clinical study. J Am Dent Assoc 1986;112:194-197.

87. Mertz-Fairhurst E, Smith C, Williams J, Sherrer J, Mackert J, Richards E, et al. Cariostatic and ultraconservative sealed restorations: Six-year results. Quintessence Int 1992;23:828-838.

88. Meryon SD, Jakeman KJ. Zinc release from dental restorative materials in vitro. J Biomed Mater Res 1986;20:285-291.

89. Meryon SD. The model cavity method incorporating dentine. Int Endod J 1988;21:79-84.

90. Miller BC, Charbeneau G. Sensitivity of teeth with and without cement bases under amalgam restorations: A clinical study. Oper Dent 1984;9:130-135.

91. Mitra SB. In vitro fluoride release from a light-cured glass-ionomer liner/base. J Dent Res 1991;70:75-78.

92. Miyauchi H, Iwaku M, Fusayama T. Physiological recalcification of carious dentin. Bull Tokyo Med Dent Univ 1978;25:169-179.

93. National Institutes of Health Consensus Development statement on dental sealants in prevention of tooth decay. J Am Dent Assoc 1984;108:233-236.

94. Newbrun E. Saliva Glands and Their Secretion. Ann Arbor, MI: University of Michigan, 1972.

95. Newbrun E. Cariology. Chicago: Quintessence, 1989.

96. Nikiforuk G. Understanding Dental Caries. 2. Prevention. Basel: Karger, 1985.

97. Nordenvall KJ, Brännström M, Torstensson B. Pulp reactions and microorganisms under ASPA and Concise composite fillings. J Dent Child 1979;46:449-453.

98. Olsen BT, Garcia-Godoy F, Marshall TD, Barnwell G. Fluoride release from glass ionomer-lined amalgam restorations. Am J Dent 1989;2:89-91.

99. Pashley DH, O'Meara JA, Williams ED, Kepler EE. Dentin permeability: Effects of cavity varnishes and bases. J Prosthet Dent 1985;53:511-516.

100. Pashley DH, Depew D. Effects of the smear layer, Copalite, and oxalate on microleakage. Oper Dent 1986;11:95-102.

101. Pashley DH. Clinical considerations of microleakage. J Endod 1990;16:70-77.

102. Paterson RC. Bacterial contamination and the exposed pulp. Br Dent J 1976;140:231-236.

103. Pereira JC, Manfio AP, Franco EB. Clinical evaluation of Dycal under amalgam restorations. Am J Dent 1990;3:67-70.

104. Peters DD, Augsberger RA. In vitro cold transference of bases and restorations. J Am Dent Assoc 1981;102:642-646.

105. Phillips RW (ed). Skinner's Science of Dental Materials. Philadelphia: Saunders, 1991:466-474.

106. Pierpont W Gray S, Hermesch C, Hilton T. Effect of various bases on the fracture resistance of amalgam [abstract 981]. J Dent Res 1993;72:226.

107. Piperno J, Barouch E, Hirsch ST, Kaim JM. Thermal discomfort of teeth related to presence or absence of cement bases under amalgam restorations. Oper Dent 1982;7:92-96.

108. Prati C. Early marginal microleakage in class II composite restorations. Dent Mater 1989;5:392-398.

109. Russell J, MacFarlane T, Aitchison T, Stephen K, Burchell C. Prediction of caries increment in Scottish adolescents. Community Dent Oral Epidemiol 1991;19:74-77.

110. Saiku JM, St Germain HA, Meiers JC. Microleakage of a dental amalgam alloy bonding agent. Oper Dent 1993;18:172-178.

111. Santos AC, Meiers JC. Fracture resistance of premolars with MOD amalgam restorations lined with Amalgambond. Oper Dent 1994;19:2-6.

112. Scheinin A, Makinen K, Tammisalo E, Rekola M. Turku sugar studies XVII- Incidence of dentinal caries in relation to 1 year consumption of xylitol chewing gum. Acta Odontol Scand 1975; 33:269-278.

113. Scherer W, Lippman N, Kaim J. Antimicrobial properties of glass-ionomer cements and other restorative materials. Oper Dent 1989;14:77-81.

114. Shklair I, Keene H, Cullen P. The distribution of *Streptococcus mutans* on the teeth of two groups of naval recruits. Arch Oral Biol 1974;19:199-202.

115. Silvestri AR, Cohen SN, Wetz JH. Character and frequency of discomfort immediately following restorative procedures. J Am Dent Assoc 1977;95:85-89.

116. Simonsen RJ. Clinical Applications of the Acid Etch Technique. Chicago: Quintessence, 1978.

117. Simonsen R. Retention and effectiveness of dental sealant after 15 years. J Am Dent Assoc 1991;122:34-42.

118. Smith GE. Surface deterioration of glass ionomer cement during acid etching: An SEM evaluation. Oper Dent 1988;13:3-7.

119. Sneed WD, Hembree JH Jr, Welsh EL. Effectiveness of three cavity varnishes in reducing leakage of a high-copper amalgam. Oper Dent 1984;9:32-34.

120. Stanley HR, Going RE, Chauncey HH. Human pulp response to acid pretreatment of dentin and to composite restoration. J Am Dent Assoc 1975;91:817-825.

121. Stanley HR. Human Response to Restorative Procedures. Gainesville, FL: Storter, 1981:9.

122. Stanley HR. Human Response to Restorative Procedures. Gainesville, FL: Storter, 1981:38.

123. Stanley HR. Human Response to Restorative Procedures. Gainesville, FL: Storter, 1981:42-43.

124. Stanley HR. Human Response to Restorative Procedures. Gainesville, FL: Storter, 1981:46.

125. Stanley HR. Human Response to Restorative Procedures. Gainesville, FL: Storter, 1981:49.

126. Stanley HR. Human Response to Restorative Procedures. Gainesville, FL: Storter, 1981:72.

127. Stanley HR. Pulpal responses to ionomer cements-biological characteristics. J Am Dent Assoc 1990;120:25-29.

128. Starr CB, Langenderfer WR. Use of a caries-disclosing agent to improve dental residents' ability to detect caries. Oper Dent 1993;18:110-114.

129. Summitt JB. On bases, liners, and varnishes [letter]. Oper Dent 1994;19:35.

130. Tam LEE, Pulver E, McComb D, Smith C. Physical properties of calcium hydroxide and glass-ionomer base and lining materials. Dent Mater 1989;5:145-149.

131. Temple-Smithson PE, Causton BE, Marshall KF. The adhesive amalgam—Fact or fiction? Br Dent J 1992;172:316-319.

132. van de Rijke JW. Use of dyes in cariology. Int Dent J 1991;41: 111-116.

133. van Houte J, Green D. Relationship between the concentration of bacteria in saliva and the colonization of teeth in humans. Infect Immun 1974;9:624-630.

134. Vojinovic O, Nyborg H, Brännström M. Acid treatment of cavities under resin fillings: Bacterial growth in dentinal tubules and pulpal reactions. J Dent Res 1973;52:1189-1193.

135. von der Fehr F, Löe H, Theilade E. Experimental caries in man. Caries Res 1970;4:131-148.

136. Watanabe I, Nakabayashi N. Bonding durability of photocured phenyl-P in TEGDMA to smear layer–retained bovine dentin. Quintessence Int 1993;24:335-342.

137. Watanabe T, Sano M, Itoh K, Wakumoto S. The effects of primers on the sensitivity of dentin. Dent Mater 1991;7:148-150.

138. Watts A, Paterson RC. Bacterial contaminations as a factor influencing the toxicity of materials to the exposed dental pulp. Oral Surg Oral Med Oral Pathol 1987;64:466-474.

139. Weine, FS. Endodontic Therapy, ed 3. St Louis: Mosby, 1982: 118.

140. Weine, FS. Endodontic Therapy, ed 3. St Louis: Mosby, 1982: 563.

141. Wright W, Mazer RB, Teixeira LC, Leinfelder KF. Clinical microleakage evaluation of a cavity varnish. Am J Dent 1992;5: 263-265.

142. Yates LY, Murray GA, Hembree JH. Cavity varnishes applied over insulating bases: Effect on microleakage. Oper Dent 1980;5:43-46.

143. Yoshiyama M, Masada J, Uchida A, Ishida H. Scanning electron microscopic characterization of sensitive vs. insensitive human radicular dentin. J Dent Res 1989;68:1498-1502.

144. Zero D, Van Houte J, Russo T. Enamel demineralization by acid produced from exogenous substrate in oral streptococci. Arch Oral Biol 1986;31:229-234.

145. Zickert I, Emilson C, Krasse B. Effect of caries preventive measures in children highly infected with the bacterium *Streptococcus mutans*. Arch Oral Biol 1982;27:661-668.

146. Zickert I, Emilson CG, Krasse B. Microbial conditions and microbial measures in Swedish teenagers. Community Dent Oral Epidemiol 1987;15:241-244.

Nomenclature and Instrumentation

James B. Summitt

Basic to any science is a language understood by the members of the community of the science. This chapter is devoted to a review of the language of operative dentistry and to the basic instrumentation of that discipline.

Nomenclature and Classification of Caries and Cavity Preparations

Systems for Naming and Numbering Teeth

Each tooth may be identified by its location in the mouth and by its individual name. Examples include the *maxillary right central incisor* and the *mandibular left second premolar.* Areas of the mouth are referred to by arch (*maxillary* or *upper* and *mandibular* or *lower*) and by the side of the patient's midline (*left* and *right*) (Fig 4-1). Each arch is divided into half at the midline, forming four quadrants (maxillary right and left quadrants and mandibular right and left quadrants). In addition, each tooth is identified as primary or permanent. Finally, the individual name of the tooth in the quadrant, eg, *molar* or *central incisor,* completes the identification of the tooth. Examples of complete tooth names are *mandibular left permanent first molar* and *maxillary right primary canine.*

Because their names are cumbersome, teeth are frequently referred to by number. The tooth-numbering systems primarily used today are the Universal system and the Fédération Dentaire Internationale (FDI) system

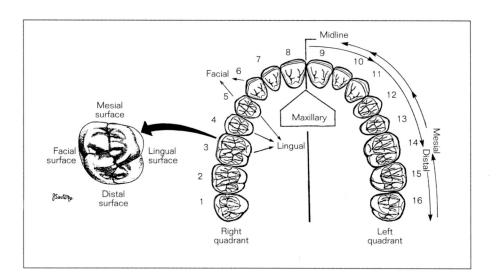

Fig 4-1 Nomenclature of directions and tooth surfaces.

Fig 4-2 Tooth-numbering systems and nomenclature.

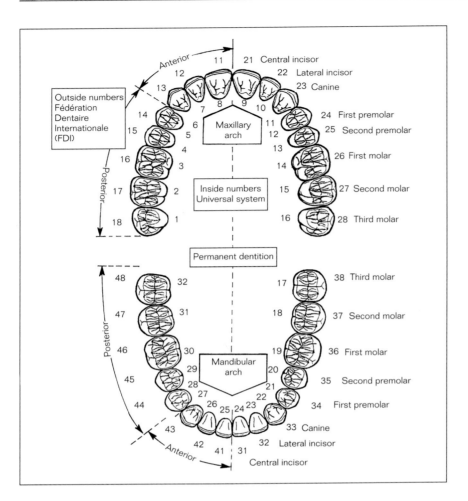

Maxillary arch

Outside numbers Fédération Dentaire Internationale (FDI)

Inside numbers Universal system

Permanent dentition

Mandibular arch

Anterior

Posterior

21 Central incisor
22 Lateral incisor
23 Canine
24 First premolar
25 Second premolar
26 First molar
27 Second molar
28 Third molar

38 Third molar
37 Second molar
36 First molar
35 Second premolar
34 First premolar
33 Canine
32 Lateral incisor
Central incisor

(Fig 4-2). In the Universal system, the numbering begins with the maxillary (upper) right third molar (tooth 1), proceeds around the arch to the maxillary left third molar (tooth 16), then to the mandibular (lower) left third molar (tooth 17) and around the mandibular arch to the mandibular right third molar (tooth 32).

In the FDI system, the first digit of the tooth number represents a quadrant (*1*, maxillary right; *2*, maxillary left; *3*, mandibular left; and *4*, mandibular right). The second digit represents the tooth (*1*, a central incisor, regardless of the arch or quadrant; *2*, lateral incisor; *3*, canine; and so on to *8*, third molar). The maxillary left first premolar would be identified as tooth 24; the mandibular right second molar would be identified as tooth 47.

Incisors and canines are referred to as *anterior teeth*, regardless of the arch; premolars and molars are *posterior teeth*.

Nomenclature of Tooth Surfaces and Cavity Preparations

The surfaces of the teeth are identified by their locations. Any surface or movement toward the midline of the arch is referred to as *mesial* (Fig 4-1). A surface or movement away from the midline is *distal*. Surfaces and movements toward the tongue are termed *lingual*; those that are in the direction of the cheek or lips are termed *facial*. For the anterior teeth, facial may be referred to as *labial* (toward the lips); for posterior teeth, facial may be referred to as *buccal* (toward the cheek).[7]

On any tooth, *gingival* refers to a surface or movement toward the gingiva (Figs 4-3 and 4-4). A distinction is made, however, between the chewing surfaces of posterior teeth, which are called *occlusal* (Figs 4-4a and 4-4b) and the biting edges of anterior teeth, which are called *incisal* (Figs 4-3a and 4-3b). A *proximal* surface is one that faces an adjacent tooth; it may be further identified as *mesial* or *distal*.[7]

Figs 4-3a and 4-3b Directions, features, and tooth surfaces of anterior teeth.

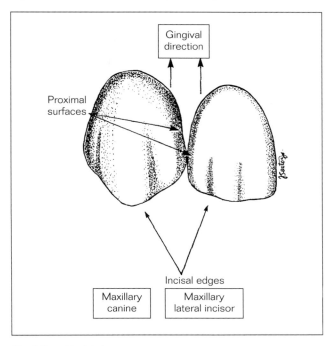

Fig 4-3a Facial view.

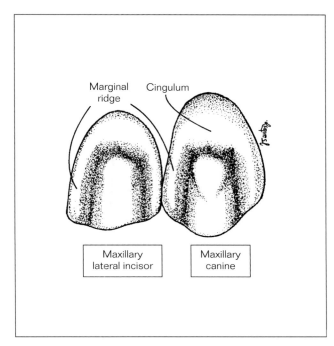

Fig 4-3b Lingual view.

Figs 4-4a and 4-4b Directions, features, and tooth surfaces of posterior teeth.

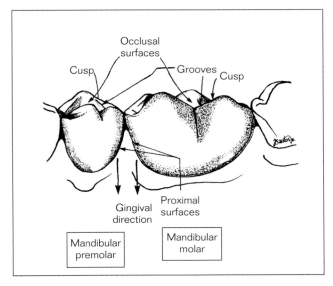

Fig 4-4a Lingual view of mandibular right second premolar and first molar.

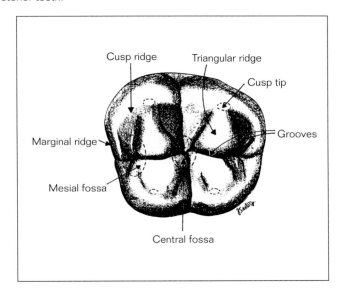

Fig 4-4b Occlusal view of mandibular right first molar.

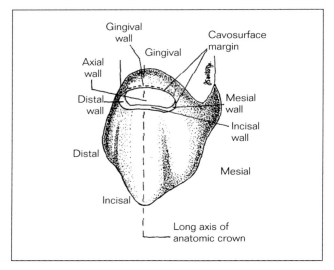

Fig 4-5 Class 5 cavity preparation in an anterior tooth (maxillary canine, facial view). In posterior teeth, there would be an occlusal wall instead of an incisal wall.

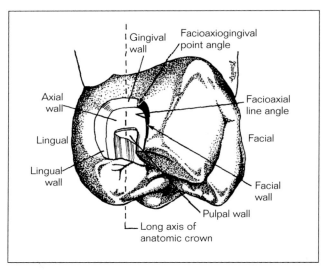

Fig 4-6 Class 2 cavity preparation (maxillary molar, proximal view).

The anatomic contour of anterior teeth is less complicated than that of posterior teeth, in which the occlusal surfaces are characterized by grooves, cusp tips and ridges, marginal ridges, and fossae. *Marginal ridges* (both mesial and distal) border the lingual surfaces of anterior teeth (Fig 4-3b) and the occlusal surfaces of posterior teeth (Fig 4-4b). A groove is a linear channel between enamel elevations, such as cusps and/or ridges. A *fissure* is a developmental linear cleft usually found at the base of a groove; it is commonly the result of the lack of fusion of the enamel of adjoining dental cusps or lobes. A *pit* is a small depression in enamel, usually located in a groove and often at the junction of two or more fissures. A *fossa* is a hollow, rounded, or depressed area in the enamel surface of a tooth. For example, a mesial fossa lies just distal to a mesial marginal ridge (Fig 4-4b).[7]

With the advent of bonding of restorative materials to teeth, walls of cavity preparations are less distinct than they are in preparations for restorations that are retained by mechanical undercuts in the preparation walls or by nonadhesive (conventional) cements. The walls of cavity preparations, however, are generally referred to by the same terms as the surface features of the teeth, for example, the gingival and distal walls (Figs 4-5 to 4-9). Exceptions are the *pulpal wall* (or floor), which is only in the occlusal portion of a preparation and is the wall adjacent or nearest to the pulp chamber of the tooth (Figs 4-6 and 4-7), and the *axial wall* which, in all other areas of a preparation, is the wall adjacent or nearest to the pulp chamber or pulp canal(s) (Figs 4-5, 4-6, and 4-9).[7]

The junction of two walls in a cavity preparation is called a *line angle*.[7] Again, in preparations for bonded restorations, line angles may not be well defined, but the names for line angles may be used to refer to general areas of the preparation. For example, the meeting of the facial and axial walls forms the facioaxial (or axiofacial) line angle (Fig 4-6). Similarly, the junction of three walls is referred to as a *point angle*. For example, the junction of the facial, axial, and gingival walls creates the facioaxiogingival (or axiofaciogingival or gingivofacioaxial) point angle. Again, the junction of two walls is often rounded, so it does not actually form a line, but it is still referred to as a line angle; likewise, a point angle is usually not a sharp point.

The *margins* (or *cavosurface angles*[7]) of a preparation, which are formed by the junction of a cavity wall and an external tooth surface, are identified by the names of the adjacent walls (eg, incisal margin, mesial margin, or gingival margin).

The *anatomic crown* of a tooth is the portion that extends from the dentinoenamel junction to the occlusal

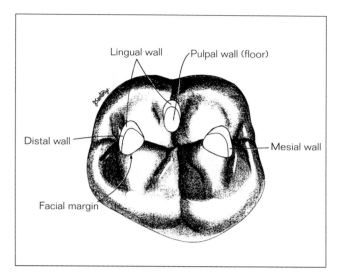

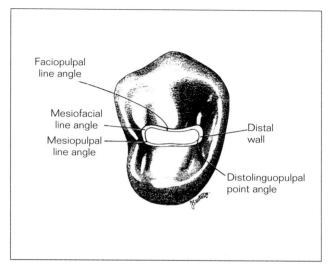

Fig 4-7 Class 1 cavity preparations in a posterior tooth. The occlusal surface of this mandibular left molar is viewed slightly from the facial aspect (occlusofacial), so the facial wall is hidden from view.

Fig 4-8 Class 1 cavity preparation in a posterior tooth (maxillary premolar, occlusal view). In a direct restoration (such as for amalgam), the facial and lingual walls would be parallel or convergent for retention of the amalgam. The walls of a preparation for bonded resin composite could diverge as shown here or by considerably more, because the restoration would be bonded to the enamel and dentin.

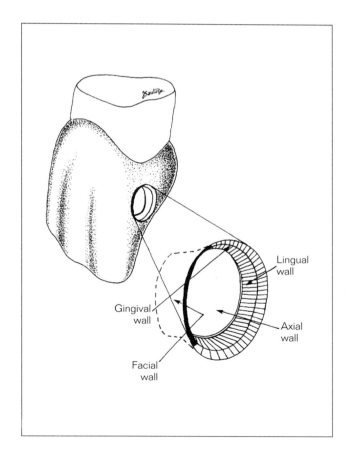

Fig 4-9 Class 3 cavity preparation (maxillary incisor, mesiofacial view). The preparation is for a bonded, tooth-colored restoration.

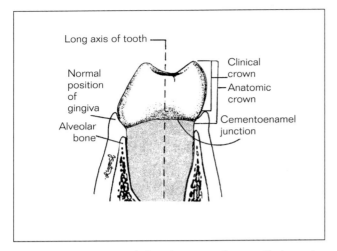

Fig 4-10 Anatomic and clinical crowns of a mandibular molar with the periodontal attachment at the normal, healthy level.

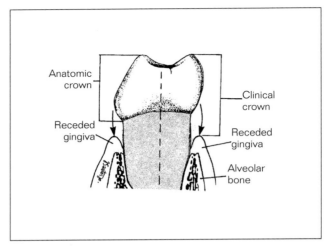

Fig 4-11 Anatomic and clinical crowns of a mandibular molar with the periodontal attachment at a more apical level (periodontal recession). With loss of gingival height comes an increase in the length of the clinical crown, but the anatomic crown, which is defined by the cementoenamel junction (or cervical line), stays constant. The occlusogingival dimension of the anatomic crown can be reduced by loss of occlusal tooth structure from wear or erosion.

surface or incisal edge; it is covered by enamel (Figs 4-10 and 4-11). The *clinical crown* is the portion that is visible in the oral cavity.[7] Depending on the tooth, the clinical crown may include only part of the anatomic crown (Fig 4-10) or it may include all of the anatomic crown and part of the root (Fig 4-11).

Classification of Carious Lesions and Tooth Preparations

Near the turn of the century, G. V. Black,[2] who is known as the father of operative dentistry, classified carious lesions into groups according to their locations in permanent teeth. The same classification is used to refer to cavity preparations, because the location of caries is a major factor in the design of the cavity preparation and the selection of instruments (Fig 4-12).

Class 1 (I) lesions occur in pits and fissures on the facial, lingual, and occlusal surfaces of molars and premolars, and, less often, the lingual surfaces of maxillary anterior teeth (most frequently lateral incisors, less frequently central incisors, rarely canines). Class 1 cavity preparations are illustrated in Figs 4-7 and 4-8.

Class 2 (II) lesions occur on the proximal surfaces of the posterior teeth (molars and premolars). If a proximal surface of a posterior tooth is involved in a restoration, it

is a Class 2 restoration. A Class 2 cavity preparation is illustrated in Fig 4-6.

Class 3 (III) lesions occur on the proximal surfaces of anterior teeth (central and lateral incisors and canines). Class 3 cavities do not involve an incisal angle. A Class 3 cavity preparation is illustrated in Fig 4-9.

Class 4 (IV) lesions occur on the proximal surfaces of anterior teeth when the incisal angle requires restoration. The angle may have to be removed because of its fragility or for proper placement of the restoration, or it may have been fractured by trauma. A Class 4 cavity preparation is illustrated in Fig 4-13.

Class 5 (V) lesions occur on smooth facial and lingual surfaces in the gingival third of teeth. Class 5 cavities begin close to the gingiva and may involve a cementum or dentinal surface as well as the enamel. A Class 5 cavity preparation is illustrated in Fig 4-5.

Class 6 (VI) lesions are pit or wear defects on the incisal edges of anterior teeth or the cusp tips of posterior teeth. Class 6 cavity preparations are illustrated in Fig 4-14.

In addition to being named for their classifications, cavity preparations and restorations are named for the tooth surfaces involved. For example, a restoration involving the mesial and occlusal surfaces of a posterior tooth is called a *mesio-occlusal Class 2 restoration;* sim-

Fig 4-12 Classification of cavity preparations.

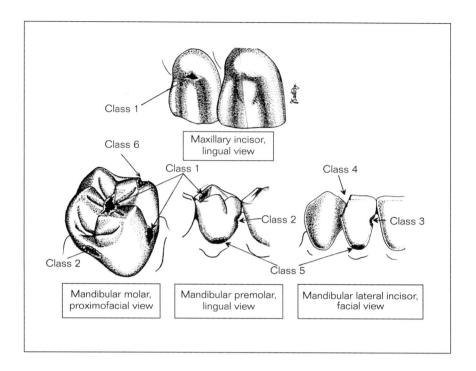

Class 1

Class 6

Class 1

Class 4

Class 2

Class 2

Class 3

Class 5

Maxillary incisor, lingual view

Mandibular molar, proximofacial view

Mandibular premolar, lingual view

Mandibular lateral incisor, facial view

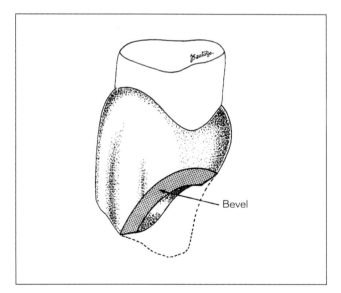

Bevel

Fig 4-13 Class 4 preparation for a bonded, tooth-colored restoration. Maxillary incisor, facial view.

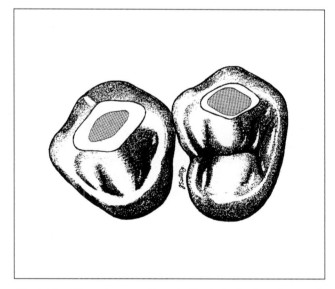

Fig 4-14 Class 6 preparations in the incisal edge of a maxillary canine and the cusp tip of a premolar (incisal/occlusal view). The dotted area of the preparation represents dentin; the clear area of the preparation represents enamel. The preparations have no mechanical, or undercut, retention; they are for bonded, tooth-colored restorations.

ply saying *mesio-occlusal restoration* identifies it as a Class 2 restoration because the proximal surface of a posterior tooth is involved. A preparation or restoration involving the mesial, occlusal, distal, and facial surfaces of a posterior tooth is called a *mesio-occlusodistofacial preparation* or *restoration.*

For the purpose of shortening the space necessary to write and the time it takes to say the surfaces involved in restorations, the names of the surfaces are often abbreviated (distal, *D;* lingual, *L;* facial, *F;* mesial, *M;* incisal, *I;* occlusal, *O*). A mesio-occlusal restoration in a posterior tooth would be abbreviated *MO,* and a distolingual restoration in an anterior tooth is abbreviated *DL.*

Black's Steps in Cavity Preparation

There are treatment modalities for dental caries other than caries removal, which are discussed in chapter 3. When it has been determined that nonsurgical means of treating caries will not suffice, however, restorative therapy is indicated. This involves the surgical removal of caries and restoration of the tooth to its original anatomic form with a suitable restorative material. The design of the cavity preparation is determined first by the location of caries in the tooth. The shape or outline of the cavity preparation, as it meets the external surface of the tooth, is referred to as *outline form.* Other factors influencing the design include the need to obtain access for the instruments as the operator is preparing or restoring the cavity (*convenience form*) and to provide retention for the restorative material (*retention form*) and resistance to stress on the restoration and the tooth to the forces of biting and chewing (*resistance form*). Because cavity preparation is a surgical procedure in which a mistake can mean injury to living tissue, it is essential that the operator be knowledgeable and highly skilled.

The steps of cavity preparation in sequence were established by Black.[2] Black's steps represent a systematic, scientific procedure for efficiency in cavity preparation. Although the technology of bonding restorative materials to enamel and dentin was not available to Black, his steps of cavity preparation are generally as appropriate today as they were when he wrote them:

1. *Establish outline form.* Outline form is based primarily on the location and extent of the carious lesion, tooth fracture, or erosion. In carious teeth, the outline form is established after penetration into carious dentin and removal of the enamel overlying the carious dentin. The extent of carious dentin should be a primary determinant of the outline form

of the preparation; the final outline is not established until carious dentin and its overlying enamel have been removed.

2. *Obtain resistance form.* Resistance for the remaining tooth structure and for the restoration must be designed in the preparation, so that the restoration is resistant to displacement and both the tooth and the restoration are resistant to fracture during function.

3. *Obtain retention form.* Retention may be obtained through mechanical shaping of the preparation to retain the restoration or etching of enamel and/or dentin for bonding procedures.

4. *Obtain convenience form.* Convenience form allows adequate observation, accessibility, and ease of operation during preparation and restoration of the tooth. Convenience form that involves the removal of sound, strong tooth structure should be limited to that which is necessary.

5. *Remove remaining carious dentin.* Removal of remaining caries applies primarily to the caries in the deepest part (pulpally) of the preparation. Other caries has been removed when the outline form was established.

6. *Finish enamel walls and cavosurface margins.* For indirect restorations (those requiring the making of an impression and fabrication of a stone duplicate of the preparation), finishing involves making the walls relatively smooth. For direct and indirect restorations not utilizing bonding, it involves removing any unsupported, weak, or fragile enamel and making the cavosurface margin smooth and continuous to facilitate finishing of restoration margins. For bonded restorations, enamel that is not supported by dentin and is not going to be exposed to significant occlusal loading is frequently allowed to remain in place and is reinforced by bonding to its internal surface.

7. *Clean the preparation.* Black called cleansing, "performing the toilet of the cavity." It includes washing or scrubbing away any debris in the preparation and drying the preparation. Afterward, the cavity is inspected for any remaining debris, caries, fragile enamel, and demineralized tooth structure.

Instrumentation

Hand Instruments

Black[2] organized the classification of cavity preparations and their parts; he also organized the naming and numbering of hand instruments. *Cutting instruments,* which

Fig 4-15 Components of a hand instrument. Although the handle is also called a *shaft*, that designation is little used.

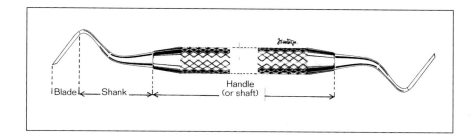

he also called *excavators*, were to be used in shaping the tooth preparation. All other hand instruments are grouped into the noncutting category.

Metals

For many years, carbon steel was the primary material used in hand instruments for operative dentistry because carbon steels were harder and maintained sharpness better than stainless steels. Stainless steels are now the preferred materials for hand instruments, because all instruments must be sterilized with steam or dry heat between patients and because the properties of stainless steels have improved. There are literally hundreds of formulas for stainless steels,[10] all incorporating a significant amount of chromium, some carbon, and iron. Chromium imparts corrosion resistance and brightness to the metal; carbon imparts hardness.

Cutting Instruments

Before rotating instruments were available, dentists could cut well-shaped cavity preparations by using sharp hand instruments alone. The process was slow. The advent of the dental handpiece in 1871,[11] at first attached to a foot-operated engine, allowed increased speed of tooth preparation. Most tooth preparation today is accomplished with rotary instruments, but hand cutting instruments are still important for finishing many tooth preparations. Few preparations involving a proximal surface can be properly completed without the use of hand cutting instruments. It is crucial that hand instruments used for cutting tooth structure or carving restorative materials be sharp.

Design. Hand cutting instruments are composed of three parts: handle (or shaft), shank, and blade[2] (Fig 4-15). The primary cutting edge of a cutting instrument is at the end of the blade (called the *working end*), but the sides of the blade are usually beveled and also may be used for cutting tooth structure (Fig 4-16). The shank joins the blade to the handle of the instrument and is angled to keep the working end of the blade within 2.0 to 3.0 mm of the axis of the handle (Fig 4-17). This

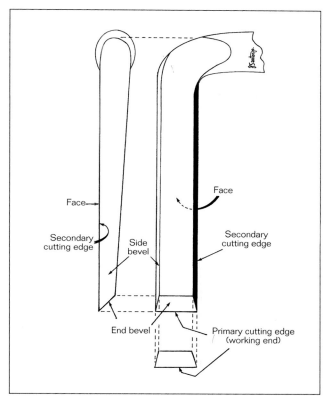

Fig 4-16 Blade bevels. Most hand cutting instruments not only have a bevel on the end of the blade but also have bevels on the sides. Although most of the work of a hand cutting instrument is accomplished with the end of the blade, the sides may also be used to plane walls and margins.

angulation is intended to provide balance in the instrument, so that when force is exerted on the instrument the instrument is not as likely to rotate, decreasing the effectiveness of the blade and possibly causing damage to the tooth. Figure 4-17a illustrates an instrument that has a single angle at the junction of the blade and the shank. Because the working end of the blade is not aligned with the handle, the instrument is said to be *out of balance*. Such an instrument may still be useful in tooth preparation. Its blade will usually be relatively

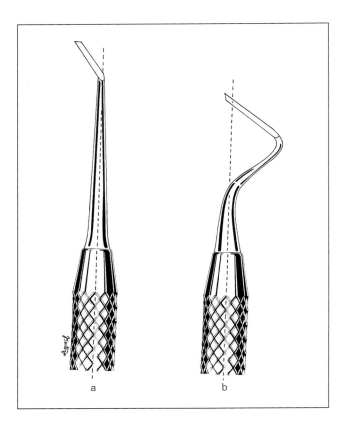

a   b

Fig 4-17 The shanks of instruments have multiple angles to keep the working end of the instrument within 2.0 to 3.0 mm of the long axis of the handle. (a) The working end of this instrument is not close to the long axis of the handle, and the instrument is, therefore, not balanced. (b) The shank of this instrument has two angles in it so that the working end is brought near to (within 2.0 mm) the long axis of the handle; this provides balance for the instrument to facilitate control of the instrument during the application of force. The instrument is said to be *contra-angled*.

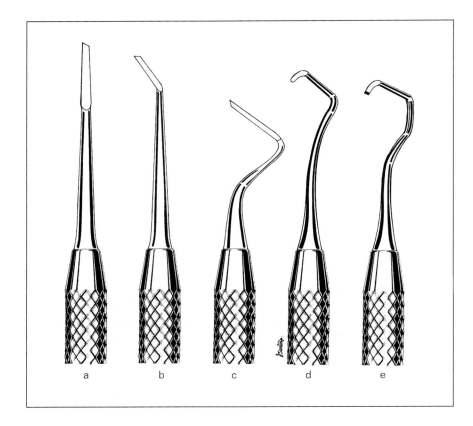

a   b   c   d   e

Fig 4-18 Instruments classified by the number of angles in the shank: (a) straight; (b) monangle; (c) binangle; (d) triple-angle; (e) quadrangle.

short and it will usually be used with low force. Figure 4-17b shows a shank that has two angles to bring the cutting edge into near alignment with the long axis of the handle to provide balance.

Nomenclature. The terminology organized by Black[2] in the early part of this century is still used today with minor modifications. Most names Black assigned to cutting instruments were based on the appearance of the instrument if it mimicked a commonly used item of the day; examples include *hatchet, hoe, spoon,* and *chisel.* For an instrument that did not have the appearance of a commonly used item, Black based the name on the intended use, for example, *gingival margin trimmer.* Black called all cutting instruments used for tooth preparation *excavators,* and he referred to instruments as *hatchet excavators, spoon excavators,* etc. The term *excavator* is still applicable, but, in the day-to-day language of operative dentistry, it is little used. In catalogs of instruments, cutting instruments are often indexed as excavators.

Black combined the name of each instrument with a designation of the number of angles in the shank of the instrument. Shanks may be straight, monangle (one angle), binangle (two angles), triple-angle (three angles), or quadrangle (four angles) (Fig 4-18). The term *contra-angled* refers to a shank in which two or more angles are necessary to bring the working end into near alignment with (within 2.0 to 3.0 mm) the axis of the handle (Fig 14-17b).

Hatchet. In a *hatchet* (also called an *enamel hatchet*) the blade and cutting edge are on a plane with the long axis of the handle; the shank has one or more angles (Figs 4-18e, 4-19a, 4-20, and 4-21). The face (Fig 4-16) of the blade of the hatchet will be directed either to the left or the right in relation to the handle, and the instrument is usually supplied in a double-ended form. Therefore, there are left-cutting and right-cutting ends on the double-ended hatchet.

Chisel. A *chisel* has a blade that is either aligned with the handle (Figs 4-18a, 4-22, and 4-23d) or is slightly angled (Figs 4-18b, 4-23a, and 4-23b) or curved (Fig 4-23c) from the long axis of the handle, with the working end at a right angle to the handle.

Hoe. A *hoe* has a cutting edge that is at a right angle to the handle, like that of a chisel. However, its blade has a greater angle from the long axis of the handle than does that of the chisel; its shank also has one or more angles (Figs 4-15, 4-18c, and 4-24). A general guideline for distinguishing between a hoe and a chisel will be given later in the chapter.

Spoon. The blade of a *spoon* is curved, and the cutting edge at the end of the blade is in the form of a semicircle (Figs 4-19b and 4-25b); this gives the instrument an outer convexity and an inner concavity that make it look somewhat like a spoon. Like the hatchet, the spoon has a cutting edge at the end of its blade that is parallel to the handle of the instrument; therefore, there are left-cutting and right-cutting spoons. The shank of some spoons holds a small circular, or disk-shaped, blade at its end, and the cutting edge extends around the disk except for its junction with the shank; these are called *discoid spoons* (Figs 4-25a and 4-25c).

Gingival margin trimmer. A *gingival margin trimmer* is similar to an enamel hatchet, except that the blade is curved, and the bevel for the cutting edge at the end of the blade is always on the outside of the curve; the face of the instrument is on the inside of the curve (Figs 4-26 and 4-27). Gingival margin trimmers, like hatchets and spoons, come in pairs (left-cutting and right-cutting) (Fig 4-26), but there are also mesial gingival margin trimmers and distal gingival margin trimmers (Fig 4-27). Thus, a set of gingival margin trimmers is composed of four instruments: left-cutting and right-cutting mesial gingival margin trimmers, and left-cutting and right-cutting distal gingival margin trimmers. Because these are usually double-ended instruments, one instrument is a mesial gingival margin trimmer (with left- and right-cutting ends), and the other is a distal gingival margin trimmer (with left- and right-cutting ends). Figure 4-27a illustrates a mesial left-cutting gingival margin trimmer. Fig 4-27b illustrates a distal left-cutting gingival margin trimmer. Contrasted with these is a right-cutting hatchet (Fig 4-27c).

Off-angle hatchet. Black's instrument names apply to instruments that have cutting edges that are either parallel or at a right angle to the handle. Instruments have been developed that have blades that are rotated 45 degrees from the plane of the long axis of the handle; these are called *off-angle hatchets.*

Usage. Hand cutting instruments are, for the most part, made in pairs, and, as with the gingival margin trimmers, most instruments used today are double-ended and will have one of the pair on each end (Figs 4-15, 4-20, and 4-26). A cutting instrument may be used with horizontal strokes, in which the long axis of the blade is directed at between 45 and 90 degrees to the

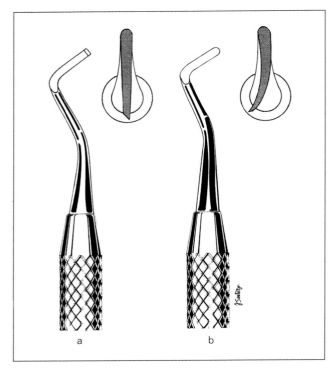

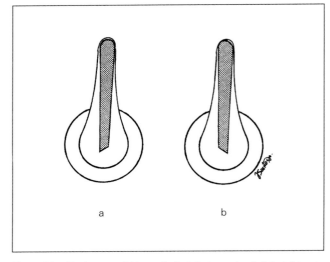

Fig 4-19 (a) Binangle hatchet. (b) Binangle spoon. A double-ended hatchet or spoon would have a left-cutting end and a right-cutting end (Fig 4-20).

Fig 4-20 End view of binangle hatchets, paired: (a) right-cutting; (b) left-cutting. A double-ended binangle hatchet has left-cutting and right-cutting ends.

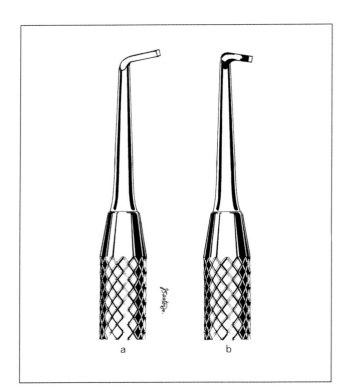

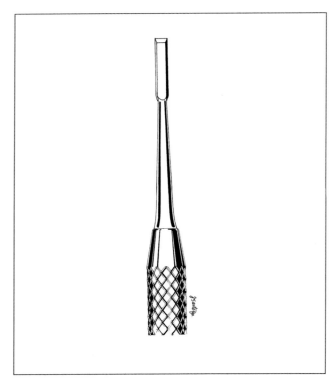

Fig 4-21 Monangle hatchets (left-cutting).

Fig 4-22 Straight chisel with bevels on the sides of the blade, to give secondary cutting edges, as well as on the end (primary cutting edge).

Fig 4-23 Chisels: (a) binangle; (b) monangle; (c) Wedelstaedt; (d) straight. The blades in a, c, and d are slightly rotated to visualize the face, as well as the side bevel.

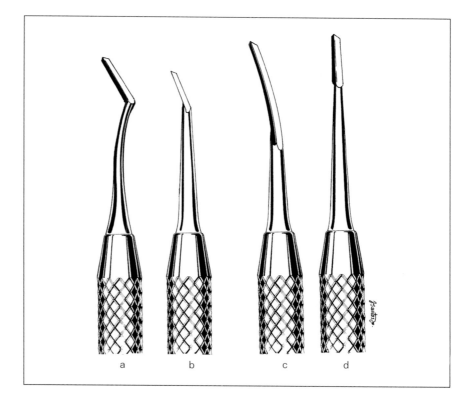

Fig 4-24 Hoes: (a) monangle; (b) binangle. The blade of a hoe has an angle from the long axis of the handle of greater than 12.5 centigrades; in contrast, the blade of a chisel will have an angle from the long axis of the handle of 12.5 centigrades or less.

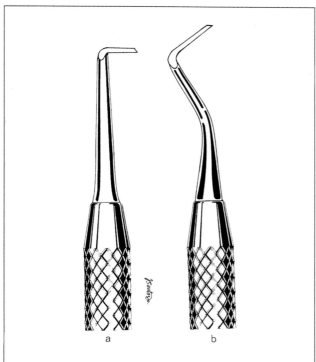

Fig 4-25 Spoons: (a) triple-angle discoid spoon; (b) binangle spoon (or regular spoon or banana spoon); (c) binangle discoid spoon. Spoons are used in tooth preparation for removing (or "spooning out") carious dentin.

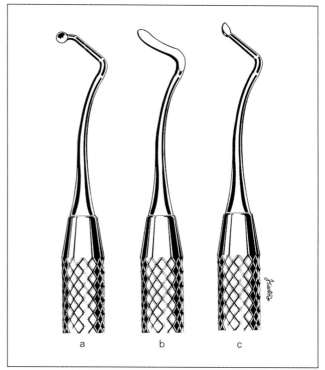

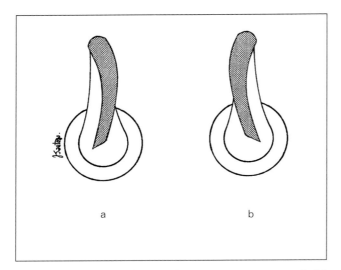

Fig 4-26 End view of gingival margin trimmers, paired; (a) right-cutting, (b) left-cutting. A double-ended gingival margin trimmer has both left-cutting and right-cutting ends, but there must be two double-ended gingival margin trimmers to complete a set, one double-ended mesial gingival margin trimmer and one double-ended distal gingival margin trimmer.

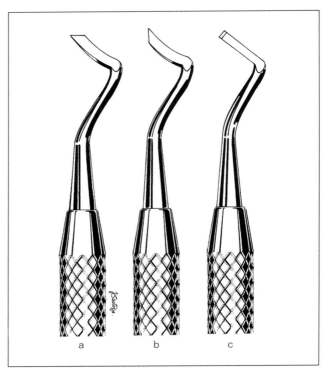

Fig 4-27 (a) Left-cutting mesial gingival margin trimmer. (b) Left-cutting distal gingival margin trimmer. (c) Right-cutting binangle hatchet.

surface being planed or scraped (Fig 4-28a); or with vertical or chopping strokes, in which the blade is nearly parallel to the wall or margin being planed (Fig 4-28b). For horizontal (scraping) or vertical (chopping) strokes, the acute angle of the cutting edge is intended to be used. The acute angle is the junction of the face of the blade with the bevel; in other words, the bevel is on the back of the blade, not the face of the blade. A double-ended hatchet, gingival margin trimmer, or spoon will have one end that is designated as right-cutting and one that is designated as left-cutting. In a double-ended hoe, in addition to allowing vertical or chopping strokes, one end is intended for pushing strokes (beveled end) and the other is intended for pulling strokes (contra-beveled end).

The cutting edges of most hand cutting instruments used today are single-beveled, as are all of those described here (Fig 4-16). Double-beveled or bi-beveled cutting edges are also available but have limited application in contemporary operative dentistry (Fig 4-29).

These instruments usually have narrow blades and are used for tasks such as adding mechanical retention points in areas of preparations that cannot be reached by a bur.

Numeric formulas. The configuration of the shanks combined with the appearance of the blade or the use of the instrument, produces names such as *straight chisel, monangle chisel, binangle hoe,* and *triple-angle hatchet.* These are descriptive terms, but they are imprecise because they do not indicate sizes or angles. For more complete identification of hand cutting instruments, Black[2] developed a system of assigning numeric formulas to instruments (Figs 4-30 and 4-31). The formulas make use of the metric system, that is, millimeters and tenths of a millimeter for instrument dimensions. For designating the degree of angulation, centigrades are used. Centigrades are based on a circle divided into 100 units (Fig 4-32), as opposed to the 360-degree circle ordinarily used to designate angles. In a centigrade circle, a right angle has 25.0 centigrades.

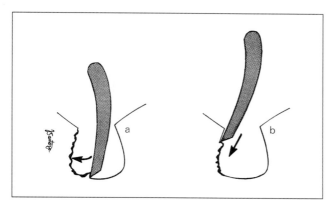

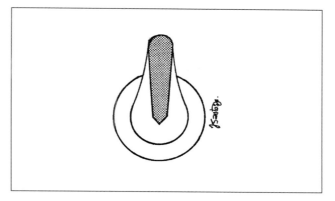

Fig 4-28 (a) Gingival margin trimmer being used in a proximal box of a Class 2 preparation with a horizontal (left or right) stroke to scrape (plane) a gingival wall and margin. (b) Gingival margin trimmer being used with a vertical, or chopping, stroke to plane a facial or lingual wall and margin. A hatchet could be used in a similar way.

Fig 4-29 Bi-beveled cutting edge, useful in placing retention points in some direct gold (gold foil) preparations, has little use in any of the preparations described in this book.

Fig 4-30 Black's three-number formula for instruments that have a primary cutting edge (working end) that is at a right angle (90 degrees) to the long axis of the blade: The first number is the width of the blade in tenths of a millimeter; the second number is the length of the blade in millimeters; and the third number is the blade angle, the angle the blade makes with the long axis of the handle, in centigrades. The complete name of the instrument illustrated would be *binangle hatchet, 10-7-14*. The formula would be the same if the blade were rotated 90 degrees on the shank to form a hoe, but the name would be different.

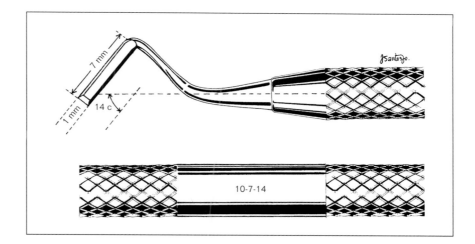

Fig 4-31 Black's four-number formula for instruments that have a primary cutting edge (working end) that is not at a right angle to the long axis of the blade: The first number is the width of the blade in tenths of a millimeter; the second number is the cutting edge angle, the angle the primary cutting edge makes with the long axis of the handle, in centigrades; the third number is the length of the blade in millimeters; and the fourth number is the blade angle, the angle the blade makes with the long axis of the handle, in centigrades. Illustrated is a right-cutting distal gingival margin trimmer, 13-95-8-14.

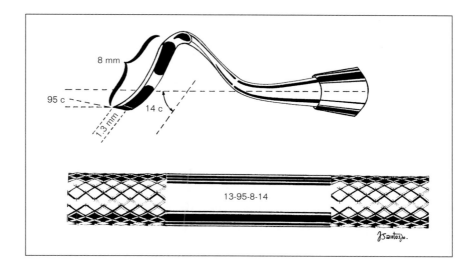

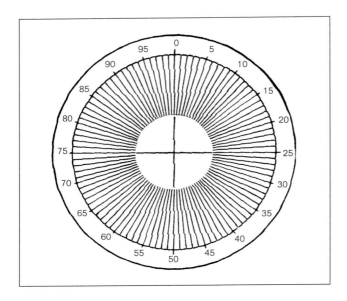

Fig 4-32 Centigrade scale. The circle is divided into 100 units.

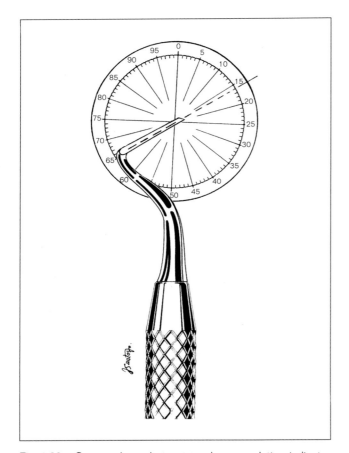

Fig 4-33 Centigrade scale inset to show angulation indicator of 16.0 centigrades for the blade angle of this hoe (three-number formula). The vertical axis (0.0 centigrades) is the axis of the instrument's handle. If the blade of the instrument were 1.4 mm wide and 10.0 mm long, the formula for the instrument would be 14-10-16.

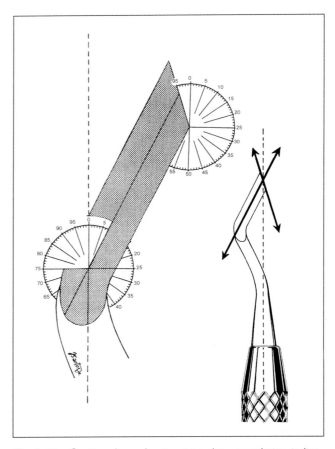

Fig 4-34 Centigrade scales inset to show angulation indicators of 7.0 centigrades for the blade angle and 95.0 centigrades for the cutting edge angle of this gingival margin trimmer (four-number formula). The vertical axis (0.0 centigrades) is the axis of the instrument's handle. If the blade were 1.5 mm wide and 10.0 mm long, the formula for the instrument would be 15-95-10-7.

Three-number formula. For instruments in which the primary cutting edge (at the end of the blade) is at a right angle to the long axis of the blade, Black developed a formula that has three numbers (Fig 4-30). The first number is the width of the blade in tenths of a millimeter; the second is the length of the blade in millimeters, and the third is the angle (in centigrades) made by the long axis of the blade and the long axis of the handle (Fig 4-33).

Four-number formula. For instruments in which the cutting edge at the end of the blade is not at a right angle to the long axis of the blade, such as the gingival margin trimmers, Black designed a four-number formula (Fig 4-31). The first number is the width of the blade in tenths of a millimeter. The second number is the angle (in centigrades) that the primary cutting edge (working end) makes with the axis of the handle (Fig 4-34), the third number is the length of the blade in millimeters, and the fourth number is the angle (in centigrades) that the long axis of the blade makes with the handle. In margin trimmers, a cutting edge angle of greater than 90 degrees is intended for distal gingival margins (Fig 4-31); an angle of 85 degrees or less is intended for mesial gingival margins.

Chisel versus hoe. Although Black defined a *chisel* as having a blade that was aligned with the handle or slightly curved from it, terminology has evolved somewhat so that a chisel may also have a blade that is angled from the handle up to 12.5 centigrades.[5] A chisel with a blade angled more than 3 or 4 centigrades from the axis of the handle must be binangle for the instrument to be balanced.

If the blade is angled greater than 12.5 centigrades, the instrument is defined as a *hoe.* In a curved or angled chisel or a hoe, a blade with its primary cutting edge (and its face) on the side of the blade toward the handle is said to be *beveled* (Figs 4-23a to 4-23c); a blade with its primary cutting edge (and its face) on the side of the blade that is away from the handle is said to be *contrabeveled* (Fig 4-18c).

Recommended instrument kit. Black recommended a long set of 96 cutting instruments, a university set of 44 cutting instruments, or a short set of 25 cutting instruments. Because bonding technology and high-speed handpieces were not available, the dental materials of the time were more limited and a primary restorative material was direct gold; the longevity of restorations depended on the retention and resistance form developed with hand cutting instruments.

With access to advanced materials and technology, current use of hand cutting instruments is greatly diminished. The kit recommended in this chapter has only 12 hand cutting instruments (six double-ended instruments). Because it is now recognized that there is no need to plane walls and floors of cavity preparations to smoothness with hand instruments for a restoration to perform well, hand cutting instruments play only a small, albeit important, part in cavity preparation. If burs alone were used for shaping proximal preparations, excessive sound tooth structure would have to be removed from the tooth being restored or the bur would damage the adjacent tooth. Hand cutting instruments enable the dentist to shape and refine small proximal boxes without damaging the adjacent tooth.

Hatchets, hoes, chisels, and gingival margin trimmers have straight cutting edges and are designed to plane enamel and dentinal walls and margins in shaping cavity preparations, especially in areas of the preparation that cannot be reached with a bur. Spoons, on the other hand, have rounded cutting edges; their intended use is the removal of carious dentin. Although slowly rotating round burs are most useful in removing carious dentin, a spoon gives more tactile sensation and is preferred by many operators.

Noncutting Instruments

Non–tooth-cutting hand instruments are similar in appearance to cutting instruments, except that the blade used for tooth preparation is replaced with a part that has a totally different use. In noncutting instruments such as burnishers and amalgam condensers, the blade is replaced by the *nib* or *point.*[2] The flat end of the nib of a condenser is called the *face.* Amalgam carvers have carving blades instead of tooth-cutting blades.

Condensers, carvers, and burnishers are used to insert dental amalgam and, to a certain extent, resin composite restorative materials. Plastic filling instruments are used for placing resin composite materials, provisional restorative materials, and sometimes cavity-basing materials into tooth preparations. Spatulas are necessary for mixing cavity-lining and -basing materials, provisional restorative materials, and cements for luting inlays, onlays, and crowns.

Amalgam carriers. For silver amalgam restorations, amalgam is placed into the preparation with an amalgam carrier, an instrument with a hollow cylinder that is filled with amalgam (Fig 4-35). A plunger operated with a finger lever pushes the amalgam out of the carrier into the preparation.

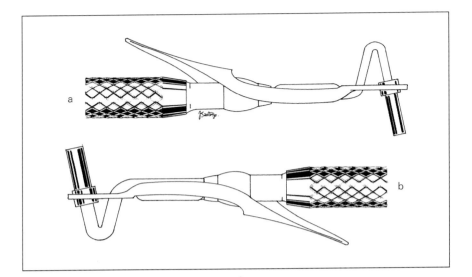

Fig 4-35 Amalgam carriers: (a) regular; (b) large. Amalgam carriers are usually supplied as a double-ended instrument. They are available in several different diameters; for example, mini is 1.5 mm; regular (medium) is 2.0 mm; large is 2.5 mm; and jumbo is 3.0 to 3.5 mm. These are the approximate inside diameters of the cylinders of amalgam carriers and may vary slightly from manufacturer to manufacturer.

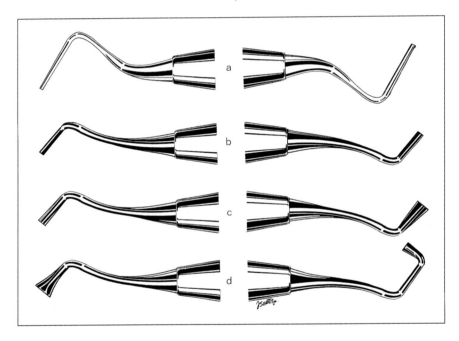

Fig 4-36 Amalgam condensers with round faces: (a) SA1, with 0.5-mm and 0.6-mm diameter faces; (b) SA2 with 0.7-mm and 1.0-mm faces; (c) SA3 with 1.5-mm and 2.0-mm faces; (d) SA4, with a 2.5-mm face on the binangle end and a 1.5-mm face on the triple-angle or back-action end.

Condensers. Amalgam condensers are used to compress the amalgam into all areas of the preparation. The working ends, or nibs, of condensers may be any shape, but usually they are round with flat ends (faces). Figure 4-36 shows four round condensers of different sizes and configurations. Other commonly used condenser nibs are triangular, rectangular, or diamond shaped. Amalgam is condensed by pushing the condenser directly into the preparation and confining the amalgam between the condenser face and the preparation floor through vertical pressure (vertical condensation). The amalgam is condensed against the vertical walls of the preparation (lateral condensation) by angling the nib and using the end for condensation, or by lateral, or side-to-side, movements of the condenser, using the sides of the nib to condense the amalgam.

The condensation pressure applied to the amalgam with a condenser depends on the size of the face and the amount of force used by the operator. For small condensers, such as the SA1 condenser (Fig 4-36a), little force is needed. The nibs of the SA1 condenser are 0.5 and 0.6 mm in diameter. For larger condensers, such as the SA3 (Fig 4-36c), with nib diameters of 1.5 and 2.0 mm, a significant amount of force (6 to 8 pounds) gives optimum condensation.

Fig 4-37a Cleoid-discoid carver: (a) cleoid end; (b) discoid end. This type of carver is a double-ended instrument. *Cleoid* means claw shaped. Both shapes are useful in carving occlusal surfaces of amalgam restorations. The point of the cleoid carver is used to carve the base of grooves in the occlusal amalgam, and the tip is usually very slightly rounded so that grooves are not sharp.

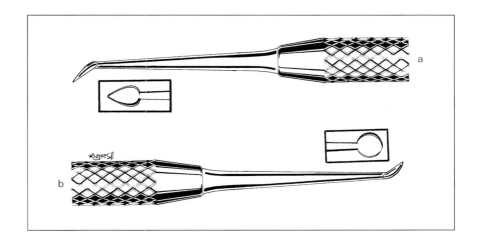

Amalgam condensers may also be used to place resin composite materials. The resin material is not actually condensed, however, but pushed or patted into all areas of the preparation with the largest condenser face that will fit into the area.

Carvers. Carvers are used to shape amalgam and resin composite (tooth-colored) materials after they have been inserted into tooth preparations. Figures 4-37a and 4-37b show the shapes of the blades of a cleoid-discoid carver. Figure 4-38 illustrates six commonly used carvers. In general, when a convex amalgam contour is being carved, a concave-shaped carver facilitates the shaping or carving. Likewise, a convex carver facilitates carving of a concave shape. A convex carver may be used to carve a convex surface; the surface is carved tangentially, with multiple strokes. Whether a carver is used to carve amalgam or resin composite, it is important that the blade be sharp.

The cleoid-discoid (or discoid-cleoid) carvers shown in Figs 4-38a and 4-38b are used primarily for occlusal carving in amalgam restorations. The Walls No. 3 carver (Fig 4-38c) is useful for carving occlusal anatomy; the end that is shaped like a hoe is also useful for shaping cusps and for carving facial and lingual surfaces of large amalgam restorations. The Hollenback No. 1/2 carver (Fig 4-38d) is useful for occlusal, interproximal, and axial (facial and lingual) surfaces; several larger Hollenback carvers, with the same general shape, are also available. The interproximal carver (IPC) (Fig 4-38e) has very thin blades and is extremely valuable for carving proximal amalgam surfaces near to the interproximal contact area. The No. 14L carver (Fig 4-38f) can be used for interproximal areas, or it may be used for carving convex facial and lingual surfaces of very large amalgam restora-

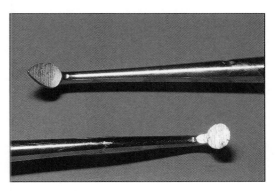

Fig 4-37b Cleoid *(top)* and discoid *(bottom)* ends of the cleoid-discoid carver.

tions. The No. 14L carver has a very strong, hollow-ground triangular blade, so it can be used to remove amalgam overhangs from completely set amalgam.

Although most of the shaping of resin composite restorations should be completed before the material is polymerized, several amalgam carvers are also useful for carving resin composite. The discoid carvers are especially useful for lingual concavities of anterior teeth; cleoid and discoid carvers and the hoe-shaped end of the Walls No. 3 carver are useful for occlusal surfaces of posterior resin composite restorations. Another carver very useful for resin composite restorations is a disposable scalpel blade (No. 12 or No. 12b blade) mounted in a scalpel handle.

Burnishers. Burnishers are used for several functions. The word *burnish* is defined as "to make shiny or lustrous, especially by rubbing; to polish;" and "to rub (a

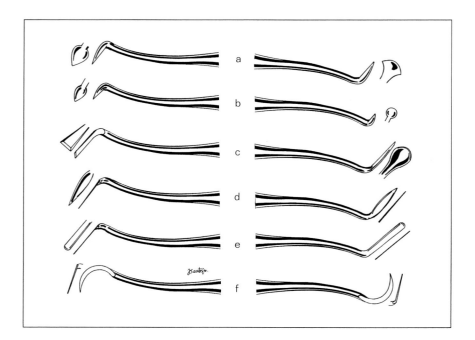

Fig 4-38 Amalgam carvers: (a) large cleoid-discoid (Tanner No. 5 [5T]) carver; (b) small cleoid-discoid (UWD5) carver; (c) Walls No. 3 carver; (d) Hollenback No. 1/2 carver; (e) interproximal carver (IPC); (f) No. 14L sickle-shaped carver.

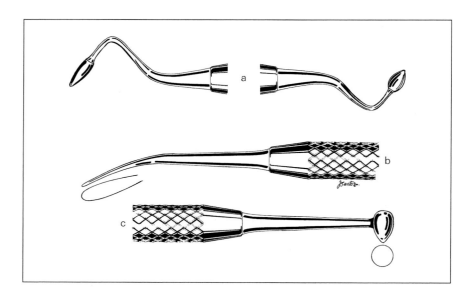

Fig 4-39 Burnishers: (a) PKT3 (rounded cone–shaped) burnisher, designed by Peter K. Thomas as a waxing instrument, but useful in placing direct restorations as well; its rounded end and cone shape allow it to serve most functions that a small ball-shaped burnisher would serve, plus others; (b) beavertail (No. 2) burnisher, (c) football or ovoid (No. 30) burnisher. The ovoid burnisher, available in various sizes (eg, 28, 29, and 31), can be used for final condensation of amalgam and the initial shaping of the occlusal anatomy in amalgam. The beavertail and ovoid burnishers are useful for burnishing margins of cast-gold restorations.

material) with a tool for compacting or smoothing or for turning an edge."[13] Burnishing is probably used in all of those ways in dentistry. Two frequently used double-ended burnishers are illustrated in Fig 4-39.

One use of burnishers is to shape metal matrix bands so that they impart more desirable contours to restorations. Large burnishers are used with considerable force to pinch off freshly condensed amalgam at the margins, or, in other words, to impart some condensation and to begin shaping the occlusal surfaces of amalgam restorations. After the amalgam has been carved, a burnisher may be used with a gentle rubbing motion to smooth the surface.

Burnishers are used to "bend" cast gold near the margin so that the gap between the gold and the tooth is narrowed. This closing of a marginal gap is best accomplished with a narrow burnisher, such as the side of a beavertail burnisher, used with heavy force in strokes parallel to the margin but about 1.0 or 1.5 mm away from it. If burnishing is accomplished directly on a thin gold margin, the gold can be bent severely and may break off.

Fig 4-40a The No. 1-2 plastic instrument, made of stainless steel, is useful for placing a rubber dam, placing and shaping resin composite and other tooth-colored restorative materials, and packing gingival retraction cord around a crown or abutment preparation before an impression is made. There are cord-packing instruments that are similar to the No. 1-2 plastic instrument but have serrated ends to provide better control of the cord.

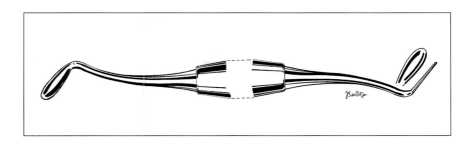

Fig 4-40b A plastic instrument made of hard plastic, rather than metal, is preferred by some operators for placing resin composites.

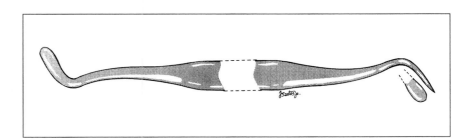

Plastic instruments. Plastic instruments (or plastic filling instruments) are so named because they were originally designed to use with plastic restorative materials, such as the silicates and acrylic resins used in the middle of this century. They are currently used to carry and shape tooth-colored restorative materials such as resin composite and glass-ionomer cements.

A commonly used plastic instrument is the No. 1-2 (Fig 4-40a). The double-ended instrument has a nib or blade on each end, one at a 90 degree angle to the other. Other double-ended plastic instruments have a blade-type nib on one end and a condenser nib on the other. The bladed plastic instruments are useful for many things in operative dentistry in addition to carrying a restorative material.

These instruments are now available in both hard plastic and metal; the original rationale for using an instrument made of plastic was to eliminate abrasion of metal by the quartz in resin composites, which caused grayness in the tooth-colored resin composite (Fig 4-40b). Because of changes in the inorganic fillers used in today's resin composites, the problem of metal abrasion and graying has been eliminated; thus, a metal instrument functions well to carry and shape resin composite.

Cement spatulas. A variety of materials in operative dentistry require mixing, some on a glass slab, others on a paper pad. Several spatulas are available, and they vary in size and thickness (Fig 4-41). The larger cement spatulas are designed for mixing luting cements and the

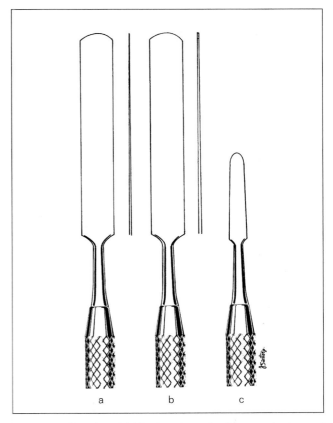

Fig 4-41 Spatulas. (a) Number 24, a flexible spatula, is used for luting cements such as zinc phosphate and glass-ionomer cements. (b) Number 24A is thicker, for more rigidity. (c) Number 313 is used for cavity liners, such as the calcium hydroxide liners.

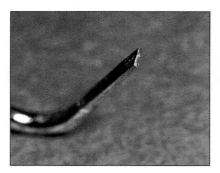

Fig 4-42a The glint from the cutting edge of this hoe indicates that the blade is quite dull.

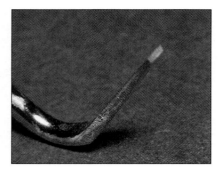

Fig 4-42b After sharpening, no glint is noticeable.

smaller for cavity liners. The thinner spatulas are flexible; the thicker ones are rigid. Selection of a rigid or flexible cement spatula is dependent on the desired viscosity of the cement and personal preference.

Sharpening of Hand Instruments

To assess sharpness, the user of the instrument should look at the cutting edge in bright light; the presence of a "glint" indicates that the edge is dull or rounded (Figs 4-42a and 4-42b). Alternatively, the dentist can pull the instrument across hard plastic, such as the handle of a plastic mouth mirror or an evacuator tip. A dull blade will slide across the plastic; a sharp blade will cut into the surface, stopping movement. A specially made, sterilizable, sharpness-testing stick is also available (Figs 4-43a and 4-43b) (Dalron Test Stick, Thompson Dental).

Sharpening is performed in different ways for different hand instruments. When chisels, hatchets, hoes, and margin trimmers are sharpened, the cutting edge bevel is placed flat against a flat stone, which is on a stable surface, and the instrument is pushed or pulled so that the acute cutting angle is moved forward, with fairly heavy force on the forward stroke, and with little or no force on the back stroke (Figs 4-44 and 4-45). Usually, unless the instrument has been badly neglected, only two or three forward strokes are required. Because the bevels of these instruments should usually make a 45 degree angle with the face of the blade, the blade should make a 45 degree angle with the surface of the sharpening stone (Fig 4-46).

When spoons, discoid carvers, and cleoid carvers are sharpened, the instrument is rotated as the blade is advanced on the flat stone (Fig 4-47). The bevel is at 45

degrees, or slightly less, to the face, and the instrument is advanced on the stone with the bevel against the surface of the stone and the cutting edge of the instrument perpendicular to the path of advancement. When a blade with a rounded edge is being sharpened, the handle cannot be simply twirled to achieve the desired rotation, but must actually be swung in an arc to keep the cutting edge of the blade perpendicular to the direction of the stroke.

The discoid carver and spoon may be sharpened with a continuous rotation of the blade; the shank moves clockwise from the 9-o'clock position to the 3-o'clock position in one motion. For the cleoid carver, however, the rotation begins with the shank in the 9-o'clock position and continues clockwise only until the bevel just next to the point is ground (Fig 4-47); to sharpen the other side of the cleoid, the rotation begins with the shank at the 3-o'clock position and continues counterclockwise to the point.

The blade of a discoid spoon may be sharpened by grinding the face of the blade with a rotating stone (Fig 4-48). This method of sharpening also thins the blade, and care must be taken to avoid using a blade that is so thin that it could easily break.

Sharpening machines are available. A slowly rotating sharpening wheel is employed by one type of machine; an oscillating flat stone, or hone, is used by another. These machines are useful for sharpening instruments between patients and prior to sterilization.

When instruments are sharpened during an operative procedure, they should be sharpened with a sterile stone. When a stone is sterilized, it should not have oil in or on it, because the oil may thicken during sterilization and form a shellac-like coating that will prevent the

Figs 4-43a and 4-43b   The sharpness testing stick is a hard plastic stick used for testing the sharpness of instruments.

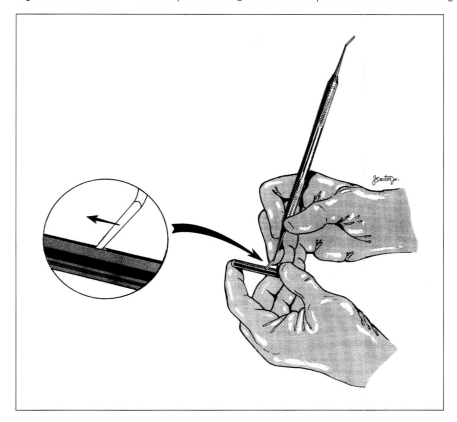

Fig 4-43a   Testing the sharpness of a monangle chisel.

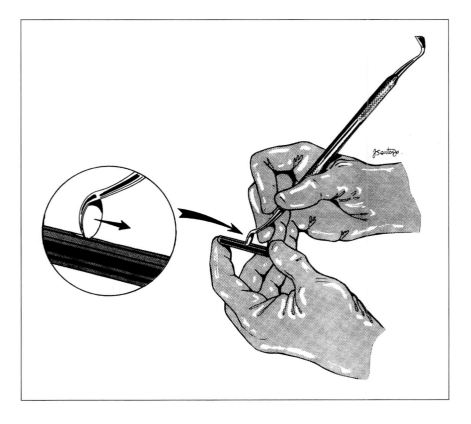

Fig 4-43b   Testing the sharpness of the discoid end of Walls No. 3 carver. For testing sharpness, the blade should be applied to the stick at an angle that is similar to that applied during use and pulled or pushed in a direction that is similar to the direction of its intended use.

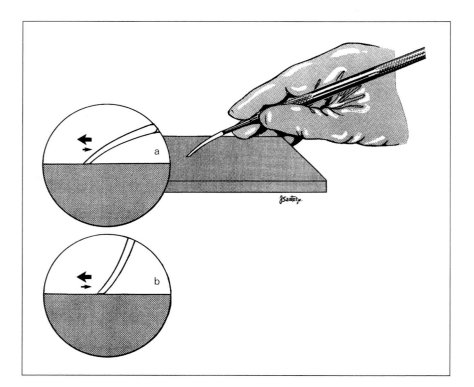

Fig 4-44 Sharpening the two ends of a double-ended Wedelstaedt chisel: (a) sharpening the contrabevel end (inside bevel); (b) sharpening the bevel end (outside bevel). The end bevel (for the primary cutting edge or working end) of each blade is placed flat on the stone; the blade will make a 45 degree angle with the stone. In the primary sharpening stroke, the cutting edge is moved forward. Unless the instrument is very dull, only two or three fairly heavy forward strokes will be necessary to sharpen the cutting edge.

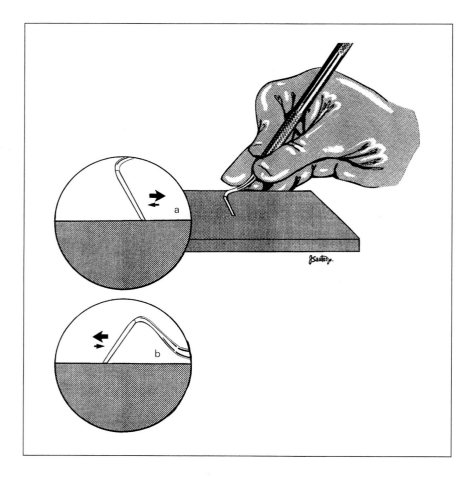

Fig 4-45 Sharpening the two ends of a double-ended binangle hoe: (a) sharpening the bevel end (outside bevel); (b) sharpening the contrabevel end (inside bevel). The primary bevel is always flat against the stone; the face of the blade is up.

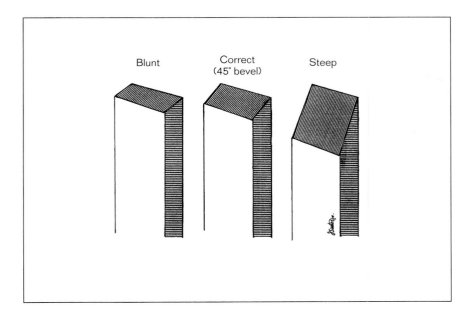

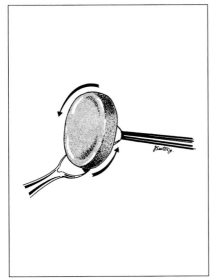

Fig 4-46 Bevels of sharpened cutting instruments. Working end bevels of chisels, hatchets, and hoes, as well as the bevels of amalgam carvers, should be at approximately 45 degrees to the face of the blade. The cutting edge at the left is too blunt, the center blade has a correctly angled cutting edge, and the cutting edge at the right is too acute and will dull rapidly.

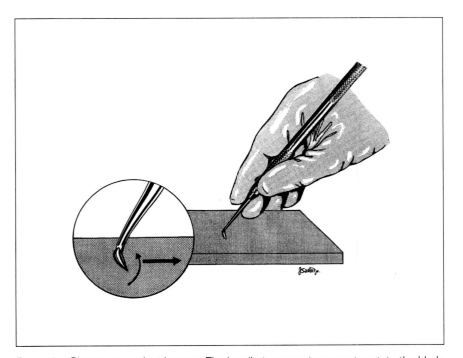

Fig 4-47 Sharpening a cleoid carver. The handle is swung in an arc to rotate the blade as the bevel is pulled forward on the stone. This movement is used to keep the cutting edge perpendicular to the direction of the stroke.

Fig 4-48 Sharpening a discoid spoon with a rotating sharpening stone. A discoid spoon may also be sharpened on a flat stone; the blade is rotated as it is pulled with the cutting edge forward. If the face is ground with a rotating stone, the blade will be thinned.

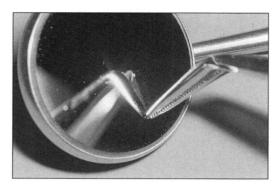

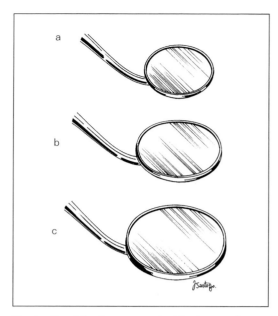

Fig 4-49a Front-surface mirror. Any object touching the mirror, such as the tips of the cotton forceps, will appear to be touching itself.

Fig 4-49b Mouth mirrors: (a) Number 2 ($^5/_8$-inch diameter); (b) Number 4 ($^7/_8$-inch diameter); (c) Number 5 ($^{15}/_{16}$-inch diameter).

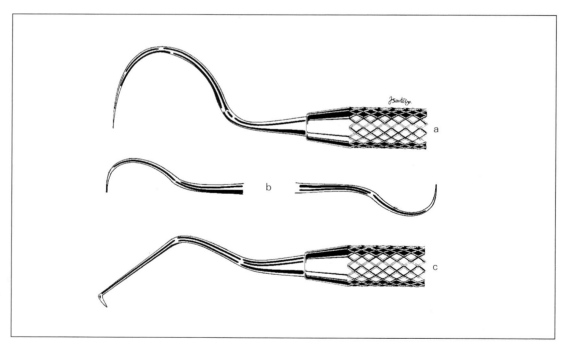

Fig 4-50 Dental explorers: (a) Number 23 explorer (shepherd's hook); (b) 3CH explorer (cowhorn or pigtail); (c) Number 17 explorer.

Fig 4-51 Periodontal probes: (a) Q-OW probe (Michigan O probe with Williams markings); (b) PCP12 probe (Marquis markings).

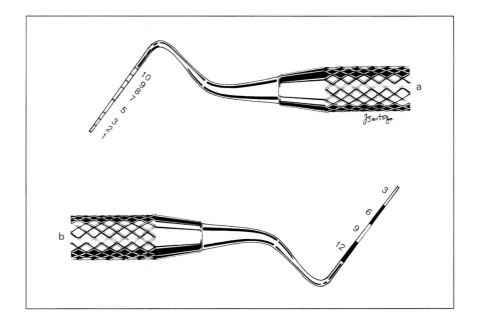

abrasion needed for sharpening. A good substitute for oil is water. Stones lubricated with water should be washed well or cleaned in an ultrasonic cleaner after use to remove the metal filings prior to sterilization. A flat, white Arkansas stone or fine synthetic sharpening stone should be made a part of the operative dentistry instrument kit so that it is available during each procedure.

Mirrors, Explorers, Periodontal Probes, and Forceps

Mirrors, explorers, periodontal probes, and forceps are basic instruments that will be needed during each appointment for diagnosis or treatment.

Mirrors. In every procedure performed in the mouth, the dentist must have clear and distinct vision of the field. Wherever possible, the field should be viewed with direct vision. When needed, the mouth mirror allows the operator to visualize areas of the mouth that he or she would not otherwise be able to see. It also allows the operator to maintain a body position that will reduce health problems associated with poor posture.

Almost as important as its allowing indirect visualization of obscure areas of the mouth is its function as a reflector of light into the area being examined or treated. A mirror that is positioned properly allows the operator to visualize the field of operation in the mirror, and, at the same time, reflects the operating light into that area. To accomplish this, the light should be positioned behind and just to the side of the operator's head.

The mouth mirror can also serve as a retractor of soft tissue (tongue, cheeks, or lips) to aid access and visualization.

For clarity of vision, the reflective surface of the mirror should be on the surface of the glass. This type of mirror is called a *front-surface mirror* (Fig 4-49a). Mouth mirrors are usually round and come in a variety of sizes (Fig 4-49b). The most widely used sizes for adults are the No. 4 and No. 5. For constricted areas in posterior regions of the mouth, when a rubber dam is in place, a smaller mirror, such as a No. 2, is helpful.

Explorers. Explorers are pointed instruments used to feel tooth surfaces for irregularities and to determine the hardness of exposed dentin. The explorer that is used most often is the shepherd's hook, or No. 23, explorer (Fig 4-50a). Another useful shape is a cowhorn explorer, which provides improved access for exploring interproximal areas (Fig 4-50b). The No. 17 explorer is also useful in interproximal areas (Fig 4-50c).

Periodontal probes. Periodontal probes are designed to detect the depth of periodontal pockets. In operative dentistry, they are also used to determine dimensions of instruments and of various features of preparations or restorations. There are many designs of periodontal probes; the differences are in the diameters, the position of the millimeter markings, and the configuration of the markings, that is, whether they are notched or painted. Two commonly used probes are illustrated in Fig 4-51.

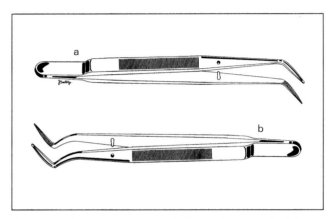

Fig 4-52 Cotton forceps: (a) College (No. 17); (b) Meriam (No. 18).

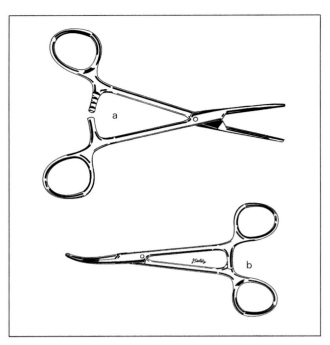

Fig 4-53 Hemostats: (a) Halstead mosquito straight, 6-inch; (b) Halstead mosquito curved, 5-inch.

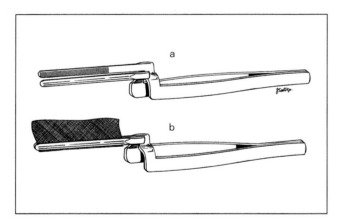

Fig 4-54 Articulating paper forceps. (a) Forceps handles provide a spring that keeps the jaws closed together; they are opened (as shown) by squeezing the handle. (b) The entire length of the piece of articulating paper or tape is supported by the jaws of the forceps.

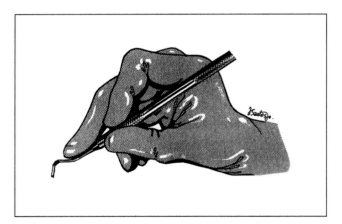

Fig 4-55 Pen grasp. The pen grasp is not actually the way a pen is held for writing. The instrument is held between the index finger and thumb, and the middle finger is placed atop the handle or shank, nearer the working end of the instrument, to provide more force, or thrust, directed toward the working end of the instrument.

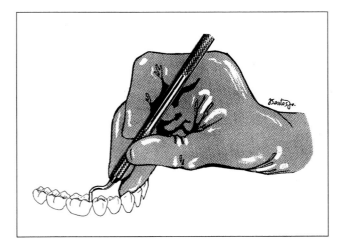

Fig 4-56a Pen grasp used in a chopping (downward) motion. The ring finger is resting on the incisal edges of the anterior teeth. During the use of any instrument in the mouth (with the exception of the mirror), a firm rest must be achieved on teeth or attached gingival tissue.

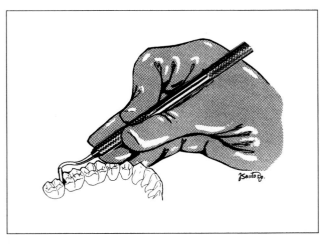

Fig 4-56b Pen grasp as the instrument is used more posteriorly and with a side-to-side or scraping motion. The small finger and ring finger are resting on surfaces, facial and occlusal, respectively.

Forceps. Forceps of various kinds are useful in operative dentistry. Cotton forceps are used for picking up various small items, such as cotton pellets (small cotton balls), and carrying them to the mouth (Fig 4-52). Other forceps useful in operative dentistry are hemostats (Fig 4-53). A hemostat locks tightly, so it is often helpful in placing or removing items used to confine amalgam for condensation. Articulating paper forceps are designed to carry an inked tape to the mouth to mark the contacts of teeth in opposing arches during closure (Fig 4-54).

Instrument Grasps

The operator should master two basic instrument grasps, the pen grasp, which provides more flexibility of movement, and the palm or palm-thumb grasp, which provides only limited movement but controlled power.

Pen grasp. This is the most frequently used instrument grasp in operative dentistry. The pen grasp is actually different from the way one would grasp a pen (Fig 4-55); the shaft of the instrument is engaged by the end, not the side, of the middle finger; this provides more finger power. The pen grasp is initiated by placement of the instrument between the thumb and index finger; the middle finger engages the handle or shank of the instrument. The ring finger is braced against the teeth to stabilize instrument movement (Figs 4-56a and 4-56b).

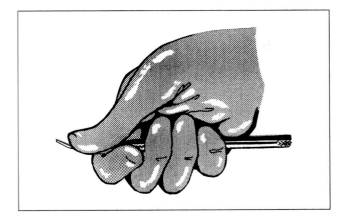

Fig 4-57 Palm-thumb grasp. The instrument is grasped much nearer to its end than in the pen grasp, so that the thumb can be braced against the teeth to provide control during movement of the instrument.

Palm or palm-thumb grasp. In this grasp, the thumb serves as a brace (Fig 4-57). Side-to-side, rotation, or thrusting movements of the instrument by the wrist and fingers are controlled by the thumb, which is firmly in contact with the teeth (Fig 4-58).

Sometimes two-handed instrumentation may be used to make refinement of a preparation more precise (Fig 4-59).

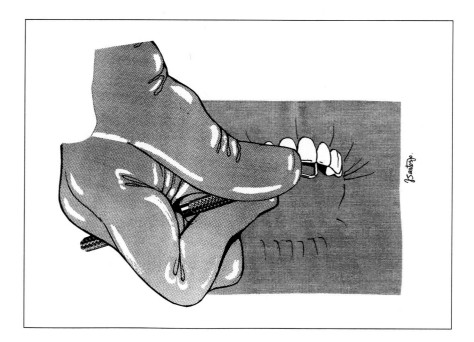

Fig 4-58 The palm-thumb grasp is used frequently when a hand cutting instrument, such as a gingival margin trimmer, is used in Class 3 preparations that have lingual access. The thumb is resting on the incisal edges of the teeth. The palm-thumb grasp is also used frequently with the Wedelstaedt chisel, usually for facial access in posterior and anterior operations, and occasionally for lingual access.

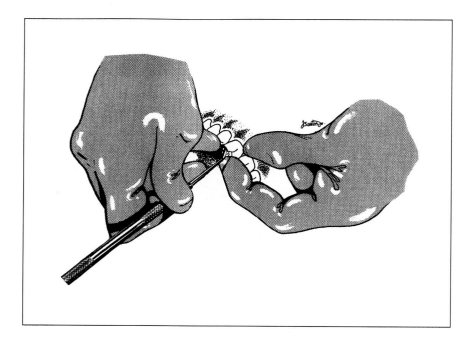

Fig 4-59 Two-handed instrumentation. The use of both hands can make refinement of a preparation more precise. The right hand is thrusting and rotating the instrument while the index finger of the left hand guides and assists the motion of the working end to refine a proximal margin of a Class 2 preparation. A similar dual-handed action is useful for condensing amalgam; it allows increased condensation force to be controlled.

Instrument Motions

The following are some of the many complex motions used with hand instruments:

- *Chopping* (in the direction of the working end of the instrument, or parallel to the long axis of the blade)
- *Pulling* (toward the operator's hand)
- *Pushing* (away from the hand)
- *Rotating*
- *Scraping* (with the blade directed at an angle between 45 and 90 degrees to the surface being scraped and moved side to side or back and forth on the surface)
- *Thrusting* (forcibly pushing against a surface)

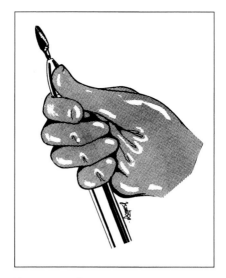

Fig 4-60 Straight handpiece. This handpiece is used occasionally in the mouth, but it is more frequently used extraorally, for tasks such as making adjustments to removable prostheses or adjusting and repolishing a cast-gold or ceramic restoration prior to insertion. The bur installed in this handpiece is a tree-shaped denture bur.

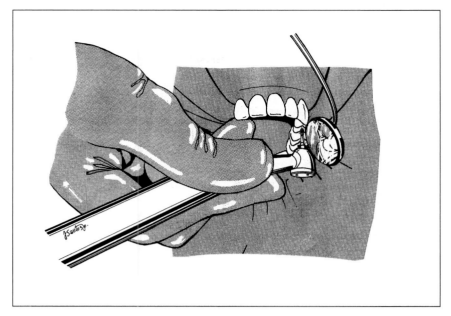

Fig 4-61 Contra-angle handpiece in use. This is a high-speed contra-angle handpiece, which is used with small diameter burs for rapid cutting of tooth structure or restorations. A low-speed contra-angle is also useful for removal of caries, with a slowly rotating round bur, and for shaping and polishing with abrasive disks and impregnated rubber polishers. Some operators also prefer the low-speed contra-angle for refining tooth preparations.

Rotating Instruments

Handpieces

In dentistry two basic types of handpiece, the straight handpiece (Fig 4-60) and the contra-angle handpiece (Fig 4-61), are used. In the straight handpiece, the long axis of the bur is the same as the long axis of the handpiece. The straight handpiece is used more frequently for laboratory work but is occasionally useful in the mouth.

The primary handpiece used in the mouth is the contra-angle handpiece. As with hand instruments, *contra-angle* indicates that the head of the handpiece is angled first away from, and then back toward, the long axis of the handle. Also as with hand instruments, this contra-angle design is intended to bring the working point (the head of the bur) to within a few millimeters of the long axis of the handle of the contra-angle handpiece to provide balance. Without balance, the handpiece would be unstable and would rotate in the hand with any application of pressure at the working point.

There are two types of contra-angle handpieces, which are classified by their speed potential. Low-speed contra-angle handpieces have a typical free-running speed range of 500 to 15,000 rpm; some are able to slow to 200 rpm and others are able to achieve speeds of 35,000 rpm. High-speed handpieces have a free-running speed range greater than 160,000 rpm, and some handpieces attain free-running speeds up to 500,000.[14] In the United States, dentists are accustomed to air-turbine high-speed handpieces; their speeds during tooth preparation are significantly less than their free-running speeds. In Europe, some handpieces powered by an electric motor can achieve free-running speeds of only around 165,000 rpm, but these handpieces are electronically regulated to maintain speed during tooth preparation.[9]

High-speed techniques are generally preferred for cutting enamel and dentin. Penetration through enamel and extension of the cavity outline are more efficient at high speed. Small-diameter burs should be used in the high-speed handpiece. High speed generates considerable heat, even with small-diameter burs, and should be used with water coolants[9] and high-efficiency evacuation. For refining preparations, a high-speed handpiece may be slowed considerably and used with only air coolant and a gentle brushing or painting motion in which each application of the bur to the tooth is brief. This technique allows visualization and prevents overheating.[4]

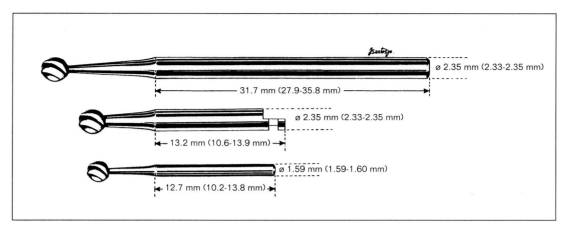

Fig 4-62 Typical dimensions (and ANSI/ADA standard dimension tolerances), in millimeters, of the three common bur designs: *(top)* straight handpiece bur; *(center)* latch-type bur for latch-type contra-angle handpiece; *(bottom)* friction-grip bur for friction-grip contra-angle handpiece.[1,12]

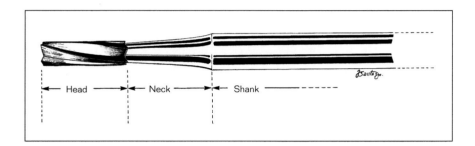

Fig 4-63 Parts of a rotary cutting instrument (bur).

Low-speed contra-angle handpieces, with round burs rotating very slowly, should routinely be used for removal of caries.

There are two types of contra-angle heads for the low-speed handpiece, a friction-grip head and a latch-type head. The shanks of the burs that fit into each of these types of contra-angle head are shown in Fig 4-62. The high-speed handpiece will receive only the friction-grip bur.

Burs

Hand-rotated dental instruments are known to have been used since the early 1700s. The foot engine came into use in dentistry in 1871 and the electric engine in 1872.[11] The most significant advance, which has made present day high-speed cutting possible, was the tungsten carbide bur, which became available in 1947.[12]

Burs have three major parts, the head, the neck, and the shank (Fig 4-63). For the different types of handpieces or handpiece heads, there are burs with different designs and dimensions (Fig 4-62).

The head of a bur is the portion of the bur that cuts. The cutting action is produced by blades on the head, and the blades are produced by cuts made into the head. The blades of a bur are usually obtuse to increase the strength and longevity of the bur. A cross section of a typical six-bladed bur is shown in Fig 4-64; the names of the faces and angles of the blades are also shown. The bur in Fig 4-64 has a negative rake angle, as do most burs used in dentistry.[12] The negative rake angle increases the life expectancy of the bur and provides for the most effective performance in low- and high-speed ranges.

A positive rake angle would produce a more acute angle on the edge of the blade (edge angle). Positive rake angles may be used to cut softer, weaker substances, such as soft dentinal caries. If a blade with a positive rake angle were used to cut a hard material, such as sound enamel or dentin, it would dig in, leaving an irregularly cut surface, and the cutting edges of the blades would chip and become dull rapidly.

The basic shapes of dental burs used in operative dentistry are shown in Fig 4-65. Many other shapes are available; most are modifications of these five. Number-

Fig 4-64 Typical bur head, viewed from end of the bur nearest the handpiece.[5,12]

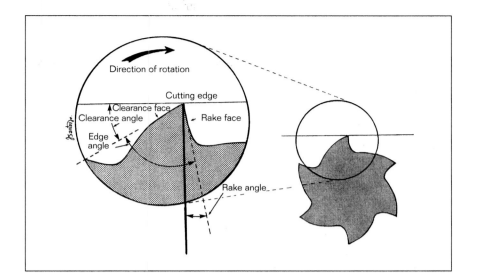

Fig 4-65 Basic bur head shapes for tooth preparation. Most burs used for tooth preparation are modifications of these burs. The primary modifications are lengthening of the bur heads and rounding ends or corners to allow preparations to be cut without sharp line angles.

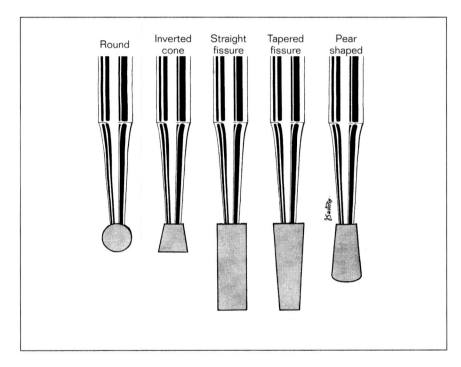

ing systems have been introduced to describe the shapes of dental burs. The original system, introduced by S.S. White Dental Manufacturing Company, had nine shapes based on the burs available at that time.[12] That system has been modified and expanded as new burs have been developed. The American National Standards Institute/American Dental Association (ANSI/ADA) specification[1] provides standard characteristics for dental burs; this specification lists both the US numbers and the International Standards Organization (ISO) numbers for dental burs.

Prior to the advent of high-speed handpieces, it was found that additional cuts across the blades of a dental bur increased cutting efficiency; these cuts were called crosscuts. Today, with high-speed handpieces, crosscut burs are not normally of any benefit.

Table 4-1 shows diagrams, US bur sizes, and the head diameters of many available regular carbide burs. International Standards Organization sizes for each type of bur can be calculated from the diameter: A bur with a diameter of 0.8 mm will have an ISO size of 008; a diameter of 1.0 mm will have an ISO size of 010. The ISO

Table 4-1 Shapes and diameters of regular carbide burs used for tooth preparation (US designations°)

Round

Bur size	¼	½	1	2	3	4	5
Diameter (mm)	.50	.60	.80	1.0	1.2	1.4	1.6

Bur size	6	7	8	9	11
Diameter (mm)	1.8	2.1	2.3	2.5	3.1

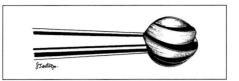

Inverted cone

Bur size	33½	34	35	36	37	39	40
Diameter (mm)	.60	.80	1.0	1.2	1.4	1.8	2.1

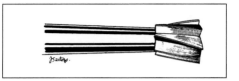

Straight fissure†

Bur size	55½	56	57	58	59	60
Diameter (mm)	.60	.80	1.0	1.2	1.4	1.6

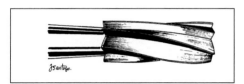

Straight fissure, rounded end (straight dome)†

Bur size	1156	1157	1158
Diameter (mm)	.80	1.0	1.2

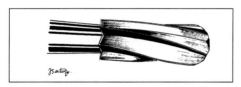

Straight fissure, crosscut†

Bur size	556	557	558	559	560
Diameter (mm)	.80	1.0	1.2	1.4	1.6

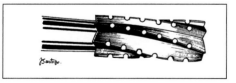

Straight fissure, rounded end, crosscut (straight dome crosscut)

Bur size	1556	1557	1558
Diameter (mm)	.80	1.0	1.2

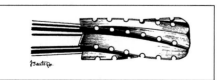

Table 4-1 (continued)

Tapered fissure†

Bur size	168	169	170	171
Diameter (mm)	.80	.90	1.0	1.2

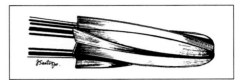

Tapered fissure, rounded end (tapered dome)†

Bur size	1169	1170	1171
Diameter (mm)	.90	1.0	1.2

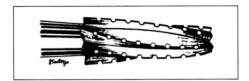

Tapered fissure, crosscut†

Bur size	699	700	701	702	703
Diameter (mm)	.90	1.0	1.2	1.6	2.1

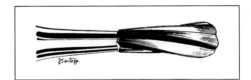

Pear†

Bur size	329	330	331	332
Diameter (mm)	.60	.80	1.0	1.2

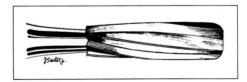

Long inverted cone, rounded corners (amalgam preparation)

Bur size	245	246
Diameter (mm)	.80	1.2

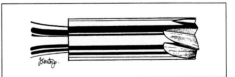

End-cutting

Bur size	956	957
Diameter (mm)	.80	1.0

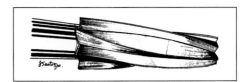

*Adapted from American National Standards Institute/American Dental Association specification 23—and catalogs of Midwest Dental Products and Brasseler.
†Some sizes available with a long head (L).

Table 4-2 Shapes and diameters of some of the available 12-bladed carbide finishing burs used for smooth cuts in tooth preparation and for finishing restorations (US designations)*

Egg

Bur size	7404	7406	7408
Diameter (mm)	1.4	1.8	2.3

Bullet

Bur size	7801	7802	7803
Diameter (mm)	.90	1.0	1.2

Needle

Bur size	7901	7902	7903
Diameter (mm)	.90	1.0	1.2

Round

Bur size	7002	7003	7004	7006
Diameter (mm)	1.0	1.2	1.4	1.8
Bur size	7008	7009	7010	
Diameter (mm)	2.3	2.7	3.1	

Flame

Bur size	7102	7104	7106	7108
Diameter (mm)	1.2	1.4	1.8	2.3

Cone

Bur size	7202	7204	7205	7206
Diameter (mm)	1.0	1.4	1.6	1.8

Table 4-2 (continued)

Long pear (inverted taper)

Bur size	7302	7303	7304
Diameter (mm)	1.0	1.2	1.4

Straight fissure

Bur size	7572	7583
Diameter (m)	1.0	1.2

Taper

Bur size	7702	7713
Diameter (mm)	1.0	1.2

*Adapted from catalogs of Midwest Dental Products and Brasseler.

sizes are combined with the shape of the bur, so an ISO *inverted cone 006* is an inverted cone bur with a 0.6-mm diameter; from Table 4-1, it can be determined that an ISO inverted cone 006 corresponds with a US No. 33½ bur.

Another type of bur that is very useful in operative dentistry is the 12-bladed trimming and finishing bur (Table 4-2). These burs are excellent for making very smooth cuts in tooth preparations, adjusting occlusion in enamel or of a restoration, and finishing restorations.

It is useful to know the diameters and lengths of the burs used in operative procedures so that they can be used as gauges of depth and distance. Bur head lengths may vary from manufacturer to manufacturer, so it is best to measure the individual burs being used and to use their dimensions as references for measuring preparation dimensions.

Diamonds. Diamonds are being used more and more in operative dentistry. They are especially useful for preparations for bonded restorations. At least one manufacturer (Brasseler) is making diamonds that mimic the shapes of many of the carbide burs. Diamonds cut tooth structure well and are acceptable substitutes for carbide burs, but many of the smaller sizes are not available as diamonds.

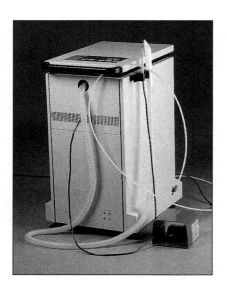

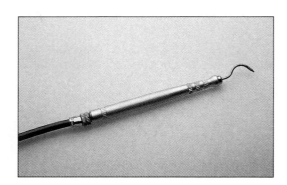

Figs 4-66a and 4-66b The KCP 2000 air-abrasion cavity preparation unit with handpiece.

Air-Abrasion Technology

In the 1940s, an instrument called the Airdent (S.S. White) was introduced to the profession as a means of cavity preparation.[3] Because all restorations placed at that time depended on cavity preparation shape for retention, and as the Airdent did not prepare undercuts in preparation, the technology soon lost favor. It was recently reintroduced, this time with a greater degree of acceptance, because bonded restorations have become routine.[8] Etched enamel and dentin, rather than the shape of the cavity preparation, give retention to many restorations. At least two air-abrasion units (KCP 2000, American Dental Technologies; MicroPrep, Sunrise Technologies) are being marketed for opening of fissures, for some cavity preparations, and to facilitate repair of existing restorations with bonding technology (Fig 4-66).

Magnifiers

The quality, and therefore the serviceability and the longevity, of restorative dentistry procedures is dependent on the ability of the operator to see what he or she is doing. One of the primary advantages of the rubber dam in operative dentistry is to improve visualization of the operating field (see chapter 5). Most current contra-angle handpieces have fiber-optic systems by which lights are placed in the contra-angle heads, again to improve visualization of the operating field.

Magnification devices are extremely helpful in restorative procedures, and some form of magnification is recommended for every dentist providing restorative dentistry services.[6] Available magnification devices run the gamut of effectiveness and expense. Among the finest magnifiers are the telescopes (Figs 4-67a and 4-67b), which are the most expensive. Less expensive loupes are available from several manufacturers (Figs 4-68a to 4-68c).

In choosing a magnification device, the operator is wise to select one that gives a focal distance in the range of 10 to 14 inches. The 2.0- to 2.5-diopter range is recommended.

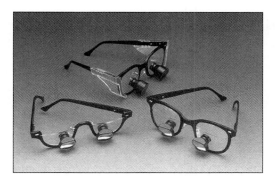

Fig 4-67a Binocular telescopes manufactured by Designs for Vision.

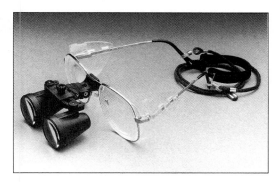

Fig 4-67b Binocular telescope manufactured by Orascoptic Research.

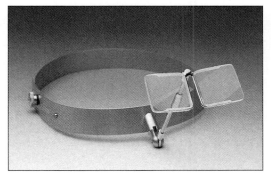

Fig 4-68a Binocular loupes manufactured by Almore International.

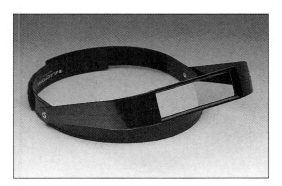

Fig 4-68b Binocular loupes manufactured by Lactona.

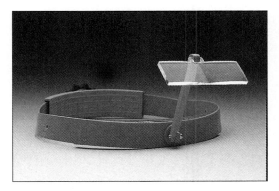

Fig 4-68c Binocular loupes manufactured by Edroy Products.

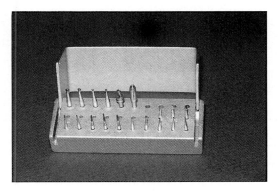

Fig 4-69 Bur block (No. A600, Brasseler), containing the burs listed in the instrument kit recommended in this chapter.

Operative Dentistry Instrument Kit

A compact assembly of hand instruments that will satisfy most operators' needs during any amalgam, resin composite, glass-ionomer cement, ceramic, or cast-gold restorative procedure is presented here. The kit has been used by dental students, residents, and practitioners, and, although another instrument may have to be added for a specific situation from time to time, the kit will more than suffice for most procedures. The kit was designed with the sequence of most operative procedures in mind. Therefore, placement of the instruments proceeds from the mirror and explorer for examination, to the plastic instrument used for dam placement as well as for placement of materials, to tooth preparation instruments, to restoration placement instruments. The kit uses a 22-slot tray with a small well (open, boxlike section) (Thompson Dental).

In slots (in this order, from left to right, with the open well to the rear):
    Mirror (No. 5 with handle)
    Explorer-periodontal probe (XP23/QOW)
    Cotton forceps (college, with serrations)
    Plastic instrument, No. 1-2
    Spoon, discoid, 11 1/2-7-14
    Hatchet, 10-7-14
    Hoe, 12-10-16
    Gingival margin trimmer, 10-80-7-14
    Gingival margin trimmer, 10-95-7-14
    Wedelstaedt chisel, 10-15-3
    TD applicator/No. 24 Spatula (Thompson Dental)
    Condenser, SA1 (Thompson Dental)
    Condenser, SA2 (Thompson Dental)
    Condenser, SA3 (Thompson Dental)
    Burnisher, beavertail-ovoid, 2/30
    Burnisher, PKT3
    Carver, cleoid-discoid, UWD5
    Carver, Walls No. 3
    Carver, Hollenback No. 1/2
    Carver, interproximal (IPC)
    Carver, No. 14L
    Articulating paper forceps

In well of tray:
    Scalpel handle, No. 3, flat
    Carrier, amalgam, medium/large
    Sharpening stone, flat, ceramic or Arkansas
    Tofflemire retainer, straight
    Tofflemire retainer, contra-angle
    Amalgam well, stainless steel, small (Thompson Dental)

Clipped to lid of tray:
    Hemostat, mosquito, 5-inch curved
    Scissors, Quimby

Sterilized separately and available for each operative procedure:
    Anesthetic syringe
    Rubber dam kit (forceps, punch, frame, clamps, W2A, W8A x 2, 27, 212SA)
    Brasseler bur block (No. A600) with burs arranged in the following order (Fig 4-69):
        Friction-grip burs, No. 1/4, 1/2, 1, 2, 33 1/2, 56, 169L, 170, 329, 330, 7404, 7803, 7901
        Latch Burs, Nos. 2, 4, 6, 8
        Mandrel for pop-on disks

Sterilized separately and available for occasional use:
    Chisel, monangle, 10-4-8
    Condenser, SA4
    Gingival margin trimmer, 13-80-7-14
    Gingival margin trimmer, 13-95-7-14
    Hemostat, mosquito, 5-inch straight
    Mirror, No. 2 (on handle)
    Proximal contact disks (Thierman Products)
    Rubber dam clamps, 00, W1A, 14A
    Scaler, McCalls, SM13s-14s
    Spatula, No. 24A (or 324)
    Spoon, discoid, 15-8-14
    Spoon, discoid, 25-9-15
    Triple angle hoe, 8-3-23
    Wedelstaedt chisel, 15-15-3

References

1. American National Standards Institute/American Dental Association Specification No. 23 (Revised) for Dental Excavating Burs. Chicago: American Dental Association, 1982.

2. Black GV. A Work on Operative Dentistry. Chicago: Medico-Dental Publishing, 1908.

3. Black RB. Technique for nonmechanical preparation of cavities and prophylaxis. J Am Dent Assoc 1945;32:955-965.

4. Bouschor CR, Matthews JL. A four-year clinical study of teeth restored after preparation with an air turbine handpiece with an air coolant. J Prosthet Dent 1966;16:306-309.

5. Charbeneau GT. Principles and Practice of Operative Dentistry, ed 3. Philadelphia: Lea & Febiger, 1988.

6. Christensen GJ. Magnification. Clin Res Assoc Newsletter 1990: 14(10):1.

7. Glossary of Operative Dentistry Terms, ed 1. Washington DC: Academy of Operative Dentistry, 1983.

8. Goldstein RE, Parkins FM. Air-abrasive technology: Its new role in restorative dentistry. J Am Dent Assoc 1994;125:551-557.

9. Lauer H, Kraft E, Rothlauf W, Zwingers T. Effects of the temperature of cooling water during high-speed and ultrahigh-speed tooth preparation. J Prosthet Dent 1990;63:407-414.

10. Metals Handbook, ed 10, vol 1. Materials Park, OH: American Society of Metals International, 1990:841-842, 908-909.

11. Ring ME. Dentistry, an Illustrated History. New York: Abrams, 1985:251.

12. Sturdevant CM, Roberson TM, Heymann HO, Sturdevant JR. The Art and Science of Operative Dentistry, ed 3. St Louis: Mosby, 1995.

13. Webster's Ninth New Collegiate Dictionary. Springfield, MA: Merriam-Webster, 1988.

14. Young JM. Dental air-powered handpieces: Selection, use, and sterilization. Compend Contin Educ Dent 1993;14:358-366.

Field Isolation

James B. Summitt

There are many ways to isolate an area of the mouth or a tooth so that a restorative service can be performed without interference from soft tissue, the tongue, saliva, or other fluids. Various tongue- and cheek- retracting devices and suction methods may be employed; some of these will be discussed later in this chapter. By far the most complete method of obtaining field isolation is the rubber dam, and this chapter will be devoted primarily to rubber dam techniques.

Rubber Dam

Sanford C. Barnum is credited with introducing the rubber dam to the profession in 1864.[6] For many years, the rubber dam has been recognized as an effective method of gaining field isolation, improving visualization, protecting the patient, and improving the quality of operative dentistry services. It has been demonstrated that most patients prefer the use of the rubber dam for restorative procedures.[10,17] In recent years, the dam has been acknowledged as an important barrier for prevention of microbial transmission from patients to members of the dental care team. In addition, it is medicolegally prudent to use a dam for procedures in which small objects, such as pin drivers or endodontic files, could be aspirated by the patient.

Christensen[7] has emphatically stated that the use of the rubber dam not only boosts quality of restorations but also increases quantity of restorative services because patients are unable to talk or expectorate when the dam is in place. He has further stated that the operating field can only be maintained free of saliva and other contaminants with the dam in place, and the field is more accessible, airborne debris is reduced, and patients feel more comfortable.

There is convincing evidence of the importance of rubber dam use during resin bonding procedures. Barghi et al[1] used cotton roll isolation or rubber dam isolation in bonding resin composite buttons to facial enamel surfaces of teeth that were to be extracted. They found shear bond strengths to be significantly greater when rubber dam isolation was used. The same group, using similar techniques, showed that rubber dam isolation significantly reduced microleakage of resin composite buttons bonded to etched enamel,[11] and that salivary contamination may affect the bond strength provided by some dentin bonding systems.[12]

Most dentists are taught the use of the rubber dam in dental school, and many suffer tremendous frustrations during rubber dam applications. For the dam to be used and to actually save chair time, the practitioner must be able to apply it quickly and easily. This chapter is designed to describe methods that facilitate use of the rubber dam.

Instruments and Materials

Rubber Dam Material

Rubber dam materials are currently available in an array of colors, ranging from green to lavender to gray to ivory. It is important in operative dentistry to use a dam color that contrasts with the color of teeth; ivory-colored dam is therefore not recommended for operative dentistry procedures. The original gray dam is still the most used, but the bright colors are gaining popularity. Some operators use the gray dam because they believe that it is better for matching shades in tooth-colored restorations. Because shades of restorative materials are selected prior to rubber dam placement, and tooth color changes with the enamel desiccation that accompanies rubber

Table 5-1 Available rubber dam thicknesses (gauges)*

Gauge	Thickness (range)*
Thin	0.006 (0.005–0.007) inch
Medium	0.008 (0.007–0.009) inch
Heavy	0.010 (0.009–0.015) inch
Extra heavy	0.012 (0.0115–0.0135) inch
Special heavy	0.014 (0.0135–0.0155) inch

*Thickness ranges listed by Hygenic.

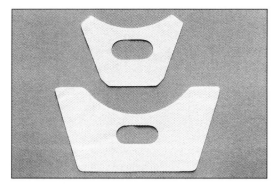

Fig 5-1 Rubber dam napkins (Hygenic) for longer procedures. Napkins provide padding between the rubber dam and the face and lips, making the dam more comfortable for the patient. The small napkin is for use with rubber dam frames. The larger napkin is for use with strap- or harness-type rubber dam holders.

dam use, the restorative shade is probably not affected by the use of a brightly colored rubber dam.

Rubber dam material is available in rolls, either 5.0 or 6.0 inches wide, from which squares may be cut. It is also available in sheets that are 5.0 inches square, usually used for children, and 6.0 inches square.

Rubber dam material is available in several thicknesses, or gauges (Table 5-1). The heavy and extra heavy gauges are recommended for isolation in operative dentistry. If the rubber of the heavier gauges is passed through the interproximal tooth contacts in a single thickness, and not bunched in the contacts, the heavy dams are no more difficult to apply than are the thinner materials, and heavier dams are less likely to tear. The heavier materials provide a better seal to teeth and retract tissues more effectively than the thinner materials.

Rubber dam material has a shelf life of more than a year, but aging is accelerated by heat. Extra boxes of dam material can be stored in a refrigerator to extend the shelf life. Dam material that has exceeded its shelf life becomes brittle and tears easily; unfortunately, this is usually noticed while the dam is being applied. A simple test for the resistance of rubber dam material to tearing is to attempt to tear a sheet grasped with thumbs and index fingers; a strong dam will be very difficult to tear. Brittle dam material should be discarded. If the material was recently purchased, it should be returned to the supplier for replacement.

Napkin

The rubber dam napkin is a piece of strong, absorbent cloth or paper placed between the rubber dam and the patient's face. The napkin provides greater comfort for the patient, especially during unusually long procedures. Napkins are available in two shapes (Fig 5-1). The smaller napkin is usually used with rubber dam frames; the larger provides padding for the side of the face when retracting straps are used.

Punch

At least two types of rubber dam punches are available (Figs 5-2a and 5-2b). The Ainsworth-type punch, which is made by several manufacturers, is excellent if it is well made. The Ivory punch (Heraeus Kulzer) is also excellent and has a self-centering coned piston, or punch point, that helps to prevent partially punched holes (Fig 5-3). Punches should have hardened steel cutting tables (or anvils) that have a range of hole sizes so that the dam will seal against teeth with various cervical diameters (Fig 5-4).

Occasionally, the rim of a hole may be damaged because the rotating cutting table wasn't snapped completely into position before an attempt was made to punch a dam. Holes must be cleanly cut; incompletely punched holes (Fig 5-3) will allow tearing of the dam during application or will affect the ability of the dam to seal.

A damaged hole rim in the cutting table will cause incomplete cutting. The damaged or dull rim can sometimes be sharpened with a mounted flat, coarse sandpaper disk or separating disk used in a low-speed handpiece or a finishing bur used in a high-speed handpiece. The level of the rim of the hole is evenly lowered to an area of the wall of the hole that is beyond the damage. The metal around that hole may then be polished with finer disks. A damaged cutting wheel should usually be replaced; a replacement wheel can be ordered from the manufacturer.

Hole-Positioning Guides

Although many operators punch the holes without a positioning aid, most find it helpful to have some form of guide to determine where the holes should be punched.

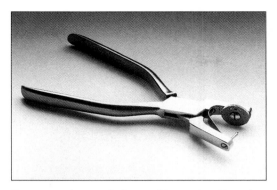

Fig 5-2a Ainsworth-design (Hygenic) rubber dam punch.

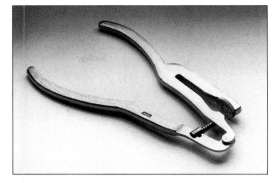

Fig 5-2b Ivory-design rubber dam punch.

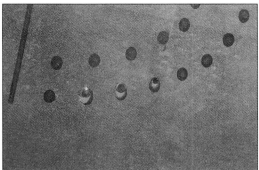
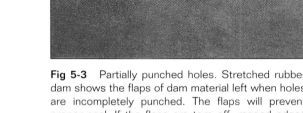

Fig 5-3 Partially punched holes. Stretched rubber dam shows the flaps of dam material left when holes are incompletely punched. The flaps will prevent proper seal. If the flaps are torn off, ragged edges can lead to tearing of the dam during application.

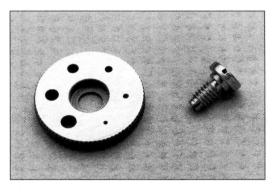

Fig 5-4 The cutting table, or anvil, of a rubber dam punch should have a range of sizes. Pictured is the cutting table from an Ivory punch.

There are several ways to mark a rubber dam so that holes can be located optimally.

Teeth as a guide. The teeth themselves can be used in marking the dam. To use the teeth, the dam is held in the desired position in the mouth over the teeth to be included in the isolation. The cusp tips of posterior teeth and incisal edges of anterior teeth can be visualized through the dam, and the centers of the teeth are marked on the dam with a pen. An advantage of this method is precise positioning of the marks even when teeth are malaligned. Its disadvantages include the time-consuming nature of the procedure and the inability to punch a dam before the patient is seated.

Template. Templates are available to guide the marking of the dam (Fig 5-5). These templates are approximately the same size and shape as the unstretched rubber dam itself. Holes in each template correspond to tooth positions. The template is laid over the dam, and a pen is

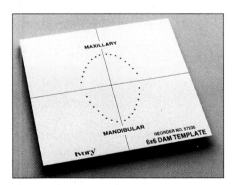

Fig 5-5 Ivory template for marking the dam. Marks corresponding to the teeth to be isolated are made on a 6.0-inch rubber dam through the holes with a felt-tipped or ballpoint pen.

used to mark through selected holes onto the dam. With the template, the dam can be marked and punched before the patient is seated.

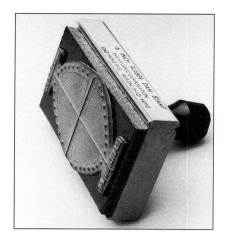 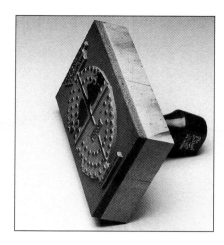

Fig 5-6a Rubber dam stamp for the adult dentition (Hygenic).

Fig 5-6b Stamp made by a rubber stamp–manufacturing company.

Rubber dam stamp. Rubber stamps provide a very convenient and efficient way of marking the dam for punching (Figs 5-6a and 5-6b). There are commercially available stamps, or stamps can be made by any rubber stamp manufacturer from a pattern such as the one shown in Fig 5-7 or any custom design. Dams should be prestamped by an assistant so that the marks for the maxillary central incisors are positioned approximately 0.9 inch from the top of the dam. Exceptions to normal tooth position are easily accommodated.

Rubber Dam Holders

Strap holders. Strap holders such as the Woodbury holder or retractor (Fig 5-8) provide the most cheek and lip retraction, access, and stability, but may cause the most discomfort to the patient. A rubber dam napkin is a necessity for patient comfort when a strap holder is used. The Woodbury retractor grasps the dam material with spring-loaded clips. When posterior teeth are isolated with a Woodbury-type holder, a tuck or fold in the dam may be needed (Fig 5-9).

Frame holders. Frame holders are exemplified by the Young frame (Young Dental) and the Nygaard-Ostby frame (Figs 5-10a to 5-10d). A U-shaped Young frame is made by several manufacturers in both metal and plastic. The Young-type frames are available in both adult and child sizes. A plastic frame is advantageous when radiographs will be a part of the procedure, because it is radiolucent. The plastic frames do not, however, stand up as well as metal frames to heat sterilization, and they have a shorter life span. Metal frames are less bulky and last for years.[16] They are available with balls on the ends to protect the patient in the event that the frame is inadvertently pushed toward the eyes.

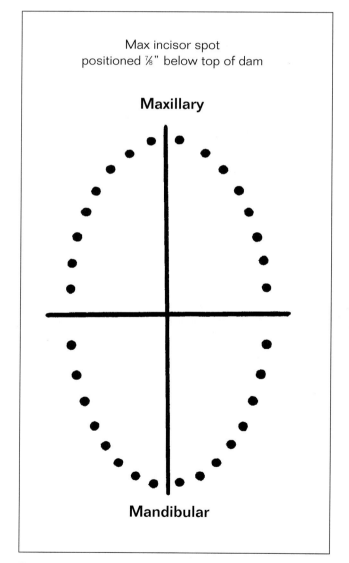

Fig 5-7 Pattern for a rubber dam stamp. This may be duplicated and taken to a rubber stamp manufacturer.

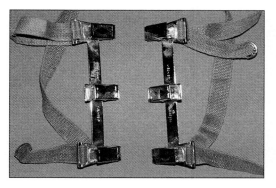

Fig 5-8 Strap- or harness-type rubber dam holders provide excellent lip and cheek retraction. Pictured is a Woodbury retractor.

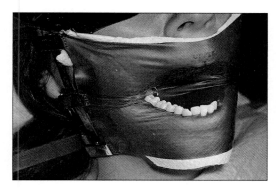

Fig 5-9 A fold or tuck is made in the rubber dam to provide an uncluttered operating field.

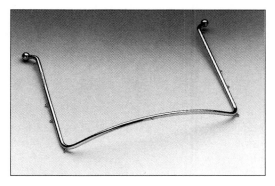

Fig 5-10a Metal Young frame with eye protectors.

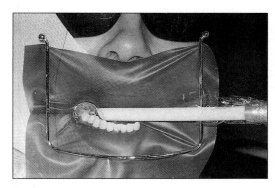

Fig 5-10b Young frame inserted into the external surface of the dam.

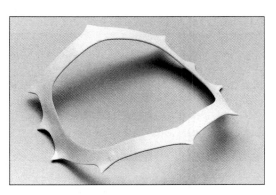

Fig 5-10c Plastic Nygaard-Ostby frame.

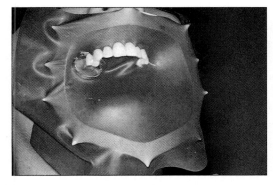

Fig 5-10d Nygaard-Ostby frame inserted into the internal surface of the dam.

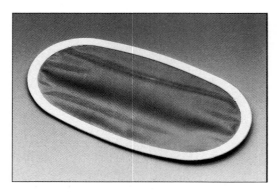

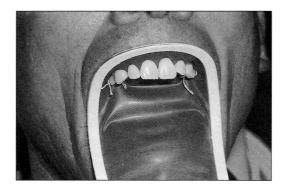

Fig 5-11a and 5-11b   Quickdam has a built-in frame or border that will fit inside or outside the mouth.

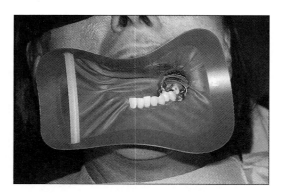

Fig 5-11c   In the HandiDam the frame is an integral part of the dam.

The Young frame is usually positioned on the outside surface of the dam so that it is not in contact with the patient's face. The Nygaard-Ostby frame is normally positioned on the tissue surface or inside surface of the dam and touches the patient's face (or the rubber dam napkin). All frames have points or pegs over which the dam material is stretched to provide a clear operating field and to hold the frame in position.

Preattached frames. One commercially available rubber dam (Quickdam, Ivoclar-Vivadent) comes with an attached flexible plastic frame or rim that is said to support the dam intraorally and eliminate the need for a frame (Figs 5-11a and 5-11b). This dam is said to provide acceptable comfort for the patient. The device is effective for saliva control in the anterior part of the mouth but less effective in the posterior area.[4] Another, larger dam (HandiDam, Aseptico), also has a built-in frame and a rod for insertion to keep the dam open (Fig 5-11c).

Clamp Forceps

Ivory-type clamp forceps are available from several manufacturers and with differently angled beaks (Fig 5-12a). Ivory forceps (Ivory, Heraeus Kulzer) have stabilizers that prevent the clamp from rotating on the beaks (Fig 5-12b). This is usually advantageous, but it limits the use of these forceps to teeth that are within a range of normal angulation.

Stokes-type clamp forceps (Fig 5-12c), which have notches near the tips of their beaks in which to locate the holes of a rubber dam clamp (Fig 5-12d), allow a range of rotation of the clamp so that it may be positioned on teeth that are mesially or distally angled.

Either of these types of clamp forceps will serve the practitioner well, and selection should be based on personal preference. The Ivory-type forceps are probably the most popular because of cost.

Clamps

Rubber dam clamps are the usual means of retaining the rubber dam. The three basic types of clamps and their parts are shown in Figs 5-13a to 5-13c. When a posterior segment is isolated, the clamp is usually placed on the distal-most exposed tooth (Fig 5-14). The clamp may also be placed on an unexposed tooth (one for which a hole has not been punched) (Fig 5-15).

There are clamps with jaw sizes to fit every tooth in the mouth. Some clamps simply have a number designation; others have a W in front of the number. The W indicates that the clamp is wingless (Fig 5-13b); those clamps that do not bear a W have wings (Fig 5-13a) so that the dam may be attached to the wings before the clamp is placed on the tooth (Fig 5-16).

Although in recent years manufacturers have reduced the number of clamps they produce, there are still many designs of clamps available. For the practice of operative dentistry, the number of clamps should be limited to a few that will satisfy most needs; these may be kept in the

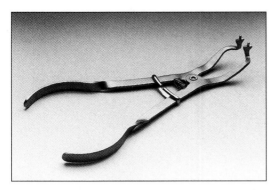

Fig 5-12a Ivory forceps.

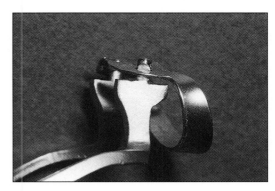

Fig 5-12b Stabilizers near the tips of the Ivory-type forceps limit rotation of the clamp when it is held by the forceps.

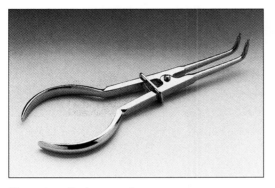

Fig 5-12c Stokes-type forceps.

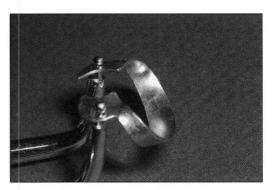

Fig 5-12d The tip design of the Stokes forceps provides more freedom for rotation of the clamp while it is held by the forceps.

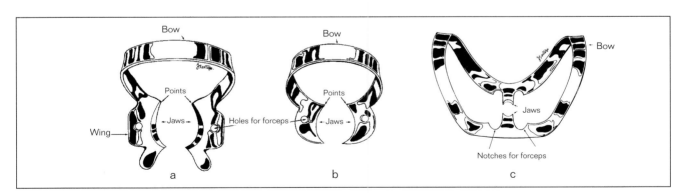

Figs 5-13a to 5-13c   (a) Winged rubber dam clamp; (b) Wingless rubber dam clamp; (c) Butterfly rubber dam clamp.

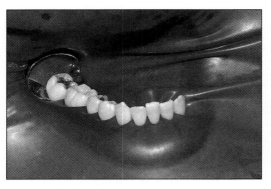

Fig 5-14 Isolated mandibular right quadrant. The clamp is positioned on the distal-most exposed tooth.

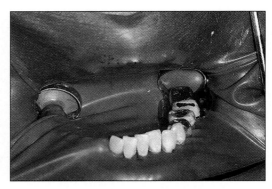

Fig 5-15 Isolated mandibular left quadrant with a second clamp placed on an unexposed molar on the right side of the mouth to give additional access to the lingual surfaces of the teeth in the left quadrant. The dam has been loosely stretched over the unexposed tooth to prevent the clamp from initiating a tear. The mirror and other instruments will now be unimpeded when the defective lingual margin of the crown on the first molar is treated.

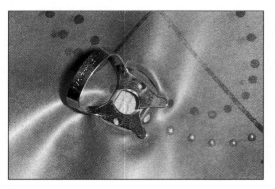

Fig 5-16 Winged clamp attached to the rubber dam. The edges of the hole are stretched over the wings of the clamp.

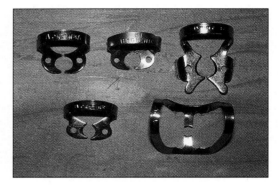

Fig 5-17 Clamps recommended for routine use: (top row [molar clamps] left to right) No. W8A, B1, 27; (bottom row) No. W2A and No. 212SA retractor.

instrument kit and sterilized along with the other operative dentistry instruments. Clamps that will serve in most situations and are recommended for inclusion in operative dentistry instrument kits are listed in Table 5-2 and shown in Fig 5-17.

Supplemental clamps, to be available on the rare occasions that the usual clamps will not suffice, should be packaged and sterilized separately. Recommended supplemental clamps are listed in Table 5-3 and shown in Fig 5-19.

Number W8A clamp. Although Ivory (Ivory, Heraeus Kulzer) has modified the design of the No. W8A clamp so that the jaw points do not extend so severely in a gingival direction, some No. W8A clamps still have points

Table 5-2 Clamps recommended for inclusion in operative dentistry instrument kits

Wingless camps	Winged clamps*	Tooth fit	Comment
W8A† or B1†	8A	Molar	
W27	27†	Molar	Bow extended distally
W2A†	2A	Premolar	
212SA†		Premolar, canine, and incisor	For Class 5 isolation

*Same clamps as in first column but with wings.
†Clamps recommended to be available for routine use.
All clamps except B1 are from Ivory catalog (Heraeus Kulzer).
B1 is from Hygenic.

Figs 5-18a to 5-18c Modification recommended for No. W8A clamps, to thin the jaws and reduce the extension of the jaw points toward gingival tissue.

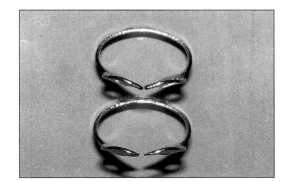

Fig 5-18a *(top)* Clamp as received from the manufacturer; *(bottom)* clamp that has been modified.

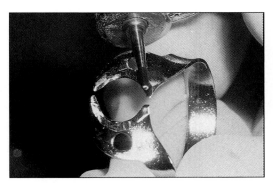

Fig 5-18b The points are trimmed from the tissue side so that gingival extension is reduced and jaws are thinned. The bur being used in the high-speed handpiece is a No. 7803 bullet-shaped finishing bur.

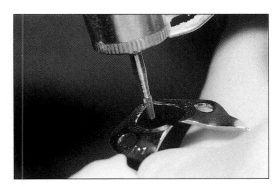

Fig 5-18c Points that have been sharpened during modification must be dulled. If the points are left sharp, they can damage the surface of the tooth.

Table 5-3 Supplemental clamps recommended for availability on request

Wingless camps	Winged clamps°	Tooth fit	Comment
W0	00†	Small incisor	
W1A†	1A	Premolar	Gingivally angled jaws
W14A†	14A†	Molar	For partially erupted molar

°Same clamps as in first column but with wings.
†Clamps recommended to be available to supplement clamps listed in Table 5-2.
All clamps are from Ivory catalog (Heraeus Kulzer).

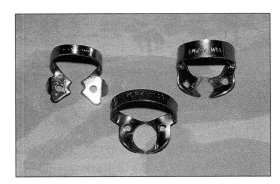

Fig 5-19 Recommended supplemental clamps: *(left to right)* Number 00 (for mandibular incisors and other small teeth), No. W14A (for partially erupted molars), and No. W1A (for premolars with subgingival margins).

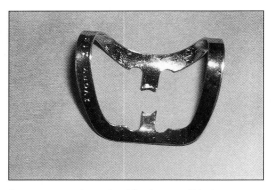
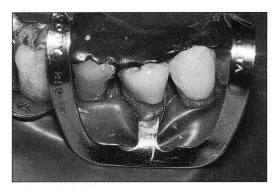

Figs 5-20a and 5-20b   Number 212SA clamp (or retractor) for retracting the gingival tissue and rubber dam.

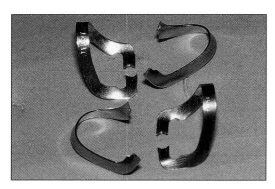
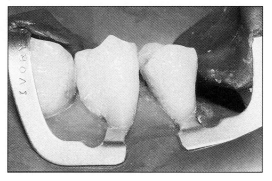

Figs 5-20c and 5-20d   Two No. 212SA retractors may be modified to give two clamps for tissue and dam retraction for side-by-side restorations. The No. 212SA and the modified No. 212SA retractors must be stabilized with modeling compound, or the jaws will damage tooth surfaces.

that extend further gingivally than is desirable. The jaws of a No. W8A clamp, for most applications, should be approximately horizontal (Fig 5-18) prior to expansion of the clamp for placement on a tooth. As the jaws are spread, the angle of the jaws will change to a gingival orientation; this is usually desirable, but before the clamp is expanded, the jaws should have little or no gingival angulation.

For No. W8A clamps in which the jaws have a significant gingival angulation, a modification procedure is recommended (Figs 5-18a to 5-18c). This modification may be made with a stone used in a low-speed handpiece or a finishing bur used in a high-speed handpiece. After the modification is made, the points, which have been sharpened by the modification procedure, must be blunted to prevent damage to tooth surfaces.

Butterfly clamps. Most of the clamps listed in Tables 5-2 and 5-3 may act as rubber dam retainers (placed on the distal tooth or teeth to hold the dam on the quadrant or arch) or as rubber dam and gingival tissue retractors (to retract the dam and tissues away from a preparation margin in the cervical area of a tooth). One clamp, however, the *butterfly clamp,* No. 212SA (Fig 5-20a), is designed to serve as a retractor only. Because of its double bow and the closeness of the points of each jaw, this clamp must be stabilized on the tooth (Fig 5-20b), or it may "seesaw" during the procedure and damage the root. Dental impression compound (such as red or green compound, Kerr/Sybron) should be used under the bows of the clamp on the occlusal (or incisal) and lingual aspects of the teeth to provide stabilization.

The double bow of the No. 212SA clamp precludes placement of two clamps on adjacent teeth. When two Class 5 restorations are to be accomplished on adjacent teeth, two No. 212SA clamps may be modified (Fig 5-20c); one of the bows of each clamp is cut off so that the remaining bow of one clamp extends to the right and the bow of the other extends to the left. If these clamps are stabilized with modeling compound, adjacent Class 5 restorations may be accomplished simultaneously (Fig 5-20d). A No. 212SA clamp or a modified No. 212SA clamp may be used on one root of a molar as well as on single-rooted teeth.

Tooth contact. An important consideration when a clamp is selected is that only its jaw points contact the tooth; this gives four-point contact (Fig 5-21). No clamp jaw can ever be contoured to fit a tooth precisely, nor is there any reason for a clamp to fit precisely because the dam, not the clamp, creates the seal. Molar clamps should have accentuated arches between the jaw points to assure that the points are in contact with the tooth, even in teeth with very convex cervical areas. The distance between the points of a jaw, along with the strength of the bow of the clamp, determines the stability of the clamp. If there is contact between the tooth and any other part of the clamp's jaw, the contact points are brought closer together, thus reducing the stability of the clamp and allowing it to rotate on the tooth and, occasionally, to be dislodged from the tooth. Four-point contact is, therefore, very desirable.

The strength or temper of the bow of the clamp should also be maintained. Clamps should be expanded with the clamp forceps no more than is necessary for the clamp to be passed over the facial and lingual heights of contour of the tooth. If a clamp has been overexpanded, it will grasp the tooth with less strength and is more likely to be dislodged. Occasionally, the jaws of clamps that have been overexpanded may be squeezed together so that enough of the strength returns, but it is usually best to discard a clamp that has been overexpanded.

Floss ligatures. Many clinicians and dental schools recommend that dental floss be attached to every clamp used in the mouth to allow retrieval if the clamp is dislodged or breaks. Certainly, it is wise to attach floss to the clamp that is positioned in the mouth prior to application of the dam. After dam placement is completed, however, the floss causes leakage if it extends under the dam or is in the way if left to dangle in the operating field. A solution is to attach the floss to the clamp during application of the dam (see Fig 5-34a) and to cut and detach the floss from the clamp after the dam is in place. If the clamp dislodges or breaks after the dam is in place, it will be either catapulted from the mouth by the tension of the dam or will be trapped by the dam so that it cannot be swallowed or aspirated.

When a winged clamp is attached to the dam during placement of the clamp onto a tooth, the attachment of a floss ligature to the clamp is redundant. Floss also need not be attached to a second clamp placed for retraction after the dam is in place.

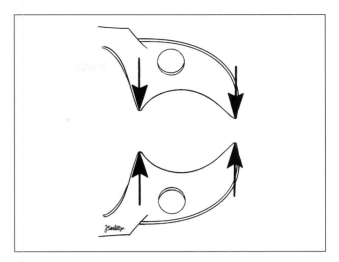

Fig 5-21 Rubber dam clamps should contact the tooth at the mesial and distal extent of the jaws. This four-point contact provides stability, or resistance to rotation or dislodgment, for the clamp.

Other Retainers

Other methods are sometimes used for rubber dam retention:

1. Dental floss or tape is placed doubly through a contact and then cut to a short length so that it does not impede access (Fig 5-22a).
2. A short strip of rubber dam material is cut from the edge of the rubber dam, stretched and carried through the contact, and then allowed to relax to retain the dam (Fig 5-22b).
3. Floss is tied to a sterilized rubber plunger from an anesthetic cartridge or similar item and then tied around the most distal isolated tooth (Fig 5-22c).
4. Elastic cord, eg, Wedjets (Hygenic), is placed interproximally to retain the dam (Figs 5-22d and 5-22e).

Modeling Compound

Modeling compound may be used as an adjunct to application of any clamp as a retainer or retractor. It is especially useful and necessary for anchoring and stabilizing the No. 212SA retainer (Figs 5-20b and 5-20d).

For stabilizing a clamp, use of modeling compound in the stick form, either red or green (Kerr/Sybron), is recommended. The clamp is positioned appropriately on the tooth and held in position with a finger until stabilization is completed. A compound stick is held over a low alcohol flame and rotated and moved back and forth so that the length to be softened is heated evenly (Fig 5-

Figs 5-22a to 5-22e Alternative methods for dam retention.

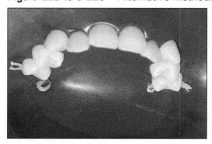

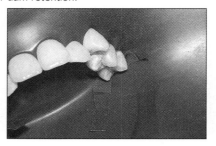

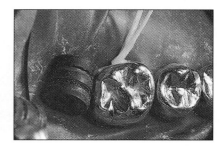

Fig 5-22a Dental tape placed doubly through the contact distal to the distal-most exposed tooth.

Fig 5-22b Short strip of rubber dam used to retain the dam.

Fig 5-22c Anesthetic cartridge plunger tied around the distal tooth with floss.

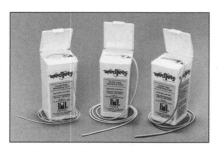

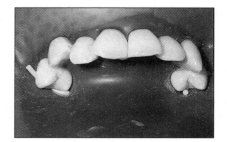

Figs 5-22d and 5-22e Elastic cord used as a rubber dam retainer.

23a). After the surface is softened, the stick is withdrawn from the flame to allow the heat to diffuse to the center of the stick. When the length is warmed to the center, there will no longer be a core of unsoftened compound to support the shape, and the softened length will sag or droop (Fig 5-23b). If the stick has been overheated, so that it elongates in addition to drooping, it should be tempered in a container of water. Before the compound is taken to the mouth, the surface should be briefly reheated to enhance adhesion of the compound to the retracting clamp and teeth.

The stick should be applied to the retainer and teeth in a location as much away from the area to be restored as possible. The stick is then twisted and pulled away, leaving softened compound in place. The compound should be shaped and molded with damp, gloved fingers into embrasures and made to contact a large area of the clamp and the lingual surfaces of the teeth. It should

then be cooled with the air syringe. Stabilization of the retracting clamp is now completed (Fig 5-23c); the finger holding the clamp may now be released, and the clamp is tested for stability.

Compound should be kept away from the planned area of operation so that it will not inhibit access; in that regard, for a facial restoration, compound should be confined to the occlusal (or incisal) and lingual surfaces. Full advantage should be taken of the lingual surfaces for maximum dependability of attachment of the compound to the teeth. When the lingual surfaces are covered by the compound, the lingual notches for the clamp forceps will be covered. To remove the clamp with forceps, the operator would have to chip away the compound to expose a lingual notch. In a simpler method, an instrument is used to pull the facial portion of the clamp away from the facial surface and then occlusally (incisally) (Figs 5-23d to 5-23i).

Figs 5-23a to 5-23i   Use of modeling compound to stabilize a No. 212SA retractor.

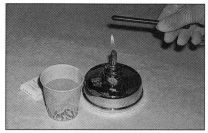

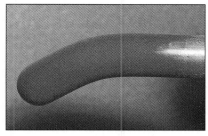

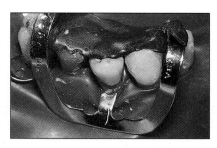

Fig 5-23a The compound stick is warmed in an alcohol flame.

Fig 5-23b After warming, the stick is removed from the flame and held until the heat has diffused to the center of the stick so that the warmed end of the stick begins to droop.

Fig 5-23c Use of compound to stabilize a No. 212SA retractor is completed.

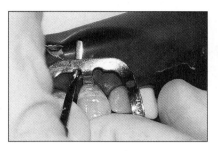

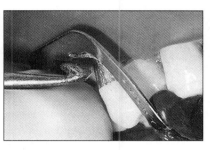

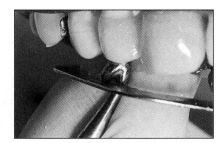

Fig 5-23d Removal of the clamp with forceps may be hampered by the compound on the lingual aspect. If so, a facial notch of the clamp may be engaged with an instrument such as a plastic instrument.

Figs 5-23e and 5-23f A No. 0 crochet hook (with handle made out of laboratory acrylic) or a No. 34 surgical elevator modified to mimic a No. 0 crochet hook may also be used to engage a notch of the clamp.

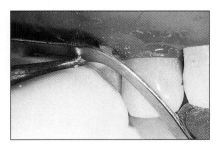

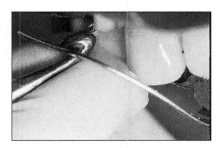

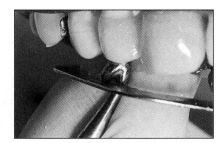

Figs 5-23g to 5-23i The facial jaw of the clamp is then pulled facially away from the tooth surface and rotated occlusally or incisally to quickly remove the clamp and the stabilizing compound.

Figs 5-24a to 5-24c Inverting instruments. Note the tip of the air syringe in each instance; a high-volume stream of air is used to dry the tooth and dam surfaces to facilitate inversion.

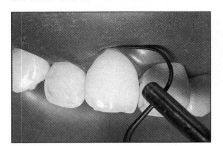

Fig 5-24a Number 23 explorer.

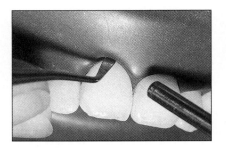

Fig 5-24b Number 1-2 plastic instrument

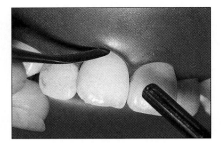

Fig 5-24c Beavertail burnisher.

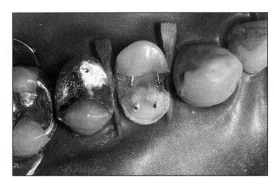

Fig 5-25 Wooden wedges are used to protect the dam from being cut during a procedure that involves the use of burs or cutting instruments near the dam.

Inverting Instrument

Almost any instrument may be used for inverting the dam. Commonly used instruments include explorers such as the No. 23 (Fig 5-24a), plastic filling instruments such as the No. 1-2 (Fig 5-24b), or a beavertail burnisher (Fig 5-24c). Dental tape or floss used interproximally is also useful for dam inversion.

Wedge

The wooden wedge, which is used to stabilize a matrix and hold it against the gingival margin of a cavity preparation involving a proximal tooth surface, is also useful for protecting the dam (Fig 5-25) when rotary cutting instruments are used in interproximal areas. Placement of water-soluble rubber dam lubricant on the wedge enhances the ease of wedge placement.

Scissors

Scissors are often useful in preparing the dam for insertion and are a necessity for cutting the dam for removal. Blunt-ended scissors are preferred by many operators, but other scissors, such as sharp crown and collar scissors

and Quimby scissors (see Fig 5-39b), will also serve well. Scissors used for cutting rubber dam must be sharp, or they will serve as a source of frustration to the operator.

Dental Tape and Floss

Waxed tape or floss, as opposed to unwaxed floss, is recommended for flossing the dam through interproximal contacts. Waxed tape, or ribbon floss (see Fig 5-34f), will carry more of a septum through a contact in a single pass than will the narrower floss, but the tape must be maintained flat and not bunched up, or it will be difficult to pass through the contact.

Proximal Contact Disk

A proximal contact disk (Thierman Products) is used to plane rough enamel, amalgam, or resin composite contacts so that the floss will go through without shredding and so that the dam can be flossed through without tearing (Figs 5-26a to 5-26c). The plane metal disk, without abrasive, is recommended. This instrument should not be used in contacts that involve a gold casting, because it can cut into the gold and produce additional obstruction to passage of the floss through the contact.

The disk is placed into the occlusal embrasure and rocked facially and lingually as it is pushed firmly, but with control, gingivally. If it cannot be worked through the contact, the teeth should be separated slightly with a plastic instrument placed snugly into the gingival embrasure and torqued slightly while the disk is being pushed into the contact from the occlusal embrasure. Several passes of the disk through the contact will usually plane it smooth.

Lubricant

Rubber dam lubricant makes a significant difference in the ease with which the dam is applied. A water-soluble lubricant is preferred. A product that has proven espe-

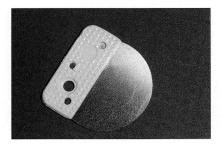
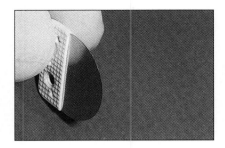

Figs 5-26a and 5-26b Proximal contact disk or plane with handle.

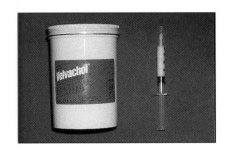

Fig 5-26c The proximal contact disk is used to plane rough contact.

Fig 5-27 A water-soluble rubber dam lubricant, such as Velvachol, can be loaded into a syringe, such as a 3.0-mL disposable syringe. From the syringe, the lubricant can be dispensed onto the tissue surface (underside) of the rubber dam or onto a glove for coating of the dam adjacent to the holes.

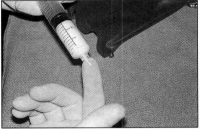

Fig 5-28a Water-soluble lubricant can be carried to the dam with a finger.

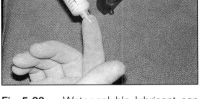

Fig 5-28b The dam lubricant is layered on the tissue surface of the dam in the area of the holes.

cially suitable for lubricating the rubber dam is Velvachol water-miscible vehicle (Galderma) (Fig 5-27); Velvachol is a pharmaceutical product, manufactured as a water-soluble ointment base, but it is an excellent dam lubricant. Petroleum-based lubricants, such as Vaseline (Chesebrough-Pond's), should be avoided as rubber dam lubricants, because they are difficult to remove from the dam after application and, therefore, can impede bonding procedures and make inversion of the dam more difficult.

Water-soluble lubricant is applied in a thin coat around the holes on the tissue surface of the dam before it is taken to the mouth (Figs 5-28a and 5-28b). The lubricant makes passage of the dam through the interproximal contacts much easier, and the dam will often pass through the contacts, in a single layer, without the

use of floss. If additional lubrication is desired, lubricant may be applied to the teeth prior to placement of the dam.

A lubricant for the lips will make the patient more comfortable during the procedure. A petroleum-based lubricant, such as Vaseline, cocoa butter, silicate lubricant, or lip balm, functions well as a lip lubricant.

Application and Removal

Preparation of the Mouth

Teeth should be cleaned, if necessary, and contacts should be checked with floss. The rapid passage of dental floss through each contact that will be involved in the isolation is very important and, if accomplished as a part

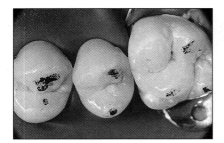

Fig 5-29 The centric occlusion markings were protected by cavity varnish during dam placement; had the markings not been protected with varnish, the placement procedure would likely have erased them.

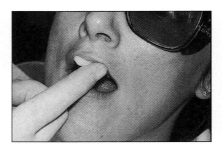

Fig 5-30 Lips are lubricated with petroleum-based lubricant prior to placement of the rubber dam.

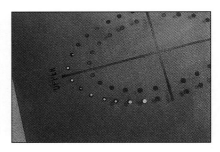

Fig 5-31 Varying hole sizes are used to seal against various sizes of teeth.

of the routine, will save chair time. Any rough contact should be smoothed with the proximal contact disk (Fig 5-26), not only to facilitate dam placement, but also to enable the patient to clean each interproximal area during routine flossing.

If a restorative procedure that involves an occlusal surface is planned, centric occlusion (maximum intercuspation) contacts should be marked with articulating paper or tape prior to application of the dam. Centric occlusion markings may be coated with a cavity varnish or light-cured resin to protect them from being rubbed off. If a cavity varnish containing a solvent is used, the cotton pellet or brush used to apply it to the centric occlusion markings should not touch the markings, or it may dissolve them and wipe them away. Instead, the pellet or brush containing the varnish is touched to the enamel adjacent to the markings, and the material is allowed to flow across the markings and dry (Fig 5-29).

If lips are to be lubricated, this should be accomplished prior to application of the dam (Fig 5-30).

Preparation of the Dam

Use of a prestamped dark (gray or green), heavy (or extra heavy) gauge dam material is recommended. Various hole sizes should be used to ensure a seal around the variety of tooth sizes (Fig 5-31). For example, an Ivory punch (Ivory, Heraeus Kulzer) has six hole sizes, numbered 1 through 6 from smallest to largest (Fig 5-4). Hole sizes recommended are 5 for clamped molars; 4 for other molars; 3 for premolars, canines, and maxillary central incisors; and 2 for lateral incisors and mandibular central incisors.

Slight variation from the recommended hole sizes may be needed, depending on the size of individual teeth, operator preference, and gauge of the dam, but a range of hole sizes should be used to prevent leakage between the dam and the teeth.

For operative procedures involving posterior teeth, the tooth or teeth to be restored should be exposed, as well as at least one tooth posterior to the most distal tooth to be restored, if possible. In addition, all teeth in the arch, around to the central or lateral incisor on the opposite side of the arch, should be exposed. This extension of the area of isolation around to the opposite side will hold the dam flat in the arch to give room for fingers and instruments in the area of the teeth to be restored. It will also expose teeth in the anterior area for finger rests during the operation (Fig 5-32).

For anterior restorations, exposure of the first premolar through the first premolar on the opposite side is recommended (Fig 5-33). This will provide room for the mirror and for hand instruments on the lingual aspect of the anterior teeth.

When a prestamped dam or a template is used, holes should be punched away from the spots to accommodate atypical alignment of teeth. In addition, when the dam is being prepared to provide isolation for Class 5 restorations, the hole for the tooth to receive a facial Class 5 restoration should be punched approximately 1.0 mm facial to the spot to allow retraction with the No. 212SA clamp. No holes should be punched for missing teeth.

After the dam is punched, the tissue side of the dam should be lubricated with a water-soluble lubricant. A small dollop of lubricant is applied to the tissue surface

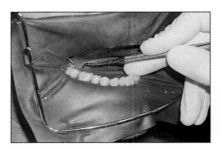

Fig 5-32 The incisal edges of the anterior teeth are used as a finger rest.

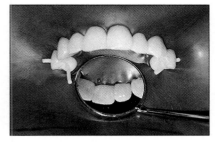

Fig 5-33 In isolation for an anterior restoration, the anterior teeth and first premolars are exposed to provide anchorage of the dam and to leave adequate working room on the lingual aspect of the anterior teeth.

and smeared over the surface of the dam in the area of the holes (Fig 5-28). The rubber dam frame should then be attached loosely to the dam to hold the edges of the dam away from the holes during application (Fig 5-34b).

Placement of the Dam

When the clamp is applied to the tooth with the clamp forceps, the clamp should be expanded only enough to allow it to pass over the crown of the tooth. Overexpansion of the clamp will permanently distort it so that it will be weak, unstable, and more likely to dislodge from the tooth.

There are several methods of dam insertion:

Dam over clamp (Figs 5-34a to 5-34h). A wingless clamp is placed on the tooth. It is recommended that a finger be maintained over the inserted clamp to prevent its dislodgment until its stability on the tooth has been confirmed. The operator checks stability by engaging the bow of the clamp with an instrument and firmly attempting to pull it occlusally (Fig 5-34a). If the clamp rotates on the tooth, it is not stable and should be repositioned or replaced.

The top and the bottom attachment points of the Young frame are engaged into the top and bottom of the dam to give a slackness or pouching of the dam (Fig 5-34b). The tissue side of the dam is lubricated in the area of the holes. Then, with a finger on each side of the distal hole in the dam, the dentist (or assistant) stretches the dam so that the hole is enlarged and appears to be an open slit; the hole is then carried over the bow and jaws of the clamp (Fig 5-34c). The hole at the opposite end of the row (usually for the lateral or central incisor on the opposite side) is then passed over the appropriate

tooth, and the septa are worked through the interproximal contacts.

A gloved fingernail used to slightly separate the anterior teeth is very helpful, and floss is rarely needed to carry the dam through anterior interproximal contacts (Fig 5-34d). Good lubrication of the dam is necessary for easy and quick application. The dam should be passed through each contact in a single layer. This may be accomplished by stretching a septum over one of the teeth adjacent to the contact, and sliding the edge of the rubber to the contact so that a leading edge of dam is touching the contact (Fig 5-34e).

In posterior areas, the leading edge should be touching the occlusal portion of the contact in the occlusal embrasure, then waxed tape (ribbon floss) or waxed floss is used to move the dam progressively through the contact (Figs 5-34e to 5-34g). Tape will carry more of the rubber through the contact in a single pass than will floss. If tape is used, it, like the rubber, should be taken through the contact in a single layer, not twisted or bunched up.

If the dam goes through with one pass of the floss, the floss may be removed from the contact without pulling the rubber back out. To accomplish this, the tail of the floss that is on the lingual side of the teeth is doubled back across the occlusal embrasure of the contact so that both ends are on the facial aspect; then the tape is pulled facially through the contact. If only a portion of the septum goes through the contact with the first pass of the floss or tape, the floss should be doubled back and passed through the contact again; it is then pulled facially out of the gingival embrasure (Fig 5-34h). The tape should be passed through repeatedly until the entire septum has been carried through the contact.

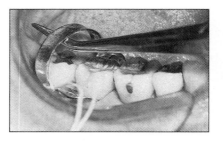

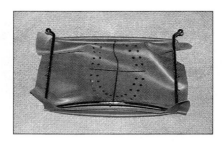

Fig 5-34a The clamp (modified No. W8A) is tested for stability. To do so, the operator attempts to pull bow occlusally.

Fig 5-34b The dam is fitted loosely on the frame.

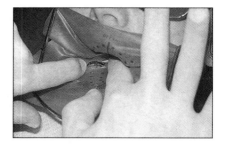

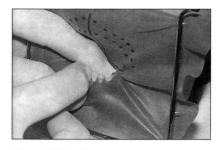

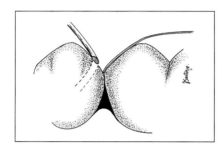

Fig 5-34c The distal hole of the dam is carried over the bow of the clamp.

Fig 5-34d The septa are worked through anterior contacts as a gloved fingernail is used to slightly separate teeth.

Fig 5-34e The leading edge of the dam is touching the occlusal aspect of the interproximal contact; floss is on the adjacent tooth.

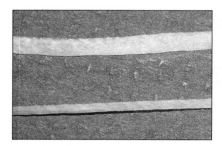

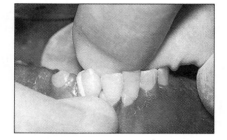

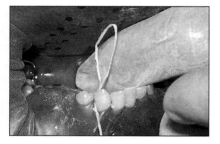

Fig 5-34f Waxed dental tape, or ribbon floss *(top)*, if it is not folded or bunched, will carry more of the dam septum through the contact in a single pass than will waxed floss *(bottom)*, but either type will serve the purpose.

Fig 5-34g The dam septum is lying on the mesial aspect of mandibular first premolar, with its leading edge at the mesial contact; the floss is lying on the distal aspect of the canine, ready to move to the contact, meeting the dam there. The floss will then carry at least a portion of the septum through the contact.

Fig 5-34h The floss has been doubled back to the facial aspect and passed through the contact again, carrying another portion of the septum through the contact. The floss is then removed from the contact; one or both of the tails of the floss are pulled facially away from the teeth.

Winged clamp in dam (Figs 5-35a to 5-35d). Prior to lubrication of the dam, the clamp is placed into the distal hole so that the hole is stretched over the wings of the clamp from its tissue side. The dam is then lubricated, and the frame is attached. The forceps are inserted into the holes of the clamp and the clamp, dam, and frame are carried as a unit to place (Figs 5-35b and 5-35c). After the stability of the clamp is confirmed, the dam is snapped off the wings of the clamp with finger tension or with a bladed instrument such as a plastic instrument (Fig 5-35d). The remainder of the dam is placed as previously described.

Wingless clamp in dam (Figs 5-36a and 5-36b). The distal hole of the lubricated dam is passed over the bow of a wingless clamp, such as the No. WSA, so that the

Figs 5-35a to 5-35d Winged clamp in dam method of dam application.

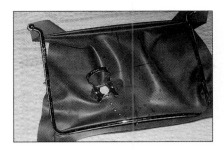

Fig 5-35a A winged clamp (No. 27) is inserted into the distal hole of the dam.

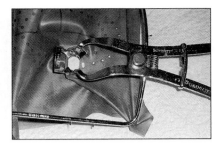

Fig 5-35b The clamp-dam-frame assembly is carried to the mouth as a unit.

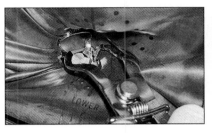

Fig 5-35c The clamp is placed on the mandibular second molar.

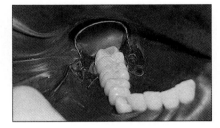

Fig 5-35d The dam has been applied to the quadrant, and a No. 1-2 plastic instrument is used to pull the edges of rubber off the wings of the clamp.

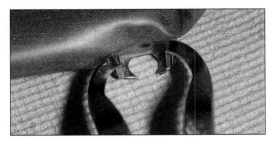

Fig 5-36a Wingless clamp in dam method of dam application. Shown is the clamp in the dam.

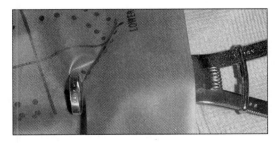

Fig 5-36b Dam and clamp with forceps in place.

hole comes to rest at the junction of the bow and the jaw arms (Fig 5-36a). The frame is not attached to the dam at this point. The dam is gathered up and elevated to expose the jaw arms of the clamp, and the forceps are then inserted into the forceps holes (Figs 5-36a and 5-36b). The gathered dam is carried to the mouth with one hand and the forceps with the other. After the clamp is applied to the distal tooth and the dam has been pulled over the jaws of the clamp, the frame is attached and the other teeth are isolated as previously described.

Clamp after dam. The dam is applied to the teeth and then the clamp is placed. This technique is occasionally necessary but is the most difficult.

Completion of Application

Application of the napkin. For longer procedures, the use of a rubber dam napkin is recommended. The napkin may be positioned before or after the dam is in place on the teeth. For placement of the napkin after the dam has been applied, the frame is removed, the napkin is placed so that the edges of the napkin remain on the skin and not in the mouth, and the frame is replaced.

Adjustment of the dam in the frame. The frame and dam are adjusted so that there is a minimum of folds and wrinkles and so that the dam does not obstruct the nostrils.

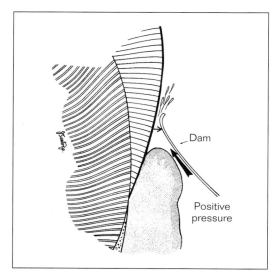

Fig 5-37a Without inversion of the dam, positive pressure under the dam, created by tongue movement, swallowing, etc, will cause leakage of saliva into the operating field.

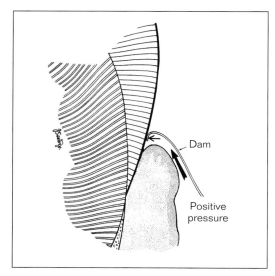

Fig 5-37b With inversion of the dam, positive pressure under the dam only causes the dam to seal more tightly against the tooth, preventing leakage.

Washing of the dam. The dam and isolated teeth are washed with an air-water spray to remove the lubricant. After they are washed, the dam and teeth should be dried with air from the air syringe.

Inversion of the dam. The dam should be inverted around the necks of the teeth, at least in the area of the tooth or teeth to be restored. The edge of the dam that is against the tooth acts as a valve. If the edge is directed occlusally (Fig 5-37a), when a positive pressure is created by the tongue and cheeks under the dam, the valve opens, and saliva and other liquids under the dam are pushed between the tooth and dam to flood the operating field; then when a negative pressure is created under the dam, the valve closes and the saliva is trapped in the field. When the dam is inverted, a positive pressure under the dam simply serves to push the valve more tightly against the tooth (Fig 5-37b) so that no flooding of the field occurs.

Almost any instrument may be used to tuck the edge of the dam gingivally (Figs 5-24a to 5-24c). A steady, high-volume stream of air should be directed at the tip of the instrument used to invert the dam, and the instrument should be moved along the margin of the dam so that the inversion is progressive.

Floss may be used to invert the dam in interproximal areas (Fig 5-38a). When it is used to carry the edge of the dam gingivally, the floss should not then be pulled occlusally for removal, because it will frequently pull the

edge of the dam with it, eliminating the inversion. Instead, the floss can be doubled over on itself on the lingual aspect and passed again through the contact. Then one end is pulled in a facial direction so that it rolls from the sulcus, leaving the dam inverted (Fig 5-38b). In this floss-facilitated inversion, a steady stream of air is as helpful as it is when inversion is accomplished with an instrument. The dam inverts more easily when the surfaces of the tooth and adjacent dam are dry.

Protection of the Dam
Torn dams provide poor isolation, so expenditure of a little effort to prevent tearing is worthwhile. An example of protection would be the use of a wedge interproximally when rotary instruments are used in the proximity of the dam. Another example is the use of a second clamp to retract the dam below a margin that is near to, or below, the level of the gingival crest (see Fig 5-45).

Removal of the Dam
The interproximal septa are stretched, one at a time, and clipped with scissors (Figs 5-39a and 5-39b). The scissors are held so that the tips are not in contact with any tissue (Fig 5-39b). When all septa are cut, the clamp is removed with the forceps and the dam is snapped from the teeth.

After the dam is free from the mouth, the teeth should be examined to assure no rubber remains around them or in the contacts. The frame should be removed

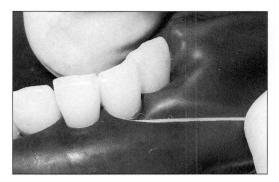

Fig 5-38a Floss is used to invert the dam in an interproximal area.

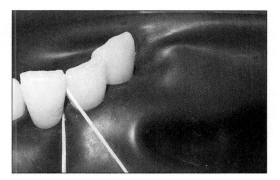

Fig 5-38b Floss is "rolled out" to the facial aspect to prevent reversal of the inversion it accomplished.

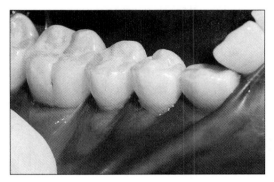

Fig 5-39a To remove the dam, the interproximal septa are stretched for cutting.

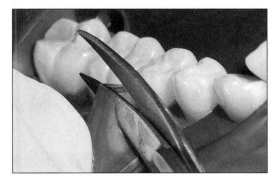

Fig 5-39b One blade of the scissors is used to pull the dam well away from any tissue before the septum is cut.

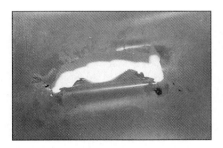

Fig 5-40a While the dam is on the frame, it is difficult to determine if any portion is missing.

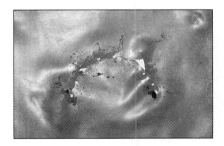

Fig 5-40b The dam is removed from the frame and laid on a flat surface. Note that a portion of dam is missing.

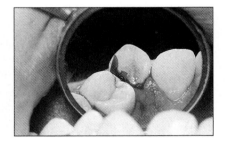

Fig 5-40c The missing piece is located in the mouth and removed.

from the dam, and the dam should be laid flat on a surface and examined to assure that no pieces are missing (Figs 5-40a and 5-40b). If a piece is missing and unaccounted for, the mouth should be reexamined in the area of the missing piece of dam; any remnant should be removed (Fig 5-40c). A small piece of dam left subgingivally can cause inflammation, gingival abscess, or even significant loss of periodontal support.

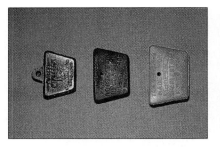
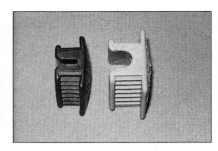
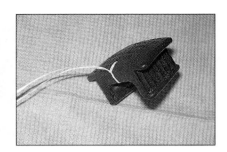

Figs 5-41a and 5-41b Rubber bite blocks are available in various sizes.

Fig 5-41c Floss is attached to the bite block for emergency retrieval if necessary.

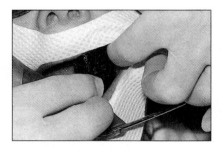
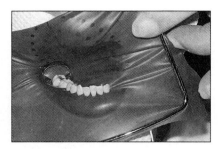

Fig 5-42a A bite block is inserted on the patient's left side after a rubber dam is applied to isolate the right quadrant.

Fig 5-42b The dam with a bite block in place aids access to the field and increases patient comfort.

Special Considerations

Bite Block

Patients often have difficulty keeping their mouths open or are uncomfortable with wide opening. A rubber bite block can relieve their discomfort, allow them to relax musculature, and permit them to keep the mouth open without constantly thinking about it. Bite blocks are available in a variety of sizes (Figs 5-41a and 5-41b). A piece of floss or tape may be attached to the bite block to allow retrieval if necessary (Fig 5-41c). Figures 5-42a and 5-42b show insertion of the bite block after the dam is in place.

Isolation for a Fixed Partial Denture

Whenever it is possible to achieve good isolation without isolating around a fixed partial denture, that is the desirable course. There are several techniques for isolating around a fixed partial denture; they are all somewhat time consuming, but are often valuable. Two methods will be described.

Cyanoacrylate method (Figs 5-43a to 5-43k). Holes for the teeth are punched in the dam. The holes for the abutment teeth are connected with a cut that is in an arc to give a "tongue" of dam material between the holes. The tongue of material is folded back, and a piece of dam material is attached with cyanoacrylate glue over the opening left when the tongue was folded back. This piece is glued into place so that there is a slit connecting the abutment holes and a tongue of material that is free to swing down over the attached piece of dam material.

The dam is inserted over all teeth for which holes have been punched, and the tongue of material is pulled under the pontic(s) and glued into place on the added piece of dam. Tension on the tongue while the glue is setting (10 to 15 seconds) will ensure that the dam is tight around the abutments after tension is released.

Figs 5-43a to 5-43k Rubber dam isolation around a fixed partial denture (cyanoacrylate method).

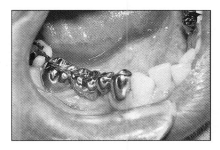

Fig 5-43a A four-unit fixed partial denture extends from the mandibular first premolar to the second molar.

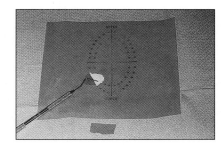

Fig 5-43b The holes for the abutment teeth are connected with an arched cut.

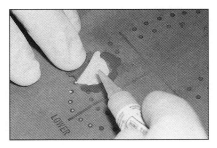
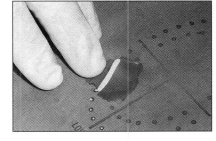

Fig 5-43c and 5-43d A small piece of dam is glued to place.

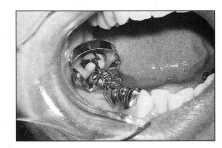

Fig 5-43e A No. W8A clamp is positioned on the second molar.

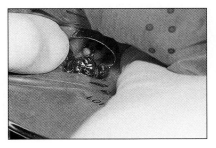

Fig 5-43f The dam is carried to place.

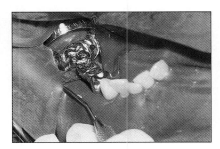

Fig 5-43g A tongue of dam material is tucked under the pontics with a periodontal probe.

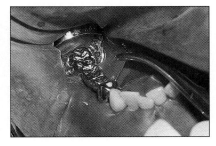

Fig 5-43h The tongue of material is grasped and pulled lingually with a hemostat.

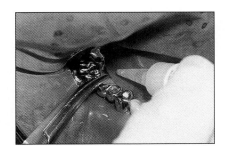

Fig 5-43i Glue is applied for the tongue attachment.

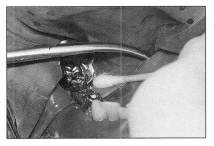

Fig 5-43j The tongue is held in place with a hemostat and a cotton-tipped applicator while the glue sets.

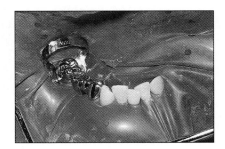

Fig 5-43k Isolation is complete.

Figs 5-44a to 5-44i   Isolation around a three-unit fixed partial denture or splinted teeth (ligation method).

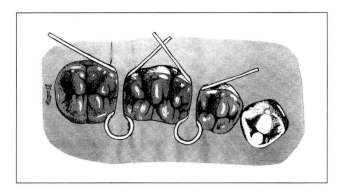

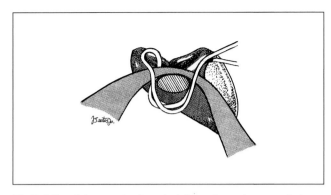

Fig 5-44a   Holes are punched for the abutment teeth and pontic, and the dam is positioned. The septa on the mesial aspect of the mesial abutment and the distal aspect of the distal abutment are flossed to place, and then the holes are stretched over the abutments and the pontic.

Fig 5-44b   A ligature is threaded through an abutment hole on the facial aspect, under the retainer-pontic connector, through the same hole again on the lingual aspect, around the septum, through the pontic hole on the lingual aspect, back under the connector to the facial aspect, and back through the pontic hole.

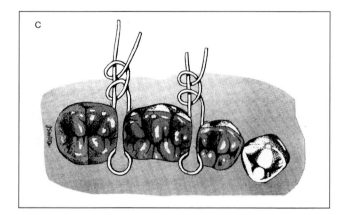

c

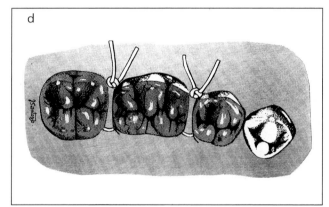

d

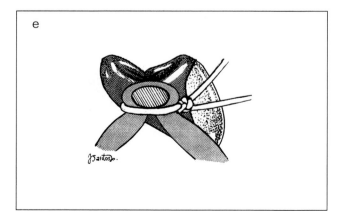

e

Figs 5-44c to 5-44e   The ends of the ligature are tied together to pull the rubber septum tightly around the connector.

Figs 5-44f and 5-44g Suture has been used for field isolation involving an anterior three-unit fixed partial denture.

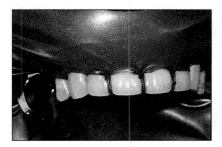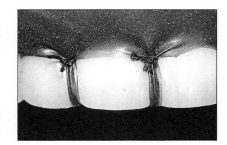

Figs 5-44h and 5-44i Floss has been used for isolation involving a cantilevered canine pontic attached to splinted premolars.

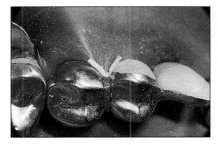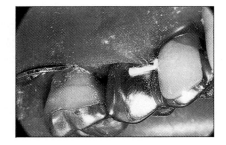

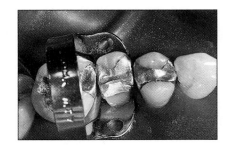

Fig 5-45 A second clamp is in place to retract the dam and give access to the gingival extent of a cusp fracture. A No. W1A clamp was used instead of a No. W2A clamp because of the need for a jaw to be apical to the fracture margin.

Ligation of septa around the retainer-pontic connectors (Figs 5-44a to 5-44i). This procedure is for three-unit fixed partial dentures or splinted teeth. Holes are punched for each abutment, and, for three-unit fixed partial dentures, another hole is punched for the pontic. A piece of floss or suture is used to tie through the holes so that the septum between adjacent holes is stretched around the retainer-pontic connector.

Facilitation of Inversion

If there is a problem with inversion, the teeth are dried and a copal resin varnish is applied to them. The tacky layer will usually allow easy inversion.

Use of Multiple Clamps

In addition to the clamp on the distal tooth, which retains the posterior portion of the dam, a second (or third) clamp is often needed. When the No. 212SA or other butterfly clamp (retractor) is used to retract tissue and dam for a Class 5 or other restoration, it is almost invariably used in addition to the posterior clamp. If a cavity that is at least partly subgingival is to be prepared, a clamp on that tooth will prevent the dam from riding up over the margin (Fig 5-45).

Placement of Clamp Over Dam

When it is desirable to clamp a tooth that was not considered when the dam was punched, the clamp may be applied over the dam (Fig 5-15). The clamp jaws should be dull, so as not to cut through the dam, and the dam should be stretched loosely over the tooth being clamped.

Gingival Relaxation Incisions

When using a No. 212 retractor for isolation for a Class 5 restoration, the jaw of the retractor should be posi-

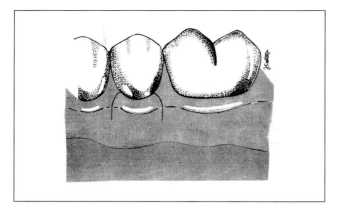

Fig 5-46a Gingival relaxation incisions are made within the keratinized gingival tissue. Either one or both can be made, depending on the amount of release needed for relaxation of the tissue.

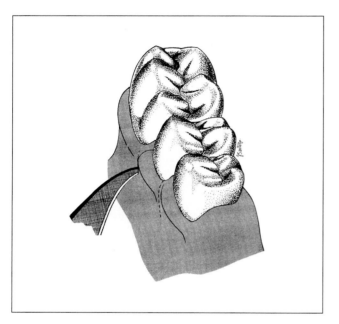

Fig 5-46b The No. 12b scalpel blade is used to make the incision.

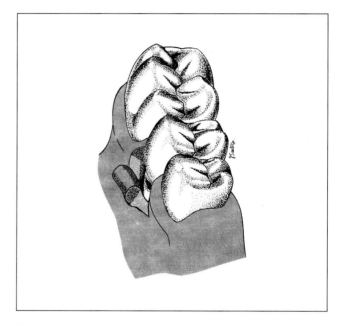

Fig 5-46c The tissue flap is reflected away from the root prior to application of the dam and No. 212 retractor. The incisions are directed slightly into the papilla and then vertically.

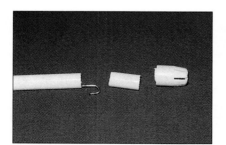

Fig 5-47a For unassisted fluid evacuation from the dam,[13] a saliva ejector is modified. First, the tip is cut off; then another 0.5 inch, except for the wire, is cut off, and the protruding wire is bent to form a hook.

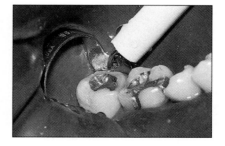

Fig 5-47b For fluid evacuation, the wire hook is attached to the forceps hole of the rubber dam clamp.

tioned at least 0.5 mm (preferably 1.0 mm) gingival to the gingival margin of the planned restoration. This can usually be accomplished without laceration of tissue, because the free gingiva is elastic enough to be retracted. If, however, the free gingival margin is fibrous and difficult to displace gingivally, forced retraction could lacerate the tissue. In such a case, it is preferable to make one or two small incisions[8,18] to allow the tissue to be displaced without tearing.

For this technique (sometimes referred to as a *mini-flap procedure*) to be successful, the peridontium must be healthy. The incisions should be confined to the keratinized gingival tissue and kept as short as possible (just long enough to allow adequate exposure for isolation). Incisions can often be limited to the free gingiva, and, although reattachment to previously unexposed cementum can be expected, unnecessary severing of attachment should be avoided. Full-thickness vertical incisions should be initiated at the mesial and/or distal aspects of the facial surface and should be directed perpendicular to the root and bony surface, first slightly toward the interproximal papilla, then apically (Figs 5-46a to 5-46c).

The blade of a plastic instrument or a beavertail burnisher may be used to push the tissue and rubber dam back while the facial jaw of the No. 212 clamp is being situated on the root of the tooth. Again, the jaw should be dull, not sharp, so that it will not damage the root surface. A finger should be used to hold the clamp in place while it is stabilized with compound (Figs 5-23a to 5-23c). After the restorative procedure is completed, the No. 212 clamp is removed (Figs 5-23d to 5-23i), and the dam is removed. Any blood in the area is washed away. The reflected gingival tissue is returned to its original location and held there with a dampened gauze sponge and finger pressure for about 2 minutes to allow initiation of a fibrin clot. As long as the incisions were confined to keratinized tissue, no sutures or periodontal dressing is needed, and healing should proceed uneventfully.

Evacuation of Fluid from Dam

If the dentist must work without an assistant, a very effective method for evacuation of fluid from the rubber dam involves the use of a suction tube anchored within the operating field.

Modified saliva ejector. One method involves the modification of a saliva ejector, as described by Lambert.[13] The molded plastic tip is cut off with a pair of crown scissors; then an additional 0.5 inch of the plastic tube is cut off without cutting the wire within the plastic. The 0.5-inch length of plastic tubing is then pulled off the wire, leaving the wire extending from the end of the tube (Figs 5-47a and 5-47b); the wire is bent at its end to form a hook. The hook is attached to the bow or a hole of the rubber dam clamp to provide anchorage of the tube within the field, and the suction is activated. This method will supply continuous fluid evacuation during the operative procedure.

Washed field apparatus. Another method employs inexpensive plastic tubing that is attached to the saliva ejector hose at one end and to the clamp or the rubber dam itself at the other (Figs 5-48a to 5-48c). Childers and Marshall[5] have recommended the use of clear vinyl tubing with an inside diameter of 0.0625 inch and an

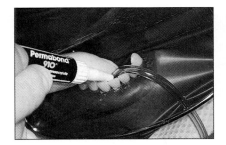
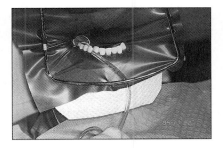
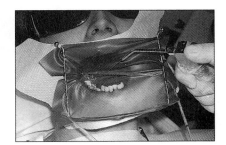

Figs 5-48a and 5-48b The washed field apparatus[2,5] is used for evacuation of fluids from the dam when no assistant is available. A small tube is attached to the dam with cyanoacrylate. (Courtesy of Dr James M. Childers and Dr Thomas D. Marshall.)

Fig 5-48c Two small tubes, extending from a Y connector, are tucked under the frame and behind the bow of the clamp to provide evacuation. (Courtesy of Dr James M. Childers and Dr Thomas D. Marshall).

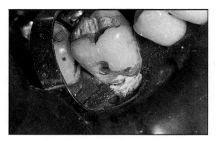

Fig 5-49 Sealing of the root concavity. The dam is retracted by the clamp to allow isolation for a large Class 5 restoration; the retraction is apical to the beginning of the root concavity of the furcation. The gap between the dam and the concave root surface is sealed with Cavit, a provisional restorative material that hardens when it comes into contact with moisture.

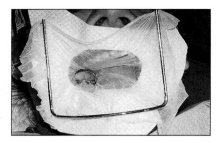

Fig 5-50 Dam fabricated from a vinyl glove for a latex-sensitive patient. (Innovation of Dr Carmen Martinez when she was a student at the University of Texas, Health Science Center at San Antonio, Dental School.)

outside diameter of 0.125 inch (No. C1001A, Mojak Plastic). As a connector for the saliva ejector hose, they recommended the use of clear vinyl tubing with an inside diameter of 0.125 inch and an outside diameter of 0.25 inch (No. C1003S, Mojak Plastic). A short section of the larger diameter tubing is cut to provide an adaptor or connector from the saliva ejector hose to the smaller tubing. A longer section of the smaller tubing is cut, and its end is fitted inside the section of larger tubing. The end of the small-diameter tube is carried under the rubber dam frame and tucked under the bow or a wing of the rubber dam clamp in the back of the dam; tubing may also be attached to the rubber dam with cyanoacrylate adhesive (Figs 5-48a and 5-48b). Small holes may be punched in the side of the tubing near the end with a rubber dam punch to provide several inlets for suctioned fluids. A similar apparatus, described by Benavides and Herrera,[2] involves a Y-type connector (DCI International) to which two small-diameter plastic tubes are attached (Fig 5-48c).

Sealing a Root Concavity

The rubber dam seals well on convex tooth surfaces. If the dam is retracted so that its edge goes across a root concavity, however, saliva will leak into the operating field. A solution is to seal the gap between the edge of the dam and the concave root surface. This may be accomplished with a provisional restorative material, such as Cavit (ESPE Premier), which is caused to harden by moisture (Fig 5-49).

Repair of a Torn Rubber Dam

A small tear in a dam may often be patched. A piece of dam material is cut to cover the tear and extend 1.0 cm or so beyond the tear on all sides. The piece is attached over the tear with cyanoacrylate.

Placement of a Second Dam Over the First

If a dam is torn beyond repair during a procedure, the dentist might choose to remove the dam and replace it, but an alternative is to place another dam over the top of the first. Brownbill[3] has also recommended that this technique be used when there is leakage around teeth through incorrectly sized holes and when strong chemicals are to be used.

Latex Allergies

There is an increasing awareness of sensitivity of dental patients to latex.[9,14,15] One survey[15] reported 3.7% of patients to have a latex allergy; the investigators recommended careful questioning of patients regarding a history of sensitivity to latex-based products, so that the use of latex products, such as gloves and the rubber dam, may be avoided with these patients.

For latex-sensitive patients, use of the latex dam should be avoided, as should other latex products. One manufacturer (Hygenic) recently introduced a non-latex dam that is fabricated from a material with elastic properties very similar to latex. It is recommended for patients with a latex allergy. Figure 5-50 shows a dam made from a vinyl glove for a latex-sensitive patient.

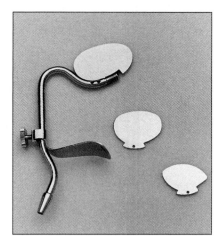

Fig 5-51a The Svedopter tongue-retracting evacuation device is supplied with three sizes of vertical blades.

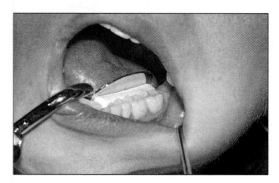

Fig 5-51b The Svedopter is used to hold the tongue away from the operating field.

Summary of Recommendations

Following are some of the procedures that facilitate rubber dam use:

1. Use a heavy gauge, prestamped dam.
2. Floss through contacts prior to dam placement, planing any contact that shreds or tears the floss.
3. Use a good water-soluble lubricant, such as Velvachol.
4. Use a clamp designed for four-point contact on the tooth and avoid overexpansion of the clamp, so that the clamp will maintain its strength and will be stable as a retainer.
5. Isolate enough teeth to hold the dam on the lingual aspect of the teeth away from the operating field and to provide exposed teeth for finger rests.
6. Floss the dam through interproximal contacts in a single layer and avoid doubling or bunching the dam in the contact.
7. Master the use of modeling compound to stabilize rubber dam retainers.

◼ Other Methods of Isolation

Svedopter

The Svedopter (E. C. Moore) is probably the most commonly used tongue retraction device (Figs 5-51a and 5-51b). It is designed so that the vacuum evacuator tube passes anterior to the chin and mandibular anterior teeth, over the incisal edges of the mandibular anterior teeth, and down to the floor of the mouth, to either the left or the right of the tongue. A mirrorlike vertical blade is attached to the evacuator tube so that it holds the tongue away from the field of operation. Several sizes of vertical blades are supplied by the manufacturer. An adjustable horizontal chin blade is attached to the evacuation tube so that it will clamp under the chin to hold the apparatus in place.

Absorbent cotton rolls are placed adjacent to the Svedopter in the floor of the mouth and in the maxillary buccal vestibule adjacent to the opening of the parotid gland (Stinson's) duct. The Svedopter is especially useful for preparation and cementation of fixed prostheses. It is less effective than the rubber dam for procedures in which total isolation from the fluids and vapors of the oral cavity is desired.

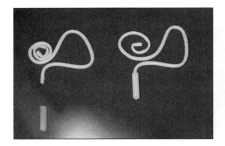 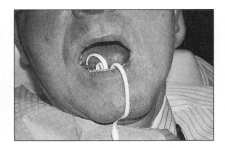 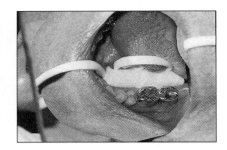

Figs 5-52a to 5-52c The Hygoformic saliva ejector should be routinely rebent to pass under the chin, over the incisal edges of the mandibular incisors, and then down to the floor of the mouth. The apparatus should usually be uncoiled slightly to extend further posteriorly. *(left)* Hygoformic saliva ejector as received; *(right)* Hygoformic saliva ejector that has been reshaped. Figs 5-52b and 5-52c show ilsolation achieved with the Hygoformic saliva ejector.

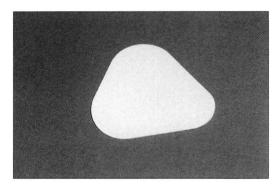 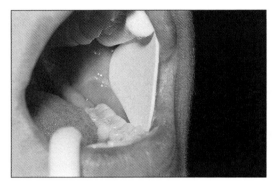

Fig 5-53a A parotid shield is a triangular absorbent paper.

Fig 5-53b A parotid shield may supplement a cotton roll in the buccal vestibule or may be used alone.

Hygoformic Saliva Ejector

This coiled saliva ejector is used in the same way as the Svedopter, but it does not have a reflective blade (Figs 5-52a to 5-52c). It is, however, usually more comfortable and less traumatic to lingual tissues than is the Svedopter. For use, the Hygoformic saliva ejector (Pulpdent) must be re-formed (rebent) so that the evacuator tube passes under the chin, up over the incisal edges of the mandibular incisors, and then down to the floor of the mouth. The tongue-retracting coil should be loosened, or partially uncoiled, so that it extends posteriorly enough to hold the tongue away from the operating field. The Hygoformic saliva ejector is also used in conjunction with absorbant cotton for maximum effectiveness.

Absorbent Paper and Cotton Products

Absorbent materials are important in dentistry. Vacuum apparatuses remove fluids from the operating field by suctioning them; cotton and paper products help control fluids by absorbing them. Several types of absorbent cotton rolls are available in various diameters and lengths. These are placed into areas of the mouth where salivary gland ducts exit to absorb saliva and prevent salivary contamination of the operating field.

Isolation using absorbent materials with suctioning devices is less effective than using the rubber dam with suction, but in many procedures, the more complete isolation provided by the dam is unnecessary. In these situations, absorbent products are useful.

Small gauze sponges may be folded or rolled to substitute for cotton rolls. In addition, absorbent paper triangles, or parotid shields, such as Dri-Aid (Lorvic), are useful on the facial aspect of posterior teeth to absorb saliva secreted by the parotid gland (Figs 5-53a and 5-53b).

References

1. Barghi N, Knight GT, Berry TG. Comparing two methods of moisture control in bonding to enamel: A clinical study. Oper Dent 1991;16:130-135.

2. Benavides R, Herrera H. Rubber dam with washed field evacuation: A new approach. Oper Dent 1992;17:26-28.

3. Brownbill JW. Double rubber dam. Quintessence Int 1987;18:699-670.

4. Champion MA, Kugel G, Gruskowski C. Evaluation of a new intraoral isolation device. Oper Dent 1991;16:181-185.

5. Childers JM, Marshall TD. Coolant evacuation; a solution for students working without dental assistance. Oper Dent 1995;20:130-132.

6. Christen AG. Sanford C. Barnum, discoverer of the rubber dam. Bull Hist Dent 1977;25:3-9.

7. Christensen GJ. Using rubber dams to boost quality, quantity of restorative services. J Am Dent Assoc 1994;125:81-82.

8. Drucker H, Wolcott RB. Gingival tissue management with Class V restorations. J Am Acad Gold Foil Oper 1970;13(1):34-38.

9. Fay MF, Beck WC, Checchi L, Winkler D. Gloves: New selection criteria. Quintessence Int 1995;26:25-29.

10. Gergely EJ. Rubber dam acceptance. Br Dent J 1989;167:249-252.

11. Knight GT, Barghi N, Berry T. Microleakage of enamel bonding as affected by moisture control methods [abstract]. J Dent Res 1991;70:561.

12. Knight GT, Barghi N. Effect of saliva contamination on dentin bonding agents in vivo [abstract 434]. J Dent Res 1992;71:160.

13. Lambert RL. Moisture evacuation with the rubber dam in place. J Prosthet Dent 1985;53:749-750.

14. March PJ. An allergic reaction to latex rubber gloves. J Am Dent Assoc 1988;117:590-591.

15. Rankin KV, Jones DL, Rees TD. Latex reactions in an adult dental population. Am J Dent 1993;6:274-276.

16. Reid JS, Callis PD, Patterson CJW. Rubber Dam in Clinical Practice, Chicago: Quintessence, 1990.

17. Reuter JE. The isolation of teeth and the protection of the patient during endodontic treatment. Int Endod J 1983;16:173-181.

18. Xhonga FA. Gingival retraction techniques and their healing effect on the gingiva. J Prosthet Dent 1971;26:640-648.

Enamel and Dentin Adhesion

Bart Van Meerbeek / Jorge Perdigão / Sonia Gladys
Paul Lambrechts / Guido Vanherle

After observing the industrial use of phosphoric acid to improve adhesion of paints and resin coatings to metal surfaces, Buonocore,[43] in 1955, applied acid to teeth to "render the tooth surface more receptive to adhesion." Buonocore's pioneering work led to major changes in the practice of dentistry. Today, we are in the age of adhesive dentistry. Traditional mechanical methods of retaining restorative materials have been replaced, to a large extent, by tooth-conserving adhesive methods. The concepts of large preparations and extension for prevention, proposed by Black[28] in 1917, have gradually been replaced by smaller preparations and more conservative techniques.

Advantages of Adhesive Techniques

Bonded restorations have a number of advantages over traditional, nonadhesive methods. Traditionally, retention and stabilization of restorations often required the removal of sound tooth structure. This is not necessary, in many cases, when adhesive techniques are used. Adhesion also reduces microleakage at the restoration-tooth interface. Prevention of microleakage, or the ingress of oral fluids and bacteria along the cavity wall, reduces clinical problems such as postoperative sensitivity, marginal staining, and recurrent caries, all of which may jeopardize the clinical longevity of restorative efforts.[70,218]

Adhesive restorations better transmit and distribute functional stresses across the bonding interface to the tooth and have the potential to reinforce weakened tooth structure.[72,126,185] In contrast, a traditional metal intracoronal restoration may act as a wedge between the buccal and lingual cusps and increase the risk of cuspal fracture. Adhesive techniques allow deteriorating restorations to be repaired and debonded restorations to be replaced with minimal or no additional loss of tooth material.

Adhesive techniques have expanded the range of possibilities for esthetic restorative dentistry.[137,253] Today's patient pays more attention to cosmetics than ever before, and teeth are a key consideration in personal appearance. Tooth-colored restorative materials are used to cosmetically restore and/or recontour teeth with little or no tooth preparation. Advances in dental adhesive technology have allowed the dentist to improve facial esthetics in a relatively simple and economic way.

Indications

Adhesive techniques with resin composites were initially employed to replace carious and fractured tooth structure or to fill erosion or abrasion defects in cervical areas. Modern adhesive techniques also allow restorative material to be added to the tooth for the correction of unesthetic shapes, positions, dimensions, or shades. Resin composite can be added in a mesiodistal direction to close diastemas, incisally to add length, or to the buccal surface to mask discoloration. Because of the alleged mercury toxicity associated with silver amalgam,[162,167] substantial research is currently focused on the development of alternatives to amalgam.[291] Posterior resin composites can be directly or indirectly bonded in Class 1 and Class 2 preparations.

Table 6-1 Bond energy and bond distance (equilibrium length)[4]

Bond type	Bond energy (kJmol⁻¹)	Equilibrium length (Å)
Primary		
Ionic	600–1200	2–4
Covalent	60–800	0.7–3
Secondary		
Hydrogen	~50	3
Dipole interactions°	~20	4
London dispersion°	~40	<10

°Dipole interactions and dispersion forces are often collectively referred to as *van der Waals forces.*

Adhesive techniques are also used to bond anterior and posterior ceramic restorations, such as veneers, inlays, and onlays, with adhesive luting resin composites. Adhesives can be used to bond silver amalgam restorations, to retain metal frameworks, to adhesively cement crowns and fixed partial dentures, to bond orthodontic brackets, for periodontal or orthodontic splints, to treat dentinal hypersensitivity, and to repair fractured porcelain, amalgam, and resin restorations. Pit and fissure sealants utilize adhesion as part of a preventive treatment program. Adhesive materials are sometimes used with core buildup foundations.

Concepts in restorative dentistry have been continually changing during the last decades, and adhesive technology has become steadily more important. Adhesion to enamel was followed by adhesion to dentin. Today, so-called universal, all-purpose, or multipurpose adhesive systems that purportedly bond to enamel, dentin, amalgam, metal, and porcelain have overwhelmed the dental market, so that it becomes difficult for the general practitioner to make an appropriate product selection for use in daily practice.

Principles of Adhesion

The word *adhesion* is derived from the Latin word *adhaerere,* which is a compound of *ad,* or *to,* and *haerere,* or *to stick.*[200] Cicero used the expression *haerere in equo,* literally *to stick to a horse,* to refer to keeping a firm seat.

In adhesive terminology, *adhesion* or *bonding* is the attachment of one substance to another. The surface or substrate that is adhered to is termed the *adherend.* The *adhesive* or *adherent,* or in dental terminology the *bond-*

ing agent or *adhesive system,* may then be defined as the material that, when applied to surfaces of substances, can join them together, resist separation, and transmit loads across the bond.[157,200] The *adhesive strength* or *bond strength* is the measure of the load-bearing capability of the adhesive. The time period during which the bond remains effective is referred to as *durability.*[2]

Adhesion refers to the forces or energies between atoms or molecules at an interface that hold two phases together.[200] In dental literature, adhesion is often subjected to tensile or shear forces in debonding tests, and the mode of failure is quantified. If the bond fails at the interface between the two substrates, the mode of failure is referred to as *adhesive.* It is referred to as *cohesive* if failure occurs in one of the substrates, but not at the interface. The mode of failure is often mixed.

Four different theories have been advanced to account for the observed phenomena of adhesion[4]:

1. Mechanical theories state that the solidified adhesive interlocks micromechanically with the roughness and irregularities of the surface of the adherend.
2. Adsorption theories encompass all kinds of chemical bonds between the adhesive and the adherend, including primary (ionic and covalent) and secondary (hydrogen, dipole interaction, and London dispersion) valence forces (Table 6-1). London dispersion forces are almost universally present, because they arise from and solely depend upon the presence of nuclei and electrons. The other bond types require appropriate chemical groups to interact.
3. Diffusion theories propose that adhesion is the result of bonding between mobile molecules. Polymers from each side of an interface can cross over and react with molecules on the other side. Eventually, the interface will disappear and the two parts will become one.
4. Electrostatic theories state that an electrical double layer forms at the interface between a metal and a polymer, making a certain, yet obscure, contribution to the bond strength.

An important requirement for any of these interfacial phenomena to take place is that the two materials being joined must be in sufficiently close and intimate relation. Besides an intimate contact, sufficient wetting of the adhesive will only occur if its surface tension is less than the surface-free energy of the adherend.[84,88,232] Wetting of a surface by a liquid is characterized by the contact angle of a droplet placed on the surface.[201] If the liquid spreads out completely on the solid surface, this indicates complete wetting or a contact angle of 0 degrees (Fig 6-1).

According to this theory of wetting and surface-free energies, adhesion to enamel is much easier to achieve than is adhesion to dentin. Enamel contains primarily hydroxyapatite, which has a high surface-free energy, whereas dentin is composed of two distinct substrates, hydroxyapatite and collagen, which has a low surface-free energy. In the oral environment, the tooth surface is contaminated by an organic saliva pellicle with a low critical surface tension of approximately 28 dynes/cm,[145] which impairs adequate wetting by the adhesive.[17] Likewise, instrumentation of the tooth substrate during cavity preparation produces a smear layer with a low surface-free energy. Therefore, the natural tooth surface should be thoroughly cleaned and pretreated prior to bonding procedures to increase its surface-free energy and hence to render it more receptive to bonding.

Several, if not all, of the mechanisms of adhesion described contribute to some extent to bond strength. Glass-ionomer cement is the only restorative material that has been reported to possess an intrinsic capacity to bond to tooth tissue without any pretreatment.[2,187] Other restorative materials with adhesive potential, such as resin composites, require the application of an intermediate resin to unite the tooth substrate with the restorative material. In the case of adhesion to enamel, a resin bonding agent is bonded primarily by micromechanical interlocking with the surface irregularities of the etched substrate. A micromechanical type of bonding is also believed to occur when dentin is involved.[31,80,189,213,283] Although there is some controversy about the contribution of primary chemical bonds to the resin-tooth bond, secondary weak London–van der Waals forces may play a contributing role because of the intimate contact between the resin and tooth substrate.[83,244,248,266,298]

Parameters Affecting Adhesion to Tooth Tissue

The strength and durability of adhesive bonds depend on several factors. Important parameters may include the physicochemical properties of the adherend and the adhesive, the structural properties of the adherend, which is heterogeneous, the formation of surface contaminants during cavity preparation, the development of external stresses that counteract the process of bonding and their compensation mechanisms, and the mechanism of transmission and distribution of applied loads through the bonded joint. Furthermore, the oral environment, subject to moisture, physical stresses, changes in temperature and pH, dietary components, and chew-

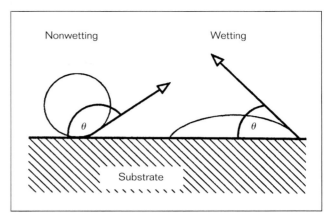

Fig 6-1 Principle of wetting measured by contact angle, θ.

ing habits, considerably influences adhesive interactions between materials and tooth tissues.[115]

Compositional and Structural Aspects of Enamel and Dentin

Because composition and structure of enamel and dentin are substantially different, adhesion to the two tooth tissues will also be quite different. The inorganic content of mature enamel is 95% to 98% by weight (wt%) and 86% by volume (vol%); the primary component is hydroxyapatite. The remainder consists of water (4 wt% and 12 vol%) and organic material (1 to 2 wt% and 2 vol%)[181] (Fig 6-2). The major inorganic fraction exists in the form of submicron crystallites, preferentially oriented in three dimensions, in which the spread and contiguous relationship of the crystallites contribute to the microscopic unit, called the *rod* or *prism*.[115,166] The natural surface of enamel is smooth, and the ends of the rods are exposed in what has been described as a keyhole pattern.[174] Operatively prepared surfaces expose rods in tangential, oblique, and longitudinal planes. Enamel is almost homogeneous in structure and composition, irrespective of its depth and location, except for some aprismatic (prismless) enamel at the outer surface,[115] in which the crystallites run parallel to each other and perpendicular to the surface.

Unlike enamel, dentin contains a higher percentage of water (12 wt%) and organic material (18 wt%), mainly type I collagen,[164] and only about 70 wt% hydroxyapatite (Fig 6-2).[181] Structurally more important to adhesion are the volumes occupied by the dentinal components. There are, combined, as much organic material (25 vol%) and water (25 vol%) as there is inorganic material (50 vol%).[181] In addition, these constituents are unevenly

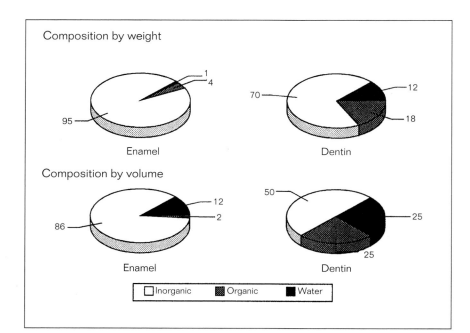

Composition by weight

95 — Enamel — 1, 4

70 — Dentin — 12, 18

Composition by volume

86 — Enamel — 12, 2

50 — Dentin — 25, 25

☐ Inorganic ▨ Organic ■ Water

Fig 6-2 Composition of enamel and dentin by weight and volume.

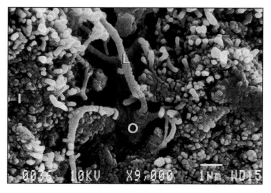

Fig 6-3 Scanning electron microscopic photomicrograph demonstrating an odontoblastic process (O) in a dentinal tubule with several lateral branches (L). (I) Intertubular dentin.

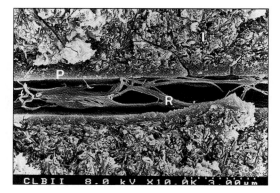

Fig 6-4 Field-emission scanning electron microscopic photomicrograph of a longitudinally fractured dentinal tubule surrounded by a collar of hypermineralized peritubular dentin (P). Note the three lateral tubule branches *(arrows)*. (I) Intertubular dentin; (R) remnants of the odontoblastic process and/or lamina limitans, exhibiting cross-banded collagen fibrils.

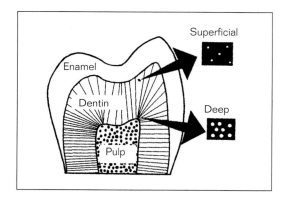

Fig 6-5 Dimension and concentration of dentinal tubules near the dentinoenamel junction (superficial dentin) and near the pulp (deep dentin). (Adapted from Heymann and Bayne.[133])

Figs 6-6a and 6-6b   Clinical views of dentin transformed by physiologic and pathologic processes.

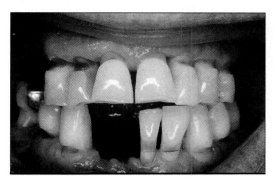

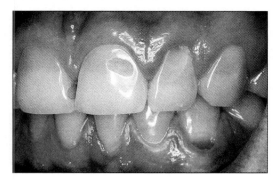

Fig 6-6a   Cervical lesions exhibiting sclerotic dentin in combined abrasive (toothbrush) and stress-induced (tooth flexure) lesions.

Fig 6-6b   Cervical lesions exhibiting sclerotic dentin in chemically induced erosive lesions.

distributed in intertubular and peritubular dentin, so the dentinal tissue is heterogeneous.

Numerous dentinal tubules radiate from the pulp throughout the entire thickness of dentin, making dentin a highly permeable tissue.[104,204] These dentinal tubules contain the odontoblastic processes as a direct connection to the vital pulp (Fig 6-3). In contrast to enamel, dentin is a vital and dynamic tissue[207,299] that is able to develop specific defense mechanisms against external injuries. The diameter of the tubuli decreases from 2.5 μm at the pulp side to 0.8 μm at the dentinoenamel junction. Likewise, the number of tubules decreases from about 45,000 per mm² near the pulp to about 20,000 per mm² near the dentinoenamel junction.[104] With an average of 30,000 tubuli per mm² in the middle part of human dentin, a considerable volume of dentin consists of their lumina. Each tubule is surrounded by a collar of hypermineralized peritubular dentin (Fig 6-4). Intertubular dentin is less mineralized and contains more organic collagen fibrils.

Because of the fan-shaped radiation of dentin tubuli (Fig 6-5), 96% of a superficial dentinal surface is composed of intertubular dentin; only 1% is occupied by fluid in the dentinal tubules, and 3% by peritubular dentin.[104,208] Near the pulp, peritubular dentin represents 66% and intertubular dentin only 12% of the surface area, while 22% of the surface area is occupied by water. Similar data demonstrate that 3% of the surface area consists of dentinal tubules in superficial dentin and 25% in deep dentin. A mean diameter of dentinal tubules ranging from 0.63 μm to 2.37 μm, depending on

depth, has been determined by using image analysis of transmission electron microscopic and scanning electron microscopic (SEM) micrographs.[168] Hence, dentin is an intrinsically wet tissue. Dentinal fluid in the tubules is under a slight, but constant, outward pressure from the pulp. The intrapulpal fluid pressure is estimated to be 25 to 30 mm Hg[281] or 34 to 40 cm water.[271]

Changes in Dentinal Structure

Dentin is a dynamic substrate subject to continuous physiologic and pathologic changes in composition and microstructure.[207,251] Dentin that has been attacked by caries or has undergone abrasion or erosion may be quite different from unaffected sound dentin (Figs 6-6a and 6-6b). Dentin undergoes *physiologic dentinal sclerosis* as an aging process and *reactive sclerosis* in response to slowly progressive or mild irritations, such as mechanical abrasion or chemical erosion.[251] *Tertiary,* or *reparative, dentin* is produced in the pulp chamber at the lesion site in response to insults such as caries, dental procedures, or attrition.[251] Hypermineralization, obstruction of tubules by whitlockite crystalline deposits, and apposition of reparative dentin adjacent to the pulp are well-documented responses to caries.[98,197] Less is known about the compositional and morphologic modifications of dentin that accompany the development of cervical abrasions and erosions.[67,68,288]

Dentinal sclerosis, or the formation of transparent, glasslike dentin, which occurs in the cervical areas of

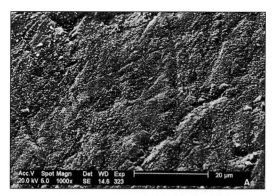

Figs 6-7a and 6-7b Scanning electron microscopic photomicrographs demonstrating heavily sclerotic dentin without exposed tubules, despite treatment with 10% citric acid. (From Van Meerbeek et al.[288] Reprinted with permission.)

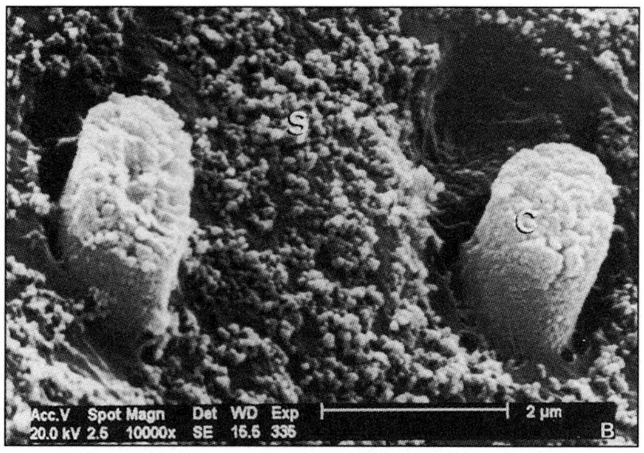

Fig 6-7b Two mineral sclerotic casts (C) extend from the tubules above the acid-etched dentinal surface, which is covered by silica particles (S) remaining from the etchant gel.[78,211]

teeth, has several common characteristics. Sclerosis is reported to result from the obstruction of dentinal tubules by apposition of peritubular dentin and precipitation of rhombohedral mineral crystals. The refractive index of the obstructed tubules is similar to that of intertubular dentin, resulting in a glasslike appearance.[68,182,300,301]

Sclerotic dentin usually contains few, if any, patent tubules, and, therefore, has low permeability[265,301] and tends to be insensitive to external stimuli.[68,288,300,301] The odontoblastic processes associated with sclerotic dentin often exhibit partial atrophy and mineralization.[95,251,299] Heavily sclerotic dentin has areas of complete hypermineralization[182,270] without tubule exposure, even when etched with an acid (Figs 6-7a and 6-7b). Some areas show abundant mineral sclerotic casts, which extend from the tubule orifices above the dentinal surface and probably represent mineralized odontoblastic processes (Fig 6-7b).

All of these morphologic and structural transformations of dentin, induced by physiologic and pathologic processes, result in a dentinal substrate that is less receptive to adhesive treatments than is normal dentin.[47,67,68,182]

The Smear Layer

When the tooth surface is instrumented with rotary and manual instruments during cavity preparation, cutting debris is smeared over the enamel and dentinal surfaces, forming what is termed the *smear layer*[76,211] (Figs 6-8a to 6-8c). The smear layer has been defined as "any debris, calcific in nature, produced by reduction or instrumentation of dentin, enamel or cementum,"[142] or

as a "contaminant"[119] that precludes interaction with the underlying pure tooth tissue. This iatrogenically produced layer of debris has a great influence on any adhesive bond formed between the cut tooth and the restorative material.[78,211]

It has been suggested that the burnishing action of the cutting instrument generates considerable amounts of frictional heat locally and shear forces, so that the smear layer becomes attached to the underlying surface in a manner that prevents it from being rinsed off or scrubbed away.[25,204,206] In an in vivo study,[175] ethylene diamine tetraacetic acid (EDTA) was found to be the most potent conditioner for removing the smear layer and opening up the orifices of the dentinal tubules. Acidic conditioners, in order of increasing potential to remove the smear layer, include citric, polyacrylic, lactic, and phosphoric acids. Cavity cleansers, such as Tubulicid (Dental Therapeutics) and hydrogen peroxide, were found to have only a slight effect.

The morphology, composition, and thickness of the smear layer are determined to a large extent by the type of instrument used, the method of irrigation employed, and by the site of dentin at which it is formed.[76,114,204,258] Its composition reflects the structure of the underlying dentin, mainly containing pulverized hydroxyapatite and altered collagen, mixed with saliva, bacteria (Figs 6-8a and 6-8b), and other grinding surface debris.[208] The thickness of the smear layer has been reported to vary from 0.5 to 5.0 μm.[76,211] Although smear debris occludes the dentinal tubules with the formation of smear plugs, the smear layer is porous and penetrated by submicron channels, which allow a small amount of dentinal fluid to pass through[212] (Figs 6-8c and 6-9). The smear layer is reported to reduce dentinal permeability by 86%.[202]

Figs 6-8a to 6-8c Field-emission scanning electron microscopic photomicrographs of the smear layer (S) covering intertubular dentin and plugging the dentinal tubules.

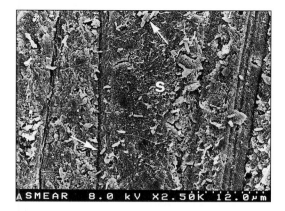

Fig 6-8a Note the bur tracks and the presence of bacteria *(arrows)*.

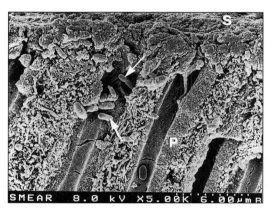

Fig 6-8b Note the presence of bacteria *(arrows)*. (P) Peritubular dentin.

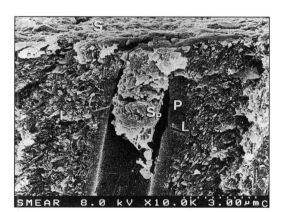

Fig 6-8c Note the smear plug (Sp). (L) Lateral tubule branch; (P) peritubular dentin; (I) intertubular dentin.

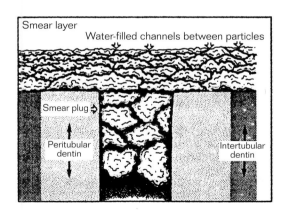

Fig 6-9 Porous smear layer with water-filled channels between the smear particles. (From Pashley et al.[212] Reprinted with permission.)

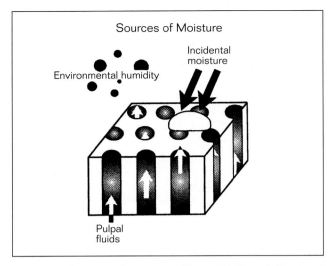

Fig 6-10 Sources of moisture. (From 3M Dental. Reprinted with permission.)

Internal and External Dentinal Wetness

The dentinal permeability and, consequently, the internal dentinal wetness depend on several factors, including the diameter and length of the tubule, the viscosity of dentinal fluid and the molecular size of substances dissolved in it, the pressure gradient, the surface area available for diffusion, the patency of the tubules, and the rate of removal of substances by pulpal circulation[203,225] (Fig 6-10). Occlusal dentin is more permeable over the pulp horns than at the center of the occlusal surface, proximal dentin is more permeable than occlusal dentin, and coronal dentin is more permeable than root dentin.[205,209] High dentinal permeability allows bacteria and their toxins to easily penetrate the dentinal tubules to the pulp, if the tubules are not hermetically sealed.[243]

The variability in dentinal permeability makes it a more difficult substrate for bonding than enamel.[207,243] Removal of the smear layer creates a wet bonding surface on which dentinal fluid exudes from the dentinal tubules. This aqueous environment affects adhesion, because water competes effectively, by hydrolysis, for all adhesion sites on the hard tissue.[66,88] Early dentin bonding agents failed primarily because their hydrophobic resins were not capable of sufficiently wetting the hydrophilic substrate.[273] In addition, bond strengths of several adhesive systems were shown to decrease as the depth of the preparation increased, because dentinal wetness was greater.[178,231,247,258,264] No significant differ-

Table 6-2 Abbreviations for chemicals used in dental adhesive technology*

AA	Acetic acid
4-AETA	4-Acryloxyethyl trimeric acid
bis-GMA	Bisphenol glycidyl methacrylate
BPDM	Biphenyl dimethacrylate
DMA	Dimethacrylate
DMAEMA	Dimethylaminoethyl methacrylate
GPDM	Glycerophosphoric acid dimethacrylate
HAMA	Hydroxyalkyl methacrylate
HDMA	Hexanediol dimethacrylate
HEMA	2-Hydroxyethyl methacrylate
HPMA	Hydroxypropylmethacrylate
MA	Methacrylate
MAC-10	11-Methacryloxy-1 1-undecadicarboxylic acid
10-MDP	10-Methacryloyloxy decyl dihydrogenphosphate
4-MET	4-Methacryloxyethyl trimellitic acid
4-META	4-Methacryloxyethyl trimellitate anhydride
MMA	Methyl methacrylate
MMEM	Mono-methacryloyloxyethylmaleat
MMEP	Mono 2-Methacryloxy ethyl phthalate
MPDM	Methacryl propane diol monophosphate
NMENMF	N-Methacryloyloxyethyl-N-methyl formamide
5-NMSA	N-Methacryloyl-5-aminosalicylic acid
NPG	N-Phenylglycine
NPG-GMA	N-Phenylglycine glycidyl methacrylate
NTG-GMA	N-Tolylglycine glycidyl methacrylate
PEG-DMA	Polyethylene glycol dimethacrylate
PENTA	Dipentaerythritol penta acrylate monophosphate
Phenyl-P	2-Methacryloxy ethyl phenyl hydrogen phosphate
PMDM	Pyromellitic acid diethylmethacrylate
PMGDM	Pyromellitic acid glycerol dimethacrylate
PMO-MA	Polymethacryloligomaleic acid
TBB	Tri-n-butyl borane
TEG-DMA	Triethylene glycol dimethacrylate
TEG-GMA	Triethylene glycol-glycidyl methacrylate
UDMA	Urethane dimethacrylate

*Adapted from Van Meerbeek et al[283] and Perdigão.[217]

ence in bond strengths is observed between deep and superficial dentin when the smear layer is left intact.[267] Bond strengths of more recent adhesive systems that remove the smear layer appear to be less affected by differences in dentinal depth,[47,233,268] probably because their increased hydrophilicity provides better bonding to the wet dentinal surface.

Besides internal dentinal wetness, external dentinal wetness, or environmental humidity, has been demonstrated to negatively affect bond strengths to dentin[97,219] (Fig 6-10). For instance, environmental humidity is affected by rubber dam use.[219] The bond strengths obtained with most adhesive systems decrease as the level of humidity in the air rises, but some systems appear to be more sensitive than others.[48,219]

Fig 6-11 Effect of polymerization contraction *(arrows)* on the resin-enamel and resin-dentin bonds when a light-curing resin composite is applied *(left)*, an autocuring resin composite *(middle)* is applied, and a light-curing resin composite is applied with an incremental layering technique *(right)* (Adapted from Davidson and de Gee,[62] Lutz et al,[165] and Imai et al.[138])

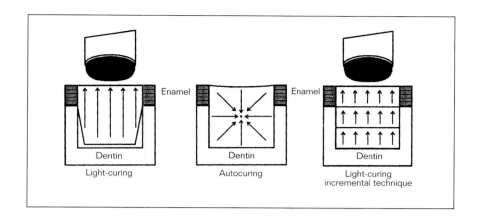

Wetting of the Adhesive

An ideal interface between dental restorative material and tooth tissue would be one that simulates the natural attachment of enamel to dentin at the dentinoenamel junction.[208] Intimate molecular contact between the two parts is a prerequisite for developing strong adhesive joints.[157] This means that the adhesive system must sufficiently wet the solid surface, have a viscosity that is low enough to penetrate the microporosities, and be able to displace air and moisture during the bonding process. The wetting characteristics of six adhesives were compared in one study, and were judged to be sufficient with contact angles of less than 15 degrees[81] (Fig 6-1). Primers in currently available systems usually contain hydrophilic monomers, such as HEMA (Table 6-2), as surface-active agents to enhance the wettability of the hydrophobic adhesive resins. In addition, solvents in modern primers, such as ethanol or acetone, assure adequate removal of air and liquid by rapid evaporation.

From polymer chemistry, it is known that polarity and solubility characterize molecular interactions that determine many physical properties, such as wetting behavior.[14,15,177] If an adhesive monomer has a polarity and a solubility similar to those of a polymer substrate, the monomer may act as a solvent for the polymer and infiltrate it. If both parameters are sufficiently different, the monomer and polymer are immiscible.[15]

Applied to dental adhesive technology, the collagen phase of dentin is a polymer and both the primer and adhesive resin contain monomers that are expected to penetrate the exposed collagen layer to form a micromechanical bond. If a given conditioner conveys to the dentinal surface a specific polarity and solubility, the primer must match these to achieve penetration. The same is true for the adhesive resin applied to the primed dentinal surface.[14,177]

Polymerization Contraction of Restorative Resins

The dimensional rearrangement of monomers into polymer chains during polymerization inevitably leads to volume shrinkage.[37,90,91] Although high filler loading of the restorative resin matrix reduces polymerization contraction, current resin composites still shrink 2.9 to 7.1 vol% during free polymerization.[90,146] Contraction stresses within resin of up to 7 MPa have been reported.[32,130]

In clinical situations, the curing contraction is restrained by the developing bond of the restorative material to the cavity walls.[153] This restriction induces polymerization contraction stress, which counteracts the developing resin-tooth bond by pulling the setting resin composite material away from the cavity walls[62,138,165] (Fig 6-11). If the weakest chain is the bonding interface with the tooth, the resin-enamel bond may survive the shrinkage, but the weaker resin-dentin interface may not.[62] No dental resin composite material that is currently available does not shrink during polymerization,[79] but research is underway to develop nonshrinking monomers. A double ring-opening polymerization process is being evaluated, which is based on high-strength expandable resin composites used in industry.[79,252]

Compensation for Polymerization Contraction

Flow

Throughout the entire polymerization process, plastic deformation, or flow, of the resin composite occurs and may partially compensate for the induced shrinkage stress.[62] This irreversible plastic deformation takes place during the early stages of the setting process, when the contraction stress exceeds the elastic limit of the restora-

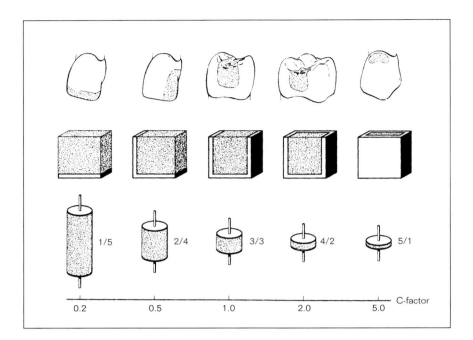

Fig 6-12 Diverse cavity configurations with different C-factors, or ratios of bonded to unbonded (free) surface, and their corresponding clinical cases. (From Feilzer et al.[89] Reprinted with permission.)

tive resin. As the setting proceeds, contraction and flow gradually decrease because stiffness increases. Fast-setting light-curing resin composites exhibit less flow-related stress relief, while self- or autocuring resin composites give the developing adhesive bond to dentin more time to survive. Only a fraction of the final stiffness is reached by most self-curing resin composites 10 minutes after mixing.[38] Consequently, the combination of a slow curing rate and rapid formation of an adhesive bond is considered favorable for the preservation of marginal integrity.[153]

The apparently superior marginal adaptation of autocuring resin composites can also be explained by the presence of air bubbles, which contribute to the amount of free surface and eventually increase the flow capacity of the resin composite.[5,92]

Restriction of flow by the configuration of the restoration, as determined by the C-factor, or the ratio of bonded (flow-inactive) to free (flow-active) surfaces, increases the contraction stress.[89] Only the free surface of a resin restoration, which is not restricted by bonding to the cavity walls, can act as a reservoir for plastic deformation in the initial stage of polymerization.[62] The higher the ratio of bonded to free resin surface, the less flow may compensate for contraction stress (Fig 6-12). In this view, a flatter and more wedge-shaped cavity design is preferred over the typical butt-joint Class 5 cavity for preserving the marginal integrity of resin composite restorations.[9,63,124]

Moreover, the use of a base material, such as glass-ionomer cement, to build up within the cavity decreases the volume of the restoration, thus generating more free restorative surface relative to the smaller amount of resin.[165] Alternatively, Bowen[34] has reported that the insertion of glass or ceramic blocks into soft resin composite before light curing, displacing as much of the resin composite as possible, results in reduced microleakage. The improvement exhibited by megafilled resin composite restorations was attributed to a decrease in the overall curing contraction of the limited amount of resin composite and a decrease in the coefficient of thermal expansion of the restoration containing the inserts.[35,65]

A prepolymerized resin composite insert technique, in which a resin composite inlay is cemented in the cavity with a luting resin composite, avoids the direct adverse effect of polymerization contraction on the developing resin-tooth bond. However, the flow-active free surface of the luting resin composite is relatively small at the narrow inlay-tooth marginal gap, yielding a high C-factor. Consequently, the luting resin composite is not likely to provide enough compensation for the shrinkage stress induced by polymerization of the luting resin composite.[89] Nevertheless, the incorporation of pores by mixing of the two components and the slow autocuring rate of the dual-cured luting resin composite, indispensable at sites inaccessible to light, such as the deep dentinal cavity wall, may still allow sufficient stress relaxation by flow.[5]

Hygroscopic Expansion

In clinical circumstances, the effect of polymerization shrinkage is also somewhat tempered by fluid absorption, which causes resin composite to swell and may offset the residual elastic stress. Again, the configuration of the cavity determines the effectiveness of this compensation mechanism.[91,154] Overcompensation may even transform contraction stress into expansion stress.

Microfilled resin composites have been shown to absorb nearly two and a half times more water than macrofilled materials, because of the greater volume of resin in the former.[8] However, hygroscopic expansion takes place during the days and weeks immediately following the placement of the resin composite restoration, after the dentin bonding may already have failed. When this has occurred, hygroscopic expansion may force a Class 5 resin composite restoration to expand beyond the margin of preparation.[154]

Elasticity

If the resin-tooth bond remains intact, the final stiffness or rigidity of a resin composite may play a compensating role in coping with remaining polymerization contraction stress. Stiffness is quantified by Young's modulus of elasticity, which represents the resistance of a material to elastic deformation.[37] The lower the Young's modulus of a restorative resin, the greater its elasticity and the more capacity it has to reduce remaining contraction stress. Resin composites with a high filler content have a higher Young's modulus of elasticity, which will reduce volumetric contraction (because of the higher filler content relative to the lower resin content), but have higher remaining contraction stress, which may affect the resin-dentin interface.

Viscous adhesive resins produce a rather thick resin bonding layer between the stiff dentinal cavity wall and the shrinking restorative resin composite. Stretching of this intermediate layer (with a low Young's modulus) may provide sufficient elasticity to relieve polymerization contraction stresses of the restorative resin composite[155,156,287] (Fig 6-13). It has been determined that a bonding layer thickness of 125 μm reduces shrinkage stresses below dentin bond strengths, so the bond is preserved.[184] A flexible intermediate resin layer may also better transmit and distribute stresses induced by thermal changes, water absorption, and occlusal forces across the interface.[287] Also, a thick adhesive resin layer permits limited inhibition of polymerization by oxygen without impairing the resin-dentin bond.[230]

Support for the elastic bonding layer concept is provided by in vitro experiments conducted with Gluma

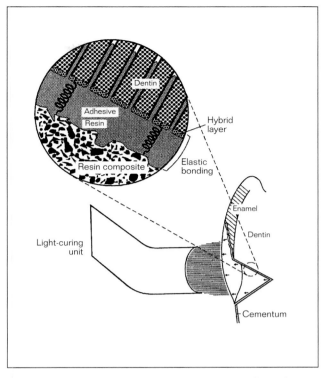

Fig 6-13 Elastic bonding area concept. Use of a relatively thick elastic adhesive may compensate for polymerization shrinkage that occurs in resin composite. Shown is an incrementally filled Class 5 resin composite restoration.

resin. When Gluma was prepolymerized in a relatively thick layer,[61,127] less microleakage occurred than when it was left uncured prior to application of the resin composite. Lack of such a built-in polymerization contraction relaxation mechanism might largely account for the high clinical failure rates recorded for Gluma, two experimental total-etch systems, and Gluma 2000.[289]

Cervical Sealing

Sealing of the cervical marginal gaps with an unfilled low-viscosity resin, after the restorative resin has been cured, is another technique to overcome the negative effects of polymerization shrinkage and obtain sealed cervical restorations.[34,152] Use of a restorative resin with high elasticity and low curing contraction in combination with such a low-viscosity resin layer may provide sufficient strain relief to deal with the small curing contraction of the unfilled resin layer.[152] However, this technique is laborious and prone to failure in the event of contamination with blood or saliva.

Initial Polymerization Site

Initiation of polymerization at the resin-tooth interface, directing the shrinking resin material toward the cavity wall rather than away from it, is advantageous.[138] Contraction occurs toward the light source in light-curing resin composites, whereas initial setting occurs in the center of the bulk of material in self-curing resin composites[165] (Fig 6-11). For both systems, tensile stresses operate across the resin composite–dentin interface, pulling the material away from the cavity walls. However, because heat accelerates the chemical reaction, Fusayama[103] argued that the initial setting of autocuring resins starts at the dentinal wall, because of the locally higher temperature of body heat, pulling the shrinking restoration toward rather than away from the cavity base. This theory, called the directed shrinkage theory, has not been substantiated, however.

For light-initiated resin composite polymerization, the unbonded resin material at the free surface of the restoration first sets when it is exposed to the light source; thus, its flow relaxation capacity is considerably diminished. The negative effects caused by light polymerization can largely be overcome by incremental layering of the resin composite material to increase the actual resin-free area relative to the resin-bonded area[125,275] (Fig 6-11). This disciplined application technique prevents the insufficient polymerization of the deepest material that may occur with bulk obturation because of the limited depth of light penetration. This technique also results in less polymerization contraction stress because the flow relaxation capacity is higher and can be used to direct polymerization shrinkage toward the cavity walls. For Class 2 resin composite restorations, the critical marginal adaptation of the gingivoproximal restoration border can be improved significantly by use of a three-sited light-curing technique with laterally light-reflecting wedges.[165]

Some adhesive systems were also designed so that resin polymerization is initiated at the surface of dentin.[11,13] For example, the simplified Gluma 2000 System attempts to impregnate the dentinal surface with an amine part of the catalytic system in the form of glycine, which is claimed to establish a chemical bond to collagen[10] (Table 6-7). Because camphoroquinone is incorporated as the other part of the catalytic system and selected methacrylic monomers, such as HEMA and bis-GMA (Table 6-2), are included in the adhesive resin, the polymerization is initiated at the adhesive interface. This simplified pretreatment technique has proved to be highly effective in reducing the marginal gap in cavities in both enamel and dentin.[12] However, several in vivo and in vitro reports on the use of amino acids have yielded contradictory results.[147,215,289]

A water-triggered polymerization has been described for the 4-META/MMA-TBB systems (Table 6-2), such as Super-Bond D Liner or Amalgambond[191] (Table 6-6). Although water and oxygen, which are omnipresent in dentin, are normally expected to affect the polymerization process of bonding agents, they may apparently also act as coinitiators of the polymerization reaction.[139] Effective water-triggered polymerization in deep, tubuli-rich dentin has been suggested to direct resin shrinkage toward the dentinal surface itself. Imai et al[138] hypothesized that the application of ferric chloride with these adhesive systems to acid-etched dentin might promote and initiate resin polymerization at the interface. More research is needed to explore these mechanisms to initiate polymerization at the interface.

Thermal Expansion Coefficient and Thermal Conductivity

Because the coefficient of thermal expansion of resin is about four times larger than that of tooth structure, any bonded resin restoration is likely to suffer from marginal gap formation.[8,227] The microfilled resin composites have a higher coefficient of thermal expansion than do hybrid-type resin composites.[37] However, Harper et al[128] suggested that the dimensional change that occurs in the clinical restoration as a result of temperature fluctuations may not be as great in magnitude as its relatively high coefficient of thermal expansion would suggest. The temperature transfer through resin composite restorations is slower and the rate of temperature change is lower than in amalgam restorations.[128] Nevertheless, marginal adaptation and microleakage studies have shown that prolonged thermocycling induces percolation under resin composite restorations.[220,227]

Transmission of Stress Across the Restoration-Tooth Interface

The adhesive bond between a restorative material and tooth has a biomechanical role in the distribution of functional stress throughout the whole tooth.[66] A true bond will transmit stress applied to the restoration to the remaining tooth structure, and bonded restorations may strengthen weakened teeth.[72,105] Displacement and bending of the cusps may compensate for the contraction stress in Class 2 posterior composite restorations,[169] but polymerization contraction may also induce cuspal fracture.[66,146,159] In general, high masticatory stresses are known to reduce the longevity of adhesively bonded restorations.[188,243]

For wedge-shaped cervical lesions, transmission of occlusal loads may affect retention of Class 5 cervical restorations. Class 5 cervical erosion and abrasion lesions have a multifactorial etiology,[39,110,159,161] including incisal or occlusal loads that induce compressive and tensile stresses at the dentinoenamel junction in the cervical region. Adhesively placed cervical restorations are subject to the same stresses,[131,132,287] which may progressively debond the resin restoration and eventually dislodge it. When resin composites with relatively low Young's moduli of elasticity, such as microfilled resin composites, are used, elastic deformation may partially compensate for the induced stress (Fig 6-14). The forces created by compression of the restoration are localized mainly in the bulk of the resin composite as compressive stress and to a lesser degree as shear stress at the adhesive interface. When more rigid, denser resin composites are placed, the shear stress at the interface might exceed the compression stress, affecting the bond of resin to dentin. Naturally, this hypothesis can only be valid when the adhesive bond is sufficiently strong. In a clinical study involving Class 5 restorations placed with diverse dentin adhesive systems, the retention rate was found to improve as the Young's moduli of the resin composites declined.[289]

A similar concept of tooth flexure has been reported by Heymann et al.[132] It has been suggested that microfilled resin composites compress rather than dislodge during tooth flexure.[22] A high correlation between the modulus of elasticity and marginal leakage was found by Kemp-Scholte and Davidson.[156] They reported that the higher the modulus of elasticity of the resin composite used, the greater the number of cervical gaps.[153] Therefore, microfilled resin composites are generally preferred for restorations in wedge-shaped cervical lesions.[152]

Biocompatibility

To the physicochemical aspects of dentin and resin composite restorative materials must be added the biologic concern of pulpal compatibility. The dissemination of residual monomer molecules to the pulp chamber via the dentinal tubules has been reported to involve a significant degree of cytotoxicity, even in low concentrations.[6] However, in vivo biocompatibility studies have demonstrated that resin composites, whether fully or partially cured, cause little pulpal irritation if the cavities are sealed to prevent ingress of bacteria from the oral environment.[58,199,250,274] Fusayama[100] has argued that the

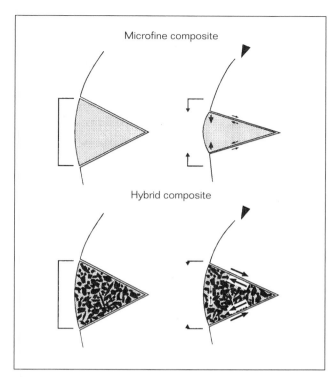

Fig 6-14 Tooth flexure concept. Microfilled resin composite flexes and absorbs some of the force, but the more rigid hybrid resin composite is more likely to be dislodged.

fundamental factor involved in pulpal irritation could also be separation of the resin from dentin (Fig 6-11). When debonding occurs, thermal and mechanical stresses on the restoration exert a pumping action on the fluid in the gap, pressing irritants or bacterial toxins into the tubules.[100,102]

Although the biological evaluation of dentin adhesive systems has received a considerable amount of attention, the results and conclusions of these biocompatibility tests widely vary and do not cover all systems. Therefore, conclusions about the influence of chemical irritants on postoperative sensitivity must still be considered premature.[243]

The use of acids on vital dentin has traditionally been avoided because of the fear of pulpal irritation, confusion over the protective function of the smear layer, and the lack in efficacy of the bonding agents.[86,101,176,224,246] Stanley et al[249] reported that acid etching of dentin causes pulpal reactions when the remaining dentin is less than 1.0 mm thick, but other histopathologic studies have shown that acid etching dentin has no adverse effects.[140,274] Fusayama stated that, in the case of carious

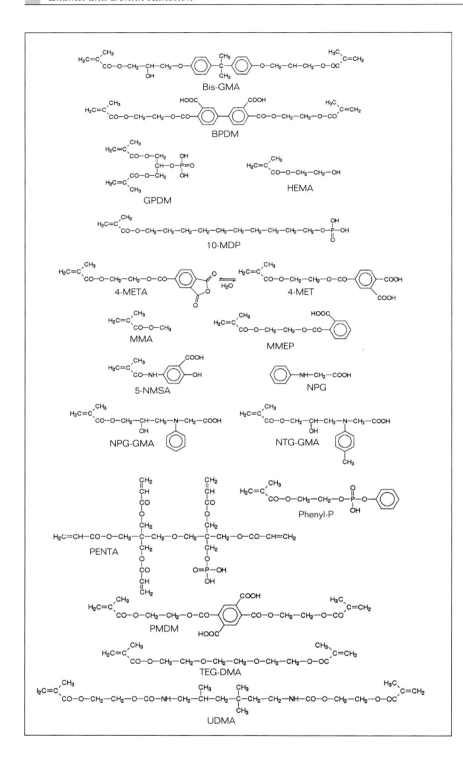

Fig 6-15 Chemical formulas of diverse monomers commonly used in dental adhesive technology.

dentin, diffusion of penetrating acid is largely limited to 10 µm, because of the blocking action of odontoblast processes in the tubules of vital teeth and intertubular crystals.[102]

Adhesion to Enamel

Enamel Acid-Etching Technique

Adhesion to enamel is achieved through acid etching of this highly mineralized substrate, which substantially enlarges its surface area for bonding. This enamel-bonding technique, known as the *acid-etching technique*, was the invention of Buonocore[43] in 1955. He demonstrated a 100-fold increase in retention of small buttons of polymethylmethacrylate to incisor teeth in vivo, when enamel was etched with 85% phosphoric acid for 2 minutes. Further research into the underlying mechanism of the bond suggested that taglike resin extensions formed and micromechanically interlocked with the enamel microporosities created by etching.[45,111,112]

Enamel etching transforms the smooth enamel surface into an irregular surface with a high surface-free energy of about 72 dynes/cm, more than twice that of unetched enamel.[145] An unfilled liquid acrylic resin with low viscosity, the enamel bonding agent wets the high-energy surface and is drawn into the microporosities by capillary attraction. Enamel bonding agents are commonly based on bis-GMA, developed by Bowen[29] in 1962, or UDMA (Fig 6-15 and Table 6-2). Both monomers are viscous and hydrophobic, and are often diluted with other monomers of higher hydrophilicity and lower viscosity, such as TEG-DMA and HEMA (Fig 6-15 and Table 6-2). The bond between enamel and the restorative material is established by polymerization of monomers inside the microporosities and by copolymerization of remaining carbon-carbon double bonds with the matrix phase of the resin composite, producing strong chemical bonds.[12] In addition, the potential for chemical interaction between specific monomers and the etched enamel surface cannot be excluded.[191]

Acid etching removes about 10 µm of the enamel surface and creates a microporous layer from 5 to 50 µm deep. Three enamel-etching patterns have been described.[113,241] These include type I, in which there is predominant dissolution of the prism cores, type II, in which there is predominant dissolution of the prism peripheries, and type III, in which no prism structures are evident (Figs 6-16a to 6-16c). Two types of resin tags have been described[21]: *Macrotags* are formed circularly between enamel prism peripheries; *microtags* are formed at the cores of enamel prisms, where the monomer cures into a multitude of individual crypts of dissolved hydroxyapatite crystals. Microtags probably contribute most to the bond strength because of their greater quantity and large surface area.

The effect of acid etching on enamel depends on several parameters[117,263]:

- The kind of acid used
- The acid concentration
- The etching time
- The form of the etchant (gel, semigel, or aqueous solution)
- The rinse time
- The way in which etching is activated (rubbing, agitation, and/or repeated application of fresh acid)
- Whether enamel is instrumented before etching
- The chemical composition and condition of enamel
- Whether enamel is on primary or permanent teeth
- Whether enamel is prism-structured or prismless
- Whether enamel is fluoridated, demineralized, or stained

An acid gel is generally preferred over a liquid because its application is more controllable.[13]

In vitro bond strengths of resin composite to phosphoric acid–etched enamel typically average 20 MPa.[19,108,118] This bond strength is thought to be sufficient to resist the shrinkage stress that accompanies the polymerization of resin composites.[63] Consequently, if the preparation is completely bordered by enamel, acid etching significantly reduces microleakage at the cavosurface interface.[60,237] Today, this enamel-etching technique has proven to be a durable and reliable clinical procedure for routine applications in modern restorative dentistry.

Complete removal of the etchant and dissolved calcium phosphates, and preservation of the clean etched field without moisture and saliva contamination are crucial to the longevity of the resin-enamel bond.[263] For this reason, isolation with a rubber dam is preferred over isolation with cotton rolls.[18]

Phosphoric Acid Etchants

Generally, use of a phosphoric acid concentration between 30% and 40%[240] (Fig 6-17), an etching time of not less than 15 seconds, and washing times of 10 to 20 seconds are recommended to achieve the most receptive enamel surface for bonding.[13,115]

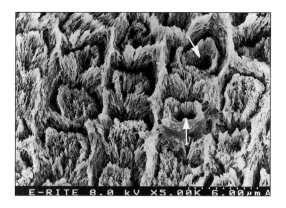

Fig 6-16a Type I enamel-etching pattern *(arrows)*. Etching of prism cores is predominant.

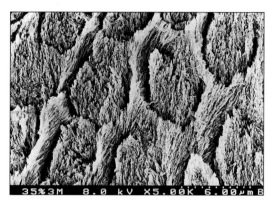

Fig 6-16b Type II enamel-etching pattern. Etching of prism peripherals is predominant.

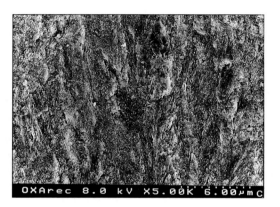

Fig 6-16c Type III enamel-etching pattern. No prism structures are evident.

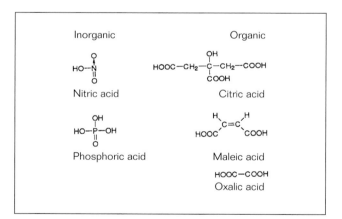

Fig 6-17 Chemical formulas of inorganic and organic acids supplied with total-etch adhesive systems.

Historically, some controversy existed about the concentration of phosphoric acid that would provide optimal etching efficacy, because some acids have been reported to form precipitates on the surface that might interfere with resin bonding.[111,151,218] One study showed that 50% phosphoric acid applied for 60 seconds on enamel produces a precipitate of monocalcium phosphate monohydrate that can be rinsed off. A precipitate of dicalcium phosphate dihydrate produced by etching with a less than 27% phosphoric acid was found not to be easily removable.[54] Calcium dissolution and etching depth increase as the concentration of phosphoric acid increases until the concentration reaches 40%; at higher concentrations, a reverse effect is obtained. Although most commercial enamel etchants have a concentration between 30% and 40%, lower concentrations are often used without compromising the enamel bond.[20,118,141,303]

The etching time has also been reduced from the traditional 60-second application with 30% to 40% phosphoric acids to etching times as brief as 15 seconds. Several laboratory and clinical studies have demonstrated bonding effectiveness to be equivalent with etching times from 15 to 60 seconds.[19,196,262]

Rinsing is important. Rinsing times of at least 15 seconds are generally required to remove dissolved calcium phosphates, which otherwise might impair infiltration of monomers into the etched enamel microporosities, from the etched surface. Recently, rinse times as brief as 1 second have been shown not to impair bond strength or promote microleakage at the enamel site.[256,257] The use of ethanol to remove residual water from the etched pattern has been reported to enhance the ability of resin monomers to penetrate the surface irregularities.[115,223] Modern primers frequently contain drying agents, such as ethanol or acetone, with a similar effect.

Alternative Enamel Etchants

Because phosphoric acid is a relatively aggressive etchant that removes substantial amounts of enamel,[303] other demineralizing agents have been tested for their etching potential. Ethylene diaminetetraacetic acid, a strong decalcifying agent, promotes only low bond strengths to enamel, probably because EDTA does not etch preferentially.[13] Pyruvic acid (10%), buffered with glycine to a pH of about 2.2, promotes high bond strengths to enamel, but has been found to be impractical because of its instability.[13]

With the introduction of total-etch systems, in which enamel and dentin are etched simultaneously, weaker acids are applied to enamel.[284] With this total-etch concept, the term *etching* is often referred to as *conditioning*, and *etchant* is referred to as the *conditioning agent*. The concentration and length of application of the conditioning agents are adapted to provide a microporous etch pattern in enamel without causing extreme demineralization of the dentinal surface. Apart from phosphoric acid, used in concentrations ranging from 10% to 40%, other inorganic acids, such as nitric acid, usually in a 2.5% concentration, have been used, as have organic acids, such as citric and maleic acids, both in a 10% concentration, and oxalic acid in a 1.6% to 3.5% concentration (Fig 6-17 and Tables 6-6 and 6-7).

Some studies have indicated that acids such as 10% phosphoric acid, 10% maleic acid, and 2.5% nitric acid etch enamel as effectively as does 37% phosphoric acid,[26,109,118,262] but data from other studies have indicated that bond strengths are significantly lower when the manufacturers' recommended application times are strictly followed.[260,277] The clinical consequences of etching enamel with weaker acids are not yet fully known, and therefore, further research concerning universal enamel-dentin conditioning agents for total-etch systems is required.[289]

A recent innovation is the use of self-etching primers, also called *condiprimers*, which serve simultaneously as conditioner and primer. The rationale behind these acidic monomer solutions is the formation of a continuum between the tooth surface and the adhesive material by the simultaneous demineralization and resin penetration of the enamel surface with acidic monomers that can be polymerized in situ. The condiprimer is applied and dispersed with air without rinsing.

One acidic monomer solution, based on a mixture of Phenyl-P, 5-NMSA, HEMA (Fig 6-15 and Table 6-2), water, and a photoinitiator, was placed on enamel for 30 seconds. The solution was found to result in bond strengths and marginal sealing efficacy equal to those obtained after the use of 40% phosphoric acid.[96,195] The acidic primer solution exhibits less demineralization of enamel than do conventional acid etchants,[195] and the resulting etch pattern differs from the one produced by conventional acids. The smear layer produced on the enamel surface is dissolved, but the outline of the enamel prisms is only slightly exposed. The grinding marks are still evident. Because this condiprimer is blown off, and not rinsed, the dissolved calcium phosphates are entrapped in the bonding resin layer. No clinical data about its enamel-bonding effectiveness are yet available, although this simplified system has recently been made commercially available as Clearfil Liner Bond 2 (Table 6-8).

Adhesion to Dentin

Successful bonding to enamel was achieved with relative ease, but the development of predictable bonding to dentin has been more problematic. Only recently have dentin adhesive systems produced laboratory results that approach those for enamel bonding,[1,47,93,94,160] and achieve a predictable level of clinical success.[71,289]

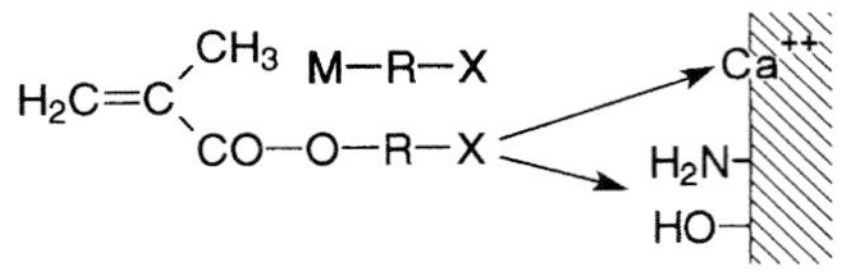

Fig 6-18 Claimed chemical bonding to inorganic and organic dentinal components. (From Asmussen and Munksgaard.[12] Reprinted with permission.)

Table 6-3 Chemical design of dentin adhesives with potential chemical bonding[*]

Potential Ca^{2+}-bonding dentin adhesives	
M-R$_1$-POYZ	Phosphate group
M-R$_2$-NZ-R$_3$-COOH	Amino acid
M-R$_3$-OH	Amino alcohol
M-R$_4$-COOH $\quad$ COOH	Dicarboxylic acid

Potential collagen-bonding dentin adhesives	
M-R$_1$-NCO	Isocyanate group
M-R$_2$-COCl	Acid chloride
M-R$_3$-CHO	Aldehyde group
M-R$_4$-CO $\quad$ COOH	Carboxylic acid anhydride

[*]M = methacrylate; R$_{1-4}$ = variable spacers; Y, Z = variable substituents. From Asmussen and Hansen.[15] Reprinted with permission.

Development of Resin Dentinal Adhesives

First-Generation Adhesives

Imitating his enamel acid-etching technique, Buonocore[44] in 1956 reported that GPDM (Fig 6-15 and Table 6-2) could bond to hydrochloric acid–etched dentinal surfaces. The bond strengths attained with this primitive adhesive technique were only 2 to 3 MPa, however, in contrast to the 15 to 20 MPa bond strengths obtained to acid-etched enamel, and the bond was unstable in water.[9] Predating the experiments of Buonocore, Hagger used the same monomer, GPDM, in the early 1950s with the introduction of Sevriton Cavity Seal (Amalgamated Dental Company), an acrylic resin material that could be catalytically polymerized by the action of sulphinic acid.[170,173]

After the failures of this early dentin–acid-etching technique, numerous dentin adhesives with complex chemical formulas were designed and developed with the objective of promoting chemical adhesion. Dentin bonding agents were no longer unfilled resins intended purely to enhance wetting of the dentinal surface prior to the application of a stiff resin composite. They became bifunctional organic monomers with specific reactive groups that were claimed to react chemically with the inorganic calcium-hydroxyapatite and/or organic collagen component of dentin[284] (Fig 6-18). The traditional concept of molecules with chemical adhesive potential is based on a bifunctional molecule with a methacrylate group, M, linked to a reactive group, X, by an intermediary group, R, or spacer[9,15] (Fig 6-18). While X is designed for reaction with and/or bonding to dentin, M allows the molecule to polymerize and copolymerize with resin composites. The spacer, R, must be of suitable length and polarity to keep the reactive groups separated.

The development of NPG-GMA (Fig 6-15 and Table 6-2) was the basis of the first commercially available dentin bonding agent, Cervident (SS White).[30] This first-generation dentin bonding agent theoretically bonded to enamel and dentin by chelation with calcium on the tooth surface and had improved water resistance.[3,36]

Second-Generation Adhesives

Clearfil Bond System F (Kuraray), introduced in 1978, was the first product of a large second generation of dentin adhesives, such as Bondlite (Kerr/Sybron), J&J VLC Dentin Bonding Agent (Johnson & Johnson Dental), and Scotchbond (3M Dental) among others. These products were based on phosphorous esters of methacrylate derivates. Their adhesive mechanism involved enhanced surface wetting as well as ionic interaction between negatively charged phosphate groups and positively charged calcium.[50,81] Although diverse chemical interactions were postulated with either the inorganic or the organic part of dentin (Fig 6-18 and Table 6-3), and are theoretically possible, primary chemical adhesion is not thought to play a major role in the bonding process.[75,79,83,84,244,245,266,286,297] The second-generation systems had modest bond strengths, seldom exceeding 5 to 6 MPa.[15] In those instances in which higher bond strengths were measured,[31,189] other bonding mechanisms that were unknown at that time were probably involved; they will be discussed later in this chapter. Clinical trials of these dentin bonding agents commonly met with poor results.[132,144,279,280,282] It was speculated that clinical failure was due to inadequate hydrolytic stability in the oral environment[82,134] and because their primary bonding was to the smear layer rather than to the underlying dentin.[302] The presence of an intermediate smear layer prevents intimate resin-dentin contact, which is a prerequisite for any chemical reaction.[157]

Table 6-4 One-step smear layer–modifying systems

Product name	Conditioner	Primer	Adhesive resin	Bonding steps*	Manufacturer
Pertac Universal Bond	—	—	carboxylic acid, MA	fgh	ESPE
Prime&Bond (no etch)	—	PENTA, TEG-DMA, elastomeric urethan-modified bis-GMA, fluoride, acetone	—	dcedce	Detrey Dentsply
Prime&Bond 2.0 (no etch)	—	PENTA, TEG-DMA, elastomeric urethan-modified bis-GMA, 2 proprietary DMA, acetone	—	dcedce	Detrey (Caulk) Dentsply
Tokuso Light Bond	—	—	MAC-10	fgh	Tokuyama Soda

The chemical abbreviations are explained in Table 6-2.

*Bonding steps: a-apply conditioner; b-rinse conditioner; c-air dry; c'-dry dentin by blot drying (wet bonding); d-apply primer; e-light cure primer; f-apply resin; g-air thin resin; h-light cure resin; i-do not cure resin; j-apply low-viscosity resin.

Table 6-5 Two-step smear layer–modifying systems

Product name	Conditioner	Primer	Adhesive resin	Bonding steps*	Manufacturer
Optec Univ. Bonding System	—	Amino acid, sodium sulfinate salt	Polycarbonate, DMA	dcfgh	Jeneric/Pentron
Pentra Bond II	—	Amino acid, sodium sulfinate salt	Polycarbonate, DMA	dcdcfgh	Jeneric/Pentrol
ProBond	—	6% PENTA, 75% acetone, 19% ethanol	56% UDMA 36% proprietary monomers, 5% PENTA, 0.7% glutaraldehyde	dcfgh	Detrey (Caulk) Dentsply
Tripton	—	0.1% polyhexanide	70% TEG-DMA, 15% UDMA, 10% MPDM, 4% aerosil	dcfgh	ICI Dental

The chemical abbreviations are explained in Table 6-2.

*Bonding steps: a-apply conditioner; b-rinse conditioner; c-air dry; c'-dry dentin by blot drying (wet bonding); d-apply primer; e-light cure primer; f-apply resin; g-air thin resin; h-light cure resin; i-do not cure resin; j-apply low-viscosity resin.

Third-Generation Adhesives

The basis for the third generation of dentin adhesives was laid when the Japanese philosophy of etching dentin to remove the smear layer gained acceptance.[99] This dentin–acid-etching technique traditionally was discouraged in America and Europe until the end of the 1980s because of concerns that acid etchants would induce pulpal inflammation.[27,59,226,249] The postulated bonding mechanism of the dentin-etching technique was that etched dentin would provide micromechanical retention for the restorative resin composite by allowing penetration of the resin bonding agent into the opened dentin tubules. However, the counterpressure of dentinal fluid and its abundant presence on the bonding site hindered the micromechanical attachment of the early hydrophobic resins.[208,273] Based on this total-etch concept, Clearfil New Bond (Kuraray) was introduced in 1984. It contained HEMA and 10-MDP (Fig 6-15 and Table 6-2), which had long hydrophobic and short hydrophilic components, as active components. The third generation adhesives are listed in Tables 6-4 to 6-7.

Removal of the smear layer by the use of acids or chelating agents reduces the availability of calcium ions for interaction with chelating surface-active comonomers, such as NPG-GMA (Fig 6-15 and Table 6-2). Bowen et al,[31] in 1982, tried to supplement the calcium

Table 6-6 Three-step smear layer–removing systems

Product name	Conditioner	Primer	Adhesive resin	Bonding steps*	Manufacturer
ABC Enhanced	2.5% nitric acid or 10% phosphoric acid	NTG-GMA, PMGDM, acetone	Bis-GMA, HDMA, DMAEMA	ac'dcfh	Chameleon
Ælitebond	10% phosphoric acid or 32% phosphoric acid	Diarylsulfone DMA, HAMA, ethanol	Bis-GMA, UDMA HAMA, Rocryl-700	abc'dcfh	Bisco Dental
All-Bond 2	10% phosphoric acid	2% NTG-GMA, 16% BPDM, ethanol, acetone	Bis-GMA, UDMA, HEMA	abc'dcfh	Bisco Dental
Amalgambond Plus	10% citric acid, 3% ferric chloride	35% HEMA, water	4-META, MMA, TBB	abcdcf	Parkell
Clearfil Liner Bond	10% citric acid, 20% CaCl$_2$	3% 5-NMSA	10-MDP	abcdcfgijh	Kuraray
Dentastic	10% phosphoric acid	NTG-GMA, PMGDM	Bis-GMA, HEMA	abcdcfh	Pulpdent
Denthesive	EDTA	Di-HEMA-phosphate, MMEM	Filled Bis-GMA	abcdcfgh	Kulzer
Experimental ESPE Bonding System	32% phosphoric acid	HEMA, HEMA-salt, water	MAC-10	abcdcfgh	ESPE
Gluma Bonding System	17% EDTA	35% HEMA, 5% glutaraldehyde	55% Bis-GMA, 45% TEG-GMA	abcdcfgi	Bayer Dental
Gluma CPS	20% phosphoric acid	35% HEMA, 5% glutaraldehyde	55% Bis-GMA, 45% TEG-GMA	abcdcfgh	Bayer Dental
Imperva Bond (total etch)	37% phosphoric acid	HEMA, 4-AETA	UDMA, 4-AETA, phosph. Bis-GMA	abcdcfh	Shofu Dental
Mirage Bond	2.5% HNO$_3$, 4% NPG	10% PMDM	Product of choice	acdcfgh	Chameleon
OptiBond (total etch)	37.5% phosphoric acid	HEMA, GPDM, MMEP, ethanol, water	Bis-GMA, HEMA, GPDM, silicate glass filler[†]	abcdcejh	Kerr/Sybron
OptiBond FL (total etch)	37.5% phosphoric acid	HEMA, GPDM, MMEP, ethanol, water	Bis-GMA, HEMA, GPDM silicate glass filler[†]	abcdcjch	Kerr/Sybron
PAAMA2	Phosphoric acid	PEGDMA	TDDDDD TEGDMA	abcdcfh	Southern Dental Industries
Permagen	10% phosphoric acid or 35% phosphoric acid	NTG-GMA, proprietary hydrophilic resin, acetone	Bis-GMA, HEMA	abc'dcfgh	Ultradent
Permaquik	35% phosphoric acid	MA-acid, ethanol	Proprietary resin	abc'dcefgh	Ultradent
Restobond 3	2.5% HNO$_3$, 4% NPG	10% PMDM	MA	acdcfh	Lee Pharmaceuticals
Scotchbond Multi-Purpose	10% maleic acid or 35% phosphoric acid	HEMA, polyalkenoic acid co-polymer, water	Bis-GMA, HEMA	abcdcfh	3M Dental
Scotchbond Multi-Purpose Plus	10% maleic acid or 35% phosphoric acid	HEMA, polyalkenoic acid co-polymer, water	Bis-GMA, HEMA	abc'dcfh	3M Dental
Super-Bond D Liner	10% citric acid, 3% FeCl$_3$	HEMA	4-META, MMA TBB	abcdcfgi	Sun Medical
Tenure S	2.5% HNO$_3$, 3.5% Al oxalate	5% NTG-GMA, 10% PMDM	Bis-GMA, HEMA	abcdcfgh	Den-Mat

The chemical abbreviations are explained in Table 6-2.

*Bonding steps: a-apply conditioner; b-rinse conditioner; c-air dry; c'-dry dentin by blot drying (wet bonding); d-apply primer; e-light cure primer; f-apply resin; g-air thin resin; h-light cure resin; i-do not cure resin; j-apply low-viscosity resin.

[†]Adhesive resin, filled with barium aluminoborosilicate glass, disodium hexafluorosilicate, fumed silica.

[‡]An unfilled or microfilled adhesive resin can be used.

Table 6-7 Two-step smear layer–removing systems

Product name	Conditioner	Primer	Adhesive resin	Bonding steps°	Manufacturer
One-Step	10% phosphoric acid	Bis-GMA, BPDM, HEMA, acetone	—	abc'dddce	Bisco Dental
Fuji Bond LC	20% polyacrylic acid 3% AlCl₃	—	Fluoroaluminosilicate glass, polyacrylic acid, HEMA, water	abcfh	GC
Gluma 2000	Oxalic acid, Al(NO₃)₃, glycine	—	NMENMF, Bis-GMA, AA	abcfgi	Bayer Dental
Prime&Bond (total-etch)	36% phosphoric acid	PENTA, TEG-DMA, elastomeric urethane-modified Bis-GMA, fluoride, acetone	—	abc'dcedce	Detrey (Caulk) Dentsply
Prime&Bond 2.0 (total-etch)	36% phosphoric acid	PENTA, TEG-DMA, elastomeric urethane-modified Bis-GMA, 2 proprietary DMA, acetone	—	abc'dcedce	Detrey (Caulk) Dentsply
Tenure Quick	37% phosphoric acid	Na-NTG-GMA		abcddci	Den-Mat

The chemical abbreviations are explained in Table 6-2.

°Bonding steps: a-apply conditioner; b-rinse conditioner; c-air dry; c'-dry dentin by blot drying (wet bonding); d-apply primer; e-light cure primer; f-apply resin; g-air thin resin; h-light cure resin; i-do not cure resin; j-apply low-viscosity resin.

ions by applying an acidic solution of 6.8% ferric oxalate to dentin as an acidic conditioner or cleanser. An insoluble precipitate of calcium oxalates and ferric phosphates was formed on the surface; the precipitate was also expected to seal the dentinal tubules and protect the pulp.[36] The subsequent application of an acetone solution of PMDM mixed with NPG-GMA or its alternative, NTG-GMA (Fig 6-15 and Table 6-2), improved bonding to levels of clinical significance.[36] Ferric oxalate sometimes caused black interfacial staining, however, and was later replaced by aluminum oxalate.[33] The microretention created by etching dentin probably contributes more to bonding than does the oxalate precipitation,[243] however, and the precipitate may, in fact, interfere with the interaction of adhesive and dentin.[213]

Extensive research in Japan has demonstrated a favorable effect of 4-META (Fig 6-15 and Table 6-2) on bonding to dentin.[189,191,192] The 4-META contains both hydrophobic and hydrophilic chemical groups. In 1982, Nakabayashi et al[189] used this system to describe the micromechanical bonding mechanism that is used by current adhesive systems. With this system, dentin is etched with an aqueous solution of 10% citric acid and 3% ferric chloride, followed by the application of an aqueous solution of 35% HEMA and a self-curing adhesive resin containing 4-META, MMA, and TBB, the last as a polymerization initiator (Fig 6-15 and Table 6-2). Based on this technology, adhesive systems

such as C&B Metabond (Sun Medical), Super-Bond D-Liner, and Amalgambond Plus are commercially available and have been reported to yield consistent results in in vitro experiments,[216,276] regardless of dentinal depth[268] (Table 6-6).

Removal of the smear layer with chelating agents such as EDTA was introduced with Gluma (Table 6-6). However, irrespective of the use of EDTA, the effectiveness of this system, as mentioned before, may have been impaired by the manufacturer's instructions to place the restorative resin composite over an uncured adhesive resin.[61,127,289] Denthesive also used EDTA to pretreat dentin prior to bonding.

Another approach to smear layer treatment was the use of Scotchprep (3M Dental), an aqueous solution of 2.5% maleic acid and 55% HEMA, followed by the application of an unfilled bis-GMA/HEMA adhesive resin (Figs 6-15 and 6-17, and Tables 6-2 and 6-8). The simultaneous etching and impregnation of the dentinal surface with this acidic hydrophilic monomer solution advanced bonding technology to a more consistent and durable result.[289] Supported by excellent clinical results in diverse clinical trials,[69,148,221] Scotchbond 2 was the first product to receive Provisional Acceptance from the American Dental Association, which was followed by Full Acceptance.[57] Other systems, such as Coltène ART Bond, Superlux Universalbond 2, and Syntac are based on this smear layer–dissolving approach (Table 6-8).

Table 6-8 Two-step smear layer–dissolving systems*

Product name	Conditioner	Primer	Adhesive resin	Bonding steps*	Manufacturer
Clearfil Liner Bond 2	—	Phenyl-P, HEMA, 5-NMSA, ethanol, water	Bis-GMA, HEMA, 10-MDP, microfiller	dcfghj	Kuraray
Coltène ART Bond	—	Maleic acid, HEMA, HPMA, PMO-MA acid, water	Bis-GMA, TEG-DMA, PMO-MA	dcfgh	Coltène
Denthesive II	—	5% maleic acid, HEMA, TEG-DMA, polymerisable poly-carboxylic acid, MMEM, water	Bis-GMA, TEG-DMA, MMEM	dcfgh	Kulzer
Imperva Bond (no etch)	—	HEMA, 4-AETA	UDMA, 4-AETA, phosphonated Bis-GMA	dcfh	Shofu Dental
OptiBond (no etch)	—	HEMA, GPDM, MMEP, ethanol, water	Bis-GMA, HEMA, GPDM silicate glass filler[†]	dcejh	Kerr/Sybron
OptiBond FL (no etch)	—	HEMA, GPDM, MMEP, ethanol, water	Bis-GMA, HEMA, GPDM silicate glass filler[†]	dcejh	Kerr/Sybron
Scotchbond 2	—	55% HEMA, 2.5% maleic acid	62.5% Bis-GMA, 37.5% HEMA	dcfgh	3M Dental
Superlux Universalbond 2	—	MA, maleic acid	Bis-GMA	dcfgh	DMG
Syntac	—	*Prim.* 25% TEG-DMA, 4% maleic acid *Adhesive* 35% PEG-DMA, 5% glutaraldehyde	60% Bis-GMA 40% PEG-DMA	dcdcfgh	Vivadent
XR-Bond	—	3.75% phosphonated DMA	60% UDMA, 30% TEG-DMA, 10% phosphonated DMA	dcefh	Kerr/Sybron

The chemical abbreviations are explained in Table 6-2.
*Bonding steps: a-apply conditioner; b-rinse conditioner; c-air dry; c'-dry dentin by blot drying (wet bonding); d-apply primer; e-light cure primer; f-apply resin; g-air thin resin; h-light cure resin; i-do not cure resin; j-apply low-viscosity resin.
[†]Adhesive resin, filled with barium aluminoborosilicate glass, disodium hexafluorosilicate, fumed silica.
*Except for Clearfil Liner Bond 2, all other systems are recommended to be used with separate enamel etching.

Fourth-Generation Adhesives

Most significant advances in adhesive dentistry have been made with the multistep dentin adhesive systems developed in the last 5 years. Essential to the enhanced adhesive capacity and responsible for the improved clinical effectiveness of today's adhesive systems is the pretreatment of dentin with conditioners and/or primers that make the heterogeneous and hydrophilic dentin substrate more receptive to bonding. A final step in the relatively complex bonding technique of modern adhesive systems involves the application of a low-viscosity adhesive resin, unfilled or semifilled, that copolymerizes with the primed dentinal surface layer and simultane-ously offers bonding receptors for copolymerization with the restorative resin composite. The term *bonding agent* no longer covers this multistep application procedure and has been replaced by *adhesive system*.

Conditioning of Dentin

Conditioning of dentin can be defined as any chemical alteration of the dentinal surface by acids or, less commonly, a calcium chelator (EDTA) with the objective to remove the smear layer and simultaneously demineralize the dentinal surface. Conditioners are most commonly

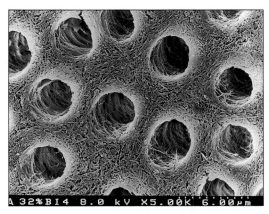

Fig 6-19a Field-emission scanning electron microscopic photomicrographs showing the effect of 32% phosphoric acid on dentin (top view). Note the microporous collagen fibril arrangement exposed by etching.

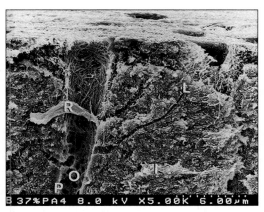

Fig 6-19b Field-emission scanning electron microscopic photomicrograph showing the effect of 37% phosphoric acid on dentin (lateral view). Intertubular dentin (I) was etched to a depth of about 2 to 3 μm. The acid penetrated the opened dentinal tubules, exposing primarily circularly oriented collagen fibrils at the dentinal tubule walls. (L) Lateral tubule branch; (O) lateral tubule branch orifice; (P) peritubular dentin; (R) remnant of odontoblastic process.

Fig 6-19c Scanning electron microscopic photomicrograph showing the effects of 10% phosphoric acid on dentin (lateral view). The effects were similar to those of 37% phosphoric acid. (I) Intertubular dentin; (L) lateral tubule; (O) lateral tubule branch orifice; (P) peritubular dentin; (R) remnant of odontoblastic process.

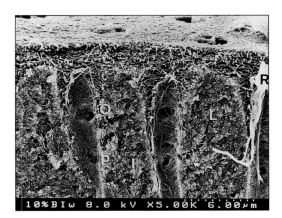

used as the initial step in the clinical application of total-etch systems and are therefore applied simultaneously to enamel and dentin. Various acids, in varying concentrations, such as citric, maleic, nitric, and phosphoric acids, are supplied by diverse adhesive systems (Fig 6-17 and Tables 6-6 and 6-8). After clinical application, these conditioners are generally rinsed off to remove any acid remnants and dissolved calcium phosphates. The only exception is the nitric acid included in ABC Enhanced; the excess etchant is blown off without rinsing. However, this procedure has been found to be unfavorable for subsequent resin infiltration.[79,217]

Besides removing the smear layer, this superficial demineralization process exposes a microporous scaffold of collagen fibrils (Figs 6-19a to 6-19c), thus increasing the microporosity of intertubular dentin.[217] Because this collagen matrix is normally supported by the inorganic dentinal fraction, demineralization causes it to collapse[254,285] (Fig 6-20). On intertubular dentin, the exposed collagen fibrils are randomly oriented and are often covered by an amorphous phase with relatively few microporosities and variable thickness (Figs 6-20 and 6-21). The formation of a relatively impermeable amorphous gel on top of the exposed collagen scaffold has been ascribed to the combined effect of denaturation and collapse of residual smear layer collagen.[79,213,285] Etchants thickened with silica leave residual silica particles deposited on the surface, but the silica does not appear to plug the intertubular microporosities[217] (Fig 6-22). Sometimes fibrous structures, probably remnants of

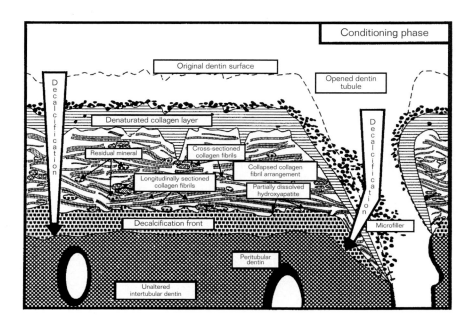

Fig 6-20 Conditioning phase of adhesive technology. (From Van Meerbeek et al.[285] Reprinted with permission.)

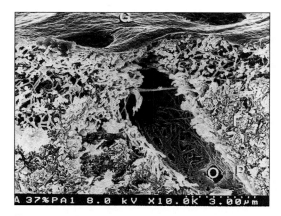

Fig 6-21a Field-emission scanning electron microscopic photomicrograph showing the formation of a residual smear gel (G) with few microporosities on top of the exposed collagen fibril scaffold.

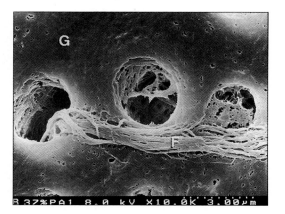

Fig 6-21b Field-emission scanning electron microscopic photomicrograph showing a fibrous structure (F), pulled out of the dentinal tubule and smeared over the surface of the smear gel (G).

odontoblastic processes, are pulled out of the tubules and smeared over the surface (Figs 6-21b and 6-23). With aggressive acid etchants, a submicron space, termed a *hiatus*, is sometimes observed at the transition between the zone of packed collagen fibrils and the unaffected dentin[217] (Fig 6-24). The cause of this hiatus has not yet been completely determined.

The depth of demineralization of the dentinal surface depends on several factors, such as the kind of acid and its application time, the acid concentration and pH, and the other components of the etchant such as surfactants, thickeners (silica versus polymer), and modifiers. Parameters such as osmolality and viscosity may also be involved in the aggressiveness of demineralization.[212,217]

The depth of demineralization also appears to be dependent on the distance between tubules. The closer the tubules, the deeper the demineralization. Because acid etching unplugs the dentinal tubules, acid is able to penetrate the tubule to a certain depth (Fig 6-20).

With increasing aggressiveness of the conditioning agent, a circumferential groove may be formed at the tubule orifice, separating a cuff of mineralized peritubular dentin from the surrounding intertubular dentin (Fig 6-22). Alternatively, the mineralized peritubular dentin may be completely dissolved to form a funnel shape. In this case, the underlying collagen network, made up primarily of circular collagen fibrils, is exposed (Fig 6-19).

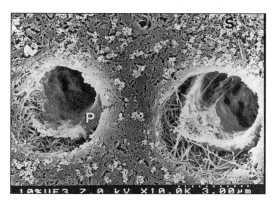

Fig 6-22 Field-emission scanning electron microscopic photomicrograph demonstrating the deposition of silica particles (S) remaining from the acid etchant on the dentinal surface. Note the preservation of a peritubular cuff (P) inside the dentinal tubule surrounded by exposed collagen fibrils.

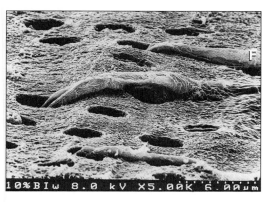

Fig 6-23 Field-emission scanning electron microscopic photomicrograph illustrating fibrous structures (F) pulled out of dentinal tubules.

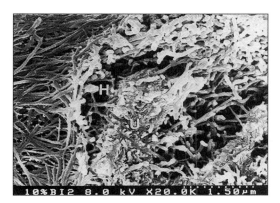

Fig 6-24 Field-emission scanning electron microscopic photomicrograph showing cross-banded collagen fibrils in the region of the dentinal tubule wall and the formation of a submicron hiatus (H) at the transition from the superficially demineralized collagen layer to the unaltered mineralized dentin (U).

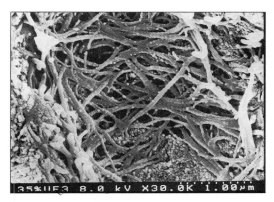

Fig 6-25 Field-emission scanning electron microscopic photomicrograph illustrating cross-banded collagen fibrils, diffusely coated with residual mineral crystals, in the wall of a dentinal tubule.

The characteristic collagen banding is most visible in the tubule wall (Figs 6-24 and 6-25).

After conditioning, maintenance of a moist dentinal surface is currently believed to be essential to optimal bonding with modern hydrophilic adhesive systems.[116,149,150,214] Desiccation of the conditioned dentin can cause collapse of the unsupported collagen web, preventing adequate wetting and infiltration of resin.[213,272] Air drying of demineralized dentin reduces its volume by 65%, but the original dimensions can be regained after reimmersion in water.[49] An appropriate amount of moisture on the dentinal surface has also been reported to promote the polymerization reaction of specific monomers.[139] The wet-bonding technique has repeatedly been reported to increase in vitro bond strengths.[116,149,150,214,259]

Clinically, a shiny, hydrated surface is seen with moist dentin. Pooled moisture should be removed by blotting or wiped off with a damp cotton pellet. Excess water might dilute the primer and render it less effective.[262] All water is then removed during the priming step by evaporation and is replaced by monomers, because water may affect resin polymerization inside the hybrid layer or at least compete for space with resin inside the demineralized dentin.[143] Alternatively, conditioned dentin may be air dried and remoistened with water or an antibacterial solution such as chlorhexidine.[126,149]

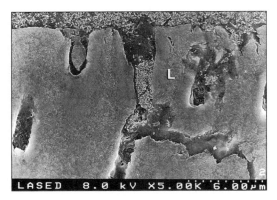

Fig 6-26 Field-emission scanning electron microscopic photomicrograph showing the surface of resin and laser-treated dentin (L). Clearfil Liner Bond System was used after preparation with a carbon dioxide laser.

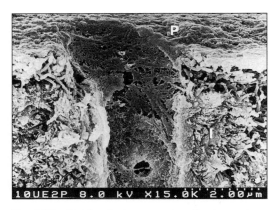

Fig 6-27 Field-emission scanning electron microscopic photomicrograph showing a dentinal surface (P) etched with 10% phosphoric acid followed by the application of Permagen primer. The primer did not plug the tubules, but the collagen fibrils appear to be coated by resin. (I) Intertubular dentin.

This demineralization process also changes the surface-free energy of dentin.[88] The high protein content exposed after conditioning with acidic agents is responsible for the low surface-free energy of etched dentin (44.8 dynes/cm), which differentiates it from etched enamel.[66] Wetting of such a low-energy surface is difficult and adhesion is hard to achieve if the dentinal surface energy is not increased by the use of surface-active promoting agents.[24]

The dentinal surface may be alternatively modified by the use of hard tissue lasers or microabrasion.[27] With laser technology, the dentinal surface is modified by microscopic explosions caused by thermal transients, increasing the bondable fraction of inorganic dentin and

micromechanical retention (Fig 6-26). Microabrasion is based on the removal of demineralized and discolored tooth tissue and results in the formation of a smear layer. It has been suggested that microabrasion may enhance the bonding capability of smear layer–mediated dentin adhesive systems. More research is needed to investigate the potential of these alternative dentinal surface treatments to enhance bonding.

Primers

Primers serve as the actual adhesion-promoting agents and contain hydrophilic monomers dissolved in organic solvents, such as acetone or ethanol. Because of their volatile characteristics, these solvents can displace water from the dentinal surface and the moist collagen network, promoting the infiltration of monomers through the nanospaces of the exposed collagen network[143] (Figs 6-19 and 6-27). Effective primers contain monomers with hydrophilic properties that have an affinity for the exposed collagen fibril arrangement and hydrophobic properties for copolymerization with adhesive resins.[88] The objective of this priming step is to transform the hydrophilic dentin surface into a hydrophobic and spongy state that allows the adhesive resin to wet and penetrate the exposed collagen network efficiently.[15,84,193,194]

2-Hydroxyethyl methacrylate, descibed as essential to the promotion of adhesion because of its excellent wetting characteristics,[193] is found in the primers of many modern adhesive systems (Tables 6-6 and 6-8). Besides HEMA, primers contain other monomers, such as NTG-GMA, PMDM, BPDM, and PENTA (Fig 6-15 and Tables 6-2 and 6-4 to 6-8). More recent primers, in All-Bond 2, OptiBond, and Clearfil Liner Bond System, also include a chemical or photopolymerization initiator, so that these monomers can be polymerized in situ. More viscous primers, such as those provided by Prime&Bond and Bisco One-Step dental adhesive, have recently been developed to combine the priming and bonding function to simplify the multistep bonding technique (Tables 6-3 and 6-7).

Primers have also been used to treat and prevent dentinal hypersensitivity.[261] Dentinal hypersensitivity is believed to be caused by pressure gradients of dentinal fluid within patent tubules that communicate with the oral environment.[41,301] Primers may induce denaturation and precipitation of proteins from the dentinal fluid and, consequently, decrease dentinal permeability and outward flow of pulpal fluid, reducing the clinical symptoms of hypersensitivity.[261]

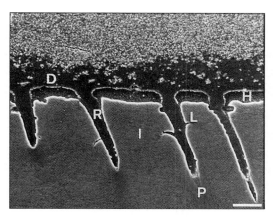

Fig 6-28a Scanning electron microscopic photomicrograph demonstrating the resin-dentin interface presented with Clearfil Liner Bond System after an argon-ion–beam etching technique.[283] (D) Dual-cured adhesive resin; (H) hybrid layer; (I) intertubular dentin; (L) lateral tubule branch; (P) peritubular dentin; (R) resin tag; (V) low-viscosity resin. Bar = 5 μm. (From Van Meerbeek et al.[285] Reprinted with permission.)

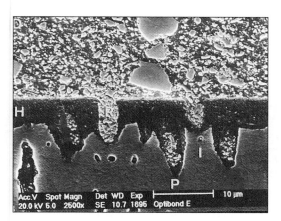

Fig 6-28b Scanning electron microscopic photomicrograph showing the resin-dentin interface presented with OptiBond after an argon-ion–beam etching technique.[283] Note the formation of particle-reinforced resin tags (R) passing through the hybrid layer (H). (D) Dual-cured adhesive resin; (I) intertubular dentin; (P) peritubular dentin.

Adhesive Resin

The adhesive resin, also called *bonding agent,* is equivalent to the enamel-bonding agent and consists primarily of hydrophobic monomers, such as bis-GMA and UDMA, and more hydrophilic monomers, such as TEG-DMA as a viscosity regulator and HEMA as a wetting agent (Fig 6-15 and Tables 6-2 to 6-8). The major role of the adhesive resin is the stabilization of the hybrid layer and the formation of resin extensions into the dentinal tubules, called *resin tags* (Figs 6-28a and 6-28b).

Adhesive resins can be light and/or autocuring. Autocuring adhesive resins have the theoretical advantage of initial polymerization at the interface by the higher temperature of the body heat,[103] but the disadvantage of being slow. For light-curing bonding agents, it is recommended that the adhesive resin be polymerized prior to the application of the restorative resin. In this way, the adhesive resin is not displaced and adequate light intensity is available to sufficiently cure and stabilize the resin-tooth bond to counteract polymerization shrinkage of the resin composite.[61,88,127] Because oxygen inhibits resin polymerization,[230] an oxygen-inhibited layer of about 15 μm will always be formed on top of the adhesive resin, even after light curing. This oxygen-inhibited layer offers sufficient double MMA bonds (Fig 6-15 and Table 6-2) for copolymerization of the adhesive resin with the restorative resin.

Clinically, brush thinning is preferred over air thinning of the adhesive resin film to prevent the film thickness from being reduced to such an extent that the air-inhibited layer permeates the resin, resulting in low bond strengths.[88,278] Furthermore, in view of the elastic bonding area concept (Fig 6-13), a sufficiently thick resin layer may absorb, by elastic accommodation, the stress induced by polymerization contraction of the resin composite.[287]

An innovative concept for relaxation of polymerization shrinkage by elastic compensation was adopted by several modern adhesive systems. Clearfil Liner Bond systems 1 and 2 provide a low-viscosity resin filled with silanated microfiller and prepolymerized filler at 42 wt%. OptiBond and Optibond FL have, respectively, a two-component dual-cured or a single-component light-cured adhesive resin that contains radiopaque, fluoride-releasing glass fillers at 48 wt% [96,287] (Fig 6-28). A filled adhesive resin is also supplied with Permaquik (Table 6-6). Also, the new glass ionomer–based adhesive system, Fuji BOND LC, provides an adhesive resin containing fluoraluminosilicate glass particles. Use of these filled adhesive resins, acting as built-in shock absorbers, has been found to result in less marginal leakage,[64] to increase bond strengths,[94] and to better retain restorations subject to occlusal stresses.[23]

Besides alleviating stress, these semifilled adhesive resins undergo less polymerization contraction. They

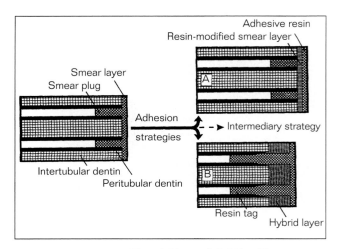

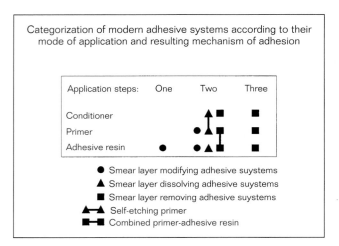

Figs 6-29a and 6-29b The two opposite adhesion strategies pursued by modern dentin adhesive systems. (From Van Meerbeek et al.[284] Reprinted with permission.)

have superior physical properties, with a compressive strength approximating that of microfilled resin composites, and a Young's modulus of elasticity closer to that of resin composites. They form particle-reinforced resin tags as anchors in the dentinal tubules (Fig 6-28). They may release fluoride to the surrounding demineralized dentin, and may provide improved esthetics by preventing the formation of a prism effect or a translucent line around the restoration's margins.[217]

Adhesion Strategies

Depending on the method of dealing with the smear layer, three adhesion strategies are currently in use with modern dentin adhesive systems[283,284] (Fig 6-29a). One strategy aims to modify the smear layer and incorporate it in the bonding process (Tables 6-4 and 6-5). The second completely removes the smear layer and concurrently demineralizes the underlying dentinal surface (Tables 6-6 and 6-7). The third adhesion strategy is a combination of these two. This system dissolves the smear layer rather than removing it and simultaneously demineralizes the underlying dentinal surface, but only superficially (Table 6-8). The currently available systems can be further subdivided into one-, two- and three-step adhesive systems (Fig 6-29b and Tables 6-4 to 6-8).

Dentin adhesives that modify the smear layer are based on the concept that the smear layer provides a natural barrier to the pulp, protecting it against bacterial invasion and limiting the outflow of pulpal fluid that might impair bonding efficiency. Efficient wetting and in situ polymerization of monomers infiltrated into the

smear layer are expected to reinforce the bonding of the smear layer to the underlying dentinal surface, forming a micromechanical and perhaps chemical bond to underlying dentin. They can be categorized in one- or two-step smear layer modifying adhesive systems when they provide solely an adhesive resin or both a primer and an adhesive resin (Tables 6-4 and 6-5). The interaction of these adhesives with dentin is very superficial, with only a limited penetration of resin into the dentinal surface (Fig 6-30).

The second adhesion strategy results in complete removal of the smear layer with acidic conditioners that are simultaneously applied to enamel and dentin utilizing a total-etch technique (Fig 6-29 and Tables 6-6 and 6-7). Their mechanism is principally based on the combined effect of hybridization and formation of resin tags. These systems are mostly applied in three consecutive steps. Because of this relatively complicated, technique-sensitive, and time-consuming clinical approach, most recent innovations are directed toward a simplified application technique by combining the primer and the adhesive resin, resulting in two-step smear layer–removing systems (Fig 6-29b and Table 6-7).

Finally, adhesive systems of the third group with an intermediary strategy provide slightly acidic primers or self-etching primers, that partially demineralize the smear layer and the underlying dentin surface without unplugging the tubule orifices (Fig 6-31 and Table 6-8). As mentioned previously, the *condiprimer* of Clearfil Liner Bond 2 contains an acidic Phenyl-P monomer and HEMA for simultaneous conditioning and priming of both enamel and dentin[195,233] (Fig 6-15 and Tables 6-2 and 6-8). Besides simplification, the rationale behind

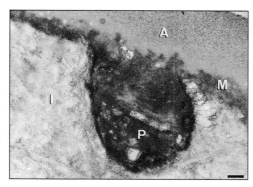

Fig 6-30 Transmission electron microscopic photomicrograph of a demineralized specimen showing the resin-dentin interface presented with ProBond. Note the formation of a superficially modified smear layer (M) and smear plug (P). (A) Adhesive resin; (I) intertubular dentin. Bar = 200 nm.

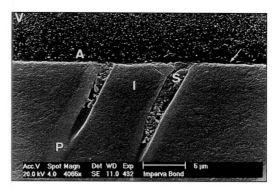

Fig 6-31 Scanning electron microscopic photomicrograph demonstrating the resin-dentin interface presented with Imperva Bond after an argon–ion–beam etching technique. Note the formation of only a slight hybrid layer *(arrow)*; the dentinal tubules remain plugged by smear debris (S). (A) Adhesive resin; (I) intertubular dentin; (P) peritubular dentin; (V) low-viscosity resin. (From Van Meerbeek et al.[283] Reprinted with permission.).

this system is to superficially demineralize dentin and simultaneously penetrate it with monomers, which can be polymerized in situ. A continuum from the unaltered dentin to the adhesive resin is created without the formation of a layer of unpolymerized hydrophilic monomers at the base of the layer of demineralized dentin, which would be highly sensitive to hydrolysis.

Hybridization

Hybridization, or the formation of a hybrid layer, occurs following an initial demineralization of the dentinal surface with an acidic conditioner, exposing a collagen fibril network with interfibrillar microporosities that subsequently becomes interdiffused with low-viscosity monomers (Figs 6-32 and 6-33). This zone, in which resin of the adhesive system micromechanically interlocks with dentinal collagen, is then termed the *hybrid layer.*

Inside the hybrid layer, three different layers have been described.[285] Depending on the adhesive system, the top of the hybrid layer consists of an amorphous electron-dense phase, such as with Clearfil Liner Bond System, that is speculated to be a zone of denatured collagen (Figs 6-32 and 6-33).[285] A more loosely arranged collagen fibril arrangement is seen with OptiBond and Super-Bond D-Liner, in which individual collagen fibrils are directed toward the adhesive resin, and the interfibrillar spaces are filled with resin (Figs 6-34 and 6-35). With Scotchbond Multi-Purpose, the hybrid layer was observed to be covered by an amorphous phase, which

may have originated in a chemical reaction of a polyalkenoic acid copolymer of the primer with residual calcium (Fig 6-36 and Table 6-6). The middle part of the hybrid layer contains cross-sectioned and longitudinally sectioned collagen fibrils separated by electron-lucent spaces (Fig 6-37). Residual mineral crystals are often found to be scattered between the collagen fibrils (Fig 6-25). The base of the hybrid layer is characterized by a gradual transition to the underlying unaltered dentin, with a partially demineralized zone of dentin containing hydroxyapatite crystals enveloped by resin (Fig 6-32b), or by a more abrupt transition (Figs 6-34 and 6-35).

This micromechanical bonding mechanism was first described by Nakabayashi et al[189] in 1982 as the formation of a resin-reinforced zone. It took researchers almost 10 years to accept this theory and to explore further details of this bonding mechanism.[79,87,213,217,285]

A number of questions remain as to which parameters are of primary importance to adhesive efficacy. First, little is known about the impact of collagen denaturation on the durability of the bond. In this respect, Nakabayashi[190] warned that denaturation of collagen by aggressive acid conditioning may cause bond failure in the long term. Evidence of such collagen denaturation was recorded by Shimokobe et al,[238] preliminarily, and by Okamoto et al,[198] when 37% and 40% phosphoric acid, respectively, were applied to demineralized dentinal collagen. Eick et al[79] related the presence of remaining cross banding of collagen fibrils inside the hybrid layer to intact undenatured collagen (Figs 6-24 and

Figs 6-32a and 6-32b Transmission electron microscopic photomicrographs of a demineralized specimen showing the resin-dentin interface produced by Clearfil Liner Bond System. (From Van Meerbeek et al.[285] Reprinted with permission.)

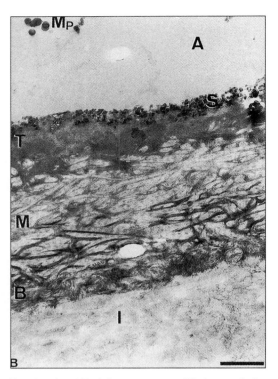

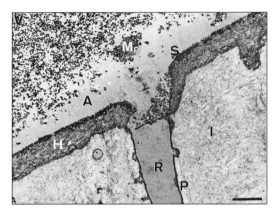

Fig 6-32a (A) Adhesive resin; (H) hybrid layer; (I) intertubular dentin; (M_P) microfiller particles of the low-viscosity resin; (P) peritubular dentin; (R) resin tag; (S) silica particles remaining from the acid etchant; (V) low-viscosity resin. Bar = 2 µm.

Fig 6-32b (A) Adhesive resin: (B) base of the hybrid layer, containing resin-enveloped hydroxyapatite crystals; (I) intertubular dentin; (M) midzone of the hybrid layer, containing cross-banded collagen fibrils separated by tunnel-like interfibrillar spaces; (M_P) microfiller particles of the low-viscosity resin; (S) silica particles remaining from the acid etchant; (T) top of hybrid layer, representing a denatured collagen smear gel. Bar = 500 nm.

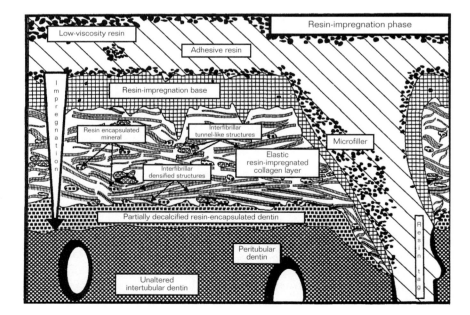

Fig 6-33 Resin-impregnation phase. (From Van Meerbeek et al.[285] Reprinted with permission.)

Figs 6-34a and 6-34b Transmission electron microscopic photomicrographs of a demineralized specimen demonstrating the resin-dentin interface produced by OptiBond.

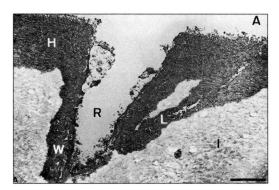

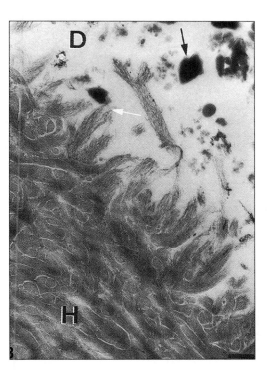

Fig 6-34a (A) Adhesive resin; (H) hybrid layer; (I) intertubular dentin; (L) hybridized lateral tubule branch; (R) resin tag; (W) hybridized tubule wall; Bar = 2 μm.

Fig 6-34b At the top of the hybrid layer (H), collagen fibrils are directed upward and appear frayed at their ends, exposing their microfibrils *(white arrow)*. At these fibril ends, crosslinks between individual collagen molecules, which are responsible for the assembly of the periodically banded collagen fibril, were probably broken during smear layer preparation and/or phosphoric acid conditioning. Note the presence of an electron lucent halo *(black arrow)* around the filler particles of the dual-cured microfilled adhesive resin (D). This halo probably represents silane, which enhances the bonding between the filler core and the resin matrix. Bar = 200 nm.

6-25). Absence of collagen banding may also indicate that the fibril structure is in a destabilized state, but not necessarily denatured to gelatin.[198,236]

Another parameter in question is the previously described formation of a relatively impermeable amorphous gel on top of the exposed collagen scaffold[79,213,217,285] that might prevent resin from fully penetrating the demineralized dentin. This gel was ascribed to the combined effect of denaturation and collapse of residual smear layer collagen.[285] A brief application of a weak sodium hypochlorite solution has been suggested to remove the gel; this has preliminarily been found to have a favorable effect on dentin bond strength.[55] Others have used sodium hypochlorite to completely dissolve and remove the collagen layer to expose the underlying pure mineralized dentin, to which adhesives could then be bonded directly.[121,290] This procedure adds another step to the already technique-sensitive and time-consuming process. Further research will be required to explore the efficacy of this approach.

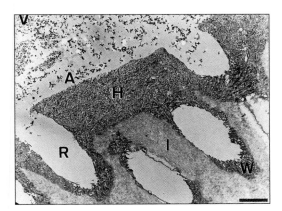

Fig 6-35 Transmission electron microscopic photomicrograph of the resin-dentin interface presented with Super-Bond D-Liner after demineralization. (A) Adhesive resin; (H) hybrid layer; (I) intertubular dentin; (R) resin tag; (V) low-viscosity resin; (W) hybridized tubule wall. Bar = 2 μm.

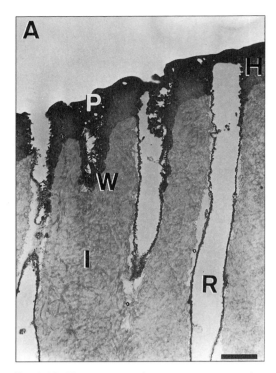

Fig 6-36 Transmission electron microscopic photomicrograph of the resin-dentin interface presented with Scotchbond Multi-Purpose after demineralization. Note the deposition of an electron-dense phase (P) on top of the hybrid layer (H). (A) Adhesive resin; (I) intertubular dentin; (R) resin tag; (W) hybridized tubule wall. Bar = 2 μm.

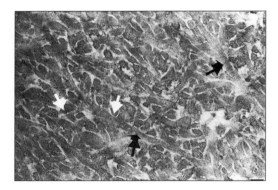

Fig 6-37 Transmission electron microscopic photomicrograph of the midzone of the hybrid layer produced by Permagen, containing cross-sectioned *(white arrows)* and longitudinally sectioned *(black arrows)* collagen fibrils with cross banding, separated by electron-lucent interfibrillar spaces. Bar = 100 nm.

Concerns have been raised that aggressive etching of dentin may cause demineralization to a depth that might be inaccessible to complete resin impregnation. If this occurred, a collagenous band at the base of the hybrid layer, not impregnated by resin, would dramatically weaken the resin-dentin bond, and, consequently, the durability of the bond.[190] Incomplete resin penetration has been described as a microporous dentinal zone at the base of the hybrid layer,[234,235] which is thought to be a pathway for nanoleakage of fluids, causing hydrolysis of collagen and shortening the longevity of the bond. Microporosities in the hybrid layer have been demonstrated by transmission electron microscopy for some of the first-generation adhesives,[79] and imperfect resin penetration has been reported for some modern adhesive systems.[79,217,266,272] Other modern adhesive systems have been reported to have completely sealed interfaces.[192,269]

Another parameter of primary importance to the strength and durability of the resin-dentin bond is the degree of polymerization conversion of resin that has infiltrated the superficially demineralized zone of dentin. Resin monomers might be able to penetrate the demineralized dentin, but, if inadequate in situ polymerization takes place, the longevity of the resin-dentin bond may be dramatically compromised. The degree of polymerization inside the hybrid layer will depend on the mode of polymerization (light-activated, or chemically activated, or both), the site of initial polymerization (interfacial or originating in the adhesive resin), and the degree of in situ available double-carbon bonds. Inadequate in situ polymerization within the hybrid layer may act as a reservoir for monomer release, and thus have cytotoxic potential.[106,107]

Finally, as mentioned before, water that is already present in the hybrid layer or introduced when a wet bonding technique is used, and residual amounts of solvents such as ethanol and acetone, if not completely evaporated, may affect resin polymerization inside the hybrid layer or at least occupy space that optimally should have been filled with resin.[143]

All of these concerns in relation to hybridization require consideration and further research, because they will eventually determine the quality of the hybrid layer and consequently the hydrolytic stability of the resin-dentin bond in the oral environment.[47]

Resin Tag Formation

Historically, the contribution of the formation of resin tag to bond strength has been a matter of speculation.[208,243,273] The finding that bond strength values drop when deeper dentin is prepared and intertubular dentin occupies less

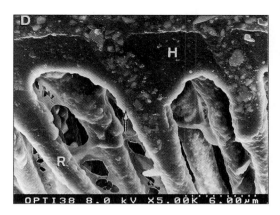

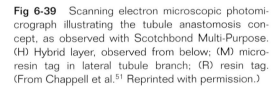

Fig 6-38a Field-emission scanning electron microscopic photomicrograph of the resin-dentin interface produced by OptiBond. The specimen was cross sectioned and subsequently polished, demineralized with hydrochloric acid, and deproteinized with sodium hypochlorite. Note the formation of particle-reinforced resin tags (R). (D) Dual-cured microfilled adhesive resin; (H) hybrid layer; *(arrow)* hybrid layer surrounding the resin tag.

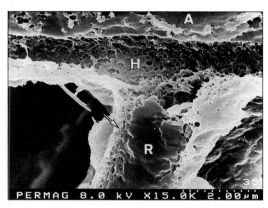

Fig 6-38b Field-emission scanning electron microscopic photomicrograph of the resin-dentin interface produced by Permagen. The specimen was cross sectioned, without polishing, demineralized with hydrochloric acid, and deproteinized with sodium hypochlorite. Note the reticular appearance of the hybrid layer (H), in which the pores may remain from collagen fibril material that was dissolved during the deproteinization step. (A) Adhesive resin; (R) resin tag; *(arrow)* hybrid layer surrounding the resin tag.

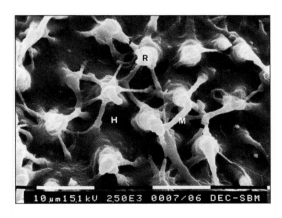

Fig 6-39 Scanning electron microscopic photomicrograph illustrating the tubule anastomosis concept, as observed with Scotchbond Multi-Purpose. (H) Hybrid layer, observed from below; (M) micro-resin tag in lateral tubule branch; (R) resin tag. (From Chappell et al.[51] Reprinted with permission.)

of the total bonding area has confirmed that the presence of intertubular dentin is more important than development of resin tags in the bonding process.[264,267]

The increased wetness of tubule-rich dentin would be expected to affect the intimate interaction of the adhesive system with the dentinal surface,[208] but the increased hydrophilicity and improved wettability of modern adhesive systems make their bond strengths less affected by the depth and wetness of dentin.[47,222,233] With the newest adhesive systems, resin tags have been observed to be intimately attached to the tubule walls with cores of resin surrounded by hybridized tubule walls (Figs 6-34a, 6-35, and 6-38). Resin even infiltrates

lateral tubule branches and hybridizes their walls, forming submicron resin tags that are attached to the walls of the lateral tubule branch (Fig 6-34a). A similar attachment of resin tags to the tubule walls through hybridization has been described to occur in vivo.[269]

The formation of submicron resin tags in lateral tubule branches has also been elegantly illustrated with the tubule anastomosis concept introduced by Chappell et al[51] (Fig 6-39). Such resin tags, which appear to adapt intimately to the inner tubule walls, probably contribute to dentin bonding.[266] In this respect, 15% of the bond strength to dentin obtained with one specific modern adhesive system was ascribed to resin tag formation.[119]

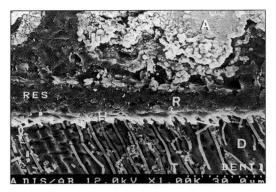

Fig 6-40a Scanning electron microscopic photomicrograph illustrating the interface of amalgam (A) and dentin (D). Note the formation of a hybrid layer (H) with resin tags when All-Bond 2 and Dispersalloy are used.

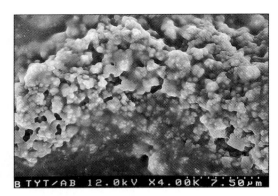

Fig 6-40b Scanning electron microscopic photomicrograph revealing the mixture of amalgam particles with resin when All-Bond 2 and Tytin are used.

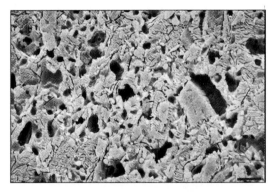

Fig 6-41 Scanning electron microscopic photomicrograph of Vita Cerec Mark-I porcelain etched with 4.9% hydrofluoric acid for 60 seconds, water sprayed, and ultrasonically cleaned. Bar = 10 μm.

Amalgam Bonding

The use of adhesive technology to bond amalgam to tooth tissue is an application of universal or multipurpose adhesive systems that has recently gained much interest. Adhesive systems such as All-Bond 2, Amalgambond Plus, Panavia, and Scotchbond Multi-Purpose Plus are advocated for bonding amalgam to enamel and dentin. The nature of the bond between resin and amalgam is yet unclear, but appears to involve at least micromechanical mixing of amalgam with resin during condensation (Figs 6-40a and 6-40b).[262] Because amalgam does not allow light transmission, these amalgam-bonding systems must have autopolymerizing capability. In vitro bond strengths of amalgam to dentin are generally less than 10 MPa, which is less than bond strengths of dentin to resin composite.[16,56,129,210] A potential problem with the incorporation of resin into amalgam is potential weakening of the mechanical properties of the bonded amalgam.[52]

The use of amalgam-bonding techniques has several potential benefits.[262] Retention gained by bonding lessens the need for removal of tooth structure to gain retention or for retentive devices such as dovetails,[28] grooves, and parapulpal pins.[53,136] Bonded amalgam may increase the fracture resistance of restored teeth,[73] and adhesive resin liners may seal the margins better than traditional cavity varnishes, with decreased risks for postoperative sensitivity and caries recurrence.[53,74,123,210] Although these amalgam-bonding techniques have also been advocated for repair of existing amalgam restorations with either resin or fresh amalgam,[255] several studies have reported poor results in strengthening of old amalgam restorations.[122,158,228]

Ceramic Bonding

Bonding resin to a ceramic surface, whether porcelain or glass ceramic, is based on the combined effects of micromechanical interlocking and chemical bonding. Porcelain and glass-ceramic surfaces are generally etched with hydrofluoric acid and ammonium bifluoride, respectively, to increase the surface area and create microporosities. The adhesive resin flows into the porosities and interlocks, forming strong micromechanical bonds (Fig 6-41).

Figs 6-42a to 6-42c Scanning electron microscopic photomicrographs of ceramic-resin interfaces. Bar = 3 µm.

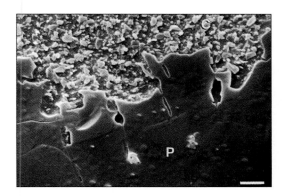

Fig 6-42a Vita Cerec Mark-I porcelain (P) was etched for 60 seconds with 4.9% hydrofluoric acid, ultrasonically cleaned, and luted with Cerec-Coltène Duo Cement.

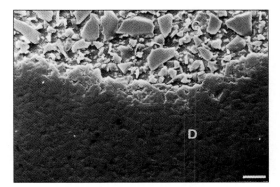

Fig 6-42b Dicor glass ceramic (D) was etched for 60 seconds with 10% ammonium bifluoride, ultrasonically cleaned, and luted with Dicor MGC. Post etching ultrasonic cleaning is necessary to remove loose and weakened crystals at the surface to prevent cohesive subsurface failure (see Fig 6-42c).

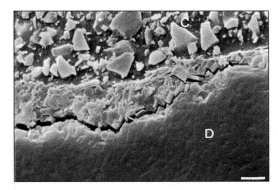

Fig 6-42c Dicor glass ceramic (D) was etched for 60 seconds with 10% ammonium bifluoride and luted with Dicor MGC (C) without ultrasonic cleaning.

Thorough rinsing followed by ultrasonic cleaning is recommended to remove any remaining acid gel, precipitates, or loose particles, which may weaken the final bond (Figs 6-42a to 6-42c). Complete drying of the etched ceramic surface can be obtained by brief immersion in a highly concentrated solution of ethanol.[229]

Chemical bonding to ceramic surfaces is achieved by silanization with a bifunctional coupling agent. A silane group at one end chemically bonds to the hydrolyzed silicon dioxide at the ceramic surface, and a methacrylate group at the other end copolymerizes with the adhesive resin (Fig 6-43). Single-component systems contain silane in alcohol or acetone and require prior acidification of the ceramic surface with hydrofluoric acid to activate the chemical reaction. With two-component silane solutions, the silane is mixed with an aqueous acid solution to hydrolyze the silane, so that it can react with the ceramic surface. If not used within several hours, the silane will polymerize to an unreactive polysiloxane[255] (Fig 6-43).

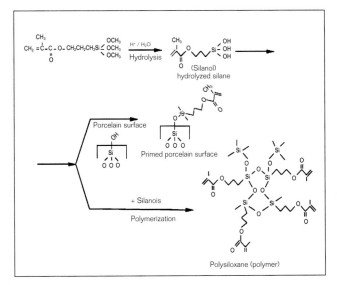

Fig 6-43 Silanization of a ceramic surface. (From Suh.[255] Reprinted with permission.)

Glass-Ionomer Cements

Conventional Glass-Ionomer Cements

Glass-ionomer cements were developed in the early 1970s by Wilson and Kent,[292,293] who combined the technology of silicate and zinc carboxylate cements (Fig 6-44). Since that time, glass-ionomer cements have undergone many improvements and modifications of their

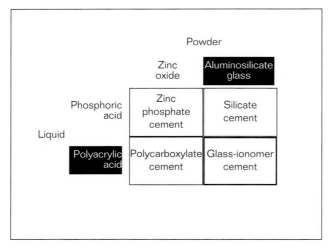

Fig 6-44 Development of glass-ionomer cements from combined technology of silicate and zinc polycarboxylate cements.

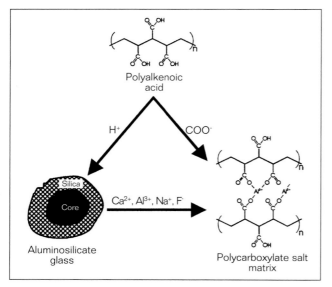

Fig 6-45 Acid-base setting reaction of conventional glass-ionomer cements.

original chemistry. Conventional glass-ionomer cements contain the ion-leachable fluoroaluminosilicate glass of the silicate cements but avoid their susceptibility to dissolution by substituting the carboxylic acids from zinc carboxylate cements for phosphoric acid.[180] As stated by McLean et al,[172] a more correct name for this type of material is *glass-polyalkenoate cement*, because chemically these cements are not true ionomers, but the term *glass-polyalkenoate cement* has never been as widely used as *glass-ionomer cement*.

The glass is high in aluminum and fluoride, with significant amounts of calcium, sodium, and silica.[239,242,295] The liquid is typically polyacrylic acid, but may contain polymers and copolymers of polyacrylic acid, itaconic, maleic, or vinyl phosphonic acid.[172,242]

The setting reaction of glass-ionomer cements has been characterized as an acid-base reaction between the glass powder and the polyacid liquid (Fig 6-45). When the powder and liquid are mixed, the fluoroaluminosilicate glass is attacked by hydrogen ions (H^+) from the polyalkenoic acid, liberating Al^{3+}, Ca^{2+}, Na^+, and F^- ions. A layer of silica gel is slowly formed on the surface of unreacted powder, with the progressive loss of metallic ions, until complete decomposition of the glass particles occurs.[46,85] When the free calcium and aluminum ions reach saturation in the silica gel, they diffuse into the liquid and cross-link with two or three ionized carboxyl groups (COO^-) of the polyacid to form a gel. As the crosslinking increases through aluminum ions and the gel is sufficiently hydrated, the cross-linked polyacrylate salt begins to precipitate until the cement is hard.

Conventional glass-ionomer cements offer several advantages over other restorative materials. They provide long-term release of fluoride ions, with cariostatic potential, and inherent adhesion to tooth tissue.[46,187,239] Because they possess a coefficient of thermal expansion closely approximating that of tooth structure and a low setting shrinkage, they are reported to provide good marginal sealing, little microleakage at the restoration-tooth interface, and a high retention rate.[46,180] They are biocompatible and have esthetic potential.[46,180]

Despite these important biotherapeutic and clinical advantages, practical difficulties have limited their clinical use.[46,135,180] The material is technically demanding and highly sensitive to changes in its water content. Early moisture contamination disrupts its surface and removes metallic ions, while desiccation causes shrinkage and crazing. Glass-ionomer cements have a short working time but a long setting time, delaying finishing of the restoration. In addition, their physical properties and esthetic potential are inferior to those of resin composites.

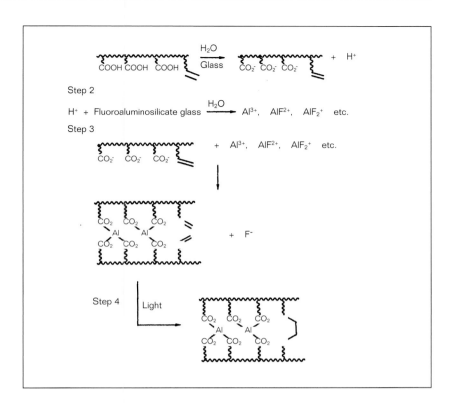

Fig 6-46 Structure of a resin-modified glass-ionomer cement and its probable setting reaction. (From Mitra.[179] Reprinted with permission.)

Resin-Modified Glass-Ionomer Cements

To overcome the practical limitations of conventional glass-ionomer cements, yet preserve their clinical advantages, conventional glass-ionomer chemistry was combined with methacrylate resin technology; this led to the creation of resin-modified glass-ionomer systems.[7,239] Often incorrectly referred to as *light-cured glass-ionomer cements,*[172,180,187] the term *dual-cured* is more appropriate, because the original acid-base reaction is supplemented by light-activated polymerization.[179,239]

Generally, these materials still have ion-leachable fluoroaluminosilicate glass in the powder, but also contain monomers, primarily HEMA (Fig 6-15 and Table 6-2), and a photoinitiator, camphorquinone, which are added to the aqueous polyacid liquid.[180,187] In the simplest form of resin-modified glass-ionomer cement, some of the water content of the conventional glass-ionomer cement is replaced by a water-HEMA mixture, while more complex formulations comprise modified polyacids with methacrylate side chains, which can be light polymerized.[239] The first setting reaction is a slow acid-base reaction, typical of conventional glass-ionomer cements (Fig 6-45). The photoinitiated setting reaction occurs much faster through homopolymerization and copolymerization of methacrylate groups grafted onto the polyacrylic acid chain and methacrylate groups of HEMA (Figs 6-15 and 6-46). With certain materials, such as Fuji II LC and Vitremer, a third polymerization initiation is claimed to occur through chemically initiated free-radical methacrylate curing of the polymer system and HEMA (Table 6-9).[46,180,262]

A diverse group of marketed materials has been placed under the term *resin-modified glass-ionomer cements* (Figs 6-47a to 6-47c and Table 6-9). The products vary from those that closely resemble conventional glass-ionomer cements to those that approximate light-curing resin composites and cure almost exclusively by light-initiated polymerization of free radicals.[46,172,262] For the latter, no or little water is present in the system to allow the acid-base reaction, typical of glass-ionomer cements.[239] A true resin-modified glass-ionomer cement, then, is defined as a two-part system, characterized by an acid-base reaction critical to its cure, diffusion-based adhesion between the tooth surface and the cement, and continuing fluoride release.[172,239]

The underlying mechanism of adhesion of glass-ionomer cements to tooth structure is thought to be an ion-exchange process, in which the polyalkenoic acid softens and infiltrates the tooth surface, displacing calcium and phosphate ions (Figs 6-48 and 6-49).[2,163,187,296] It has been postulated that an intermediate adsorption layer of calcium and aluminum phosphates and polyacrylates is formed at the glass-ionomer cement—hydroxyapatite interface.[186,239,294] A reversible breaking and reforming of calcium-carboxyl complexes in the presence of water is suggested to form a dynamic bond.[42]

Clinically, glass-ionomer cement can be used as a luting agent, as a cavity liner or base, as a core buildup material, as a direct restorative material in permanent and primary teeth, as a pit and fissure sealant, as a provisional restorative material, and as retrograde root filling material.[171,239,262]

Table 6-9 Grouping of resin-modified glass-ionomer cements according to their setting mechanism

| | | Setting mechanism | | |
		Acid-base	Visible light	Chemical
Material	Manufacturer			
Compoglass	Vivadent	☐	■	
Dyract	DeTrey Dentsply	☐	■	
Fuji II LC	GC	■	■	■
Geristore	Den-Mat	■	■	
Ionosit	DMG	■	■	
Photac-Fil	ESPE	■	■	
Variglass	DeTrey Dentsply		■	
Vitremer	3M	■	■	■

☐ Questionable

Figs 6-47a to 6-47c Scanning electron microscopic photomicrographs of resin-modified glass-ionomer cements after argon-ion–beam etching.[283]

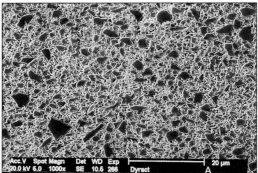

Fig 6-47a Dyract.

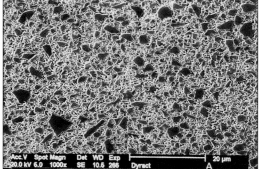

Fig 6-47b Photac Bond.

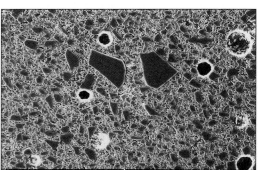

Fig 6-47c Vitremer.

Figs 6-48a and 6-48b Scanning electron microscopic photomicrographs of the resin-modified glass-ionomer cement–dentin interface.

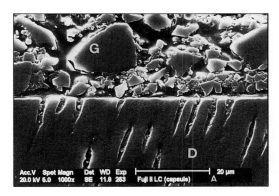

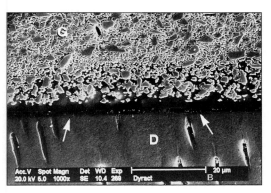

Fig 6-48a Fuji II LC. The dentinal tubules appear to be occluded by smear debris. (D) Dentin; (G) resin-modified glass-ionomer cement.

Fig 6-48b Dytract. A hybridlike structure *(arrows)* is formed and covered by an adhesive resin layer. (D) Dentin; (G) resin-modified glass-ionomer cement.

Resin-modified glass-ionomers are easier to use than conventional glass-ionomer cements. The supplementary light polymerization allows a longer working time, a rapid hardening on command, and a more rapid early development of strength and resistance against aqueous attack than are found with conventional glass-ionomer cements.[239,262] Mechanical properties, such as compressive, tensile, and flexural strengths, fracture toughness, wear resistance, fatigue resistance, bond strengths to enamel, dentin, and other resin-based restorative materials, marginal adaptation, and microleakage, are reported to be improved over the mechanical properties of conventional glass-ionomer cements.[40,46,239,262] They appear to be less sensitive to water, are radiopaque, and offer better esthetic possibilities than conventional glass-ionomer cements. The fluoride release of resin-modified glass-ionomer cements is reported to be equal to or higher than that of conventional glass-ionomer cements, and fluoride potential may even be rechargeable.[183,239] However, their physical properties are still inferior to those of resin composites. At this time, long-term clinical trials with these resin-modified glass-ionomer cements are lacking. Although the future of resin-modified glass-ionomer cements is still unclear, currently available materials appear promising.

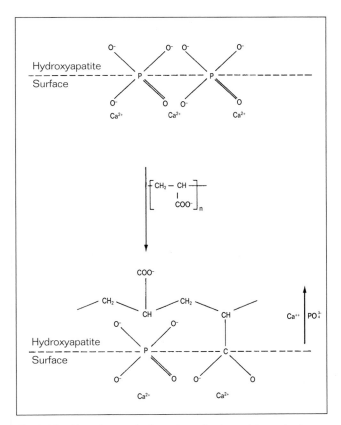

Fig 6-49 Hypothesized adsorption of polyacrylate on hydroxyapatite. (From Wilson and Nicholson.[296] Reprinted with permission.)

References

1. Abdalla AI, Davidson CL. Shear bond strength and microleakage of new dentin bonding systems. Am J Dent 1993;6:295.

2. Akinmade AO, Nicholson JW. Glass-ionomer cements as adhesives. Part I. Fundamental aspects and their clinical relevance. J Mater Science Mater Med 1993;4:95.

3. Alexieva C. Character of the hard tooth tissue-polymer bond. II. Study of the interaction of human tooth enamel and dentin with N-phenylglycine-glycidyl methacrylate adduct. J Dent Res 1979;58:1884.

4. Allen KW. Adsorption Theory of Adhesion. Theories of adhesion. In: Packham DE (ed). Handbook of adhesion, ed 1. Essex, England: Longman, 1992:39,473.

5. Alster D, Feilzer AJ, de Gee AJ, Mol A, Davidson CL. The dependence of shrinkage stress reduction on porosity concentration in thin resin layers. J Dent Res 1992;71:1619.

6. Anderson DAF, Ferracane JL, Zimmerman E, Kaga M. Cytotoxicity of variably cured light-activated dental composites [abstract 905]. J Dent Res 1988;67:226.

7. Antonucci JM, McKinney JE, Stansbury JW. Resin-modified glass-ionomer cement. US patent application, 160856, 1988.

8. Asmussen E. Clinical relevance of physical, chemical, and bonding properties of composite resins. Oper Dent 1985;10:61.

9. Asmussen E, Munksgaard EC. Adhesion of restorative resins to dentinal tissues. In: Vanherle G, Smith DC (eds). Posterior Composite Resin Dental Restorative Materials, ed 1. Utrecht, The Netherlands: Peter Szulc, 1985:217.

10. Asmussen E, Bowen RL. Adhesion to dentin mediated by Gluma: Effect of pretreatment with various amino acids. Scand J Dent Res 1987;95:521.

11. Asmussen E, Antonucci JM, Bowen RL. Adhesion to dentin by means of Gluma resin. Scand J Dent Res 1988;96:584.

12. Asmussen E, Munksgaard EC. Bonding of restorative resins to dentine: Status of dentine adhesives and impact on cavity design and filling techniques. Int Dent J 1988;38:97.

13. Asmussen E, de Araujo PA, Peutzfeldt A. In-vitro bonding of resins to enamel and dentin: An update. Trans Acad Dent Mater 1989;2:36.

14. Asmussen E, Uno S. Solubility parameters, fractional polarities, and bond strengths of some intermediary resins used in dentin bonding. J Dent Res 1993;72:558.

15. Asmussen E, Hansen EK. Dentine bonding agents. In: Vanherle G, Degrange M, Willems G (eds). State of the Art on Direct Posterior Filling Materials and Dentine Bonding. Proceedings of the International Symposium Euro Disney, ed 2. Leuven, Belgium: Van der Poorten, 1994:33.

16. Bagley A, Wakefield CW, Robbins JW. *In vitro* comparison of filled and unfilled universal bonding agents of amalgam to dentin. Oper Dent 1994;19:97.

17. Baier RE. Principles of adhesion. Oper Dent 1992;suppl 5:1.

18. Barghi N, Knight GT, Berry TG. Comparing two methods of moisture control in bonding to enamel: A clinical study. Oper Dent 1991;16:130.

19. Barkmeier WW, Shaffer SE, Gwinnett AJ. Effects of 15 vs 60 second enamel acid conditioning on adhesion and morphology. Oper Dent 1986;11:111.

20. Barkmeier WW, Erickson RL. Shear bond strength of composite to enamel and dentin using Scotchbond Multi-Purpose. Am J Dent 1994;7:175.

21. Bayne SC, Flemming JE, Faison S. SEM-EDS analysis of macro and micro resin tags of laminates [abstract 1128]. J Dent Res 1982;61:304.

22. Bayne SC, Heymann HO, Sturdevant JR, Wilder AD, Sluder TB. Contributing co-variables on clinical trials. Am J Dent 1991;4:247.

23. Bayne SC, Wilder AD, Heymann HO, Sturdevant JR, Roberson TM. 1-year clinical evaluation of stress-breaking class V DBA design. Trans Acad Dent Mater 1994;7:91.

24. Benediktsson S, Retief DH, Russel CM, Mandras RS. Critical surface tension of wetting of dentin [abstract 777]. J Dent Res 1991;70:362.

25. Berry EA III, von der Lehr WN, Herrin HK. Dentin surface treatments for the removal of the smear layer: An SEM study. J Am Dent Assoc 1987;115:65.

26. Berry TG, Barghi N, Knight GT, Conn LJ. Effectiveness of nitric-NPG as a conditioning agent for enamel. Am J Dent 1990;3:59.

27. Bertolotti RL. Conditioning of the dentin substrate. Oper Dent 1992;suppl 5:131.

28. Black GV. A Work on Operative Dentistry in Two Volumes, ed 3. Chicago: Medico-Dental Publishing, 1917.

29. Bowen RL. Dental filling material comprising vinyl silane, treated fused silica and a binder consisting of the reaction product of bisphenol and glycidyl acrylate. U.S. Patent 3066.112,1962.

30. Bowen RL. Adhesive bonding of various materials to hard tooth tissues. II. Bonding to dentin promoted by a surface-active comonomer. J Dent Res 1965;44:895.

31. Bowen RL, Cobb EN, Rapson JE. Adhesive bonding of various materials to hard tooth tissues: Improvement in bond strength to dentin. J Dent Res 1982;61:1070.

32. Bowen RL, Nemoto K, Rapson JE. Adhesive bonding of various materials to hard tooth tissue: Forces developing in composite materials during hardening. J Am Dent Assoc 1983;106:475.

33. Bowen RL, Tung MS, Blosser RL, Asmussen E. Dentine and enamel bonding agents. Int Dent J 1987;37:158.

34. Bowen RL. Bonding agents and adhesives: Reactor response. Adv Dent Res 1988;2:155.

35. Bowen RL, Eichmiller FC, Marjenhoff WA. Glass-ceramic inserts anticipated for "megafilled" composite restorations. J Am Dent Assoc 1991;122:71.

36. Bowen RL, Marjenhoff WA. Development of an adhesive bonding system. Oper Dent 1992;suppl 5:75.

37. Braem M. An In-Vitro Investigation into the Physical Durability of Dental Composites [thesis]. Leuven, Belgium, 1985.

38. Braem M, Lambrechts P, Vanherle G, Davidson CL. Stiffness increase during the setting of dental composite resins. J Dent Res 1987;66:1713.

39. Braem M, Lambrechts P, Vanherle G. Stress-induced cervical lesions. J Prosthet Dent 1992;67:718.

40. Braem MJA, Gladys S, Lambrechts P, Davidson CL, Vanherle G. Flexural fatigue limit of several restorative materials [abstract 47]. J Dent Res 1995;74:17.

41. Brännström M, Linden LA, Astrom A. The hydrodynamics of the dentinal tubule and of pulp fluid. A discussion of its significance in relation to dentinal sensitivity. Caries Res 1967;1:310.

42. Brook IM, Craig GT, Lamb DJ. Initial in-vitro evaluation of glass-ionomer cements for use as alveolar bone substitutes. Clin Mater 1991;7:295.

43. Buonocore MG. A simple method of increasing the adhesion of acrylic filling materials to enamel surfaces. J Dent Res 1955;34:849.

44. Buonocore M, Wileman W, Brudevold F. A report on a resin composition capable of bonding to human dentin surfaces. J Dent Res 1956;35:846.

45. Buonocore MG, Matsui A, Gwinnett AJ. Penetration of resin dental materials into enamel surfaces with reference to bonding. Arch Oral Biol 1968;13:61.

46. Burgess J, Norling B, Summitt J. Resin ionomer restorative materials: The new generation. J Esthet Dent 1994;6:207.

47. Burrow MF, Takakura H, Nakajima M, Inai N, Tagami J, Takatsu T. The influence of age and depth of dentin on bonding. Dent Mater 1994;10:241.

48. Burrow MF, Taniguchi Y, Nikaido T, Satoh M, Inai N, Tagami J, Takatsu T. Influence of temperature and relative humidity on early bond strengths to dentine. J Dent 1995;23:41.

49. Carvalho RM, Pashley EL, Yoshiyama M, Wang G, Pashley DH. Dimensional changes in demineralized dentin [abstract 171]. J Dent Res 1995;74:33.

50. Causton BE. Improved bonding of composite restorative to dentine. Br Dent J 1984;156:93.

51. Chappell RP, Cobb CM, Spencer P, Eick JD. Dentinal tubule anastomosis: A potential factor in adhesive bonding? J Prosthet Dent 1994;72:183.

52. Charlton DG, Murchison DF, Moore BK. Incorporation of adhesive liners in amalgam: Effect on compressive strength and creep. Am J Dent 1991;4:184.

53. Charlton DG, Moore BK, Swartz ML. *In vitro* evaluation of the use of resin liners to reduce microleakage and improve retention of amalgam restorations. Oper Dent 1992;17:112.

54. Chow LC, Brown WE. Phosphoric acid conditioning of teeth for pit and fissure sealants. J Dent Res 1973;52:1158.

55. Ciucchi B, Sano H, Pashley DH. Bonding to sodium hypochlorite treated dentin [abstract 1556]. J Dent Res 1994;73:296.

56. Cooley RL, Tseng EY, Barkmeier WW. Dentinal bond strengths and microleakage of a 4-META adhesive to amalgam and composite resin. Quintessence Int 1991;22:979.

57. Council on Dental Materials, Instruments, and Equipment. ADA Clinical Protocol Guidelines for Dentin and Enamel Adhesive Restorative Materials. Chicago: American Dental Association, 1987.

58. Cox CF, Keall CL, Keall HJ, Ostro E, Bergenholtz G. Biocompatibility of surface-sealed dental materials against exposed pulp. J Prosthet Dent 1987;57:1.

59. Cox CF. Effects of adhesive resins and various dental cements on the pulp. Oper Dent 1992;suppl 5:165.

60. Crim GA, Shay JS. Effect of etchant time on microleakage. J Dent Child 1987;54:339.

61. Crim GA. Prepolymerization of Gluma 4 sealer: Effect on bonding. Am J Dent 1990;3:25.

62. Davidson CL, de Gee AJ. Relaxation of polymerization contraction stress by flow in dental composites. J Dent Res 1984;63:146.

63. Davidson CL, de Gee AJ, Feilzer A. The competition between the composite-dentin bond strength and the polymerization contraction stress. J Dent Res 1984;63:1396.

64. Davidson CL, Abdalla AI. Effect of occlusal load cycling on the marginal integrity of adhesive class V restorations. Am J Dent 1994;7:111.

65. Donly KJ, Wild TW, Bowen RL, Jensen ME. An in vitro investigation of the effects of glass inserts on the effective composite resin polymerization shrinkage. J Dent Res 1989;68:1234.

66. Douglas WH. Clinical status of dentine bonding agents. J Dent 1989;17:209.

67. Duke ES, Lindemuth JS. Polymeric adhesion to dentin: Contrasting substrates. Am J Dent 1990;3:264.

68. Duke ES, Lindemuth JS. Variability of clinical dentin substrates. Am J Dent 1991;4:241.

69. Duke ES, Robbins JW, Snyder DE. Clinical evaluation of a dentinal adhesive system: Three-year results. Quintessence Int 1991;22:889.

70. Duke ES. Adhesion and its application with restorative materials. Dent Clin North Am 1993;37:329.

71. Duke ES, Robbins JW, Trevino D. The clinical performance of a new adhesive resin system in class V and IV restorations. Compend Contin Educ Dent 1994;15:825.

72. Eakle WS. Fracture resistance of teeth restored with Class II bonded composite resin. J Dent Res 1986;65:149.

73. Eakle WS, Staninec M, Lacy AM. Effect of bonded amalgam on the fracture resistance of teeth. J Prosthet Dent 1992;68:257.

74. Edgren BN, Denehy GE. Microleakage of amalgam restorations using Amalgambond and Copalite. Am J Dent 1992;5:296.

75. Edler TL, Krikorian E, Thompson VP. FTIR surface analysis of dentin and dentin bonding agents [abstract 1534]. J Dent Res 1991;70:458.

76. Eick JD, Wilko RA, Anderson CH, Sorenson SE. Scanning electron microscopy of cut tooth surfaces and identification of debris by use of the electron microprobe. J Dent Res 1970;49:1359.

77. Eick JD, Cobb CM, Chappell RP, Spencer P, Robinson SJ. The dentinal surface: Its influence on dentinal adhesion. Part I. Quintessence Int 1991;22:967.

78. Eick JD. Smear layer–materials surface. Proc Finn Dent Soc 1992;88(suppl 1):8.

79. Eick JD, Robinson SJ, Byerley TJ, Chappelow CC. Adhesives and nonshrinking dental resins of the future. Quintessence Int 1993;24:632.

80. Eick JD, Robinson SJ, Chappell RP, Cobb CM, Spencer P. The dentinal surface: Its influence on dentinal adhesion. Part III. Quintessence Int 1993;24:571.

81. Eliades GC, Caputo AA, Vougiouklakis GJ. Composition, wetting properties and bond strength with dentin of 6 new dentin adhesives. Dent Mater 1985;1:170.

82. Eliades GC, Vougiouklakis GJ. ^{31}P-NMR study of P-based dental adhesives and electron probe microanalysis of simulated interfaces with dentin. Dent Mater 1989;5:101.

83. Eliades G, Palaghias G, Vougiouklakis G. Surface reactions of adhesives on dentin. Dent Mater 1990;6:208.

84. Eliades G. Clinical relevance of the formulation and testing of dentine bonding systems. J Dent 1994;22:73.

85. Ellison S, Warrens C. Solid-State NMR Study of Aluminosilicate Glasses and Derived Dental Cements. Report of the Laboratory of the Government Chemist. 1987.

86. Ericksen HM. Protection against harmful effects of a restorative procedure using a acid cavity cleanser. J Dent Res 1976;55:281.

87. Erickson RL. Mechanism and clinical implications of bond formation for two dentin bonding agents. Am J Dent 1989;2:117.

88. Erickson RL. Surface interactions of dentin adhesive materials. Oper Dent 1992;suppl 5:81.

89. Feilzer AJ, de Gee AJ, Davidson CL. Setting stress in composite resin in relation to configuration of the restoratives. J Dent Res 1987;66:1636.

90. Feilzer AJ, de Gee AJ, Davidson CL. Curing contraction of composites and glass ionomer cements. J Prosthet Dent 1988;59:297.

91. Feilzer AJ. Polymerization Shrinkage Stress in Dental Composite Resin Restorations—An In-Vitro Investigation [thesis]. Amsterdam, 1989.

92. Feilzer AJ, de Gee AJ, Davidson CL. Increased wall-to-wall curing contraction in thin bonded resin layers. J Dent Res 1989;68:48.

93. Fortin D, Perdigao J, Swift EJ Jr. Microleakage of three new dentin adhesives. Am J Dent 1994;7:315.

94. Fortin D, Swift EJ, Denehy GE, Reinhardt JW. Bond strength and microleakage of current dentin adhesives. Dent Mater 1994;10:253.

95. Frank RM, Voegel JC. Ultrastructure of the human odontoblast process and its mineralization during dental caries. Caries Res 1980;14:367.

96. Fujitani M, Hosoda H, Yamauchi J. Advanced bonding system using salicylic acid derivative and phosphate monomers [abstract 1211]. J Dent Res 1992;71:667.

97. Fundingsland JW, Aasen SM, Bodger PD, Cernhous JJ. The effect of high humidity on adhesion to dentine [abstract 1199]. J Dent Res 1992;72:665.

98. Fusayama T. Two layers of carious dentin: Diagnosis and treatment. Oper Dent 1979;4:63.

99. Fusayama T, Nakamura M, Kurosaki N, Iwaku M. Non-pressure adhesion of a new adhesive restorative system. J Dent Res 1979;58:1364.

100. Fusayama T. Factors and prevention of pulp irritation by adhesive composite resin restorations. Quintessence Int 1987;18:633.

101. Fusayama T. The problems preventing progress in adhesive restorative dentistry. Adv Dent Res 1988;2:158.

102. Fusayama T. A new dental caries treatment system developed in Japan. Proc Jpn Acad 1990;66:121.

103. Fusayama T. Biological problems of the light-cured composite resin. Quintessence Int 1993;24:225.

104. Garberoglio R, Brännström M. Scanning electron microscopic investigation of human dentinal tubules. Arch Oral Biol 1976;21:355.

105. Gelb MN, Barouch E, Simonsen RJ. Resistance to cusp fracture in class II prepared and restored premolars. J Prosthet Dent 1986;55:184.

106. Gerzina TM, Hume WR. Effect of dentine on release of TEGDMA from resin composite in vitro. J Oral Rehabil 1994;21:463.

107. Gerzina TM, Hume WR. Effect of hydrostatic pressure on the diffusion of monomers through dentin in vitro. J Dent Res 1995;74:369.

108. Gilpatrick RO, Ross JA, Simonsen RJ. Resin-to-enamel bond strengths with various etching times. Quintessence Int 1991;22:47.

109. Glasspoole EA, Erickson RL. The effect of various acids on enamel: Determination, SEM, and bond strength [abstract 2281]. J Dent Res 1994;73:387.

110. Goel VK, Khera SC, Ralston JL, Chang KH. Stresses at the dentinoenamel junction of human teeth—A finite element investigation. J Prosthet Dent 1991;66:451.

111. Gwinnett AJ, Buonocore MG. Adhesion and caries prevention. A preliminary report. Br Dent J 1965;119:77.

112. Gwinnett AJ, Matsui A. A study of enamel adhesives. The physical relationship between enamel and adhesive. Arch Oral Biol 1967;12:1615.

113. Gwinnett AJ. Histologic changes in human enamel following treatment with acidic adhesive conditioning agents. Arch Oral Biol 1971;16:731.

114. Gwinnett AJ. Smear layer: Morphological considerations. Oper Dent 1984;suppl 3:3.

115. Gwinnett AJ. Interactions of dental materials with enamel. Trans Acad Dent Mater 1990;3:30.

116. Gwinnett AJ. Moist versus dry dentin: Its effect on shear bond strength. Am J Dent 1992;5:127.

117. Gwinnett AJ. Structure and composition of enamel. Oper Dent 1992;suppl 5:10.

118. Gwinnett AJ, Kanca J. Micromorphology of the bonded dentin interface and its relationship to bond strength. Am J Dent 1992;5:73.

119. Gwinnett AJ. Quantitative contribution of resin infiltration/hybridization to dentin bonding. Am J Dent 1993;6:7.

120. Gwinnett AJ. Dentin bond strength after air drying and rewetting. Am J Dent 1994;7:144.

121. Gwinnett AJ. Altered tissue contribution to interfacial bond strength with acid conditioned dentin. Am J Dent 1994;7:243.

122. Hadavi F, Hey JH, Ambrose ER, Elbadrawy HE. The influence of an adhesive system on shear bond strength of repaired high copper amalgams. Oper Dent 1991;16:175.

123. Hadavi F, Hey JH, Ambrose ER, Elbadrawy HE. Effect of different adhesive systems on microleakage at the amalgam/composite resin interface. Oper Dent 1993;18:2.

124. Hansen EK, Asmussen E. Cavity preparation for restorative resins used with dentin adhesives. Scand J Dent Res 1985;93:474.

125. Hansen EK. Effect of cavity depth and application technique on marginal adaptation of resins in dentin cavities. J Dent Res 1986;65:1319.

126. Hansen EK. In vivo cusp fracture of endodontically treated premolars restored with MOD amalgam or MOD resin fillings. Dent Mater 1988;4:169.

127. Hansen SE, Swift EJ. Microleakage with Gluma: Effects of unfilled resin polymerization and storage time. Am J Dent 1989;2:266.

128. Harper RH, Schnell RJ, Swartz ML, Phillips RW. In vivo measurements of thermal diffusion through restorations of various materials. J Prosthet Dent 1980;43:180.

129. Hasegawa T, Retief DH, Russell CM, Denys FR. A laboratory study of the Amalgambond Adhesive System. Am J Dent 1992;5:181.

130. Hegdahl T, Gjerdet NR. Contraction stresses of composite filling materials. Acta Odontol Scand 1987;35:191.

131. Heymann HO, Sturdevant JR, Brunson WD, Wilder AD, Sluder TB, Bayne SC. Twelve-month clinical study of dentinal adhesives in Class V cervical lesions. J Am Dent Assoc 1988;116:179.

132. Heymann HO, Sturdevant JR, Bayne S, Wilder AD, Sluder TB, Brunson WD. Examining tooth flexure effects on cervical restorations: A two-year clinical study. J Am Dent Assoc 1991;122:41.

133. Heymann HO, Bayne SC. Current concepts in dentin bonding: Focusing on dentinal adhesion factors. J Am Dent Assoc 1993;124:27.

134. Huang GT, Söderholm K-JM. In vitro investigation of shear bond strength of a phosphate based dentinal bonding agent. Scand J Dent Res 1989;97:84.

135. Hunt PR (ed). Glass Ionomers: The Next Generation. Proceedings of the 2nd International Symposium on Glass Ionomers. Philadelphia: International Symposia in Dentistry, 1994.

136. Ianzano JA, Mastrodomenico J, Gwinnett AJ. Strength of amalgam restorations bonded with Amalgambond. Am J Dent 1993;6:10.

137. Ibsen R, Ouellet D, Strassler H. Clinically successful dentin and enamel bonding. Am J Dent 1991;2:125.

138. Imai Y, Kadoma Y, Kojima K, Akimoto T, Ikakura K, Ohta T. Importance of polymerization initiator systems and interfacial initiation of polymerization in adhesive bonding of resin to dentin. J Dent Res 1991;70:1088.

139. Imai Y, Suzuki A. Effects of water and carboxylic acid monomer on polymerization of HEMA in the presence of N-phenylglycine. Dent Mater 1994;10:275.

140. Inokoshi S, Iwaku M, Fusayama T. Pulp response to a new adhesive restorative resin. J Dent Res 1982;61:1014.

141. Inoue M, Finger WJ, Mueller M. Effect of filler content of restorative resins on retentive strength to acid-conditioned enamel. Am J Dent 1994;7:161.

142. Ishioka S, Caputo AA. Interaction between the dentinal smear layer and composite bond strengths. J Prosthet Dent 1989;61:180.

143. Jacobsen T, Ma R, Söderholm K-J. Dentin bonding through interpenetrating network formation. Trans Acad Dent Mater 1994;7:45.

144. Jendresen MD. Clinical performance of a new composite resin for class V erosion [abstract 1057]. J Dent Res 1978;57:339.

145. Jendresen MD, Glantz P-O. Microtopography and clinical adhesiveness of an acid etched tooth surface. Acta Odontol Scand 1981;39:47.

146. Jensen ME, Chan DCN. Polymerization shrinkage and microleakage. In: Vanherle G, Smith DC (eds). Posterior Composite Resin Dental Restorative Materials, ed 1. Utrecht, The Netherlands: Szulc, 1985:243.

147. Jordan RE, Suzuki M, MacLean DF. Early clinical evaluation of Tenure and Scotchbond 2 for conservative restoration of cervical erosion lesions. J Esthet Dent 1989;1:10.

148. Jordan RE, Suzuki M, Davidson DF. Clinical evaluation of a universal dentin bonding resin: Preserving dentition through new materials. J Am Dent Assoc 1993;124:71.

149. Kanca J III. Effect of resin primer solvent and surface wetness on resin composite bond strength to dentin. Am J Dent 1992;5:213.

150. Kanca J III. Resin bonding to wet substrate. I. Bonding to dentin. Quintessence Int 1992;23:39.

151. Kellar M, Duke ES. Neutralizing phosphoric acid in the acid etch resin technique. J Oral Rehabil 1988;15:625.

152. Kemp-Scholte CM, Davidson CL. Marginal sealing of curing contraction gaps in class V composite resin restorations. J Dent Res 1988;67:841.

153. Kemp-Scholte CM. The Marginal Integrity of Cervical Composite Resin Restorations [thesis]. Amsterdam, 1989.

154. Kemp-Scholte CM, Davidson CL. Overhang of Class V composite resin restorations from hygroscopic expansion. Quintessence Int 1989;20:551.

155. Kemp-Scholte CM, Davidson CL. Complete marginal seal of class V resin composite restorations effected by increased flexibility. J Dent Res 1990;69:1240.

156. Kemp-Scholte CM, Davidson CL. Marginal integrity related to bond strength and strain capacity of composite resin restorative systems. J Prosthet Dent 1990;64:658.

157. Kinloch AJ. Adhesion and Adhesives. Science and Technology, ed 1. London: Chapman and Hall, 1987.

158. Lacy AM, Rupprecht R, Watanabe L. Use of self-curing composite resins to facilitate amalgam repair. Quintessence Int 1992;23:53.

159. Lambrechts P, Braem M, Vanherle G. Evaluation of clinical performance for posterior composite resins and dentin adhesives. Oper Dent 1987;12:53.

160. Lee S-Y, Greener EH, Mueller HJ, Chiu C-H. Effect of food and oral simulating fluids on dentine bond and composite strength. J Dent 1994;22:352.

161. Lee WC, Eakle WS. Possible role of tensile stress in the etiology of cervical erosive lesions of teeth. J Prosthet Dent 1984;52:374.

162. Leinfelder KF. After amalgam, what? Other materials fall short. J Am Dent Assoc 1994;125:586.

163. Lin A, McIntyre NS, Davidson RD. Studies on the adhesion of glass ionomer cements to dentin. J Dent Res 1992;71:1836.

164. Linde A. The extracellular matrix of the dental pulp and dentin. J Dent Res 1985;64:523.

165. Lutz F, Krejci I, Oldenburg TR. Elimination of polymerization stresses at the margins of posterior composite resin restorations: A new restorative technique. Quintessence Int 1986;17:659.

166. Lyon D, Darling AI. Orientation of the crystallites in human dental enamel. Br Dent J 1957;102:483.

167. Mackert JR. Dental Amalgam and mercury. J Am Dent Assoc 1991;122:54.

168. Marchetti C, Piacentini C, Menghini P. Morphometric computerized analysis on the dentinal tubules and the collagen fibers in the dentine of human permanent teeth. Bull Group Int Rech Sci Stomatol Odontol 1992;35:125.

169. McCullock AJ, Smith BGN. In vitro studies of cuspal movement produced by adhesive restorative materials. Br Dent J 1986;161:405.

170. McLean JW, Kramer IRH. A clinical and pathological evaluation of a sulphinic acid activated resin for use in restorative dentistry. Br Dent J 1952;93:255.

171. McLean JW. Clinical applications of glass-ionomer cements. Oper Dent 1992;suppl 5:184.

172. McLean JW, Nicholson JW, Wilson AD. Proposed nomenclature for glass-ionomer dental cements and related materials [guest editorial]. Quintessence Int 1994;25:587.

173. McLean JW. Bonding to enamel and dentin [letter]. Quintessence Int 1995;26:234.

174. Meckel AH, Grebstein WJ, Neal RJ. Structure of mature human enamel as observed by electron microscopy. Arch Oral Biol 1965;10:775.

175. Meryon SD, Tobias RS, Jakeman KJ. Smear removal agents: A quantitative study in vivo and in vitro. J Prosthet Dent 1987;57:174.

176. Michelich V, Schuster GS, Pashley DH. Bacterial penetration of human dentin, in vitro. J Dent Res 1980;59:1398.

177. Miller RG, Bowles CQ, Chappelow CC, Eick JD. Solubility parameters and dentin bonding agents. J Biomed Mater Res (in press).

178. Mitchem JC, Gronas DG. Effects of time after extraction and depth of dentin on resin dentin adhesives. J Am Dent Assoc 1986;113:285.

179. Mitra SB. Adhesion to dentin and physical properties of a light-cured glass-ionomer liner/base. J Dent Res 1991;70:72.

180. Mitra S. Curing reactions of glass ionomer materials. In: Hunt PR (ed). Glass Ionomers: The Next Generation. Proceedings of the 2nd International Symposium on Glass Ionomers. Philadelphia: International Symposia in Dentistry, 1994:13.

181. Mjör IA, Fejerskov O (eds). Human Oral Embryology and Histology, ed 1. Copenhagen: Munksgaard, 1986.

182. Mjör I. Reaction patterns of dentin. In: Thylstrup A, Leach SA, Qvist V (eds). Dentine and Dentine Reactions in the Oral Cavity. Oxford, England: IRL Press, 1987:27.

183. Momoi Y, McCabe JF. Fluoride release from light-activated glass ionomer restorative cements. Dent Mater 1993;9:151.

184. Moon PC, Chang YH. Effect of DBA layer thickness on composite resin shrinkage stress [abstract 1357]. J Dent Res 1992;71:275.

185. Morin D, DeLong R, Douglas WH. Cusp reinforcement by the acid-etch technique. J Dent Res 1984;63:1075.

186. Mount GJ. An Atlas of Glass-Ionomer Cements. London: Martin Dunitz, 1990.

187. Mount GJ. Glass-ionomer cements: Past, present and future. Oper Dent 1994;19:82.

188. Munksgaard EC, Itoh K, Jorgensen KD. Dentin-polymer bond in resin fillings tested in vitro by thermo- and load-cycling. J Dent Res 1985;64:144.

189. Nakabayashi N, Kojima K, Masuhara E. The promotion of adhesion by the infiltration of monomers into tooth substrates. J Biomed Mater Res 1982;16:265.

190. Nakabayashi N. Bonding of restorative materials to dentine: The present status in Japan. Int Dent J 1985;35:145.

191. Nakabayashi N, Nakamura M, Yasuda N. Hybrid layer as a dentin-bonding mechanism. J Esthet Dent 1991;3:133.

192. Nakabayashi N. Adhesive bonding with 4-META. Oper Dent 1992;suppl 5:125.

193. Nakabayashi N, Takarada K. Effect of HEMA on bonding to dentin. Dent Mater 1992;8:125.

194. Nikaido T, Burrow MF, Tagami J, Takatsu T. Effect of pulpal pressure on adhesion of resin composite to dentin: Bovine serum versus saline. Quintessence Int 1995;26:221.

195. Nishida K, Yamauchi J, Wada T, Hosoda H. Development of a new bonding system [abstract 267]. J Dent Res 1993;72:137.

196. Nordenvall K-J, Brännström M, Malmgren O. Etching of deciduous teeth and young and old permanent teeth. A comparison between 15 and 60 seconds of etching. Am J Orthod 1980;78:99.

197. Ogawa K, Yamashita Y, Ichijo T, Fusayama T. The ultrastructure and hardness of the transparent layer of human carious dentin. J Dent Res 1983;62:7.

198. Okamoto Y, Heeley JD, Dogon IL, Shintani H. Effects of phosphoric acid and tannic acid on dentine collagen. J Oral Rehabil 1991;18:507.

199. Otsuki M. Histological study on pulpal response to restorative composite resins and their ingredients. J Stomatol Soc Jpn 1988;55:203.

200. Packham DE. Adhesion. In: Packham DE (ed): Handbook of Adhesion, ed 1. Essex, England: Longman, 1992:18.

201. Padday JF. Contact angle measurement. In: Packham DE (ed). Handbook of Adhesion, ed 1. Essex, England: Longman, 1992:88.

202. Pashley DH, Livingstone MJ, Greenhill JD. Regional resistances to fluid flow in human dentin in vitro. Arch Oral Biol 1978;23:807.

203. Pashley DH. The influence of dentin permeability and pulpal blood flow on pulpal solute concentrations. J Endod 1979;5:355.

204. Pashley DH. Smear layer: Physiological considerations. Oper Dent 1984;suppl 3:13.

205. Pashley DH, Andringa HJ, Derkson GD, Derkson ME, Kalathoor SR. Regional variability in the permeability of human dentine. Arch Oral Biol 1987;32:519.

206. Pashley DH, Tao L, Boyd L, King GE, Horner JA. Scanning electron microscopy of the substructure of smear layers in human dentine. Arch Oral Biol 1988;33:265.

207. Pashley DH. Dentin: A dynamic substrate—A review. Scan Microsc 1989;3:161.

208. Pashley DH. Interactions of dental materials with dentin. Trans Acad Dent Mater 1990;3:55.

209. Pashley DH, Pashley EL. Dentin permeability and restorative dentistry: A status report for the *American Journal of Dentistry*. Am J Dent 1991;4:5.

210. Pashley EL, Comer RW, Parry EE, Pashley DH. Amalgam buildups: Shear bond strength and dentin sealing properties. Oper Dent 1991;16:82.

211. Pashley DH. Smear layer: An overview of structure and function. Proc Finn Dent Soc 1992;88:215.

212. Pashley DH, Horner JA, Brewer PD. Interactions of conditioners on the dentin surface. Oper Dent 1992;suppl 5:137.

213. Pashley DH, Ciucchi B, Sano H, Horner JA. Permeability of dentin to adhesive agents. Quintessence Int 1993;24:618.

214. Perdigão J, Swift EJ, Cloe BC. Effects of etchants, surface moisture, and composite resin on dentin bond strengths. Am J Dent 1993;6:61.

215. Perdigão J, Swift EJ. Analysis of dentin bonding systems using the scanning electron microscope. Int Dent J 1994;44:349.

216. Perdigão J, Swift EJ, Denehy GE, Wefel JS, Donly KJ. In vitro bond strengths and SEM evaluation of dentin bonding systems to different dentin substrates. J Dent Res 1994;73:44.

217. Perdigão J. An Ultra-Morphological Study of Human Dentine Exposed to Adhesive Systems [thesis]. Leuven, Belgium, 1995.

218. Phillips RW. Skinner's Science of Dental Materials, ed 8. Philadelphia: Saunders, 1982:25.

219. Plasmans PJJM, Reukers EAJ, Vollenbrock-Kuipers L, Vollenbrock HR. Air humidity: A detrimental factor in dentine adhesion. J Dent 1993;21:228.

220. Porte A, Lutz F, Lund MR, Swartz ML, Cochran MA. Cavity designs for composite resins. Oper Dent 1984;9:50.

221. Powell LV, Gordon GE, Johnson GH. Clinical comparison of class 5 resin composite and glass ionomer restorations. Am J Dent 1992;5:249.

222. Prati C. Reaction paper: Mechanisms of dentine bonding. In: Vanherle G, Degrange M, Willems G (eds). Proceedings of the International Symposium on State of the Art on Direct Posterior Filling Materials and Dentine Bonding, ed 2. Leuven, Belgium: Van der Poorten, 1994:171.

223. Qvist V, Qvist J. Effect of ethanol and NPG-GMA on replica patterns on composite restorations performed in vivo in acid-etched cavities. Scand J Dent Res 1985;93:371.

224. Qvist V, Thylstrup A. Pulpal reactions to resin restorations. In: Anusavice KJ (ed). Quality Evaluation of Dental Restorations. Criteria for Placement and Replacement. Chicago: Quintessence, 1989:291.

225. Reeder OW, Walton RE, Livingston MJ, Pashley DH. Dentin permeability: Determinants of hydraulic conductance. J Dent Res 1978;57:187.

226. Retief DH, Austin JC, Fatti LP. Pulpal response to phosphoric acid. J Oral Pathol 1974;3:114.

227. Retief DH. Dentin bonding agents: A deterrent to microleakage? In: Anusavice KJ (ed). Quality Evaluation of Dental Restorations. Criteria for Placement and Replacement. Chicago: Quintessence, 1989:185.

228. Roeder LB, Deschepper EJ, Powers JM. In vitro bond strength of repaired amalgam with adhesive bonding systems. J Esthet Dent 1991;3:126.

229. Roulet J-F, Herder S. Bonded Ceramic Inlays. Chicago: Quintessence, 1991.

230. Rueggeberg FA, Margeson DH. The effect of oxygen inhibition on an unfilled/filled composite system. J Dent Res 1990;69:1652.

231. Rueggeberg FA. Substrate for adhesion testing to tooth structure—Review of literature: A report of the ASC MD156 Task Group on test methods for the adhesion of restorative materials. Dent Mater 1991;7:2.

232. Ruyter IE. The chemistry of adhesive agents. Oper Dent 1992;suppl 5:32.

233. Sano H, Shono T, Sonoda H, Takatsu T, Ciucchi B, Carvalho R, Pashley DH. Relationship between surface area for adhesion and tensile bond strength—Evaluation of a micro-tensile bond test. Dent Mater 1994;10:236.

234. Sano H, Shono T, Takatsu T, Hosoda H. Microporous dentin zone beneath resin-impregnated layer. Oper Dent 1994;19:59.

235. Sano H, Takatsu T, Ciucchi B, Horner JA, Matthews WG, Pashley DH. Nanoleakage: Leakage within the hybrid layer. Oper Dent 1995;20:18.

236. Scott PG, Leaver AG. The degradation of human collagen by trypsin. Connect Tissue Res 1974;2:299.

237. Shaffer SE, Barkmeier WW, Kelsey WP. Effects of reduced acid conditioning time on enamel microleakage. Gen Dent 1987;35:278.

238. Shimokobe H, Honda T, Kobayashi Y, Nakamura H, Takita H, Kuboki Y. Denaturation of dentin collagen by phosphoric acid treatment [abstract 908]. J Dent Res 1988;67:226.

239. Sidhu SK, Watson TF. Resin-modified glass ionomer materials. A status report for the *American Journal of Dentistry*. Am J Dent 1995;8:59.

240. Silverstone LM. Fissure sealants: Laboratory studies. Caries Res 1974;8:2.

241. Silverstone LM, Saxton CA, Dogon IL, Fejerskov O. Variation in pattern of etching of human dental enamel examined by scanning electron microscopy. Caries Res 1975;9:373.

242. Smith DC. Polyacrylic acid–based cements: Adhesion to enamel and dentin. Oper Dent 1992;suppl 5:177.

243. Söderholm K-JM. Correlation of in vivo and in vitro performance of adhesive restorative materials: A report of the ASC MD156 Task Group on test methods for the adhesion of restorative materials. Dent Mater 1991;7:74.

244. Spencer P, Byerley TJ, Eick JD, Witt JD. Chemical characterization of the dentin/adhesive interface by Fourier Transform Infrared Photoacoustic Spectroscopy. Dent Mater 1992;8:10.

245. Spencer P, Wieliczka DM, Meeske J, Adams SE, Eick JD. The resin-dentin interface—Morphological and chemical characterization [abstract 44]. J Dent Res 1994;73:107.

246. Stanford JW. Bonding of restorative materials to dentine. Int Dent J 1985;35:133.

247. Stanford JW, Sabri Z, Jose S. A comparison of the effectiveness of dentine bonding agents. Int Dent J 1985;35:139.

248. Stangel I, Ostro E, Domingue A, Sacher E, Bertrand L. Photoacoustic Fourier transform IR spectroscopic study of polymer-dentin interaction. In: Pireaux JJ, Bertrand P, Bredas JL (eds). Polymer-Solid Interfaces, Philadelphia: Institute of Physics Publishing, 1991:157.

249. Stanley HR, Going RE, Chauncey HH. Human pulp response to acid pretreatment of dentin and to composite restoration. J Am Dent Assoc 1975;91:817.

250. Stanley HR, Bowen RL, Folio J. Compatibility of various materials with oral tissues. II. Pulp responses to composite ingredients. J Dent Res 1979;58:1507.

251. Stanley HR, Pereira JC, Spiegel E, Broom C, Schultz M. The detection and prevalence of reactive and physiologic sclerotic dentin, reparative dentin and dead tracts beneath various types of dental lesions according to tooth surface and age. J Oral Pathol 1983;12:257.

252. Stansbury JW. Synthesis and evaluation of new oxaspiro monomers for double ring-opening polymerization. J Dent Res 1992;71:1408.

253. Strassler HE. Insights and innovations. J Esthet Dent 1991;3:114.

254. Sugizaki J. The effect of the various primers on the dentin adhesion of resin composites—SEM and TEM observations of the resin-impregnated layer and adhesion promoting effect of the primers. Jpn J Conserv Dent 1991;34:228.

255. Suh BI. All-Bond—Fourth generation dentin bonding system. J Esthet Dent 1991;3:139.

256. Summitt JB, Chan DCN, Burgess JO, Dutton FB. Effect of air/water rinse versus water only and of five rinse times on resin-to-etched enamel shear bond strength. Oper Dent 1992;17:142.

257. Summitt JB, Chan DCN, Dutton FB, Burgess JO. Effect of rinse time on microleakage between composite and etched enamel. Oper Dent 1993;18:37.

258. Suzuki T, Finger WJ. Dentin adhesives: Site of dentin vs bonding of composite resins. Dent Mater 1988;4:379.

259. Swift EJ, Triolo PT. Bond strengths of Scotchbond Multi-Purpose to moist dentin and enamel. Am J Dent 1992;5:318.

260. Swift EJ, Cloe BC. Shear bond strengths of new enamel etchants. Am J Dent 1993;6:162.

261. Swift EJ, Hammel SA, Perdigão J, Wefel JS. Prevention of root surface caries using a dental adhesive. J Am Dent Assoc 1994;125:571.

262. Swift EJ, Perdigão J, Heymann HO. Bonding to enamel and dentin: A brief history and state of the art, 1995. Quintessence Int 1995;26:95.

263. Tagami J, Hosoda H, Fusayama T. Optimal technique of etching enamel. Oper Dent 1988;13:181.

264. Tagami J, Tao L, Pashley DH. Correlation among dentin depth, permeability, and bond strength of adhesive resin. Dent Mater 1990;6:45.

265. Tagami J, Hosoda H, Burrow MF, Nakajima M. Effect of aging and caries on dentin permeability. Proc Finn Dent Soc 1992;88(suppl 1):149.

266. Tam LE, Pilliar RM. Fracture surface characterization of dentin-bonded interfacial fracture toughness specimens. J Dent Res 1994;73:607.

267. Tao L, Pashley DH. Shear bond strengths to dentin: Effects of surface treatments, depth and position. Dent Mater 1988;4:371.

268. Tao L, Tagami J, Pashley DH. Pulpal pressures and bond strengths of Superbond and Gluma. Am J Dent 1991;4:73.

269. Tay FR, Gwinnett AJ, Pang KM, Wei SHY. Structural evidence of a sealed tissue interface with a total-etch wet-bonding technique in vivo. J Dent Res 1994;73:629.

270. Ten Cate JM, Jongebloed WL, Simons YM. Adaptation of dentin to the oral environment. In: Thylstrup A, Leach SA, Qvist V (eds). Dentine and Dentine Reactions in the Oral Cavity. Oxford, England: IRL Press,1987:67.

271. Terkla LG, Brown AC, Hainisch AP, Mitchem JC. Testing sealing properties of restorative materials against moist dentin. J Dent Res 1987;66:1758.

272. Titley K, Chernecky R, Maric B, Smith D. Penetration of a dentin bonding agent into dentin. Am J Dent 1994;7:190.

273. Torney D. The retentive ability of acid-etched dentin. J Prosthet Dent 1978;39:169.

274. Torstenson BC, Nordenvall KJ, Brännström M. Pulpal reaction and microorganisms under Clearfil composite resin in deep cavities with acid etched dentin. Swed Dent J 1982;6:167.

275. Torstenson BC, Odén A. Effects of bonding agent types and incremental techniques on minimizing contraction gaps around resin composites. Dent Mater 1989;5:218.

276. Triolo PT, Swift EJ. Shear bond strengths of ten dentin adhesive systems. Dent Mater 1992;8:370.

277. Triolo PT, Swift EJ, Mudgil A, Levine A. Effect of etching time on enamel bond strengths. Am J Dent 1993;6:302.

278. Tsai YH, Swartz ML, Phillips RW, Moore BK. A comparative study: Bond strength and microleakage of dentin bond systems. Oper Dent 1990;15:53.

279. Tyas MJ, Burns GA, Byrne PF, Cunningham PJ, Dobson BC, Widdop FT. Clinical evaluation of Scotchbon: Three-year results. Aust Dent J 1989;34:277.

280. Tyas MJ. Three-year clinical evaluation of dentine bonding agents. Aust Dent J 1991;36:298.

281. Van Hassel HJ. Physiology of the human dental pulp. Oral Surg Oral Med Oral Pathol 1971;32:126.

282. Vanherle G, Lambrechts P, Braem M. An evaluation of different adhesive restorations in cervical lesions. J Prosthet Dent 1991;65:341.

283. Van Meerbeek B, Inokoshi S, Braem M, Lambrechts P, Vanherle G. Morphological aspects of the resin-dentin interdiffusion zone with different dentin adhesive systems. J Dent Res 1992;71:1530.

284. Van Meerbeek B, Vanherle G, Lambrechts P, Braem M. Dentin- and enamel-bonding agents. Curr Opin Dent 1992;2:117.

285. Van Meerbeek B, Dhem A, Goret-Nicaise M, Braem M, Lambrechts P, Vanherle G. Comparative SEM and TEM examination of the ultrastructure of the resin-dentin interdiffusion zone. J Dent Res 1993;72:495.

286. Van Meerbeek B, Mohrbacher H, Celis JP, Roos JR, Braem M, Lambrechts P, Vanherle G. Chemical characterization of the resin-dentin interface by micro-Raman spectroscopy. J Dent Res 1993;72:1423.

287. Van Meerbeek B, Willems G, Celis JP, Roos JR, Braem M, Lambrechts P, Vanherle G. Assessment by nano-indentation of the hardness and elasticity of the resin-dentin bonding area. J Dent Res 1993;72:1434.

288. Van Meerbeek B, Braem M, Lambrechts P, Vanherle G. Morphological characterization of the interface between resin and sclerotic dentine. J Dent 1994;73:141.

289. Van Meerbeek B, Peumans M, Verschueren M, Gladys S, Braem M, Lambrechts P, Vanherle G. Clinical status of ten dentin adhesive systems. J Dent Res 1994;73:1690.

290. Wakabayashi Y, Kondou Y, Suzuki K, Yatani H, Yamashita A. Effect of dissolution of collagen on adhesion to dentin. Int J Prosthod 1994;7:302.

291. Willems G. Multistandard Criteria for the Selection of Potential Posterior Composites [thesis]. Leuven, Belgium, 1985.

292. Wilson AD, Kent BE. The glass-ionomer cement, a new translucent cement for dentistry. J Appl Chem Biotechnol 1971;21:313.

293. Wilson AD, Kent BE. A new translucent cement for dentistry. The glass ionomer cement. Br Dent J 1972;132:133.

294. Wilson AD, Prosser HJ, Powis DM. Mechanism of adhesion of polyelectrolyte cement to hydroxyapatite. J Dent Res 1983;62:590.

295. Wilson AD, McLean JW. Glass ionomer cement. Chicago: Quintessence, 1988.

296. Wilson AD, Nicholson JW. Acid-base Cements. Their Biomedical and Industrial Applications. Cambridge, England: Cambridge University Press, 1993.

297. Wolinsky LE, Armstrong RW, Seghi RR. The determination of ionic bonding interactions of N-phenyl glycine and N-(2-hydroxy-3-methacryloxypropyl)-N-phenyl glycine as measured by carbon-13 NMR analysis. J Dent Res 1993;72:72.

298. Xu J, Butler IS, Gilson DFR, Stangel I. The HEMA interface with dentin and collagen by FT-Raman spectroscopy [abstract 615]. J Dent Res 1995;74:88.

299. Yamada T, Nakamura K, Iwaku M, Fusayama T. The extent of the odontoblast process in normal and carious human dentin. J Dent Res 1983;62:798.

300. Yoshiyama M, Masada J, Uchida A. Scanning electron microscope characterization of sensitive vs. insensitive human radicular dentin. J Dent Res 1989;68:1398.

301. Yoshiyama M, Noiri Y, Ozaki K, Uchida A, Ishikawa Y, Ishida H. Transmission electron microscopic characterization of hypersensitive human radicular dentin. J Dent Res 1990;69:1293.

302. Yu XY, Joynt RB, Wieczkowski G, Davis EL. Scanning electron microscopic and energy dispersive x-ray evaluation of two smear layer–mediated dentinal bonding agents. Quintessence Int 1991;22:305.

303. Zidan O, Hill G. Phosphoric acid concentration: Enamel surface loss and bonding strength. J Prosthet Dent 1986;55:388.

Direct Anterior Restorations

Daniel C.N. Chan / Robert L. Cooley

Patients demand superior esthetics from restorations placed in anterior teeth. An esthetic restorative material must simulate the appearance of the tooth in color, translucence, and texture,[5] yet must have adequate strength and wear characteristics, good marginal adaptation and sealing, insolubility, and biocompatibility.[36] This chapter will address the materials and clinical procedures used to place direct esthetic restorations in anterior teeth.

By far the most commonly used restorative materials in the anterior part of the mouth are resin composites (also called composite resins or just composites). Composites are currently the materials that best fulfill the requirements of excellent esthetics and durability. The longevity of anterior composite restorations has been reported to range from 3.3 to 16 years.[33,42,43,55] Using actuarial methods to assess the clinical longevity of these restorations, van Noort and Davis[57] calculated the overall probability of survival at 5 years to be 62.9% for Class 3 and 71.8% for Class 5 composite restorations. The length of service of composite restorations is generally shorter than that of amalgam restorations.[49]

Material Considerations

By definition, a composite contains four structural components: polymer matrix, filler particles, a coupling agent, and an initiator. The *matrix* is the continuous phase to which the other ingredients are added. Most composite matrices are based on the bis-GMA (bisphenol-A–glycidyl methacrylate) resin developed by R. L. Bowen of the National Institute of Standards and Technology and patented in 1962. Some composites use urethane dimethracrylate instead of bis-GMA, while others use a combination of the two materials.

Filler particles are usually a type of glass (such as barium glass) or silicon dioxide added to the matrix to improve its physical properties. The filler improves translucency, reduces the coefficient of thermal expansion, reduces polymerization shrinkage, and makes the material harder, denser, and more resistant to wear. Generally, the greater the percentage of filler added (by volume or weight), the better are the physical properties of the composite. Filler loading has an upper limit, after which the material becomes too viscous for clinical use.

The filler particles are coated with *silane*, a *coupling agent*, to promote adhesion to the matrix. Without a coupling agent, the composite is not as strong, and the filler particles tend to pop out of the matrix as they come to the surface.

The *initiator* activates the polymerization reaction of composites. Activation may be initiated by chemical reaction or exposure to light of the proper wavelength.

Most current composite restorative materials rely on polymerization initiated upon exposure to visible light in the range of 460 to 480 nm (blue light).

Physical Characteristics of Composites

Composites have steadily improved in recent years, and have progressed so that they are now durable, esthetic, and predictable. Used in combination with an adhesive system, composites form a reliable, durable bond to enamel. Although adhesion to dentin is not yet as reliable as that to enamel, dentin adhesive systems have also improved steadily in the last several years.

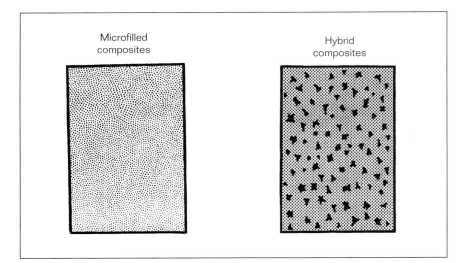

Microfilled
composites

Hybrid
composites

Fig 7-1 Most commonly used classes of resin composite. The microfilled resins contain only submicron particles, while the hybrids contain a combination of submicron particles and particles up to 4 μm in diameter.

Composites have several undesirable characteristics that must be overcome to achieve long-term clinical success. Volumetric shrinkage during polymerization can be as great as 7%[22] and can generate contraction forces of 4.0 to 7.0 MPa,[11,15,19,29,38] leading to cracking and crazing at the enamel margins. Polymerization shrinkage tends to cause gap formation between the composite and the walls of the preparation with the weakest bonds (usually dentin or cementum). Gap formation may result in microleakage, sensitivity, and recurrent caries.[39] Incremental curing techniques are often used in an attempt to compensate for polymerization shrinkage.[46]

Composites have a coefficient of thermal expansion that is two to six times higher than that of tooth structure.[9] This means that composite expands and contracts at a greater rate than does tooth structure in response to changes in temperature, such as when hot coffee or ice cream is consumed. This mismatch contributes to loss of adhesion and greater microleakage.[39]

The steady improvement in adhesive systems has helped offset some of the inherent problems associated with composites. Nonshrinking composites are under development and appear to be the next advance in resin composite technology.[20]

Microfilled Resin Composites

When microfilled composites are manufactured, submicron inorganic filler particles (averaging 0.04 μm) are added to the matrix until the composite is very viscous.

The composite is then polymerized and ground into 5- to 50-μm blocks, which are incorporated into additional microfilled material to form the restorative material for clinical use (Fig 7-1). In this way, filler content is maximized, polymerization shrinkage is minimized, and the composite remains highly polishable.[6]

Microfilled composites can be polished to the highest luster and smoothest surface of all the resin composites, and their primary indication is for esthetic areas where a high luster is required, such as Class 5 restorations or direct composite veneers. Microfilled composites in general are not as strong as other classes of composites, however, and are not usually recommended for Class 4 restorations. When a highly polished Class 4 restoration is needed, a hybrid material may be used as a substructure that can be veneered with a microfilled composite.

Hybrid Resin Composites

As the name implies, hybrid resins contain a blend of submicron (0.04 μm) and small-particle (1- to 4-μm) fillers (Fig 7-1). The combination of medium and small filler particles allows the highest levels of filler loading among composites, and a corresponding improvement in physical properties. They can be polished to a fairly high luster, but not to the extent of a microfilled material. Hybrid composites are a combination of conventional and microfill technology and are often the material of choice for Class 3 and Class 4 restorations.

Fig 7-2 Saucer-shaped preparation in enamel. The carious lesion is usually located slightly gingival to the contact area. Every attempt should be made to maintain natural tooth contact between the adjacent teeth when restoring these lesions. If no cavitation is present, remineralization is preferable to restoration.

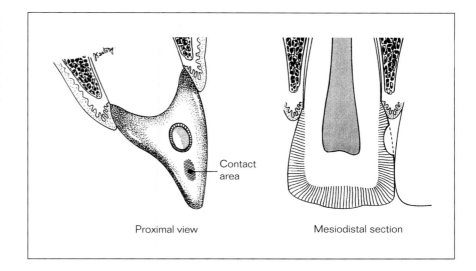

Proximal view   Mesiodistal section

Glass-Ionomer Restorative Materials

Glass-ionomer restorative materials are not commonly used in anterior teeth, but are sometimes recommended for patients with high rates of caries. The traditional chemically cured glass-ionomer material is not very esthetic, but the esthetics of some of the resin-modified glass-ionomer materials are quite good and are suitable for use in visible anterior areas. Glass-ionomer restorative materials are discussed in more depth in chapters 6 and 11.

Class 3 Restorations

Class 3 caries is smooth-surface caries that is found on the proximal surfaces of anterior teeth, usually slightly gingival to the proximal contact, but does not involve the incisal angle of the tooth. It can usually be detected with an explorer, radiographically, or with transillumination. Clinical changes in translucency may be evident and may be enhanced if a light source is placed against the proximal area (transillumination). An area of caries appears more opaque than does sound enamel.

The penetration through the enamel and the pattern of spread is typical of smooth-surface lesions. Incipient lesions tend to be V-shaped and confined to enamel; deeper lesions tend to spread laterally along the dentinoenamel junction, and penetrate dentin.

Incipient Enamel Caries

The proximal lesion that is located within enamel, is not cavitated, and is barely detectable on radiographs may not need a restoration. Although there is no doubt that the lesion is pathologic, research and clinical experience have shown that this lesion is often dormant. Charting it as a potential lesion is a valid and acceptable procedure.[18,40] With proper home care, there is evidence that enamel caries can be remineralized.[53] Chapter 3 contains a more complete discussion of caries and remineralization.

Cavitated Enamel Caries

When the enamel surface is cavitated, it is past the point of remineralization. A cavity preparation may be made with a round tungsten carbide or diamond bur used in a high-speed handpiece. The finished preparation resembles a saucer and has no retentive undercuts (Fig 7-2). Adhesion to acid-etched enamel provides the necessary retention. Both laboratory and 3-year clinical data have demonstrated the durability of these saucer-shaped restorations.[35,51]

Dentinal Caries with All-Enamel Margins

The preparation for dentinal caries is similar to that for enamel caries except that the pulpal floor extends into dentin and the external enamel margins receive a bevel

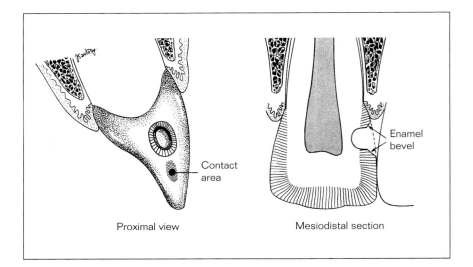

Fig 7-3 This preparation is similar to that in Fig 7-2, except that the axial wall is extended into dentin and the external enamel margins are beveled.

Contact area

Enamel bevel

Proximal view

Mesiodistal section

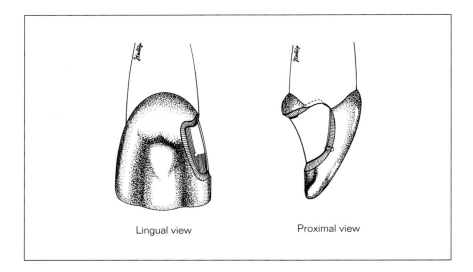

Fig 7-4 Mechanical retention is not necessary, but can be added if desired. A retentive groove may be placed with a No. ¼ round bur on the gingival floor, and a retentive point may also be placed at the same depth at the facioincisioaxial point angle. Reinforcement of remaining dental structure, eg, thinned incisal edge, may be obtained from internal etching and bonding to the composite material.

Lingual view

Proximal view

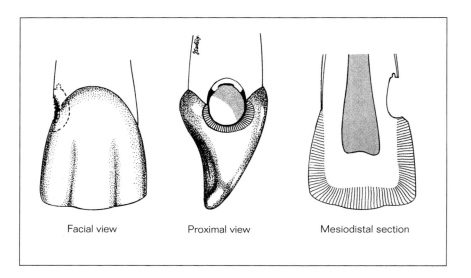

Fig 7-5 Caries extending to the dentin-cementum surface. A retentive groove is placed 0.5–0.7 mm from the external surface of the root.

Facial view

Proximal view

Mesiodistal section

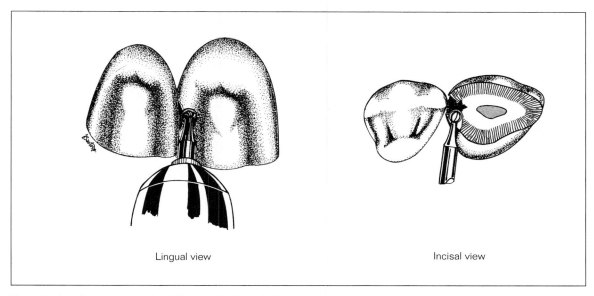

Lingual view

Incisal view

Fig 7-6 Initial penetration should be made through the marginal ridge, away from the adjacent tooth surface. Note the angulation of the long axis of the bur in relation to the location of the lesion.

(Fig 7-3). When only structureless enamel and carious dentin are removed, the resultant adhesive preparation has better margins than do cavities with right-angled butt-joint margins or cavities with concave bevels.[24,47] When the cavity margins are on sound enamel, usually no undercuts are required because the restoration will be retained by adhesion.[57] Conservative retentive points and grooves may be added to enhance retention if desired (Fig 7-4).

Dentinal Caries with Margin Extending onto the Root Surface

In areas where there is little or no enamel for bonding, placement of a retentive groove is recommended. This may be placed to the depth of a No. ¼ round bur, 0.5 to 1.0 mm inside the cementoenamel junction (Fig 7-5). The gingival groove helps minimize gap formation at the gingival margin.[8] A more complete discussion of gap formation may be found in chapters 6 and 8. As dentin bonding agents continue to improve, mechanical undercut retention may become unnecessary.

Preparation Approach and Instrumentation

Resin Composite Restorations
Outline form for composite restorations is determined solely by access and the extent of the caries. There is

no need for either extension for prevention or to remove sound tooth structure to gain mechanical retention. The lingual approach is preferred, but not always possible, depending on the location of the carious lesion. The number of burs used for cavity preparation should be kept to the minimum. A No. 2 round bur or a No. 329 pear-shaped carbide bur in a high-speed handpiece can be used for initial access to the lesion. Initial penetration should be made through the marginal ridge, away from the adjacent tooth surface (Fig 7-6). The outline form of the preparation is then extended to provide access to the carious lesion. A larger round bur may be used in the low-speed handpiece to excavate caries.

For beveling, a flame-shaped finishing bur or a gingival margin trimmer may be used. All accessible enamel margins should be beveled to remove loose enamel rods and expose the ends of the enamel rods to the adhesive. If possible, the facial bevel should barely break contact so that the restoration will be nearly invisible from the facial aspect (Figs 7-7a and 7-7b). Unsupported enamel can be left for internal etching and bonding to composite.[21]

The facial approach is only indicated when caries already involves the labial surface or when the adjacent tooth overlaps, preventing a lingual approach. The outline should be as conservative as possible, preserving the facial enamel. Enamel is more natural and esthetic than the best restorative materials.

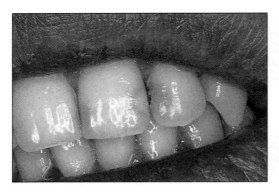

Fig 7-7a Moderate-sized Class 3 carious lesions on the mesial and distal surfaces of the maxillary left central incisor and mesial surface of the lateral incisor.

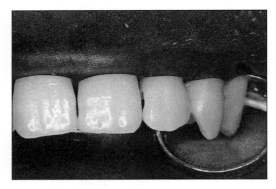

Fig 7-7b After cavity preparation, the labial margins are only slightly visible, and the labial enamel is unsupported by dentin.

Glass-Ionomer Cement Restorations

Because of its anticaries potential, glass-ionomer restorative materials may be utilized for Class 3 lesions in patients with a high risk of caries. Because of the brittleness of glass-ionomer cement, cavity preparations for this material should have butt-joint margins without bevels. Only enough tooth structure should be removed to allow access for excavation of caries. Because glass-ionomer cement bonds to enamel and dentin, placement of retention grooves or points is optional. Preparations for resin-modified glass-ionomer materials should resemble those for resin composite.

Class 4 Restorations

Class 4 restorations are usually necessitated by fracture of an incisal angle. The situation is plainly visible on clinical examination. If caries is present, radiographs may be helpful to determine the extent of the carious lesion and its proximity to the pulp chamber.

Etiology and Treatment Rationale

Caries-induced Class 4 restorations are usually large Class 3 lesions that have undermined the incisal edge. Traumatic fracture-related Class 4 lesions are often found in children or young adults. The frequency of fractures of permanent incisors in children is reported to range from 5%[30] to 20%.[31] The loss of tooth substance in these situations is likely to be more horizontal than vertical.

For Class 4 carious lesions, the cavity design follows the conventional form of the Class 3 preparation and includes a portion of the incisal edge. Caries and weak incisal enamel are removed, and all enamel margins are beveled (Fig 7-8). A modified Class 4 preparation with extensive loss of incisal enamel is shown in Fig 7-9.

For fractures, if there is no caries or pulpal involvement, a bevel is often the only preparation necessary[3] (Fig 7-10). An enamel bevel of at least 1.0 mm should be placed around the periphery of the cavity where enamel thickness allows. Increasing the length of the bevel beyond 1.0 mm has been shown to provide no additional strength,[1] but a longer bevel can achieve a more harmonious esthetic blend between the composite and enamel. If the original tooth fragment is available after the trauma, the fragment may be reattached to the tooth in some instances by etching and bonding the fractured surfaces.[13,54]

Use of Pins

Generally, retentive pins are not needed because the adhesive technique provides sufficient retention for the restoration. A recent study concluded that there was only a small (10%) increase in fracture toughness of large Class 4 composite restorations if pins were added to supplement the acid-etching technique.[44] Some clinicians argue that, if the adhesion is broken, it is better to lose the restoration than to have it held in place by the pins. Such a scenario is illustrated in Figs 7-11a and 7-11b.

Fig 7-8 Typical Class 4 preparation. Incisal fracture caused by undermining associated with a Class 3 lesion may necessitate a Class 4 cavity preparation, which is similar to a Class 3 preparation but includes the incisal edge.

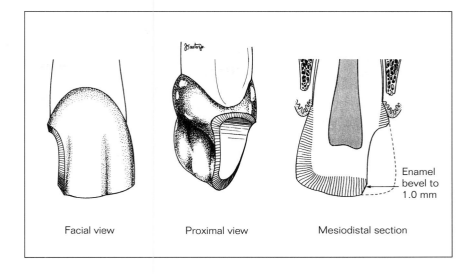

Facial view   Proximal view   Mesiodistal section

Enamel bevel to 1.0 mm

Fig 7-9 Class 4 preparation when loss of incisal enamel is extensive.

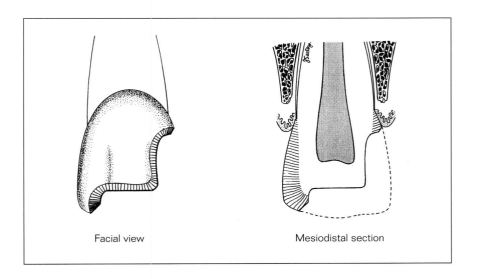

Facial view   Mesiodistal section

Fig 7-10 Fractures often require no preparation other than an external bevel.

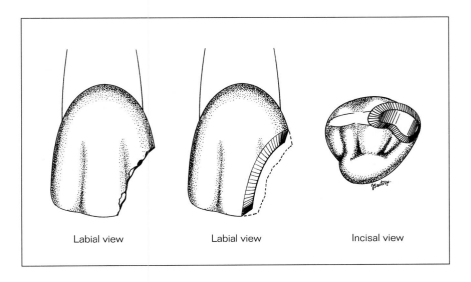

Labial view   Labial view   Incisal view

Figs 7-11a and 7-11b Pins add minimal retention to a Class 3 or Class 4 composite restoration when adequate enamel is present and can create an esthetic problem if not masked with opaque resin.

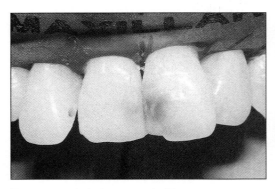

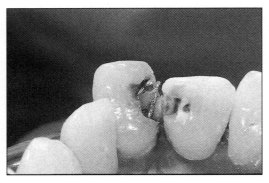

Fig 7-11a Labial view of Class 4 composite restoration retained with two pins. Note the wear and color change of composite material and the recurrent caries.

Fig 7-11b Lingual view after removal of composite material.

In rare situations, when little enamel is available for bonding, and composite is the only viable treatment option, pins may be used for additional retention. They should be placed about 1.0 mm inside the dentinoenamel junction.

Commercial products are available to mask pins. They contain dentin-colored opaques that are painted onto the pins and bond to composite.

Direct Resin Composite Veneers

Resin composite may be used for closing diastemas and/or veneering the labial surfaces of teeth. Direct composite veneers offer several advantages over ceramic veneers. Direct composite veneers can generally be placed in one visit without laboratory involvement or laboratory fees. Although the chair time required for placement of direct veneers is considerable, the cost to the patient is generally less than for ceramic veneers. In many cases, little or no enamel must be removed. The technique is shown in Figs 7-12a and 7-12b. Achieving natural esthetics is difficult with composite, however, and these veneers do not maintain their appearance as well as ceramic restorations. The percentage of practitioners providing direct (freehand) resin veneers has declined in recent years.

Direct composite veneers are placed in layers. The tooth surface is etched, and an adhesive system is applied. If dark tooth structure is present, an opaque layer may be placed and polymerized. To add a natural look to a direct composite veneer, orange or brown composite may be added to the cervical or proximal surfaces, and translucent composite may be added to the incisal aspect. The composite is built to slightly oversized proportions, and is then finished and polished to the proper contours (Fig 7-13).

Diastema Closure

The technique for closure of diastemas is similar to that for placement of direct veneers, and the two techniques may be used in combination. In most cases, no tooth structure has to be removed, and the restorations are retained solely by adhesives. For small diastemas, resin composite added to the proximal surfaces of adjacent teeth will usually suffice (Fig 7-14). If the diastema exceeds 2.5 mm, it may be necessary to use a combination of direct veneering and orthodontic movement.

When diastema closure is performed, occlusal relationships, as well as the overall facial esthetics, must be considered. When anterior teeth are widened, it may also be necessary to lengthen them to preserve natural anatomic proportions. If occlusal relationships and esthetics will allow it, the proper tooth length can be established by

Figs 7-12a and 7-12b Direct composite veneering technique with the body shade deposited in bulk and distributed by plastic instrument. A brush slightly wetted with liquid resin adhesive may also be used for contouring.

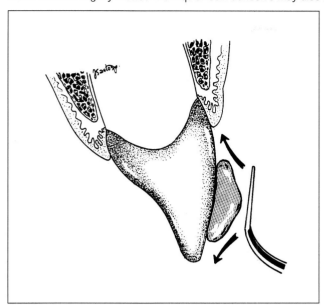

Fig 7-12a Side view.

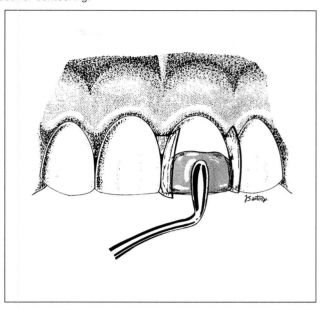

Fig 7-12b Labial view showing the use of Mylar matrix strips in both proximal areas.

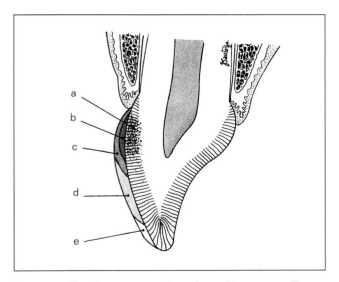

Fig 7-13 Facial veneering and masking of heavy stain/fluorosis using a combination of opaque, cervical, body, and translucent shades. a = stain/fluorosis; b = opaque shade; c = cervical shade; d = body shade; e = translucent shade.

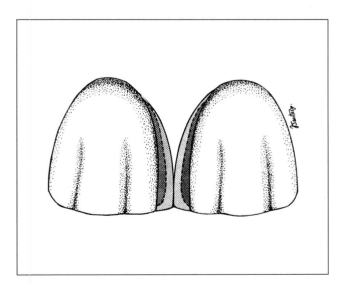

Fig 7-14 Labial view of finished diastema closure showing the use of body and translucent shades to simulate natural tooth color and translucency.

Clinical Steps for a Direct Resin Composite Veneer

1. Select a basic shade prior to initiation of dehydration.
2. Place a rubber dam and No. 212 retainer if desired. If a rubber dam is not used, place gingival retraction cord to control sulcular fluid and retract the gingival tissue.
3. In most cases, the composite material is bonded directly to the tooth surface. If it is necessary to remove tooth structure to establish proper tooth alignment or to create space to mask dark tooth structure, a blunt diamond bur is recommended. Remove as little tooth structure as necessary to achieve the desired objective.
4. Etch the tooth surface with an appropriate etchant, such as 37% phosphoric acid. Protect the adjacent teeth with Mylar strips.
5. Rinse the tooth thoroughly and dry the etched tooth surface with a stream of air.
6. Place a Mylar strip or other matrix and wedge interproximally.

7. Apply opaque resin if indicated and light cure.
8. Add the selected composite and adapt and contour the material. Light cure for at least 40 seconds.
9. Add additional composite as necessary to achieve the proper shape, color, and translucency. Light cure each increment for at least 40 seconds.
10. Contour the gingival margins and remove flash with a No. 12 or 12b scalpel blade.
11. Contour and finish the composite material with a carbide or diamond finishing bur.
12. Repeat the above process on adjacent teeth if indicated.
13. Remove the rubber dam, if used.
14. Check the occlusion and adjust as necessary with finishing burs.
15. Finish and polish with discs, rubber points, etc.
16. Use aluminum oxide polishing paste for final polishing.

Table 7-1 Dimensional averages (in mm) for maxillary incisors and canines*

Tooth	Males Length/Width		Females Length/Width	
Central incisor	10.7	9.4	9.6	9.1
Lateral incisor	9.1	7.5	8.2	7.1
Canine	10.7	8.5	9.2	8.0

*From Gillen et al.[28] Reprinted with permission.

Table 7-2 Length/width and width/width ratios for maxillary incisors and canines*

	Males			
	Length/ Width	Width/Width Central	Width/Width Lateral	Width/Width Canine
Central incisor	1.15:1	—	1.25:1	1.1:1
Lateral incisor	1.2:1		—	
Canine	1.25:1	—	1.15:1	—
	Females			
	Length/ Width	Width/Width Central	Width/Width Lateral	Width/Width Canine
Central Incisor	1.05:1	—	1.3:1	1.15:1
Lateral Incisor	1.15:1		—	
Canine	1.15:1	—	1.15:1	—

The length-to-width ratios are for the teeth in the first column.

The width-to-width ratios are between different teeth. Only the larger-to-smaller ratios are listed. For example, the central incisor–to–lateral incisor width ratio is listed, but not the lateral incisor–to–central incisor ratio.

*From Gillen et al.[28] Reprinted with permission.

adding to the incisal edge. If not, gingival tissue may be surgically removed or apically repositioned. The desired lengths and widths should be worked out with study casts before the treatment is begun. A trial run with composite on the patient's unetched teeth may be helpful in evaluating the esthetics.

Maintenance of the proper length and width relationships in anterior teeth is very important to achieving an esthetic result for composite veneers, porcelain veneers, and diastema closures. A study evaluating the length and width of anterior teeth revealed that, on average, central incisors and canines are approximately equal in length and are 20% longer than lateral incisors. The proper dimensions, length-to-width ratios, and width-to-width ratios are shown in Tables 7-1 and 7-2.[28]

Proximal additions of composite can be difficult to match to the rest of the tooth because of differences in the optical properties between composite and tooth structure. Even when diastema closure is combined with direct facial veneering, the proximal additions tend to be more translucent. To avoid this shine-through effect, an opaque dentin shade or a heavily filled composite may be used to build up the lingual portion of the proximal addition. The facial and incisal contours and the incisal margin can then be established with an enamel shade to reproduce the surface gloss and translucency of a natural tooth. The composite on one proximal surface should be contoured and polished before the adjacent tooth is restored.

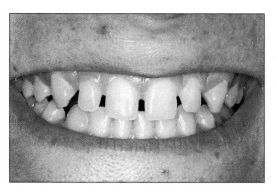 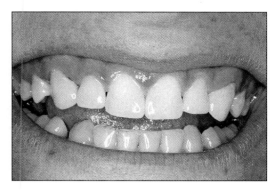

Figs 7-15a and 7-15b Diastema closures frequently require bonding of two to six teeth to achieve proper esthetic relationships. Multiple veneers were needed in this case.

Factors Influencing Shade Selection

Proper Lighting

One of the first requirements for a good color match is proper lighting. Commonly used fluorescent tubes emit light with a green tint that can distort color perception. Color-corrected fluorescent tubes that approximate natural daylight are available and are recommended for dental operatories. The objective is to obtain a shadow-free, color-balanced illumination that is without distracting glare or false colors (see box).[60,10]

If this lighting is not available, color selection can be made near a window. However, even daylight varies considerably from day to day and throughout the day. It is wise to use multiple light sources when the shade is determined.

Color Acuity and Eye Fatigue

When selecting a color or shade, the operator should avoid staring at the tooth and shade guide for long periods of time. Staring at these objects during shade selection will cause the colors to blend, resulting in a loss of color acuity. The shade guide should be placed adjacent to the tooth to be restored and then viewed briefly to determine which shades match the tooth; then the eyes should be moved away. Ideally, the eyes should be "rested" by viewing the horizon through a window or by looking at an object with muted blue or violet colors.

The dental assistant and patient can also assist in shade selection. By viewing the shade guide and tooth from several positions and accepting input from the assistant and patient, the dentist can achieve an acceptable color match.

Color-Corrected Lighting[58]

Overhead lights (Fluorescent tube)

Color Rendering Index (CRI): 90 or higher

Spectral energy distribution (SED): Natural daylight

Color temperature: 5,500° K

Illumination intensity: approximately 150 to 200 foot-candles at 30 inches above floor

Dental operating light

Illumination Intensity: 1,000 to 2,000 foot-candles

Color temperature: optimum 5,000° K, should be adjustable from 4,500° K to 5,500° K to assist in color matching

---

A periodontal probe or caliper may be used as a measuring device to evenly divide the space to be restored. Diastema closures frequently require bonding of two to six teeth to achieve proper esthetic relationships (Figs 7-15a and 7-15b).

■ Shade or Color Selection

Selection of the shade or color of the resin composite restorative material is an important and sometimes difficult step in completing an anterior restoration.

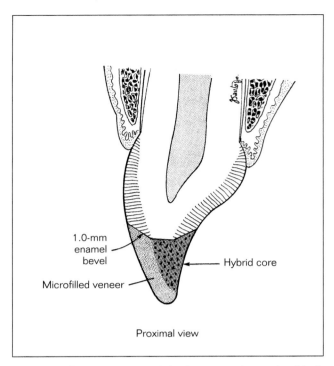

1.0-mm enamel bevel

Microfilled veneer

Hybrid core

Proximal view

Fig 7-16 Opaque resin or a hybrid core may be used to block the shine-through effect.

Achieving Optimal Color Match

The color or shade selection should be accomplished before the restorative procedure is initiated. Therefore, selection is made while the tooth is moist, before the cavity preparation, and before the rubber dam is placed. Desiccation of the tooth causes significant lightening of the shade, and the presence of a rubber dam can distort color perception.

Most manufacturers of composite provide or recommend a shade guide for their products to provide an approximation of the colors available. The selected shade can be confirmed with a small amount of composite (test shade) placed directly on or adjacent to the tooth and cured. This procedure should be performed on an unetched tooth surface to make removal easy after shade verification. For Class 4 restorations and others in which no tooth structure is remaining lingual to the composite, the test shade should be placed in the approximate thickness of the tooth structure to be replaced to assure adequate opacity, or color density.

Tinting and Opaquing

Many manufacturers of composite resins provide accessory shades that contain a number of intense colors and opaques, premixed in syringes or ampules. These materials are normally not necessary in conservative Class 3 restorations, but can play an important role in large Class 4 restorations, diastema closures, and direct veneers. Opaque shades, or hybrid resin materials, can be used to block the reflection of darkness from the mouth that may cause a Class 4 restoration to appear too dark or low in value (Fig 7-16). Opaque resins may also be needed to mask discolored tooth structure.

Use of the proper accessory shades can create the appearance of dentin overlaid with enamel. Accessory shades can also be used to recreate the yellow color seen in cervical areas or the translucency that appears in incisal areas. Tints may be used to imitate white or brown spots that appear on adjacent teeth.

Mixing Resin Composites

Often the shade selection from one single commercial brand of composite does not meet the demanding needs of esthetic dentistry. In such a case, the dentist is faced with the dilemma of using more than one resin system to achieve an acceptable and shade match.

Contrary to some manufacturers' claims, different types and brands of composites can be used together. The two common types of composite, bis-GMA and urethane dimethacrylate, are polymerizable by a free-radical system, and are capable of high cross-linking. Both have identical reactive groups. It is probably best to use layering rather than mixing to integrate shades, because mixing can incorporate air and cause voids in the polymerized resins.

■ Matrices

For Class 3 Restorations

With Class 3 restorations, the most commonly used matrix is the Mylar strip (Fig 7-17). The Mylar matrix, when properly wedged, will reduce flash (excess material) at the gingival margin. It is placed between the teeth and adjacent to the cavity preparation. The resin composite may be shaped with the plastic instrument, or the Mylar strip may be pulled snugly around the tooth and held in place manually to provide shape to the restoration. An excellent contouring instrument for resin composite is the interproximal carver described in chapter 4.

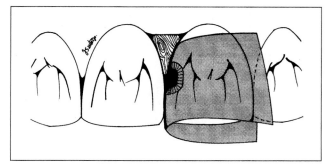

Fig 7-17 Lingual view of matrix and wedge placement for a typical Class 3 composite restoration.

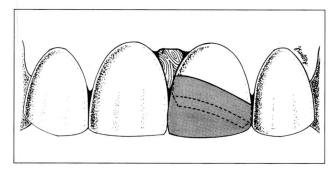

Fig 7-18 Crown form and wedge in place for a Class 4 restoration. If this technique is used, the matrix should be thinned in the contact area and polymerization time should be extended.

For Class 4 Restorations

The majority of Class 4 restorations must be built up incrementally, to avoid resin thicknesses of greater than 2.0 mm that would prevent adequate polymerization. This method usually requires placement of several increments. A Mylar strip and wedge may be used to achieve proximal contact and contours.

For small Class 4 preparations, some clinicians prefer to use a celluloid crown form (Fig 7-18). The crown form should be trimmed to fit 1.0 mm past the prepared margins. The contact area of the crown form should be thinned with an abrasive disk to allow contact of the restoration with the adjacent tooth.

Wedging

Wooden wedges are inserted between the teeth and against the matrix to seal the gingival margin, separate the teeth, assure proximal contact, and push the rubber dam and proximal tissue gingivally to open the gingival embrasure.

Prewedging, or placement of the wedge prior to tooth preparation, may be helpful in some situations. This is generally not a problem with Class 3 restorations, but may be with Class 4 preparations. Prewedging allows greater separation of the teeth and more space to build a contact. Resin composites cannot be condensed against the adjacent tooth, as can amalgam, and depend on the space created by the wedge for achieving contact with the adjacent tooth.

Insertion and Curing of Resin Composite Restorations

Light-cured resin composites are packaged in bulk form in syringes or in unit-dose ampules. The main advantage of purchasing material in bulk is that it costs less. However, for direct placement into the preparation, bulk material requires more handling because it must be dispensed and then loaded into a composite syringe. Unit-dose ampules allow ejection of composite directly into the preparation, minimizing entrapped air bubbles in the material.[41] The ampules also make infection control easier because they are discarded after use and require no disinfection.

Incremental Placement and Curing

Incremental placement and curing of the resin composite may be necessary for large light-cured restorations. Most resin composites should not be placed in thicknesses of greater than 2.0 mm. In restorations greater than 2.0 mm in thickness, incremental placement will produce a more thoroughly cured material. Incremental insertion also offsets some of the effects of polymerization shrinkage.[12]

Incremental placement is possible because of a phenomenon referred to as the *air-* (or *oxygen-*) *inhibited layer.* Polymerization of resin composites is initiated and progresses because of free radicals that are formed in the resin monomers. These free radicals are highly reactive to oxygen; when they come in contact with air at the surface of the composite, an unpolymerized air-inhibited

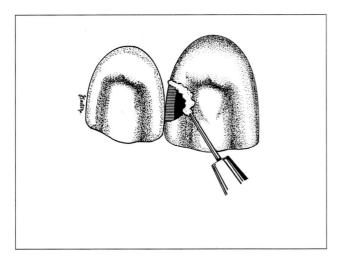

Fig 7-19 Application of gel etchant using a syringe tip. A matrix strip should be placed first to protect the adjacent tooth from the acid.

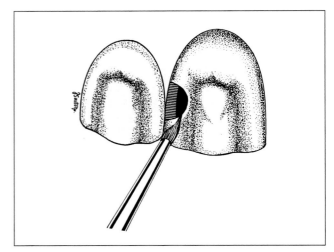

Fig 7-20 The primer and adhesives are placed with disposable brushes and light cured in accordance with the manufacturer's protocol.

layer is formed.[52] The air-inhibited layer is reactive to new composite, however, and forms a cohesive bond to additional increments.

Insertion Technique

Class 3 Restorations

The enamel margins are etched, usually with phosphoric acid. Phosphoric acid is most easily dispensed in a gel form with a small syringe (Fig 7-19). The dentin may also be etched, depending on the adhesive system used. (See chapter 6 for a discussion of dentin adhesives.) The dentin adhesive system may be applied and polymerized either before or after the Mylar matrix and wedge have been placed (Fig 7-20).

The composite-dispensing tip should be inserted in the preparation and the composite slowly injected until there is a slight overfill. Small Class 3 preparations can be restored in a single step without incremental placement. For larger Class 3 restorations placement of multiple increments is recommended to minimize the effects of polymerization shrinkage and assure complete polymerization in deep areas (Figs 7-21a and 7-21b).

After placement, the composite is shaped with a plastic instrument or by pulling the Mylar matrix strip tight. The resin is polymerized for a minimum of 40 seconds. Sixty seconds of polymerization is recommended for deeper preparations or those receiving a darker shade of composite. When the material has set, the wedge and matrix strip are removed, and the restoration is inspected for voids. If voids are present, they can be filled with the resin, which is then polymerized.

Class 4 Restorations

Etching procedures are performed and a dentin primer and adhesive are applied. In most cases, composite is built up incrementally and polymerized. Each increment should be polymerized for a minimum of 40 seconds from the facial aspect and 40 seconds from the lingual aspect. Short curing times will result in composite restorations with inferior physical properties. The cavity should be slightly overfilled to allow contouring and finishing.

If a crown form is to be used, it is filled with composite, placed over the preparation, and wedged in place. After the crown form and wedge are in position, excess material is removed with an explorer. The restoration is then polymerized for a minimum of 60 seconds on the facial aspect and 60 seconds on the lingual aspect.

An overlay technique may be used for Class 4 restorations to obtain both strength and a very smooth surface.[61] The bulk of the restoration is built up with a hybrid resin composite to provide strength. The final layer is a veneer of microfilled resin composite to provide a smooth, shiny surface. The final layer should be contoured and shaped prior to polymerization until it closely resembles the desired shape of the tooth. It is then polymerized with a visible light source. After any voids are eliminated, the restoration is contoured, finished, and polished.

Figs 7-21a and 7-21b   Incremental insertion of composite in a Class 3 restoration.

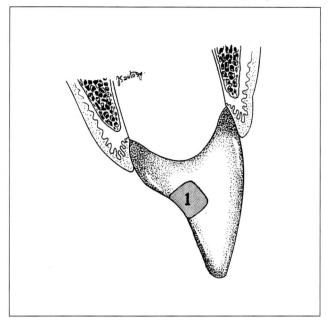

Fig 7-21a   Small restorations may be filled in a single increment.

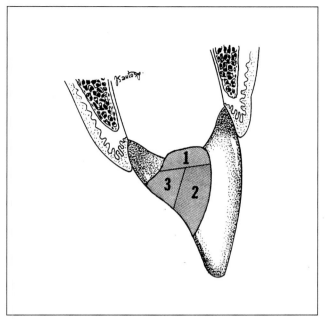

Fig 7-21b   Large cavities require multiple increments to minimize the effects of polymerization shrinkage and assure adequate polymerization.

Visible Light–Curing Units

Any visible light–curing unit may be used with any resin composite. However, the various commercially available units do not have the same capacity to cure resin composites. Some units have been shown to cure greater thicknesses of material than others.[60] A light's effectiveness depends on three factors: *(1)* the wavelength of the emitted light (it should be 460 to 480 nm), *(2)* the intensity of the bulb, and *(3)* curing time. Studies of light-curing units have found some do not have the correct wavelength, which reduces the curing ability of the unit.[45]

As curing units age, the bulb and its reflector degrade, reducing light output and curing ability. Friedman[23] examined 67 curing lights in use by dentists around the country and found bulb blackening in 21 lamps, frosted glass envelopes in 33 lamps, and reflector degradation in three lamps.

Light-curing units can rapidly lose their effectiveness. The bulb and reflector should be examined regularly for signs of degradation, and the light tip should be checked for clarity. Some authorities recommend that bulbs be replaced periodically or when any discoloration is noted. Every office should have a light analyzer (curing radiometer) to evaluate curing lights at least weekly.

Lasers have been evaluated for curing resin composites. *Laser* is an acronym for *light amplification by stimulated emission of radiation.* Lasers have the ability to cure much faster and to a greater depth than the regular halogen light-curing units.[4] However, at present, lasers are relatively expensive and not practical for everyday use for curing resin composites.

Finishing and Polishing

Finishing includes the shaping, contouring, and smoothing of the restoration, while polishing imparts a shine or luster to the surface. Sharp amalgam carvers and scalpel blades, such as the No. 12 or 12b, are useful for shaping polymerized resins (Fig 7-22). There are many products on the dental market for finishing and polishing. These include diamond and carbide burs, various types of flexible disks, impregnated rubber points and cups, metal and plastic finishing strips, and polishing pastes. The smoothest possible surface is obtained, however, when the composite polymerizes against a Mylar strip without finishing or polishing.[48,56]

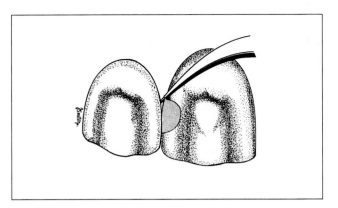

Fig 7-22 Gingival flash is removed with a No. 12 or 12b scalpel blade.

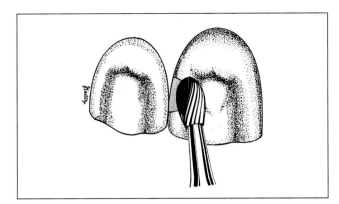

Fig 7-23 A finishing bur or fine diamond bur is used for gross finishing.

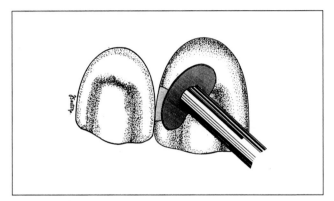

Fig 7-24 Polishing of the final restoration may be accomplished with flexible disks or impregnated rubber points.

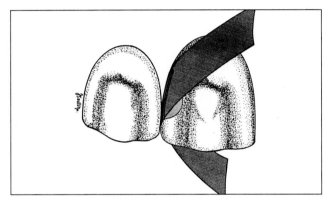

Fig 7-25 Polishing strips are used to contour and polish the proximal surface and margin.

The finishing and polishing process can affect the wear characteristics of the composite. A traumatic finishing technique or overheating can damage the surface of a composite[37,59] and result in accelerated wear characteristics.[37,50] The finishing technique may be one reason that wear of composites is often reported to be greatest in the first 6 to 12 months after placement.

Instruments

Diamond vs Carbide Burs

The 12-fluted carbide burs have traditionally been used to perform gross finishing of resin composites (Fig 7-23). These finishing burs may be used to develop the proper anatomy for the tooth being treated. The transition from resin to enamel should be slowly smoothed until it is undetectable. These burs can be used dry to better visualize the margins and anatomy that are being developed but should be used with light pressure to avoid overheating and possibly damaging the composite surface.

Fine diamond finishing burs are also available for finishing composite restorations. They are used in a series of progressively finer particle sizes.

Disks

One brand of flexible disk (Sof-Lex, 3M Dental) has practically become the standard in finishing and polishing. These disks have a soft, flexible backing and a series of grits that can provide a smooth, even finish. When all four grits are used in sequence, Sof-Lex disks are reported to provide the best surface of any finishing system.[2,6] Sequential use of disks to a fine grit produces a smooth, durable finish (Fig 7-24).

Dry finishing with disks used in sequence is reported to be superior or equal to wet finishing for smoothness, hardness, and color stability.[17] The composite surface should be rinsed before a finer disk is used to remove the larger particles from the previous disk.

Clinical Steps for a Class 3 or Class 4 Resin Composite Restoration

1. Select a shade before initiation of dehydration.
2. Place a rubber dam.
3. Prewedge if you anticipate difficulty in achieving proximal contact.
4. Initiate the cavity preparation by accessing the caries through the marginal ridge with a No. 329 or 330 bur in a high-speed handpiece. Remove the proximal plate of enamel. Be careful to avoid damaging the adjacent tooth.
5. Remove the caries with a round bur in a low-speed handpiece.
6. Remove unsupported enamel if appropriate, and place bevels with a finishing bur and/or gingival margin trimmer.
7. Etch the enamel. Be careful not to etch the adjacent tooth; protect it with a Mylar strip.
8. Place the primer and adhesive, following the manufacturer's instructions.
9. Light cure as indicated.
10. If the preparation is large, place composite into the deep areas.
11. Light cure for at least 40 seconds
12. Place a Mylar strip or other matrix and wedge.
13. Add composite and contour the Mylar strip to contain the material in the proper shape.
14. Light cure for at least 40 seconds.
15. Remove the wedge and Mylar strip, and inspect the restoration for voids. Add composite if necessary.
16. Remove gingival flash with a No. 12 or 12b scalpel blade.
17. Remove flash from the other margins, and contour the restoration with a finishing bur or diamond.
18. Remove the rubber dam.
19. Check the occlusion and adjust as necessary.
20. Finish and polish with disks, rubber points, etc.
21. Use aluminum oxide polishing paste for final polishing.

Impregnated Rubber Points and Cups

A wide variety of rubber points and cups are available that are impregnated with abrasive materials. Like disks, rubber cups and points are used sequentially from coarse to fine grit. The coarse grits are effective for gross reduction and finishing, while the fine grits create a smooth, shiny surface. The primary advantage of rubber points and cups over disks is for accessing grooves and the concave lingual surfaces of anterior teeth.

Finishing Strips

Finishing strips are used to contour and polish the proximal surfaces and margins gingival to the contact (Fig 7-25). They are available with metal or plastic backings. Most metal strips are used for gross reduction, but care must be taken not to over-reduce the restoration, because they will also remove enamel. Plastic strips come in various widths and grits and can be used for both finishing and polishing.

Procedures

A No. 12 or 12b scalpel blade is effective for removing interproximal flash, carving the proximal margins, and otherwise shaping the polymerized resin. Gross reduction and shaping are then performed with diamonds or carbide burs. Finishing should be done carefully, while water or air is applied as a coolant, to avoid damaging the surface of the composite. Finishing strips can be used on the proximal surfaces and margins so that floss snaps through the contact smoothly without shredding. After the composite is polished with fine disks or rubber cups, a high shine can be added with aluminum oxide pastes.

Rebonding (Glazing)

Rebonding (also called *glazing*) is an advisable procedure that involves re-etching the enamel margins of a polished composite restoration and placing a coat of unfilled or lightly filled resin. Rebonding has been reported to improve marginal integrity,[25] lessen microleakage, improve wear characteristics, and help reduce staining of the restoration.[16,26,27,34] The long-term benefits of rebonding have been questioned,[32] but a clinical study reported that glazed restorations show less discoloration after 5 years than unglazed restorations.[16]

References

1. Bagheri J, Denehy GE. Effect of enamel bevel and restoration length on Class 4 acid-etch retained composite resin restorations. J Am Dent Assoc 1983;107:951-953.

2. Berastegui E, Canalda C, Brau E, Miquel C. Surface roughness of finished composite resins. J Prosthet Dent 1992,68:742-790.

3. Black JB, Retief DH, Lemmons JE. Effect of cavity design on the retention of Class 4 composite resin restorations. J Am Dent Assoc 1981;103:42-46.

4. Blankenau RJ, Kelsey WP, Powell GL, Shearer GO, Barkmeier WW, Cavel WT. Degree of composite resin polymerization with visible light and argon laser. Am J Dent 1991;4:40-42.

5. Buda M. Form and color reproduction for composite resin reconstruction of anterior teeth. Int J Periodont Rest Dent 1994;14:34-47.

6. Chen RCS, Chan DCN, Chan KC. A quantitative study of finishing and polishing techniques for a composite. J Prosthet Dent 1988;59:292-298.

7. Cipalla AJ. Laser Curing of Photoactivated Restorative Materials. Salt Lake City: ILT Systems, 1994.

8. Coli P, Blixt M, Brännström M. The effect of cervical grooves on the contraction gap in Class 2 composites. Oper Dent 1993;18:33-36.

9. Craig RG. Restorative Dental Materials, ed 9. St. Louis: Mosby, 1993:256-257.

10. Crigger LP, Foster CD, Young JM, Stockman TD. Visible-Light Curing Units. Aeromedical Review, San Antonio, TX:USAF School of Aerospace Medicine, Oct 1984.

11. Crim G, Chapman K. Effect of placement techniques on microleakage of a dentin-bonded composite resin. Quintessence Int 1986;17:21-24.

12. Crim GA. Microleakage of three resin placement techniques. Am J Dent 1991;4:69-72.

13. Croll TP. Emergency repair followed by complete-coronal restoration of a fractured mandibular incisor. Quintessence Int 1992; 23:817-822.

14. Darveniza M. Cavity design for Class 4 composite resin restorations—a systematic approach. Aust Dent J 1987;32:270-275.

15. Davidson CL, DeGee AJ. Relaxation of polymerization contraction stresses by flow in dental composites. J Dent Res 1984;63:16-48.

16. Dickinson GL, Leinfelder KF. Assessing the long term effects of a surface penetrating sealant. J Am Dent Assoc 1993;124:68-72.

17. Dodge WW, Dale RA, Cooley RL, Duke ES. Comparison of wet and dry finishing of resin composites with aluminum oxide discs. Dent Mater 1991;7:18-20.

18. Eames WB. When not to restore. J Am Dent Assoc 1988;117:429-432.

19. Eick JD, Welch F. Polymerization shrinkage of posterior composite resins and its possible influence on postoperative sensitivity. Quintessence Int 1986;17:103-111.

20. Eick JD, Robinson SJ, Byerley TJ, Chappelow CC. Adhesives and nonshrinking dental resins of the future. Quintessence Int 1993;24:632-640.

21. Espinosa HD. In vitro study of resin-supported internally etched enamel. J Prosthet Dent 1979;40:526-529.

22. Feilzer AJ, Degee AJ, Davidson CL. Curing contraction of composites and glass-ionomer cements. J Prosthet Dent 1988;59:297-300.

23. Friedman J. Variability of lamp characteristics in dental curing lights. J Esthetic Dent 1990;1:189-190.

24. Fusayama T. Ideal cavity preparation for adhesive composites. Asian J Aesthet Dent 1993;1:55-62.

25. Galan JR, Mondelli J, Coradazzi JL. Marginal leakage of two composite restorative systems. J Dent Res 1976: 55:74-76.

26. Garman TA, Fairhurst CW, Hewer GA, Williams HA, Beglau DL. A comparison of glazing materials for composite restorations. J Am Dent Assoc 1977;95:950-956.

27. Gibson GB, Richardson AS, Patton RE, Waldman R. A clinical evaluation of occlusal composite and amalgam restorations: One-year and two-year results. J Am Dent Assoc 1992;104:335-337.

28. Gillen RJ, Schwartz RS, Hilton TJ, Evans DB. Analysis of selected normative tooth proportions. Int J Prosthodont 1994;7:410-417.

29. Gordon M, Plasschaert A, Saiku J, Plezner R. Microleakage of posterior composite resin materials and an experimental urethane restorative material, tested in vitro above and below the cementoenamel junction. Quintessence Int 1986;17:11-15.

30. Grundy JR. Incidence of fractured incisors. Br Dent J 1959;106: 312-314.

31. Gutz DP. Fractured permanent incisors in a clinical population. J Dent Child 1971;38:94-95.

32. Itoh K, Iwaku M, Fusayama T. Effectiveness of glazing composite resin restorations. J Prosthet Dent 1981;45:606-613.

33. Jokstad A, Mjör IA, Qvist V. The age of restorations in situ. Acta Odontol Scand 1994;52:234-242.

34. Kawai K, Leinfelder KF. Effect of surface-penetrating sealant on composite wear. Dent Mater 1993;9:108-113.

35. Kidd EAM, Roberts GT. The saucer preparation. Part 2. Laboratory evaluation. Br Dent J 1982;153:138-140.

36. Lambrechts PP, Willems G, Vanherle G, Braem M. Aesthetic limits of light-cured composites in anterior teeth. Int Dent J 1990; 40:149-158.

37. Leinfelder KF, Wilder AD, Teixeira AC. Wear rates of posterior composite resins. J Am Dent Assoc 1986;112:829-833.

38. Lutz F, Krejci I, Oldenburg TR. Elimination of polymerization stresses at the margins of posterior composites resin restorations: A new restorative technique. Quintessence Int 1986;17:777-784.

39. Lutz F, Krejci I, Barbakow F. Quality and durability of marginal adaptation in bonded composite restorations. Dent Mater 1991;7: 107-113.

40. McDonald SP, Sheiham A. A clinical comparison of non-traumatic methods of treating dental caries. Int Dent J 1994;44:465-470.

41. Medlock JW, Zinck JH, Norling BK, Sisca RF. Composite resin porosity with hand and syringe insertion. J Prosthet Dent. 1985; 54:47-51.

42. Mjör IA. Placement and replacement of restorations. Oper Dent 1981;6:49-54.

43. Mjör IA, Toffenetti F. Placement and replacement of resin-based restorations in Italy. Oper Dent 1992;17:82-85.

44. Nuemeyer S, Wolfgang G, Kappert HF, Hellekes E, Botsch H. PCR pin-anchored anterior fracture restorations. Gen Dent 1992; 40:200-202.

45. Newman SM, Murray GA, Yates JL. Visible lights and visible light–activated composite resins. J Prosthet Dent 1983;50:31-35.

46. Podshadley AG, Gullett G, Crim G. Interface seal of incremental placement of visible light-cured composite resins. J Prosthet Dent 1985;53:625-626.

47. Porte A, Lutz F, Lund MR, Swartz ML, Cochran MA. Cavity designs for composite resins. Oper Dent 1984;9:50-55.

48. Pratten DH, Johnson GH. An evaluation of finishing instruments for an anterior and posterior composite. J Prosthet Dent 1988;60: 154-158.

49. Qvist V, Thystrup A, Mjör IA. Restorative treatment pattern and longevity of resin restorations in Denmark. Acta Odontol Scand 1986;44:351-356.

50. Ratanapridakul K, Leinfelder KF, Thomas J. Effect of finishing on the in vivo wear rate of a posterior composite resin. J Am Dent Assoc 1989;118:524-526.

51. Roberts GT. The saucer preparation. Part 1: Clinical evaluation over 3 years. Br Dent J 1982;153:96-98.

52. Ruyter IE. Unpolymerized surface layers on sealants. Acta Odontol Scand 1981;39:27-32.

53. Silverstone LM. Fluorides and Remineralization: Clinical Uses of Fluorides. Philadelphia: Lea & Febiger 1985:153-175.

54. Simonsen RJ. Restoration of a fractured central incisor using the original tooth fragment. J Am Dent Assoc 1982;105:646-648.

55. Smales RJ. Effects of enamel bonding, type of restoration, patient age and operator on the longevity of an anterior composite resin. Am J Dent 1991;4:130-133.

56. Stoddard JW, Johnson GH. An evaluation of polishing agents for composite resins. J Prosthet Dent 1991;65:491-495.

57. Summitt JB, Chan DCN, Dutton FB. Retention of Class 3 composite restorations: Retention grooves versus enamel bonding. Oper Dent 1993;18:88-93.

58. van Noort R, Davis LG. A prospective study of the survival of chemically activated anterior resin composite restorations in general practice: 5-year results. J Dent 1993;21:209-215.

59. Wu W, Toth EE, Ellison JA. Subsurface damage layer of in vivo worn dental composite restorations. J Dent Res 1984;63:675-680.

60. Young JM, Satrom KD, Berrong JM. Intraoral dental lights: Test and evaluation. J Prosthet Dent 1987;57:99-107.

61. Zalkind M, Heling I. Composite resin layering: An esthetic technique for restoring fractured anterior teeth. J Prosthet Dent 1992;68:204-205.

Direct Posterior Composite Restorations

Thomas J. Hilton

The use of resin composite as a material for restoring posterior teeth has increased greatly in recent years. Patients are attracted to a restoration that matches the shade of the natural tooth.[82,98] Resin composite meets this demand and has become the most frequently used esthetic restorative material in dentistry.[100] In addition, resin composites contain no mercury, are thermally nonconductive,[82] and bond to tooth structure with the use of adhesive agents.[40,84,116] There are problems associated with utilizing resin composite for posterior restorations, however, including shrinkage that occurs on setting,[54] postoperative sensitivity,[143] questions about long-term durability,[17] and problems with wear resistance.[71,88,101,103,110] To minimize these negative properties requires meticulous operative procedures. Technique is the most important variable governing the success of posterior resin composite restorations.[52,99]

This chapter will examine the advantages, disadvantages, and most appropriate indications for resin composite as a posterior restorative material and will describe clinical placement techniques.

▓ Advantages of Resin Composite as a Posterior Restorative Material

Esthetics

Manufacturers have developed sophisticated resin composite systems with multiple shades, tints, and opaquers that allow the practitioner to provide a restoration that is highly esthetic. Clinical studies often report an excellent color match with tooth structure; one study found that 98% of composite restorations still provided an excellent color match at 2 years.[113] Visible light–cured (VLC) composites have less amine content than the autocured systems, resulting in less yellowing of the restoration and greater color stability over time.[172] Microfilled composites have the smoothest surface finish of all the systems, and tend to stain less than other systems.[172] Because they are more heavily filled, hybrid composites tend to result in a restoration with a more opaque appearance.[168]

Conservation of Tooth Structure

Although it is still recommended by some that preparation design for posterior resin composite restorations be patterned after the traditional amalgam preparation,[99] most researchers now recommend a more conservative approach.[22,146,161] To take advantage of resin composite's positive properties and to minimize its negative ones, the *adhesive preparation* has evolved. This design limits the removal of tooth structure to the amount needed to eliminate caries and severely thinned enamel[75] (Figs 8-1a to 8-1f).

The adhesive preparation for posterior Class 2 resin composite restorations differs from the traditional amalgam design of G. V. Black in several ways[15]:

1. The preparation tends to be shallower. Because retention is provided through bonding to tooth structure rather than mechanical undercuts, there is no need to penetrate enamel if the caries does not.

Figs 8-1a to 8-1f Posterior resin composite restorations differ from the traditional Class 2 preparation. In general, they can be prepared more conservatively because it is not necessary to remove sound tooth structure to create mechanical retention.

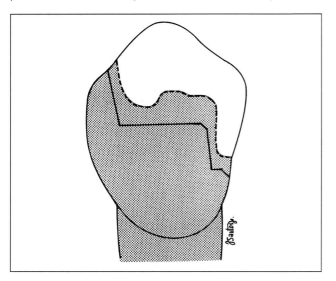

Fig 8-1a The adhesive preparation (*dotted line*) is extended only enough to provide access and to remove caries, unlike the traditional preparation (*solid line*).

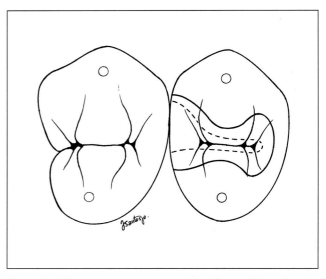

Fig 8-1b The more conservative outline form of the adhesive resin composite restoration (*dotted line*) is compared to that of the traditional restoration (*solid line*).

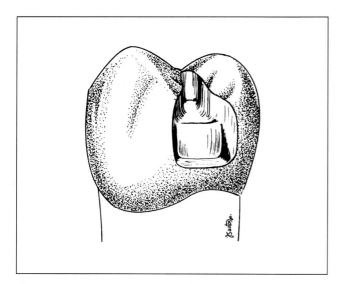

Fig 8-1c In the adhesive preparation, internal angles are rounded.

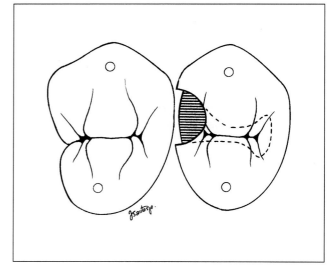

Fig 8-1d If no occlusal caries is present, a Class 2 preparation for a resin composite restoration can be very conservative, similar to a Class 3 preparation. The occlusal grooves and fissures (*dotted line*) can be sealed after placement of the restoration.

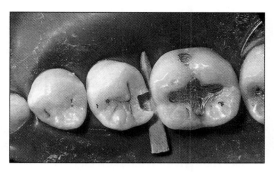

Fig 8-1e A conservative Class 2 preparation has been made. The occlusal fissures are stained but not carious.

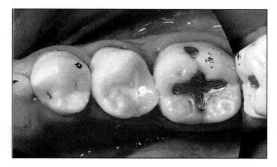

Fig 8-1f After the restoration is completed, a sealant is placed in fissures.

This conserves tooth structure and expands the area of enamel available for bonding (Fig 8-1a).

2. The preparation tends to be narrower, which allows less occlusal contact on the restoration and reduces wear.[11,63,103,135,174] A less bulky restoration helps to decrease the adverse affects of composite polymerization shrinkage, resulting in improved marginal integrity[75] and less cuspal deflection[145] (Fig 8-1b).

3. The preparation has rounded internal line angles, which conserves tooth structure, decreases stress concentration associated with sharp line angles,[172] and enhances resin adaptation during placement[39,78] (Fig 8-1c).

4. There is no extension for prevention. The occlusal pits and grooves are included in the preparation only if the presence of caries dictates this need. Extending the preparation across the occlusal surface does not make the restoration more resistant to fracture than a slot preparation.[146] Adjacent pits and fissures can be treated with sealants to enhance caries prevention[172] (Figs 8-1d to 8-1f).

Adhesion to Tooth Structure

The clinical success of bonded resin composite restorations is well documented.[1,30,67,122] The bond between composite and tooth structure achieved with bonding systems offers the potential to seal the margins of the restoration[57] and reinforce remaining tooth structure against fracture.[40,84,116] Although not all studies have found them to have an increased resistance to fracture,[83,142] and the longevity of the bond is shortened by increased occlusal forces,[55] it has been suggested that less cuspal flexure occurs with bonded resin composite

restorations under subcatastrophic occlusal loads, providing protection against the propagation of cracks, which ultimately result in fatigue failure.[142]

Low Thermal Conductivity

Because resin composites do not readily transmit temperature changes, there is an insulating effect that helps to reduce postoperative temperature sensitivity.[54]

Elimination of Galvanic Currents

Resin composite does not contain metal and so will not initiate or conduct galvanic currents.[172]

Radiopacity

Radiopaque restorative materials are necessary to allow the practitioner to evaluate the contours and marginal adaptation of the restoration as well as to distinguish among restoration, caries, and tooth structure.[45,155] Most modern resin composites have a radiopacity in excess of that of enamel[154] and greater than that of an equal thickness of aluminum,[2] the criterion the American Dental Association uses to allow a manufacturer to claim its material is radiopaque.

Alternative to Amalgam

Amalgam, despite being a restorative material with a long track record of clinical success,[32,89,134] has become increasingly controversial because of its mercury content. Although concerns about mercury in amalgam are more psychologic than scientific, there is an increasing desire to find mercury-free alternatives.[16] Patients are aware of indictments against amalgam, and some express concern over potential health hazards.[22] Amalgam is also less attractive to dental professionals as government agencies consider classifying it as hazardous waste[38] and requiring that dental offices install expensive systems to remove mercury from waste water.[6,16] As amalgam comes under closer scrutiny, resin composite will be increasingly looked to as an alternative material for posterior restorations.

Disadvantages of Resin Composite as a Posterior Restorative Material

Polymerization Shrinkage

Despite improvements in resin composite formulations over the years, modern systems are still based on variations of the bis-GMA molecule, which has been in existence for more than 30 years.[17] One of the major drawbacks of this material is the polymerization shrinkage that occurs during the setting reaction. Modern composites undergo volumetric polymerization shrinkage of 2.6% to 7.1%.[48]

Most of the problems associated with posterior composite restorations can be related directly or indirectly to polymerization shrinkage. During polymerization, composite may pull away from the least retentive cavity margins (usually the gingival margin), resulting in gap formation.[42,93,106] Tensile forces developed in enamel margins can result in marginal degradation from mastication.[113] Contraction forces on cusps can result in cuspal deformation,[121] enamel cracks and crazes[112] (Figs 8-2a and 8-2b), and ultimately decreased fracture resistance of the cusps.[165]

Polymerization shrinkage occurs regardless of the system used to initiate the setting reaction, but there is a significant difference in the direction of the force vectors developed (Figs 8-3a and 8-3b). Autocured composite polymerizes toward the center of the mass of the resin composite, while VLC composite polymerizes toward the light source.[54,106]

A number of techniques have been suggested to decrease the adverse affects of polymerization shrinkage. The most commonly used is incremental placement

of VLC composite, which decreases the overall setting contraction by reducing the bulk of composite cured at one time.[106] In addition, the ratio of bonded to unbonded surface area is decreased, which helps to relieve the stress developed at the bond between tooth and composite.[47] The incremental placement technique will be discussed at length later in this chapter.

Beta-quartz inserts that may be incorporated into the composite during insertion have been developed to reduce the bulk of composite and resultant polymerization shrinkage.[41] While little research is available on the efficacy of the inserts, early indications are that cuspal strain is reduced[37] without adversely affecting the wear properties of the restoration.[85]

Autocured composites are sometimes recommended for posterior restorations because they tend to induce less polymerization stress than does a comparable bulk of VLC composite. This is because greater porosity is incorporated into the autocured resin composite as a result of mixing. The incorporated oxygen inhibits the set of resin immediately adjacent to the voids and decreases the ratio of bonded to unbonded surface area.[5] In addition, the voids increase the free surface area for stress compensation by flow of the composite during the setting reaction.[49] However, a number of problems associated with the use of autocured composites in posterior restorations argue against their use. These will be discussed in subsequent sections.

The best hope for overcoming the problems of polymerization shrinkage lies in the development of future composites that do not contract on setting. This is an area of vigorous research.[43,79,169]

Secondary Caries

Several clinical studies have demonstrated that secondary caries is a significant cause of failure in posterior resin composite restorations.[10,101,127] It is believed that the marginal gap formed at the gingival margin as a result of polymerization shrinkage allows the ingress of cariogenic bacteria[101] (Figs 8-4a to 8-4c). Because marginal degradation has been demonstrated to increase with time,[10,11,34,164] the risk of secondary caries increases with time.

Studies have shown that levels of mutans streptococci, the organisms linked most closely to the incidence of dental caries,[178] are significantly higher in the plaque adjacent to interproximal posterior composite restorations than in plaque adjacent to either amalgam or glass-ionomer restorations. A retrospective study by Qvist et al[127] revealed that less secondary caries occurred in all

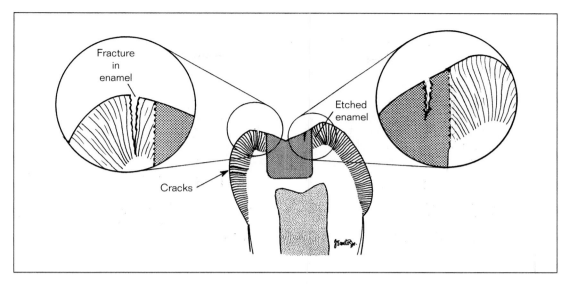

Fig 8-2a   Polymerization shrinkage can cause crazing in the enamel or fractures within the resin composite.

Fig 8-2b Craze lines are evident in the lingual cusp of the maxillary right second premolar after placement of a Class 2 resin composite restoration.

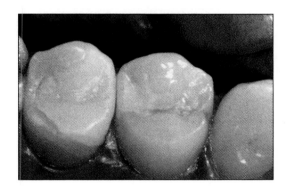

Fig 8-3a   Polymerization shrinkage occurs toward the center of the mass of resin in autocuring resin composites.

Fig 8-3b   Polymerization shrinkage occurs toward the light in light-curing resin composites.

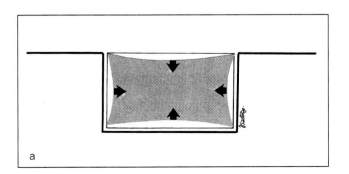

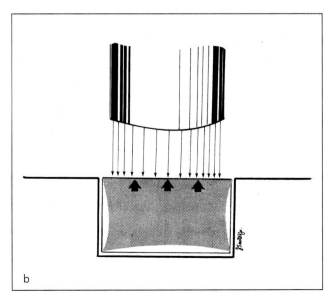

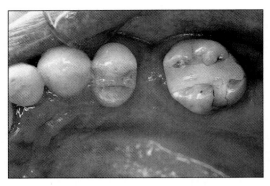

Fig 8-4a In the existing posterior resin composite restorations, the dark shadowing adjacent to the occlusal margins indicates the presence of caries.

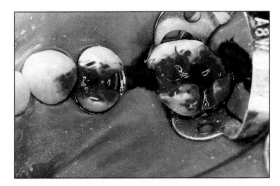

Fig 8-4b After placement of a rubber dam, the resin composite restorations are removed and caries-detecting solution is placed.

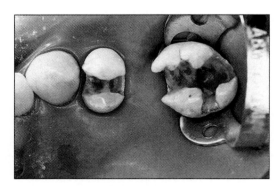

Fig 8-4c Stained areas confirm the presence of caries.

classes of amalgam restorations than in resin composite restorations. In addition, the organic acids of plaque have been demonstrated to soften bis-GMA polymers, which in turn could have an adverse effect on wear and surface staining.[8] These facts emphasize the need for good recall and close follow-up of posterior composite restorations.

Postoperative Sensitivity

Postoperative sensitivity has been associated with the placement of posterior composite restorations. One clinical study noted that 29% of teeth suffered from sensitivity following placement of the restoration.[143] Reports of postoperative sensitivity have diminished somewhat with improvements in dentin adhesives.[13]

A number of reasons have been postulated for the occurrence of postoperative sensitivity, but the most commonly accepted theories relate to polymerization shrinkage. As previously discussed, polymerization shrinkage results in gap formation, which allows bacterial penetration and fluid flow under the restoration. The bacteria may enter the dentinal tubules and cause pulpal inflammation and sensitivity.[19] Gap formation also allows a slow, continuous outflow of dentinal fluid from the pulp, through the tubules, to the gap. Cold or other stimuli may cause a contraction of fluid in the gap, leading to a sudden, rapid outflow of fluid, which the pulp interprets as painful.[18]

Contraction forces of polymerization shrinkage may also result in cuspal deformation, with resultant cracking and crazing of remaining tooth structure (Fig 8-2b), which can cause a tooth to be sensitive.[112] Flexure of resin composite under an occlusal load may cause hydraulic pressure in the tubular fluid to be transmitted to the odontoblastic processes.[21,42]

Awareness of the potential for postoperative sensitivity allows the practitioner to forewarn the patient of this possibility. Careful adherence to the guidelines for restoration placement will help to reduce this problem.

Decreased Wear Resistance

The wear resistance of posterior composite restorations has been the subject of considerable attention. Although this characteristic has improved as refinements in materials have taken place,[13] it is still a concern for restoration longevity.[168,170] Composite wear results from the combination of chemical damage to the surface of the material and mechanical breakdown.[9,53,72,176]

Composites undergo wear by two different mechanisms. *Abrasion,* generalized wear across the entire occlusal surface caused by the abrasive action of particles during mastication, occurs in all areas of the restoration (Fig 8-5). *Attrition* is the loss of material that occurs as a result of direct contact with opposing tooth surfaces in the occlusal contact areas of the restoration.[110] Generally, wear can be related to either material or clinical factors.

Material problems relate to the resin composite's filler content, particle size, and distribution.[81] Clinical studies have shown less heavily filled composites (less than 60% by volume) to exhibit unacceptable wear.[168,170] Because of their generally lower filler content (30% to 50%), microfill composites are more subject to attrition[113] and marginal breakdown,[34,143,164] especially in those areas adjacent to occlusal contact areas.[113] However, they are more resistant to abrasion because of their smoother surface, decreased interparticle spacing, and decreased friction to food particles.[12,143] The more heavily filled hybrid resin composites are more resistant to attrition than are the microfilled materials.[103] However, resin composites that have a larger mean particle size (greater than 3 µm) tend to have significantly higher abrasion wear.[63,103,168–170] This is due to the loss of the larger filler particles, leading to three-body wear[103,170] and increased stress transfer from the filler particles to the resin matrix, which results in formation of cracks during mastication.[7]

The rate of wear varies with particle size as well. As mean filler size decreases (below 1 µm), the wear rate tends to be linear with time. Conversely, composites with increased mean filler size tend to have more rapid wear initially but slower wear with time.[34,62,114,164,169]

Clinically related wear factors include the size of the restoration, its location in the arch, and the occlusal load it must withstand. As the surface area and length of cavosurface margins increase, so does the exposure to occlusal forces, with a resultant increase in wear.[11,63,103,135,174] The more posteriorly a tooth is located, the greater are the masticatory forces and the more rapid is the wear of resin composites.[10,11,13,94,174] Fracture resistance decreases as a result of fatigue from chewing,[51] and increased chewing pressure will result in increased wear.[107]

Interproximal surfaces are subjected to the forces of abrasion during function as well. As a result, interproximal wear of posterior composite restorations is significantly greater than that of unrestored surfaces[10,11,31,160] (Fig 8-5).

At the present time, the best wear characteristics for posterior use are generally exhibited by heavily filled composite (more than 60% by volume) with a mean filler particle size between 1 and 3 µm.[96,103,169] Clinical studies are showing that current composite formulations have

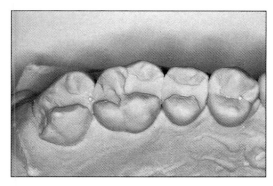

Fig 8-5 Wear has traditionally been a problem with posterior resin composite restorations. A cast reveals generalized wear of the posterior resin composite restorations in the maxillary right first and second molars and second premolar. In addition, proximal wear has resulted in broad, flat contacts and loss of arch length.

acceptable wear characteristics at 3 years.[13] In fact, some studies have indicated that posterior resin composite restorations wear as well as amalgam.[71,135] However, other studies report that composites have significantly higher wear rates than amalgam,[71,88,101,103,110] and no composite has been demonstrated to exhibit less wear than amalgam. It should also be noted that 3 years may not be long enough to adequately assess the wear characteristics of composite as a posterior restorative material.[169]

Other Physical Properties

Generally, the closer the physical properties of a restorative material simulate those of enamel and dentin, the better the restoration's longevity.[100,169,173] A number of the physical properties of resin composite are inferior to those of tooth structure and other restorative materials. These inferior properties can have an adverse effect on the durability of the restoration.

Composite has low tensile strength relative to its compressive strength, resulting in low fracture toughness.[93,101] Indeed, fracture of posterior composites has been noted as a significant cause of failure in some clinical studies.[13,174] Increased filler loading of composite leads to improved fracture toughness.[51,53]

Resin composite has a relatively high degree of elastic deformation (ie, low modulus of elasticity) that exceeds that of amalgam by six to eight times.[21] Failures of resin composite restorations associated with its high elastic deformation have included bulk fracture,[93] microcrack formation,[53] and relatively low resistance to occlusal loading.[143] As with fracture resistance, more highly filled composites exhibit less elastic deformation than their less filled counterparts.[169]

The coefficient of thermal expansion of composite is another property that differs significantly from that of tooth structure.[29] Because the coefficient of thermal expansion of composite is higher than tooth structure, composite tends to expand and contract more than enamel and dentin when subjected to variations in temperature. This can increase marginal gap formation and exacerbate the effects of polymerization shrinkage on cuspal deformation and may result in the fracture of composite or enamel.[93,173] It has been demonstrated that, as the mismatch in thermal expansion properties between restorative material and the tooth structure increases, so does marginal leakage.[24] As the filler content of composite increases, however, the mismatch decreases.[29]

Water Sorption

Water sorption is another factor in the clinical performance of resin composites. Water is absorbed preferentially into the resin component of composite and is therefore greater when resin content is increased.[17,93] Because of the swelling of the resin matrix, the filler particle–resin bond is weakened. If the resulting stress is greater than the bond strength, the resulting debond is referred to as *hydrolytic breakdown*.[93,140] Incompletely cured resin composite will exhibit more water sorption and greater resultant hydrolytic degradation.[115]

It has been suggested that the swelling of composite caused by water sorption can be beneficial by closing the marginal gap caused by polymerization shrinkage. However, studies have shown that the swelling from moisture absorption usually is not enough to overcome the polymerization shrinkage gap.[6,113] Even if water sorption did result in a closed marginal gap, it would only be a close adaptation without adhesion between the composite and tooth.[91]

It has been demonstrated that composites containing strontium and barium, added to increase radiopacity, tend to have an increased incidence of hydrolytic breakdown and crack formation.[140]

Variable Degrees of Polymerization

Analysis of the polymerization, or cure, of resin composites reveals that certain characteristics of this material are at odds with one another. As the polymerization of composite increases, the physical properties improve.[5,12,17] However, polymerization shrinkage also increases with more thorough cure.[158] Resins with decreased filler content exhibit decreased viscosity and improved diffusion of reactive groups during the polymerization reaction, and, thereby, improved cure.[50] However, a decreased filler content also results in inferior physical properties,[29,51,53,169] and poorer clinical performance.[34,103,113,143,164] Achieving the best balance among these traits is a challenge for both the manufacturers of composites and clinicians.

Visible light–cured (VLC) composites have been shown to achieve a somewhat higher degree of polymerization than autocured materials.[7,50] However, the best degree of polymerization that can be achieved with modern composites is in the range of 73% to 74%.[102]

Several factors influence the degree of polymerization of VLC composites. Lighter shades cure more easily and in less time than darker shades.[54] Resin composites with larger filler particles tend to transmit light throughout the material more effectively than those with smaller filler particles.[136] The longer the composite is subjected to the VLC unit, the more effective the cure,[123] but the thickness of each increment should be limited to 2.0 mm.[54] The degree of cure is inversely related to the distance of the light tip from the resin composite[123,137] and the condition of the curing unit can impact the effectiveness of the cure.[56]

Inconsistent Dentin Bonding (Marginal Leakage)

Polymerization shrinkage causes the composite to pull away from cavity margins, resulting in gap formation.[42,93,106] Despite advances in dentin bonding agents, they still do not consistently and reliably achieve bond strengths to dentin and cementum that are high enough to prevent this occurrence.[132,141,157] This sometimes results in open margins, sensitivity, and bacterial invasion.[27] In addition, the bond between adhesive and tooth has been demonstrated to degrade with aging, both in vitro[163] and in vivo.[66]

Technique Sensitivity

Because of the aforementioned negative aspects of using composite as a posterior restorative material, the most important variable in clinical success is the placement technique.[168] There is little room for error.[52] This may account for the great variability reported in clinical success rates for posterior composite restorations.[101]

Questionable Durability

The lack of durability of posterior composite restorations has been a major shortcoming.[17,53] Resin composite lasts significantly longer in anterior teeth than in posterior teeth.[13] Similarly, amalgam shows significantly better clinical longevity as a posterior restorative material than resin composite.[13] It is apparent that posterior composite restorations demand meticulous operative procedures to achieve long-term clinical success.

Autocured Versus Light-Cured Resin Composites

Autocured composite restorative materials largely disappeared from clinical practice in the 1980s because of the popularity of the light-cured materials. In recent years, some practitioners have started recommending the use of autocured composites, either alone or in combination with VLC resin composites, for posterior applications.[14,58,59] The primary advantage of a autocured material is that it can be placed in bulk, saving time compared to the incremental insertion technique used with VLC materials.

Although more time consuming, utilization of VLC resin composites has a number of advantages over use of autocured resin composites. Visible light–cured composites achieve more complete polymerization,[7] resulting in superior physical properties[5,17,137] and exhibit better color stability.[5,156] Visible light–cured composites better resist the early stress on the bond to tooth structure caused by polymerization shrinkage than autocured composites.[49] Autocured composites tend to incorporate voids as a result of mixing in two-paste systems,[49] and the increased porosity decreases tensile strength and surface smoothness,[33] accelerating wear.[96] Mixing interrupts the polymerization process and may compromise the size and configuration of the final polymer molecule, resulting in reduced strength and wear resistance.[166]

Visible light–cured composites should be used with an incremental placement technique to reduce the overall polymerization shrinkage of the final restoration.[152] This technique allows the practitioner to build up and sculpt the restoration. Research has shown VLC increments to have adequate interfacial strength.[124]

Perhaps most importantly, VLC composites performed better in clinical trials than autocured over 1 year[103] and 3 years.[31]

Indications for Utilizing Resin Composite as a Posterior Restorative Material

Based on the foregoing discussion, several factors should be considered before a posterior composite restoration is recommended to a patient. Esthetics should be a prime consideration.[161] There are few indications for composite in nonesthetic areas. The buccolingual width of the cavity preparation should be restricted to one-third of the intercuspal distance,[52] and, if possible, the gingival cavosurface margin (in Class 2 restorations) should be located on intact enamel.[161,171] Centric occlusal stops should be located primarily on tooth structure.[161] There should be no signs of excessive wear resulting from clenching or grinding,[52] and the tooth should be amenable to rubber dam isolation.[52]

Direct Posterior Resin Composite Restorations

Preoperative Evaluation

Several factors should be considered in the preoperative evaluation. The esthetic demands of the patient should be weighed against the strengths and weaknesses of composite as a posterior restorative material. The patient's occlusion should be evaluated for excessive wear and to determine if the majority of occlusal forces can be supported by tooth structure rather than restorative material. The occlusion should be marked with articulating paper as a guide to preparation design. Finally, the best type of composite for the restoration should be chosen. At present, the heavily filled hybrid composites are considered best suited for posterior use, with a mean particle size of 1 to 3 μm.[103,169]

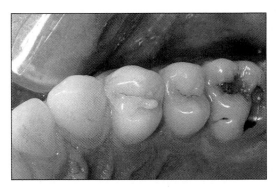

Fig 8-6 A small amount of resin composite is placed on the unprepared tooth to verify the shade prior to isolation with a rubber dam.

Shade selection should always be performed before isolation of the tooth causes dehydration. A shade is chosen from the shade guide that accompanies the composite, and then a small portion of the composite is placed on the unprepared tooth and polymerized (Fig 8-6). Some clinicians prefer to quickly rough out the preparation and polymerize a small portion of the composite to check the shade. In both cases, the resin can be easily removed because the tooth is not etched or primed.

Isolation

Placement of a rubber dam is mandatory; failure to maintain a dry field will result in clinical failure.[99] In a clinical study, the margins of all Class 2 composite restorations placed without a rubber dam demonstrated marginal leakage 4 to 6 weeks after placement.[1] The rubber dam prevents moisture contamination and protects gingival tissues.[1]

Prewedging

Resin composite does not have the condensability that permits amalgam to deform a matrix band and maintain close adaptation to an adjacent tooth. This makes obtaining an adequate interproximal contact one of the more difficult aspects of placing a Class 2 composite restoration. Placement of an interproximal wedge at the start of the procedure is recommended to open the contact with the adjacent tooth and to compensate for the thickness of the matrix band.[161] It has been demonstrated that multiple wedging, ie, inserting a wedge initially and then reapplying seating pressure several times during the

course of the procedure, is more effective at opening the contact than is a single placement of a wedge.[160] In addition, the wedge can protect the rubber dam and gingival tissues from laceration and reduce leakage into the operative site.[161]

Preparation

The conservative adhesive preparation, referred to previously, should be utilized. Bevel placement is a point of controversy with this preparation. When used in conjunction with adhesive agents and composite, bevels in enamel provide more area for acid etching and bonding. In addition, the bevel is designed to expose enamel rods transversely (cross cut, or "end on") to achieve a more effective etching pattern. Research has shown that etching of transversely exposed enamel results in a bond that is significantly greater than that attained with a longitudinal etching (lengthwise) pattern (Figs 8-7a and 8-7b). Clinical research has demonstrated favorable results with the use of acid-etched beveled preparations in Class 3 composite restorations.[128] The disadvantage to beveling is the exposure of thin portions of composite to occlusal stresses.

The following recommendations regarding bevel placement in Class 2 preparations for posterior composite restorations should be followed:

Facial and Lingual Margins of the Proximal Box
Conservative bevels (0.5 to 1.0 mm) are placed on the facial and lingual cavosurface margins of the proximal box preparation. This will achieve the previously mentioned benefits of beveling, as well as aid in placing the margins in a more accessible location for finishing and polishing.

Gingival Margin
The decision to place a gingival margin bevel requires clinical judgment. As the preparation nears the cementoenamel junction, the enamel layer is thinner than other regions of the crown, and beveling the preparation increases the potential of removing the little enamel that remains. Because of the presence of prismless enamel in this region, acid etching is often less effective.[111] The gingival margin should be beveled only if the margin is well above the cementoenamel junction and an adequate band of enamel remains. A groove at the gingivoaxial line angle has been demonstrated to reduce microleakage if the gingival margin lies below the cementoenamel junction, and addition of the groove should be considered if this situation should arise.[26]

Fig 8-7a When needed, a bevel is placed on enamel to expose the ends of enamel rods for etching.

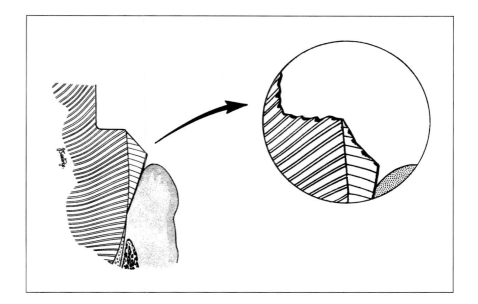

Fig 8-7b Longitudinal etching of enamel rods has been shown to be less effective. However, if only a small amount of enamel is present at the gingival margin, it should not be beveled.

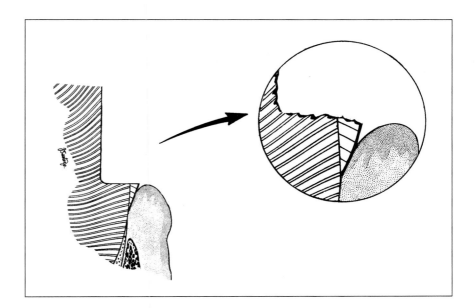

Occlusal Margin

Proponents of beveling the occlusal cavosurface margin argue that doing so maximizes the exposure of end-cut enamel prisms.[111] However, it has been noted that a normal preparation in the occlusal surface will result in end-cut enamel prisms as a result of the orientation of the enamel rods in cuspal inclines[79] (Fig 8-8). Avoidance of bevels on the occlusal surface prevents the loss of sound tooth structure, decreases the surface area of the final restoration, lessens the chance of occlusal contact on the restoration, eliminates a thin area of composite that would be more susceptible to fracture, and presents a well-demarcated marginal periphery at which composite can be more precisely finished.[10,82,99,171]

Placement of occlusal bevels has demonstrated no benefit to clinical longevity of class 2 posterior composite restorations.[174] The most significant factor predicting the survivability of posterior resin composite restorations is the proportion of the occlusal surface restored; this factor is increased by occlusal beveling.[174] Therefore, occlusal bevels should not be utilized for posterior composite preparations.

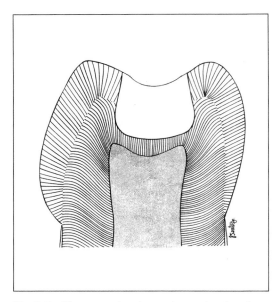

Fig 8-8 The enamel rods on the occlusal surface are oriented in such a way that the ends are exposed without beveling.

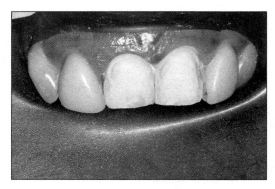

Fig 8-9 The appearance of the central incisors is characteristic of etched enamel. Note the difference between the "frosted" appearance of the central incisors and the enamel of the other teeth. Exposed dentin is present in the cervical and incisal areas.

Pulpal Protection

If used, calcium hydroxide should be limited to those areas of the preparation in which there is the potential for pulpal exposure.[13] Placement of a calcium hydroxide liner over an extensive area of dentin provides no benefit to the pulp and decreases the surface area for adhesion, and dissolution of the liner during acid etching can interfere with a sound bond to enamel and dentin.[101] If the preparation is conservative in size, no liner in addi-

tion to adhesive agent is required. In deeper preparations and those that approach or extend beyond the cementoenamel junction, a glass-ionomer liner or base may be considered. Pulpal considerations are discussed in depth in chapter 3.

Glass-ionomer liners and bases are reported to offer a number of potential advantages when used in posterior composite restorations. Glass-ionomer bonds to both tooth structure and composite (via a bonding adhesive).[142] Glass ionomer introduces less polymerization stress into tooth structure than resin composite.[48] It releases fluoride into adjacent tooth structure,[23] which may be advantageous because of the tendency for secondary caries to form around posterior composite restorations.[99] Use of a glass-ionomer liner has been demonstrated to improve marginal integrity[104] and decrease marginal leakage.[1,70,125] Less bulk of composite is required to fill the preparation, reducing the amount of polymerization shrinkage,[11,92] and improving marginal adaptation.[106] Glass-ionomer liners, particularly the autocuring versions, have excellent rigidity,[25] which helps to decrease deformation of resin composite under load. This results in improved wear and marginal integrity. Glass-ionomer cement can reinforce the preparation walls by adhering to dentin and minimizing cuspal deformation under loading.[92] Glass-ionomer liners also reduce the rise in pulpal temperature associated with application of the curing light during incremental insertion procedures.[64] However, with improvements in dentin adhesives, the use of glass ionomer under posterior composite restorative has been greatly reduced in recent years.

Acid Etching

The enamel walls of the preparation should be etched with 37% phosphoric acid for 15 to 30 seconds and rinsed.[23] The enamel is examined for the frosted matte appearance to confirm proper enamel conditioning (Fig 8-9).

Bonding Agent Application

The manufacturer's instructions for the particular bonding system should be followed. In most adhesive systems, a primer is placed first, followed by an adhesive. The primer is usually a hydrophilic resin contained in a volatile carrier liquid. After application of the primer, the carrier evaporates, leaving behind a very thin layer of resin. The adhesive (bonding agent) is then applied in a

Figs 8-10a to 8-10c Three common matrices are shown for posterior resin composite restorations.

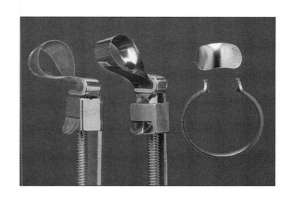

Fig 8-10a Clear and metal matrix bands are shown with Tofflemire retainers, and a Bitine ring is shown with a sectional metal matrix.

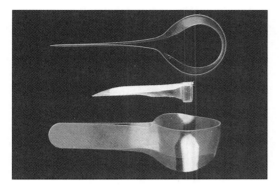

Fig 8-10b The clear matrix is usually used with a reflecting wedge.

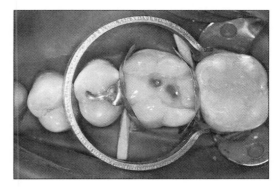

Fig 8-10c A Bitine ring can be used to stabilize a sectional matrix and is effective in creating slight separation between the teeth to assure tight interproximal contacts.

thin layer and thinned further with a dry brush. A layer of adhesive that is too thick can reduce bond strength.[95] Air should not be used to thin the adhesive agent, however, because this has been demonstrated to significantly reduce bond strength.[74]

If the etchant and bonding agent are placed before application of the matrix, visualization and access to all areas of the preparation are better and it is easier to brush thin the adhesive and avoid pooling. However, placement of a matrix after the adhesive sometimes results in contamination of the preparation with blood or saliva. Enamel and dentin adhesives are discussed at length in chapter 6.

Matrix Application

Several useful matrices are available (Fig 8-10a), including the clear plastic matrix, the ultrathin (0.001-inch) Tofflemire metal matrix, and the thin (0.0015-inch) sectional matrix.

The clear matrix can be used in conjunction with a transparent reflecting wedge (Fig 8-10b) and offers the advantage of allowing penetration of the curing light from multiple directions. This allows the clinician to cure the increments of composite from the proximal and gingival directions, rather than from the occlusal aspect, to more favorably direct the polymerization shrinkage of the composite. However, the clear matrix is thicker than the thinnest metal matrices and its lack of rigidity makes placement through tight interproximal contacts difficult.[10]

Tight proximal contacts are more easily developed with the ultrathin metal matrices than the clear matrices, because they are easier to place, maintain their shape better, and can be burnished against the adjacent tooth.[10] One disadvantage of the metal matrices is that increments must be initially cured only from the occlusal aspect. After removal of the band, the proximal box is further polymerized from the facial and lingual directions. Metal bands should be precontoured before placement to avoid flat interproximal contours.

Another device that is helpful in developing adequate interproximal contact is the Bitine ring (Fig 8-10c). After the matrix band is placed, the Bitine ring is placed between the teeth adjacent to the box preparation with a rubber dam forceps. The engaged ring exerts a continuous separating force that aids in the development of adequate interproximal contact.

Composite Insertion: Incremental Technique

Visible light–cured composite should be inserted in successive, laminated increments to ensure proper curing and prevent excessive polymerization shrinkage.[11,139] Incremental curing decreases the effects of polymerization shrinkage, enhances marginal adaptation, reduces marginal leakage, decreases cuspal deformation, and makes the cusps more resistant to subsequent fracture.[30,37,42,105,106,165]

First Increment

Some general guidelines should be followed for insertion of the resin composite. The gingival margin is critical, because of the tendency for microleakage to occur in this area.[125] Thus, techniques must be utilized to enhance the bond and reduce the adverse effects of polymerization shrinkage. First, a composite increment no thicker than 1.0 mm is placed against the floor of the proximal box.[23] A thin layer will ensure proper light irradiation throughout the increment. A light, translucent shade should be used in the box to maximize the polymerization.[172] Because this portion of the restoration is rarely critical from an esthetic standpoint, a shade mismatch with the tooth will not adversely affect the final appearance of the restoration.

If a clear matrix and reflecting wedge are being used, the initial curing should be directed through the flat end of the wedge. It has been shown that a transparent reflecting wedge will transmit approximately 90% to 95% of the incident light.[104] This will draw the curing light to the gingival margin of the restoration and direct the polymerization shrinkage toward the margin. This method will result in better marginal adaptation than curing from an occlusal direction.[104–106,108,109]

Because the plastic wedges are so smooth, they may slip out of proper position easily and may not maintain the pressure necessary to ensure proper adaptation of the gingival aspect of the matrix band and separation from the adjacent tooth. Two suggestions may help to overcome this problem. After the plastic wedge is positioned, a wooden wedge is inserted beside it on the side away from the tooth being restored. Alternatively, the plastic wedge can be maintained in proper position with the light curing tip during curing of the initial incre-

ment. After this is completed, the plastic wedge has accomplished its purpose and may be replaced with a wooden wedge.

If a metal matrix has been chosen, then all increments must be cured from the occlusal direction. The tip of the light should be positioned as close as possible to the resin being cured.[12,54] After the metal mixture is removed, all proximal areas of the restoration should receive additional curing with the light.

Vertical Increments

Subsequent increments should be placed vertically in thicknesses of no greater than 2.0 mm. If a metal matrix is utilized, an occlusogingival layering technique should be utilized (Fig 8-11a), and the restoration should be cured from the buccal and lingual aspects after removal of the band. If a clear matrix is used, an oblique or vertical technique should be used (Figs 8-11b and 8-11c). Use of these techniques allows initial curing to occur from the facial or lingual direction, to direct polymerization shrinkage toward the facial or lingual proximal preparation margin. This has been shown to improve marginal integrity[65,152] and decrease cuspal deformation.[93,139] When the proximal boxes have been filled and polymerized, the occlusal channel, if present, is filled and cured incrementally.

An alternative to the layering techniques is the use of a conical light-curing tip. The proximal box is filled with composite to just short of the contact area and the conical tip is wedged into the composite. The cone is used to apply pressure to the matrix band against the adjacent tooth during curing. Subsequent increments restore the cone-shaped gap formed by the tip. This technique is designed to ensure adequate interproximal contact and to minimize the thickness of composite that must be cured through. While the technique is relatively untested, initial study results have shown formation of fewer marginal gaps than in the more traditional incremental technique,[44] as well as improved hardness and decreased porosity.[159]

The use of prepolymerized composite has also been suggested to aid in establishing interproximal contact. The normal incremental technique is used until the proximal box is filled to just short of the proximal contact. A small, slightly flattened ball of composite is precured on the tip of an instrument (eg, No. ½ Hollenback). An additional increment of uncured composite is placed into the proximal box. The precured ball is placed into this increment and utilized to wedge the matrix band tightly against the adjacent tooth, while the recently placed composite is cured.[162]

Figs 8-11a to 8-11c   The incremental fill technique varies depending on the type of matrix used.

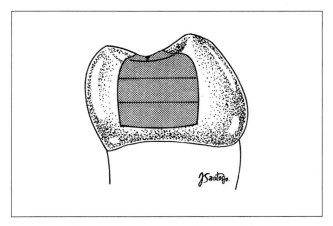

Fig 8-11a   If a metal matrix is used with a light-curing resin composite, the material is layered vertically in increments of 2.0 mm or less.

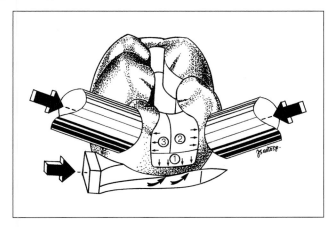

Fig 8-11b   If a clear matrix is used with a light-reflecting wedge, increments are placed as pictured, gingival increment first, followed by wide then narrow increments. The light is used to "pull" each increment toward the adjacent margin.

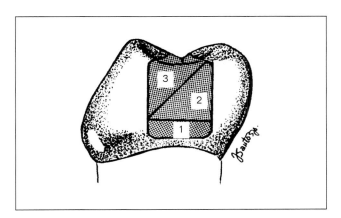

Fig 8-11c   Alternating oblique increments can also be used after placing and curing the gingival increment. As in Fig 8-11b, the light is used to direct polymerization toward the preparation margin. Additional increments may be required to ensure that no increment exceeds 2.0 mm in thickness.

It is sometimes difficult to obtain adequate interproximal separation if both interproximal surfaces are wedged simultaneously. When a mesio-occlusodistal preparation is restored, one proposed remedy is to remove the wedge from one interproximal area, reapply pressure to the remaining wedge to maximize separation, and incrementally place composite to fill that box only. The wedge is removed from the interproximal area of the restored surface, reapplied to the unrestored surface, and composite is added to restore the remainder of the preparation. Bitine rings may be used in a similar manner, or simultaneously on the mesial and distal surfaces.

Final Increment

Careful control of the final increment will minimize the amount of finishing. A conical instrument (eg, PKT No. 3) moistened with some dentin adhesive, may be used to shape and form the occlusal surface before curing. Some clinicians recommend use of a composite that has a slightly different shade from the tooth to aid in locating margins during finishing procedures.[58]

Composite Insertion: Other Techniques

Materials other than VLC composite have been suggested for placement in the box preparation. Autocured (also called *self-cured*) composites are available for this purpose in both low- and high-viscosity formulations. It has been suggested that the portion of the autocured composite adjacent to the gingival margin cures first, especially if used in conjunction with an autocured (or dual-cured) adhesive. The shrinkage of the autocured composite is supposedly directed toward the gingival margin due to initiation of the curing reaction by the ongoing polymerization of the adhesive and accelerated by the higher temperature in that area. This supposedly results in less marginal stress by reducing polymerization shrinkage away from the floor[14,58] and improves marginal adaptation.

Another class of materials that is sometimes suggested for use in the proximal box is the autocured or dual-cured resin modified–glass ionomers. They are placed in a manner similar to that used for the chemically cured composites and allowed to polymerize. All of the self-

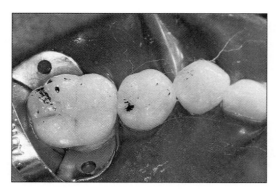

Fig 8-12a Preoperatively, the rubber dam is in place and the occlusion is marked.

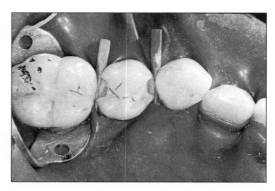

Fig 8-12b Conservative mesio-occlusal and disto-occlusal preparations have been made in the maxillary left second premolar. Wooden wedges are in place for prewedging.

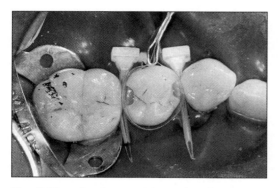

Fig 8-12c A clear matrix and reflecting wedges in place.

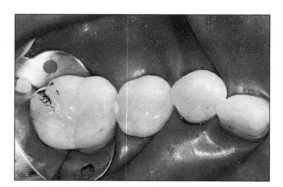

Fig 8-12d When the resin composite restorations are completed, an occlusal surface sealer is placed.

curing materials should be veneered occlusally with a VLC composite. Although using an autocuring material in this way is theoretically appealing, clinical research has not verified the success of the technique.

Finishing

Placement procedures that minimize the need for finishing and polishing should be utilized. The smoothest surface that can be obtained is unfinished resin composite formed against a smooth matrix.[126] Polishing procedures are inherently destructive to the restored surface[4] and may result in formation of microcracks below the surface of the composite.[97,175] Because cracks may also be produced or exacerbated during mastication, the fracture toughness of the composite may be significantly reduced by destructive finishing techniques.[51]

Early finishing of resin composite (3 minutes after placement) has been shown to significantly increase microleakage.[57] Therefore, finishing should be delayed as long as possible to minimize adverse effects. Delaying finishing for 10 to 15 minutes will allow approximately 70% of maximal polymerization to occur during the "dark-curing" phase following application of the curing light.[3,4]

The finishing and polishing process for posterior composite restorations is similar to that for other composites. Excess material can be removed from the occlusal surface with multifluted carbide finishing burs or fine diamonds. A No. 12 or 12b scalpel blade is useful for removing flash from the proximal and gingival margins. The composite material can then be finished and blended to the tooth with successively finer grades of polishing points, cups, or disks. Aluminum oxide–impregnated finishing strips can be used to finish the proximal surfaces. The final high polish can be accomplished with aluminum oxide polishing pastes. Some of the clinical steps involved in placement of a posterior composite restoration are shown in Figs 8-12a to 8-12d.

Rebonding and Final Cure

As previously mentioned, finishing procedures are destructive to the composite restoration and have been shown to adversely affect wear in clinical studies.[129] In addition, the composite surface closest to the light tip during curing, which has the best physical properties, is removed during finishing procedures. Finishing procedures can also exacerbate the marginal gaps formed during polymerization.[42,93,106]

For these reasons, the occlusal surface and all accessible restoration margins should be rebonded with an unfilled VLC resin. The lower the viscosity of the rebonding agent, the more effective it will be in penetrating interfacial gaps and subsurface microcracks.[131,151] Several new low-viscosity resins called surface sealers are being marketed for use in rebonding. Rebonding has been shown to improve the marginal integrity of composite restorations in vitro[35] and in vivo,[86] significantly reduce microleakage in vitro,[60,131,151,153] and reduce marginal staining in vivo.[63] Rebonding has been demonstrated in clinical studies to significantly reduce wear, but must be reapplied yearly for maximal effectiveness.[35,63,86]

Although the need for etching prior to rebonding is somewhat controversial, phosphoric acid is usually applied to the marginal areas for 10 seconds. The adhesive is placed, thinned with a brush, and light cured for 40 to 60 seconds. This will not only polymerize the rebonding agent, but may also provide additional polymerization to the new surface of the composite.[12,136,137]

The Tunnel Preparation

An alternative to the traditional approach to accessing interproximal caries has been termed the *tunnel preparation*. It was first suggested by Jinks[80] in 1963 as a method for placing a silver alloy mixed with sodium silicofluoride in the distal aspect of primary second molars to "inoculate" permanent first molars with fluoride as they erupted. Hunt[76] and Knight[90] later modified this procedure to be utilized as a conservative technique for restoring small interproximal carious lesions.

Advantages

There are several proposed advantages to this technique. The outer surface of the interproximal enamel is removed only if cavitated by caries, so there is less potential for a restorative overhang. Overhangs have been shown to occur 25% to 76% of the time with traditional Class 2 restorations, resulting in bleeding, gingivitis, and bone loss.[20] With an occlusal approach, the proximal ridge is preserved, and destruction of tooth structure is minimized. A two-surface cavity preparation has been shown to reduce tooth stiffness by 46%; only a 20% reduction occurs with an occlusal preparation.[130] The perimeter of the restoration is reduced, decreasing the potential for microleakage.[118] Because minimal preparation is required interproximally, the potential for disturbance of the adjacent tooth is reduced. If the caries is more extensive than originally thought and greater access is required, the preparation can easily be extended into a more traditional Class 2 design.[77]

Disadvantages

Despite these seemingly attractive benefits of the tunnel procedure, it remains largely unused in practice. It is highly technique sensitive, demanding careful control of the preparation by the operator. The angulation of the preparation often passes close to the pulp. Studies have shown that the tunnel preparation often passes within 1.0 mm of the pulp. A typical Class 2 preparation tends to leave greater remaining dentinal thickness than does the tunnel procedure.[119,144] Because of the conservative nature of the preparation, visibility is decreased, and caries removal is more uncertain.[76,77,177] In vitro studies on the effectiveness of caries removal in the tunnel preparation have shown that a high rate of residual caries is left behind.[120,144] For this reason, caries-detecting solution should be used to disclose remaining caries.

There is also concern that the marginal ridge strength is reduced because of undermining. As the diameter of the preparation increases, the marginal ridge strength decreases.[2,46,73] Although use of an adhesive restorative material has been shown to restore much of the strength of the marginal ridge,[2,46,73] this is not always the case,[119] and the degree to which marginal ridge strength is restored can depend on the size of the preparation.[46]

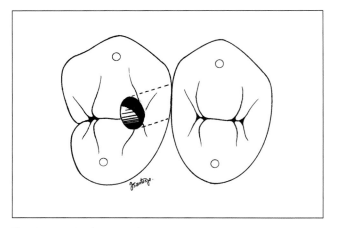

Fig 8-13a In the tunnel preparation, access is made in the occlusal fossa adjacent to the marginal ridge.

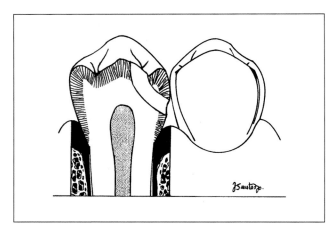

Fig 8-13b A "tunnel" is made under the marginal ridge to the carious lesion, usually just below the proximal contact.

Indications and Contraindications

Use of the tunnel preparation can be considered when small, proximal carious lesions necessitate restoration and esthetic demands are high. This preparation should be avoided when large carious lesions are diagnosed, where access is particularly difficult, or when the overlying marginal ridge is subjected to heavy occlusion or demonstrates a crack.

Preoperative Evaluation

The above factors, along with the patient's oral hygiene status, must be assessed before the tunnel preparation is initiated. The occlusion should be marked with articulating paper.

Rubber Dam Isolation

For the reasons mentioned previously, use of a rubber dam should be considered very important for this procedure.

Preparation

Access may be gained through the occlusal surface with a No. 2 round bur used in a high-speed handpiece and directed toward the carious lesion. The preparation should be started about 2.0 mm from the marginal ridge (Figs 8-13a and 8-13b). Caries removal can be accom-

plished with a No. 2 round bur in a low-speed handpiece. Because of the limited access, caries-disclosing solution is needed to improve visibility for caries removal.[77] Dentin stained with a caries-disclosing solution is removed to assure complete removal of infected carious dentin.[138] Magnifying loupes may also be useful in helping the clinician to ascertain the completeness of caries removal.

After the dentinal caries is removed, the proximal enamel lesion is evaluated. If it is weak or porous, the enamel is punched or drilled through; if it is intact, it is left alone.[77] The early enamel lesion is more resistant to carious attack than sound enamel[87] and should be left alone and allowed to remineralize. If the enamel is to be removed, a matrix band is placed to protect the adjacent tooth. If the clinician determines that the marginal ridge has been undermined, the tunnel preparation can be converted to a traditional Class 2 preparation at this time.

Restoration

Glass ionomer has been the suggested restorative material of choice. Cermet–glass ionomers were originally used because of their radiopacity and fluoride release. Compared to amalgam, they have been shown to reduce recurrent caries around the restoration as well as adjacent tooth surfaces.[150] In addition, mutans streptococci levels in plaque adjacent to interproximal glass-ionomer restorations are lower than levels adjacent to either composite or amalgam restorations.[148,149] Although one study showed good sealing of tunnel preparations with a glass-ionomer cermet,[61] another did not.[133] Resin-modified–glass ionomers are the current materials of choice for this restoration. They are radiopaque, and have been shown to prevent microleakage.[36] The glass ionomer should be placed in accordance with the manufacturer's recommendations, to approximately the level of the dentinoenamel junction.

The occlusal 1.5 to 2.0 mm of the preparation should be restored with a VLC resin composite utilizing the techniques previously described for incremental insertion. Glass ionomer has shown a marked propensity to fail under occlusal stress.[167] Resin composites are more wear resistant than glass ionomer and may help to increase the fracture resistance of the restored tooth.[7] Finishing and rebonding should be accomplished as described previously in this chapter.

Clinical studies have shown variable results, ranging from no failures[77] to 48% failure at 2 years,[167] although the latter was due to a failure of the restorative material (Ketac-Silver, ESPE) on the occlusal surface rather than to failure of the tunnel procedure itself. Marginal ridge failure has ranged from 0% to 5%.[68,167,177] Higher incidences of marginal ridge failure are associated with undermining of the marginal ridge or punching through the proximal enamel.[68] Early results seem to indicate that clinical success is possible with discriminating case selection.

References

1. Abdalla AI, Davidson CL. Comparison of the marginal integrity of in vivo and in vitro Class II composite restorations. J Dent 1993;21:158-162.

2. Akerboom HBM, Kreulen CM, van Amergongen WE, Mol A. Radiopacity of posterior composite resins, composite resin luting cements, and glass ionomer lining cements. J Prosthet Dent 1993;70:351-355.

3. Albers HF (ed). Direct composite restoratives. ADEPT Report 1991;2:53-64.

4. Albers HF (ed). Finishing direct restoratives. ADEPT Report 1992;3:1-16.

5. Alster K, Feilzer AJ, deGee AJ, Mol A, Davidson CL. The dependence of shrinkage stress reduction on porosity concentration in thin resin layers. J Dent Res 1992;71:1619-1622.

6. Amalgam update. FDI Dent World, 1992 (Sept-Oct):14-15.

7. Asmussen E. Factors affecting the quantity of remaining double bonds in restorative resin polymers. Scand J Dent Res 1982; 90:490-496.

8. Asmussen E. Softening of BISGMA-based polymers by ethanol and by organic acids of plaque. Scand J Dent Res 1984;92:257-261.

9. Bailey SJ, Swift EJ. Effects of home bleaching products on composite resins. Quintessence Int 1992; 23:489-494.

10. Barnes DM, Holston AM, Strassler HE, Shires PJ. Evaluation of clinical performance of twelve posterior composite resins with a standardized placement technique. J Esthet Dent 1990;2:36-43.

11. Barnes DM, Blank LW, Thompson VP, Holston AM, Gingell JCP. A 5- and 8-year clinical evaluation of a posterior composite resin. Quintessence Int 1991;22:143-151.

12. Bayne SC, Taylor DF, Heymann HO. Protection hypothesis for composite wear. Dent Mater 1992;8:305-309.

13. Bayne SC, Heymann HO, Swift EJ. Update on dental composite restorations. J Am Dent Assoc 1994;125:687-701.

14. Bertolotti RL. Posterior composite technique utilizing directed polymerization shrinkage and a novel matrix. Aesthet Chron 1991;3:53-58.

15. Black GV. A Work on Operative Dentistry. Chicago: Medico Dental Publishing, 1908;143-177.

16. Bonner P. Advances in dental materials: An exclusive interview with Dr. Karl Leinfelder. Dent Today 1994 (Mar):32-34.

17. Bowen RL, Marjenhoff WA. Dental composites/glass ionomers: The materials. Adv Dent Res 1992;6:44-49.

18. Brännström M. Hydrodynamic theory of dentinal pain: Sensation in preparations, caries and the dentinal crack syndrome. J Endod 1986;12:453-457.

19. Brännström M. Infection beneath composite resin restorations: Can it be avoided? Oper Dent 1987;12:158-163.

20. Brunsvold MA, Lane JJ. The prevalence of overhanging dental restorations and their relationship to periodontal disease. J Clin Periodontol 1990;17:67-72.

21. Bryant RW, Mahler DB. Modulus of elasticity in bending of composites and amalgams. J Prosthet Dent 1986;56:243-248.

22. Bryant RW. Direct posterior composite resin restorations: A review. 1. Factors influencing case selection. Aust Dent J 1992; 37:81-87.

23. Bryant RW. Direct posterior composite resin restorations: A review. 2. Clinical technique. Aust Dent J 1992;37:161-171.

24. Bullard RH, Leinfelder KF, Russell CM. Effect of coefficient of thermal expansion on microleakage. J Am Dent Assoc 1988; 116:871-874.

25. Burgess JO, Barghi N, Chan D, Hummert T. A comparative study of three glass ionomer base materials. Am J Dent 1993;6:137-141.

26. Coli P, Blixt M, Brännström M. The effect of cervical grooves on the contraction gap in Class 2 composites. Oper Dent 1993;18:33-36.

27. Coli P, Brännström M. The marginal adaptation of four different bonding agents in Class II composite resin restorations applied in bulk or in two increments. Quintessence Int 1993;24:583-591.

28. Covey D, Schulein TM, Kohout FJ. Marginal ridge strength of restored teeth with modified class II cavity preparations. J Am Dent Assoc 1989;118:199-202.

29. Craig RG (ed). Dental Restorative Materials, ed 8. St Louis: Mosby, 1989:262.

30. Crim GA. Microleakage of three resin placement techniques. Am J Dent 1991;4:69-72.

31. Cunningham J, Mair LH, Foster MA, Ireland RS. Clinical evaluation of three posterior composite and two amalgam restorative materials: 3 year results. Br Dent J 1990;169:319-323.

32. Dawson AS, Smales RJ. Restoration longevity in an Australian Defense Force population. Aust Dent J 1992;37:196-200.

33. deGee AJ. Some aspects of vacuum mixing of composite resins and its effects on porosity. Quintessence Int 1979;10(7):69-75.

34. Dickinson GL, Gerbo LR, Leinfelder KF. Clinical evaluation of a highly wear resistant composite. Am J Dent 1993;6:85-87.

35. Dickinson GL, Leinfelder KF. Assessing the long-term effect of a surface penetrating sealant. J Am Dent Assoc 1993;124:68-72.

36. Doerr CL, Hilton TJ, Hermesch C. Thermocycling effect on microleakage of conventional and VLA glass ionomer [abstract 765]. J Dent Res 1995;74:107.

37. Donly KJ, Wild TW, Bowen RL, Jensen ME. An in vitro investigation of the effects of glass inserts on the effective composite resin polymerization shrinkage. J Dent Res 1989;68:1234-1237.

38. Douglas DD. Environmental cops hot on the trail of mercury discharge; dentists avert mercury pollution rules. AGD Impact 1995;23:8-12.

39. Douvitsas G. Effect of cavity design on gap formation in class II composite resin restorations. J Prosthet Dent 1991;65:475-479.

40. Eakle WS. Fracture resistance of teeth restored with class II bonded composite resin. J Dent Res 1986;65:149-153.

41. Eichmiller FC. Clinical use of beta-quartz glass-ceramic inserts. Compend Contin Educ Dent 1992;13:568-574.

42. Eick JD, Welch FH. Polymerization shrinkage of posterior composite resins and its possible influence on postoperative sensitivity. Quintessence Int 1986;17:103-111.

43. Eick JD, Robinson SJ, Byerley TJ, Chappelow CC. Adhesives and nonshrinking dental resins of the future. Quintessence Int 1993;24:632-640.

44. Ericson D, Derand T. Reduction of cervical gaps in class II composite resin restorations. J Prosthet Dent 1991;65:33-37.

45. Espelid I, Tveit AB, Erickson RL, Keck SC, Glasspoole EA. Radiopacity of restorations and detection of secondary caries. Dent Mater 1991;7:114-117.

46. Fasbinder DJ, Davis RD, Burgess JO. Marginal ridge strength in class II tunnel restorations. Am J Dent 1991;4:77-82.

47. Feilzer AJ, deGee AJ, Davidson CL. Setting stress in composite resin in relation to configuration of the restoration. J Dent Res 1987;66:1636-1639.

48. Feilzer AJ, deGee AJ, Davidson CL. Curing contraction of composites and glass-ionomer cements. J Prosthet Dent 1988;59:297-300.

49. Feilzer AJ, deGee AJ, Davidson CL. Setting stresses in composites for two different curing modes. Dent Mater 1993;9:2-5.

50. Ferracane JL Greener EH. Fourier transform infrared analysis of degree of polymerization in unfilled resins: Methods comparison. J Dent Res 1984;63:1093-1095.

51. Ferracane JL, Antonio RC, Matsumoto H. Variables affecting the fracture toughness of dental composites. J Dent Res 1987;66:1140-1145.

52. Ferracane JL. Using posterior composites appropriately. J Am Dent Assoc 1992;123:53-58.

53. Ferracane JL, Marker VA. Solvent degradation and reduced fracture toughness in aged composites. J Dent Res 1992;71:13-19.

54. Ferracane JL. Materials in Dentistry. Principles and Applications. Philadelphia: Lippincott 1995:88-102.

55. Fissore B, Nicholls JI, Yuodelis RA. Load fatigue of teeth restored by a dentin bonding agent and a posterior composite resin. J Prosthet Dent 1991;65:80-85.

56. Friedman J. Variability of lamp characteristics in dental curing lights. J Esthet Dent 1989;1:189-190.

57. Fusayama A, Kohno A. Marginal closure of composite restorations with the gingival wall in cementum/dentin. J Prosthet Dent 1989;61:293-296.

58. Fusayama T. Indications for self-cured and light-cured adhesive composite resins. J Prosthet Dent 1992;67:46-51.

59. Fusayama T. Biologic problems of the light-cured composite resin. Quintessence Int 1993;24:225-226.

60. Garcia-Godoy F, Malone WFP. Microleakage of posterior composite restorations after rebonding. Compend Contin Educ Dent 1987;8:606-609.

61. Garcia-Godoy F, Marshall TD, Mount GJ. Microleakage of glass ionomer tunnel restorations. Am J Dent 1988;1:53-56.

62. Gerbo L, Leinfelder KF, Mueninghoff L, Russell C. Use of optical standards for determining wear of posterior composite resins. J Esthet Dent 1990;2:148-152.

63. Gibson GB, Richardson AS, Patton RE, Waldman R. A clinical evaluation of occlusal composite and amalgam restorations: One and two year results. J Am Dent Assoc 1982;104:335-337.

64. Goodis HE, White JM, Marshall SJ, Koshrovi P, Watanabe LG, Marshall GW. The effect of glass ionomer liners in lowering pulp temperatures during composite placement, in vitro. Dent Mater 1993;9:146-150.

65. Hansen EK. Effect of cavity depth and application technique on marginal adaptation of resins in dentin cavities. J Dent Res 1986;65:1319-1321.

66. Hansen EK. In vivo cusp fracture of endodontically treated premolars restored with MOD amalgam or MOD resin fillings. Dent Mater 1988;4:169-173.

67. Hansen EK, Asmussen E. Marginal adaptation of posterior resins: Effect of dentin-bonding agent and hygroscopic expansion. Dent Mater 1989;5:122-126.

68. Hasselrot L. The tunnel preparation. Traditional and alternative methods. Tandlakartidningen 1990;82:1114-1126.

69. Hellie CM, Charbeneau GT, Craig RG, Brandau HE. Quantitative evaluation of proximal tooth movement effected by wedging: A pilot study. J Prosthet Dent 1985;53:335-341.

70. Hembree JH. Microleakage at the gingival margin of class II composite restorations with glass-ionomer liner. J Prosthet Dent 1989;61:28-30.

71. Hendriks FHJ, Letzel H, Vrijhoef MMA. Composite versus amalgam restorations: A three year clinical evaluation. J Oral Rehabil 1986;13:401-411.

72. Hengchang X, Tong W, Vingerling RA, Shiqing S. A study of surfaces developed on composite resins in vivo during 4-5 years: Observations by SEM. J Oral Rehabil 1989;16:407-416.

73. Hill FJ, Halaseh FJ. A laboratory investigation of tunnel restorations in premolar teeth. Br Dent J 1988;165:364-367.

74. Hilton TJ, Schwartz RS. The effect of air thinning on dentin adhesive strength. Oper Dent 1995;20:133-137.

75. Hinoura K, Setcos JC, Phillips RW. Cavity design and placement techniques for class 2 composites. Oper Dent 1988;13:12-19.

76. Hunt PR. A modified Class II cavity preparation for glass ionomer restorative materials. Quintessence Int 1984;15:1011-1018.

77. Hunt PR. Microconservative restorations for approximal carious lesions. J Am Dent Assoc 1990;120:37-40.

78. Jacobsen PH. The restoration of Class II cavities by polymeric materials. J Dent 1984;12:47-52.

79. Jendresen MD. Clinical behavior of 21st century adhesives and composites. Quintessence Int 1993;24:659-662.

80. Jinks GM. Fluoride-impregnated cements and their effect on the activity of interproximal caries. J Dent Child 1963;30:87-92.

81. Johnson WW, Dhuru VB, Brantley WA. Composite microfiller content and its effect on fracture toughness and diametral tensile strength. Dent Mater 1993;9:95-98.

82. Jordan RE, Suzuki M. Posterior composite restorations; where and how they work best. J Am Dent Assoc 1991;122:31-37.

83. Joynt RB, Wieczkowski G, Klockowski R, Davis EL. Effects of composite restorations on resistance to cuspal fracture in posterior teeth. J Prosthet Dent 1987;57:431-435.

84. Kasloff Z, Galan D, Williams PT. Cuspal deflection studies using an electronic probe [abstract 2264]. J Dent Res 1993;72:386.

85. Kawai K, Leinfelder KF. Effect of glass inserts on wear of composite resins [abstract 81]. J Dent Res 1993;72:114.

86. Kawai K, Leinfelder KF. Effect of surface-penetrating sealant on composite wear. Dent Mater 1993;9:108-113.

87. Kidd EAM, Joyston-Bechal S. Susceptibility of natural carious lesions in enamel to an artificial caries-like attack in vitro. Br Dent J 1986;160:345-348.

88. Kilpatrick NM. Durability of restorations in primary molars. J Dent 1993;21:67-73.

89. Klausner LH, Green TG, Charbeneau GT. Placement and replacement of amalgam restorations: A challenge for the profession. Oper Dent 1987;12:105-111.

90. Knight GM. The use of adhesive materials in the conservative restoration of selected posterior teeth. Aust Dent J 1984;29:324-331.

91. Koike T, Hasegawa T, Manabe A, Itoh K, Wakumoto S. Effect of water sorption and thermal stress on cavity adaptation of dental composites. Dent Mater 1990;6:178-180.

92. Krejci I, Lutz F, Krejci D. The influence of different base materials on marginal adaptation and wear of conventional Class II composite resin restorations. Quintessence Int 1988;19:191-198.

93. Lambrechts P, Braem M, Vanherle G. Evaluation of clinical performance for posterior composite resins and dentin adhesives. Oper Dent 1987;12:53-87.

94. Lambrechts P, Braem M, Vuylsteke-Wauters M, Vanherle G. Quantitative in vivo wear of human enamel. J Dent Res 1989;68:1752-1754.

95. Langdon RS, Moon PC, Barnes RF. Effect of dentin bonding adhesive thickness on bond strength [abstract 244]. J Dent Res 1994;73:132.

96. Leinfelder KF. Composite resins. Dent Clin North Am 1985;29:359-371.

97. Leinfelder KF, Wilder AD, Teixeira AC. Wear rates of posterior composite resins. J Am Dent Assoc 1986;112:829-833.

98. Leinfelder KF. Posterior composite resins. J Can Dent Assoc 1989;55:34-39.

99. Leinfelder KF. Using composite resin as a posterior restorative material. J Am Dent Assoc 1991;122:65-70.

100. Leinfelder KF. Composite resin systems for posterior restorations. Caulk Restorative Supplement 1993;(Apr):23-27.

101. Letzel H. Survival rates and reasons for failure of posterior composite restorations in multicentre clinical trial. J Dent 1989;17:S10-S17.

102. Lundin SA. Studies on posterior composite resins with special reference to class II restorations. Swed Dent J 1990;73(suppl):6-33.

103. Lutz F, Phillips RW, Roulet J-F, Setcos JC. In vivo and in vitro wear of potential posterior composites. J Dent Res 1984;63:914-920.

104. Lutz F, Krejci I, Luescher B, Oldenburg TR. Improved proximal margin adaptation of Class II composite resin restorations by use of light-reflecting wedges. Quintessence Int 1986;17:659-664.

105. Lutz F, Krejci I, Oldenburg TR. Elimination of polymerization stresses at the margins of posterior composite resin restorations: A new restorative technique. Quintessence Int 1986;17:777-784.

106. Lutz F, Krejci I, Barbakow F. Quality and durability of marginal adaptation in bonded composite restorations. Dent Mater 1991;7:107-113.

107. Lutz F, Krejci I, Barbakow F. Chewing pressure vs. wear of composites and opposing enamel cusps. J Dent Res 1992; 71:1525-1529.

108. Lutz F, Krejci I, Barbakow F. The importance of proximal curing in posterior composite resin restorations. Quintessence Int 1992;23:605-609.

109. Lutz F, Krejci I, Barbakow F. Restoration quality in relation to wedge-mediated light channeling. Quintessence Int 1992;23:763-767.

110. Mair LH, Vowles RW, Cunningham J, Williams DF. The clinical wear of three posterior composites. Br Dent J 1990;169:355-360.

111. Martin FE, Bryant RW. Acid-etching of enamel cavity walls. Aust Dent J 1984;29:308-314.

112. Marzouk MA, Ross JA. Cervical enamel crazings associated with occluso-proximal composite restorations in posterior teeth. Am J Dent 1989;2:333-337.

113. Mazer RB, Leinfelder KF, Russell CM. Degradation of micro-filled posterior composite. Dent Mater 1992;8:185-189.

114. Mitchem JC, Gronas DG. In vivo evaluation of the wear of restorative resin. J Am Dent Assoc 1982;104:333-335.

115. Mitchem JC. The use and abuse of aesthetic materials in posterior teeth. Int Dent J 1988;38:119-125.

116. Morin D, DeLong R, Douglas WH. Cusp reinforcement by the acid-etch technique. J Dent Res 1984;63:1075-1078.

117. Munechika T, Suzuki K, Nishiyama M, Ohashi M, Horie K. A comparison of the tensile bond strengths of composite resins to longitudinal and transverse sections of enamel prisms in human teeth. J Dent Res 1984;63:1079-1082.

118. Papa J, Wilson PR, Tyas MJ. Tunnel restorations: A review. J Esthet Dent 1992;4 (suppl):4-9.

119. Papa J, Cain C, Messer HH, Wilson PR. Tunnel restorations versus Class II restorations for small proximal lesions: A comparison of tooth strengths. Quintessence Int 1993;24:93-98.

120. Papa J, Cain C, Messer HH. Efficacy of tunnel restorations in the removal of caries. Quintessence Int 1993;4:715-719.

121. Pearson GJ, Hegarty SM. Cusp movement of molar teeth with composite filling materials in conventional and modified MOD cavities. Br Dent J 1989;166:162-165.

122. Penning C, van Amerongen JP. Microleakage of extended and nonextended class I composite resin and sealant restorations. J Prosthet Dent 1990;64:131-134.

123. Pires JAF, Cvitko E, Denehy GE, Swift EJ. Effects of curing tip distance on light intensity and composite resin microhardness. Quintessence Int 1993;24:517-521.

124. Podshadley AG, Gullett CE, Binkley TK. Interface strength of incremental placement of visible light-cured composites. J Am Dent Assoc 1985;110:932-934.

125. Prati C. Early marginal microleakage in Class II resin composite restorations. Dent Mater 1989;5:392-398.

126. Pratten DH, Johnson GH. An evaluation of finishing instruments for an anterior and a posterior composite. J Prosthet Dent 1988;60:154-158.

127. Qvist V, Qvist J, Mjör IA. Placement and longevity of tooth-colored restorations in Denmark. Acta Odontol Scand 1990;48:305-311.

128. Qvist V, Strom C. 11-year assessment of class III resin restorations completed with two restorative procedures. Acta Odontol Scand 1993;51:253-262.

129. Ratanapridakul K, Leinfelder KF, Thomas J. Effect of finishing on the in vivo wear rate of a posterior composite resin. J Am Dent Assoc 1989;118:524-526.

130. Reeh ES, Messer HH, Douglas WH. Reduction in tooth stiffness as a result of endodontic and restorative procedures. J Endod 1989;15:512-516.

131. Reid JS, Saunders WP, Yick YC. The effect of bonding agent and fissure sealant on microleakage of composite resin restorations. Quintessence Int 1991;22:295-298.

132. Retief DH, Mandras RS, Russell CM. Shear bond strength required to prevent microleakage at the dentin/restoration interface. Am J Dent 1994;7:43-46.

133. Robbins JW, Cooley RL. Microleakage of Ketac Silver in the tunnel preparation. Oper Dent 1988;13:8-11.

134. Robbins W, Summitt JB. Longevity of complex amalgam restorations. Oper Dent 1988;13:54-57.

135. Rowe AHR. A five year study of the clinical performance of a posterior composite resin restorative material. J Dent 1989;17:S6-S9.

136. Rueggeberg FA, Caughman WF, Curtis JW, Davis HC. Factors affecting cure at depths within light-activated resin composites. Am J Dent 1993;6:91-95.

137. Rueggeberg FA, Jordan DM. Effect of light-tip distance on polymerization of resin composite. Int J Prosthodont 1993;6:364-370.

138. Sato Y, Fusayama T. Removal of dentin by fuchsin staining. J Dent Res 1976;55:678-683.

139. Segura A, Donly KJ. In vitro posterior composite polymerization recovery following hygroscopic expansion. J Oral Rehabil 1993;20:495-499.

140. Soderholm KJ, Zigan M, Ragan M, Fischlschweiger W, Bergman M. Hydrolytic degradation of dental composites. J Dent Res 1984;63:1248-1254.

141. Sorenson JA, Dixit NV, White SN, Avera SP. In vitro microleakage of dentin adhesives. Int J Prosthodont 1991;4:213-218.

142. Stamplia LL, Nicholls JI, Brudvik JS, Jones DW. Fracture resistance of teeth with resin-bonded restorations. J Prosthet Dent 1986;55:694-698.

143. Stangel I, Barolet RY. Clinical evaluation of two posterior composite resins: Two-year results. J Oral Rehab 1990;17:257-268.

144. Strand GV, Tveit AB. Effectiveness of caries removal by the partial tunnel preparation. Scand J Dent Res 1993;101:270-273.

145. Suliman AA, Boyer DB, Lakes RS. Cusp movement in premolars resulting from composite polymerization shrinkage. Dent Mater 1993;9:6-10.

146. Summitt JB, Della Bona A, Burgess JO. The strength of Class II composite restorations as affected by preparation design. Quintessence Int 1994;25:251-257.

147. Suzuki M, Jordan RE. Glass ionomer–composite sandwich technique. J Am Dent Assoc 1990;120:55-57.

148. Svanberg M, Krasse B, Ornerfeldt HO. Mutans streptococci in interproximal plaque from amalgam and glass ionomer restorations. Caries Res 1990;24:133-136.

149. Svanberg M, Mjör IA, Orstavik D. Mutans streptococci in plaque from margins of amalgam, composite, and glass-ionomer restorations. J Dent Res 1990;69:861-864.

150. Svanberg M. Class II amalgam restorations, glass-ionomer tunnel restorations, and caries development on adjacent tooth surfaces: A 3-year clinical study. Caries Res 1992;26:315-318.

151. Tjan AHL, Tan DE. Microleakage at gingival margins of Class V composite resin restoration rebonded with various low-viscosity resin systems. Quintessence Int 1991;22:565-573.

152. Tjan AHL, Bergh BH, Lidner C. Effect of various incremental techniques on the marginal adaptation of class II composite resin restorations. J Prosthet Dent 1992;67:62-66.

153. Torstenson B, Brännström M, Mattsson B. A new method for sealing composite resin contraction gaps in lined cavities. J Dent Res 1985;64:450-453.

154. Toyooka J, Taira M, Wakasa K, Yamaki M, Fujita M, Wada T. Radiopacity of 12 visible-light-cured dental composite resins. J Oral Rehabil 1993;20:615-622.

155. Tveit AB, Espelid I. Radiographic diagnosis of caries and marginal defects in connection with radiopaque composite fillings. Dent Mater 1986;2:159-162.

156. Tyas MJ. Colour stability of composite resins: A clinical comparison. Aust Dent J 1992;37:88-90.

157. Tyas MJ. Clinical evaluation of five adhesive systems. Am J Dent 1994;7:77-80.

158. Venhoven BAM, deGee AJ, Davidson CL. Polymerization contraction and conversion of light-curing BisGMA-based methacrylate resins. Biomater 1993;14:871-875.

159. Von Beetzen M, Li J, Nicander I, Sundstrom F. Microhardness and porosity of Class 2 light-cured composite restorations cured with a transparent cone attached to the light-curing wand. Oper Dent 1993;18:103-109.

160. Wang JC, Charbeneau GT, Gregory WA, Dennison JB. Quantitative evaluation of approximal contacts in Class 2 composite resin restorations: A clinical study. Oper Dent 1989;14:193-202.

161. Warren JA, Clark NP. Posterior composite resin: Current trends in restorative techniques, Part I. Pre-preparation considerations, preparation, dentin treatment, etching/boding. Gen Dent 1987;(Sept-Oct):368-372.

162. Warren JA, Clark NP. Posterior composite resin: Current trends in restorative techniques, Part II. Insertion, finishing, and polishing. Gen Dent 1987;(Nov-Dec):497-499.

163. Watanabe I, Nakabayashi N. Bonding durability of photocured phenyl-P in TEGDMA to smear layer-retained bovine dentin. Quintessence Int 1993;24:335-342.

164. Wendt SL, Leinfelder KF. Clinical evaluation of a posterior resin composite: 3-year results. Am J Dent 1994;7:207-211.

165. Wieczkowski F, Joynt RB, Klockowski R, Davis EL. Effects of incremental versus bulk fill technique on resistance to cuspal fracture of teeth restored with posterior composites. J Prosthet Dent 1988;60:283-287.

166. Wilder AD, May KN, Leinfelder KF. Three-year clinical study of UV-cured composite resins in posterior teeth. J Prosthet Dent 1983;50:26-30.

167. Wilkie R, Lidums A, Smales R. Class II glass ionomer cermet tunnel, resin sandwich and amalgam restorations over 2 years. Am J Dent 1993;6:181-184.

168. Willems G, Lambrechts P, Braem M, Vanherle G. Three-year follow up of five posterior composites: In vivo wear. J Dent 1993;21:74-78.

169. Willems G, Lambrechts P, Braem M, Vanherle G. Composite resins of the 21st century. Quintessence Int 1993;24:641-658.

170. Willems G, Lambrechts P, Lesaffre E, Braem M, Vanherle G. Three-year follow-up of five posterior composites: SEM study of differential wear. J Dent 1993;21:79-86.

171. Williams PT, Johnson LN. Composite resin restoratives revisited. J Can Dent Assoc 1993;59:538-543.

172. Wilson EG, Mandradjieff M, Brindock T. Controversies in posterior composite resin restorations. Dent Clin North Am 1990;34:27-44.

173. Wilson HJ. Resin-based restoratives. Br Dent J 1988;164:326-330.

174. Wilson NHF, Wilson MA, Wastell DF, Smith GA. Performance of occlusion in butt-joint and bevel-edged preparations: Five-year results. Dent Mater 1991;7:92-98.

175. Wu W, Cobb EN. A silver staining technique for investigating wear of restorative dental composites. J Biomed Mater Res 1981;15:343-348.

176. Wu W, Toth EE, Ellison JA. Subsurface damage layer of in vivo worn dental composite restorations. J Dent Res 1984;63:675-680.

177. Zenkner JEA, Baratieri LN, Monteiro S, Andrada MAC, Vieira LCC. Clinical and radiographic evaluation of cermet tunnel restorations on primary molars. Quintessence Int 1993;24:783-791.

178. Zickert I, Emilson CG, Krasse B. Correlation of level and duration of streptococcus mutans infection with incidence of dental caries. Infect Immun 1983;39:982-985.

Posterior Inlays and Onlays

J. William Robbins / Dennis J. Fasbinder / John O. Burgess

There are several treatment options for esthetic Class 1 and Class 2 restorations, in addition to direct resin composite restorations. This chapter will discuss tooth-colored inlays and onlays fabricated in resin composite and in ceramic materials. Restorations fabricated with computer-assisted design/computer-assisted manufacture (CAD/CAM) technology will also be discussed.

Esthetic inlays and onlays have a number of characteristics in common, whether they are resin, ceramic, or fabricated with CAD/CAM technology. Common features will be discussed first, followed by details of the individual restorations.

General Considerations

Preparations

The preparations for ceramic and resin composite inlays and onlays are the same. Preparations for CAD/CAM restorations differ somewhat and will be discussed in a later section.

There is minimal research to support the efficacy of any preparation design.[2] However, based on knowledge of the materials and clinical experience, the divergent, relatively nonretentive preparation is most commonly advocated because of ease of placement during the fitting process (Figs 9-1a to 9-1h). Resistance form may be incorporated with rounded proximal boxes, but grooves should not be used. Resistance and retention are provided primarily by adhesion to enamel and dentin. The walls and floors of the preparation should be smooth and flat, and the internal angles should be rounded to enhance adaptation of the restorative material.

There is no benefit to placement of bevels at the occlusal or gingival margins, and bevels should be avoided because both resin composite and porcelain are susceptible to chipping at try-in or cementation.[58,80] A 90-degree butt joint minimizes the chipping problem, but will result in a visible demarcation between the tooth and the restoration. Therefore, when the esthetic blend of the restoration and the tooth is important, such as on the facial surface of a maxillary tooth, a long chamfer may be placed (Fig 9-2). A minimum 2-mm thickness of resin or ceramic is recommended in all other areas for strength[11] (Fig 9-3).

Bases and Liners

The use of bases and liners is somewhat controversial. Initially, glass-ionomer bases were used for dentinal protection and to base the preparation to ideal form. However, it has been shown that it is not necessary to protect the dentin from the phosphoric acid etchant.[27,71] Therefore, currently glass-ionomer cement is only recommended for routine blockout of undercuts.

Provisional Restoration

Provisional restorations can be a challenge with esthetic inlays and, particularly, onlays because of the nonretentive design of the preparations. Provisional restorations can be made in the usual manner with acrylic resin or resin composite and cemented with temporary cement. It is commonly stated that a eugenol-containing cement should not be used with the provisional restoration when the final restoration will be bonded with a resin cement.[2,52] However, this assertion is generally not sup-

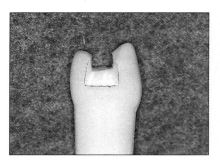

Fig 9-1a Simulation of amalgam preparation after removal of the amalgam.

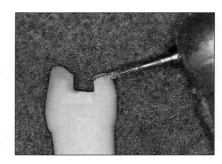

Fig 9-1b Use of a diamond of known diameter to make the first depth cut of 1 mm.

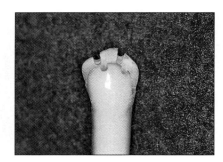

Fig 9-1c First depth cuts of 1 mm.

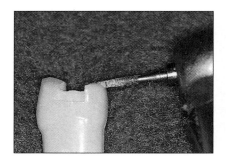

Fig 9-1d Use of a diamond of known diameter to make the second depth cuts of 1.0 mm.

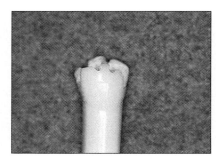

Fig 9-1e Second depth cuts of an additional 1 mm.

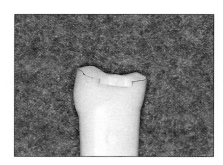

Fig 9-1f Occlusal reduction of 2 mm completed; however, sharp line angles remain in the box area.

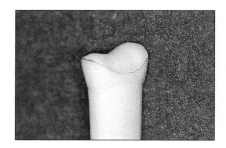

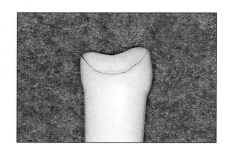

Figs 9-1g and 9-1h Completed smooth, flowing preparation without sharp angles.

ported by the literature.[64,65] Because of the nonretentive design of the onlay preparation, polycarboxylate cement is the temporary luting cement of choice. If adjacent teeth are being restored, the provisional restorations can be connected to improve retention.

For inlay preparations, flexible light-cured materials, such as Fermit (Vivadent) or Barricade (Dentsply), may be used. To provide retention and to decrease sensitivity, a dentin primer can be placed in the preparation and air dried or a small amount of resin-modified glass-ionomer cement liner can be placed on the pulpal floor and polymerized. The preparation is filled with the provisional material, and the patient is instructed to bite into maximum intercuspation to develop the occlusion. Excess

material is removed with an explorer, and the provisional restoration is light cured. This technique is only recommended for short-term use in small preparations.[8]

Cementation

Resin luting cement is the only material recommended for cementation, because it bonds to enamel, dentin, and the restorative material. Resin cement limits microleakage, enhances the strength of the restoration,[17] and provides at least short-term strengthening of the tooth.[12,59] Dual-cured resin cement, which combines light-curing and chemical-curing components, should be

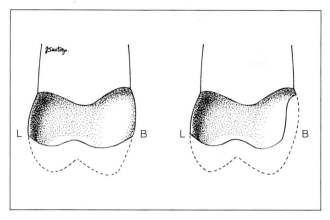

Fig 9-2 Standard onlay preparation *(left)* and modified onlay preparation *(right)* that includes coverage of facial surface to achieve a superior esthetic blend with the natural tooth color. (L) Lingual; (B) buccal.

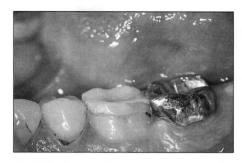

Fig 9-3 Inadequate occlusal reduction for porcelain onlay, resulting in fractured porcelain.

used to cement all indirect posterior bonded restorations. The light-curing component polymerizes rapidly on exposure to light of the proper wavelengths, while the chemical-curing component undergoes a slow polymerization process in those areas to which the light does not penetrate. It is important that the curing light be applied to dual-cured resin for an adequate period of time, because the dual-cure process results in more complete polymerization than is achieved with the chemical polymerization alone.[24] The shelf life of dual-cured resins is shorter than that of conventional light-cured resin composites. Therefore, a test batch of dual-cured resin cement should periodically be mixed and allowed to cure in a dark environment to ensure that it will polymerize in the absence of light. It should polymerize in the dark within 10 minutes.

Preparing the Restoration for Cementation

Adhesion is more easily and reliably achieved to ceramic materials than to resin composite. Ceramics can be etched, creating durable micromechanical retention.[1] The ceramic onlay is prepared for cementation by etching of the internal surface, usually with hydrofluoric acid. This is generally done at the laboratory, but may be done chairside. Shortly before cementation, silane is applied to the etched surface to enhance wetting by the adhesive cement.

Bonding to resin composite restorations is more difficult. In most cases, the resin surface has no air-inhibited layer and relatively few unreacted methacrylate groups, so a reliable chemical bond does not form between the inlay and the resin cement.[77]

Because the resin composite–cement interface may be the weak link, several procedures have been recommended to enhance the bond to resin. With hybrid resin composite, the resin surface to receive the cement should be carefully air abraded with 50-µm aluminum oxide (avoiding the margins)[43] and then cleaned with a steam cleaner or in an ultrasonic bath. The air abrasion provides a rough surface for frictional retention. The cleaned surface should be treated with an agent to allow better wetting by the cement. Silane is sometimes recommended, as is Special Bond II (Vivadent), a mixture of methacrylates in a solvent.[41] Treatment with hydrofluoric acid has also been recommended to etch the glass particles in the hybrid resin composite, but the efficacy of this method has not been verified.

Bonding to microfilled resin composite is even more problematic. Neither air abrasion nor hydrofluoric acid etching is effective in preparing the surface for bonding.[18] Although only minimally effective, use of Special Bond II on the microfilled material prior to bonding is the best method of surface preparation. No method to obtain a true chemical bond to either hybrid or microfilled resin inlays and onlays is currently available.

Preparing the Tooth for Cementation

The rubber dam is placed to ensure an isolated field (Fig 9-4a). Once the restoration is ready for cementation, the tooth is prepared in the usual manner for bonded restorations. The enamel and dentinal surfaces are etched and rinsed. A primer is applied, followed by a dual-cured adhesive. The dual-cured adhesive is also applied on the inner surface of the restoration. Use of an

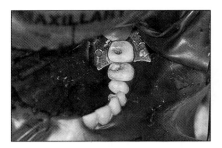

Fig 9-4a Rubber dam isolation for cementation of a quadrant of porcelain onlays.

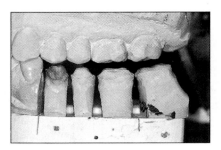

Fig 9-4b Master cast of a quadrant of porcelain onlay preparations. Note the amount of occlusal reduction.

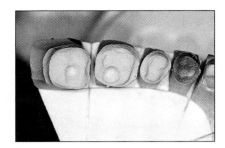

Fig 9-4c Occlusal view of onlay preparations.

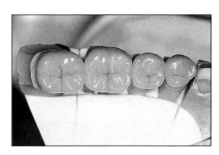

Fig 9-4d Porcelain onlays on master cast.

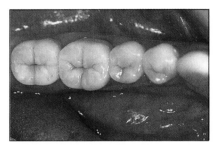

Fig 9-4e Porcelain onlays after insertion.

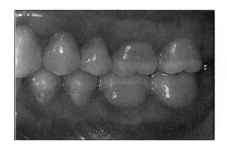

Fig 9-4f

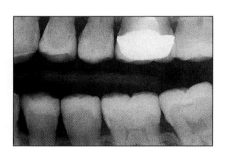

Fig 9-4g

Fig 9-4f Lateral view of the maxillary and mandibular quadrants of porcelain onlays. The esthetic blend on the facial aspect of the maxillary premolars is better because the preparations were taken farther gingivally than on the molars.

Fig 9-4g Bitewing radiograph showing porcelain onlays on all teeth except the maxillary first molar, which has a ceramometal crown.

adhesive system with resin cements is reported to decrease microleakage[6] and increase bond strength.[45]

Light-cured adhesive should not be used under indirect posterior bonded restorations. The light-cured adhesive must be air thinned prior to polymerization to ensure that there is no pooling of the adhesive that would prevent complete seating of the restoration. However, it has been shown that air thinning of the light-cured adhesive significantly decreases the bond strength.[25] Therefore, only dual-cured adhesive should be used under indirect posterior bonded restorations because it is not necessary to polymerize this type of adhesive prior to cementation of the restoration.

The dual-cured cement is mixed and placed into the preparation and restoration, and the restoration is seated. Excess cement should be removed prior to light polymerization. The gingival margins must be completely cleaned with floss and interproximal instruments prior to polymerization of the resin cement. Some clinicians recommend placement of a clear gel, such as glycerin, on the margins prior to polymerization to prevent the formation of an air-inhibited layer in the cement at the margin.[3] The margins may be finished with microfine diamonds or finishing burs and a No. 12 scalpel blade and can be polished with disks, rubber points, or cups. The final step is rebonding, as described in chapter 8, with an unfilled or lightly filled resin (Figs 9-4b to 9-4g).

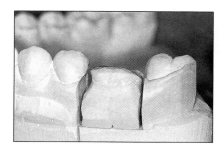

Fig 9-5a Master die of a preparation for a ceramic onlay on a mandibular first molar.

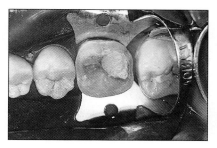

Fig 9-5b Onlay preparation isolated for bonding of the onlay.

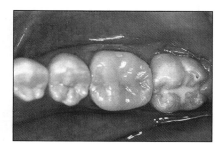

Fig 9-5c Completed Empress onlay on mandibular first molar.

Wear

There is a significant difference in the wear characteristics of composite and porcelain. Wear is not a significant factor in a porcelain restoration,[10,11] but porcelain is highly abrasive and can cause significant wear of the opposing dentition. Composites, in contrast, do not cause significant wear to the opposing dentition but can undergo significant wear themselves.[73]

The data about the wear of resin composite materials are somewhat contradictory,[9,22] but there have been significant improvements in this area. Enamel is reported to wear at a rate of 20 to 40 µm a year.[42] Most modern composites fall within that range.[73]

Maintenance

Maintenance is a very important factor in the longevity of esthetic inlays and onlays. As with all types of restorative dentistry, poor oral hygiene can cause the finest dentistry to fail.

Use of devices such as an ultrasonic scaler or air-abrasive polisher on these restorations should be avoided, because they can cause surface and marginal damage. Hand instruments should be carefully used to remove calculus. When scalers are used around the bonded inlay or onlay, care must be taken not to chip the margins. Surface stain may be removed from a restoration with aluminum oxide polishing paste or diamond polishing paste on a felt wheel or rubber cup. Acidulated phosphate fluoride should not be used intraorally in patients with ceramic restorations, because of its ability to etch porcelain.

The patient should be advised that foods and liquids with a high potential for staining, such as coffee and tea, increase the potential for marginal staining. The patient must be made aware of the potential for the restoration to fracture. Activities such as ice chewing and nail biting must be absolutely avoided. When a patient has a history of a parafunctional habit, a protective appliance should be fabricated to protect both the inlay or onlay and the opposing teeth.

Longevity

Results of short-term clinical studies of resin inlays are encouraging, but there are, as yet, no long-term results. Bishop[5] reported one failure out of 92 resin inlays that had been in place for 7 months to 4 years. A Swedish study[4] reported 29 of 30 resin inlays were excellent or acceptable at 17 months. An American study[78] reported no failures among 60 resin inlays after 3 years. There have been no published clinical studies of resin onlays.

A few clinical studies have evaluated ceramic inlays. One study[38] evaluated 10 inlays made of a pressed glass-ceramic material (Empress, Ivoclar) (Figs 9-5a to 9-5c) and reported that they were performing well after 1.5 years. Another reported satisfactory results after 2 years for traditional ceramic inlays.[33] In both 3-year[29] and 5-year clinical evaluations,[51] CAD/CAM restorations have performed satisfactorily.

Failures

Two types of failure are most common with esthetic inlays and onlays, bulk fracture (Fig 9-3) and marginal breakdown (Fig 9-6). Bulk fracture sometimes occurs in areas of cuspal coverage, particularly if the restorative material is thinner than 2.0 mm. It also occurs at the isthmus adjacent to marginal ridges, where the porcelain is poorly supported by tooth structure.

Marginal ditching is a common finding in esthetic inlays and onlays.[40,41,53,72] Because resin cements tend not to be heavily filled, they wear more quickly than the adja-

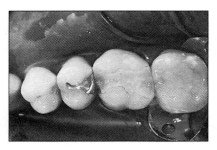

Fig 9-6 Maxillary first molar with a 7-year-old Dicor (Dentsply) inlay that is demonstrating marginal ditching and a small fracture of the marginal ridge.

cent restorations or tooth structure. This is particularly true if the marginal fit is poor.[53,79] Kawai and others[36] demonstrated a linear relationship between wear of resin cement and the horizontal marginal gap. They concluded that reduction of the marginal gap is an important clinical consideration in minimizing the wear of the resin cement. They also found that hybrid resin cements wear faster than microfilled resins. Isenberg et al[29] reported 3-year results of a clinical study of 121 Cerec inlay and onlay restorations. None of the restorations exhibited any evidence of interfacial staining, discoloration, or caries, but about 50% of the restorations exhibited gap dimensions sufficiently large to be detected with an explorer. The rate of wear of the resin composite luting agent was linear over the first year, but no further vertical wear was noted over the course of the investigation. The depth-width ratio of the gap generally did not exceed 50%.

Resin Composite Inlays and Onlays

Inlays and onlays made of resin composite are quite popular in Europe, but have not gained wide acceptance in the United States. They may be fabricated intraorally or on a cast. After polymerization, the restoration is bonded in place with a resin luting cement. Resin composite inlays can be highly esthetic and have certain advantages over direct resin composite and bonded ceramic restorations.

Advantages Over Direct Resin Composite Restorations

As discussed in chapter 8, inadequate proximal contours and open contacts are common problems of direct composite restorations. These are rarely problems with resin inlays, because contours and contacts can be developed outside of the mouth. If a contact is inadequate, it can easily be corrected prior to cementation.

Several problems associated with direct resin composite restorations are the result of polymerization shrinkage. During polymerization, resin composite shrinks on the order of 2% to 4%,[21] causing a gap to form at the least retentive marginal interface, which is usually the gingival margin. Microleakage and bacterial ingress into the marginal gap sometimes cause pulpal irritation and tooth sensitivity.[7] Current dentin adhesives have lessened the problem, but a bond strength of approximately 21 MPa is necessary to prevent microleakage.[60] None of the current dentin adhesives consistently achieves a bond strength of 21 MPa to dentin. Polymerization shrinkage can also cause cuspal flexure, which is sometimes associated with craze lines in the enamel (see Fig 8-2b) and postoperative sensitivity.[31,32]

In theory, polymerization shrinkage should be less of a problem with resin inlays because they are polymerized prior to cementation. The only polymerization shrinkage that occurs at the time of cementation is in the thin layer of resin cement. Resin inlays are reported to have less microleakage,[23,61,67] greater strength and hardness,[34,74,75] and result in less postoperative sensitivity than direct resin composite restorations.[78]

Secondary Polymerization

The superior physical properties of resin inlays are primarily due to more complete polymerization resulting from secondary polymerization procedures. Resin composites harden through a process of free-radical polymerization of methacrylate groups. The polymerization reaction is initiated (in most cases) when a molecule within the resin composite (camphorquinone) forms free radicals when exposed to light of the appropriate wavelength (about 470 nm). The radicals react with a photoreducer (an aromatic or aliphatic amine) to initiate chain formation of the methacrylate groups. As polymerization progresses, the methacrylate chains grow and the material loses its fluidity. A hard surface forms and spreads progressively deeper into the resin composite. The reaction stops when the light is removed, the thickness is too great to allow adequate light penetration, or there are no more reactive molecules in close proximity to each other. Even with long curing times and powerful lights, incomplete polymerization occurs, particularly below the surface.[44]

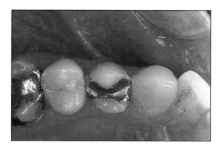

Fig 9-7a Preoperative view of a maxillary first premolar with an amalgam restoration that must be replaced.

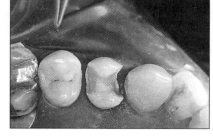

Fig 9-7b Preparation for a direct mesio-occlusodistal resin composite inlay.

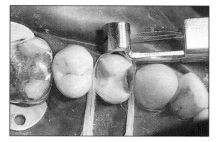

Fig 9-7c Placement of a matrix for a direct resin composite inlay.

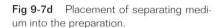

Fig 9-7d Placement of separating medium into the preparation.

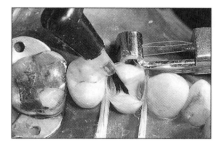

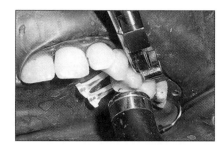

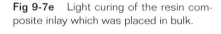

Fig 9-7e Light curing of the resin composite inlay which was placed in bulk.

Fig 9-7d

Fig 9-7e

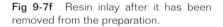

Fig 9-7f Resin inlay after it has been removed from the preparation.

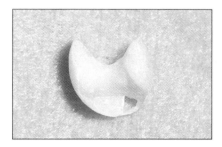

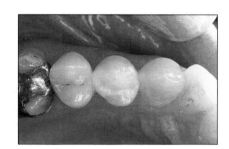

Fig 9-7g Two-year postoperative view of the direct mesio-occlusodistal resin composite inlay in the maxillary first premolar.

Fig 9-7f

Fig 9-7g

Light-cured resin composite inlays undergo this initial polymerization, but then are further polymerized in an oven or pressure pot with a combination of intense light, heat, and/or pressure. The postcure can be performed in a postcure unit specifically made for this purpose, in a toaster oven at approximately 250°F for 7 minutes,[34] or with a curing light or light box. Studies[74,75] have shown that the secondary polymerization results in improved physical properties but no clinical difference in wear characteristics.[76] The secondary curing procedures are recommended with all indirect resin systems, although they may not be mentioned in all manufacturers' instructions.

There are many resin composite inlay systems on the market. For the purposes of this chapter, they will be classified as direct (made on the tooth) or indirect (made on a cast).

Direct Resin Inlays

Inlays can be fabricated directly on the tooth (Figs 9-7a to 9-7g). After preparation, a water-soluble separating medium and a matrix are placed on the tooth. The preparation is bulk filled with resin composite and light cured from all directions. The matrix is removed and the inlay is teased out of the preparation. Because the resin composite shrinks during polymerization, the inlay is slightly smaller than the preparation and will come out easily if no undercuts are present. The inlay is then postcured. Finally, it is tried in, adjusted, and bonded into the preparation (see box on p. 236 for the direct resin inlay technique).

Direct Resin Inlay Technique

Fabrication

1. Choose a shade of composite.
2. Place rubber dam to isolate tooth to be restored.
3. Remove restoration and/or caries and make preparation with 8 to 10 degrees of occlusal divergence. The preparation should be smooth, with rounded line angles and without marginal bevels.
4. Coat preparation with a thin layer of water-soluble lubricant (Velvachol).
5. Place matrix and interproximal wedge(s).
6. Bulk fill preparation with composite.
7. Light cure for 60 seconds.
8. Remove wedges and matrix and remove the resin inlay with a spoon excavator.
9. Post cure inlay.

Insertion

10. Return the inlay to the preparation and check for complete seating. As a result of postcure shrinkage, a three-surface inlay will commonly not seat completely. When this occurs, the inner surfaces of both proximal boxes are lightly reduced with a microfine diamond. Try-in the inlay again, and repeat the process until the inlay seats completely.
11. Check interproximal contacts. If contact is light, roughen proximal surface of the inlay, wash surface, place light-cured adhesive and resin composite, and light cure. Return inlay to the preparation, make necessary adjustments and polish the repaired proximal surface.
12. Air abrade inner surface of the resin inlay with 50-µm aluminum oxide and wash or steam clean.

13. Place strips to protect the proximal surfaces of adjacent teeth, and place 37% phosphoric acid in the preparation for 20 seconds and rinse.
14. Place dentin primer on the prepared tooth according to manufacturer's instructions.
15. Place silane on the inner surface of the inlay and air dry.
16. Mix dual-cured adhesive resin and place a thin coat on the inner surface of the inlay and a thin layer into the preparation.
17. Mix dual-cured resin cement and place into the preparation with a syringe.
18. Place inlay in the preparation, almost completely seat, and remove excess resin cement.
19. Completely seat inlay, leaving a bead of resin cement at all accessible margins, and light cure for 5 seconds from the occlusal direction.
20. Completely clean out excess resin cement from the proximal surfaces with floss and interproximal instruments.
21. Light cure for 90 seconds from the occlusal aspect and 30 seconds from each interproximal direction.

Finishing

22. Finish occlusal margins with a 12-fluted pear-shaped finishing bur, and interproximal margins with a 12-fluted flame-shaped finishing bur and a No. 12 or 12b scalpel blade.
23. Remove the rubber dam and adjust the occlusion.
24. Smooth and polish with a composite-finishing kit.
25. Etch with phosphoric acid for 5 to 10 seconds and rebond.

Direct/Indirect Resin Inlay Technique

Fabrication

1. Choose a shade of composite.
2. Remove restoration and/or caries and make a preparation with 8 to 10 degrees of occlusal divergence. Preparation should be smooth, with rounded line angles and without marginal bevels.
3. Make impression.
4. Pour impression.
5. Remove master cast from the impression and lubricate with stone separator.
6. Place composite in the preparation, shape, and contour.
7. Light cure for 60 seconds.
8. Saw die from master cast and remove resin inlay.
9. Finish resin margins and contours on the die.
10. Postcure inlay.

Insertion

11. Place rubber dam to isolate the tooth to be restored.
12. Place inlay in the preparation and check for complete seating. Because of postcure shrinkage, a three-surface inlay commonly will not seat completely. When this occurs, the inner surfaces of both proximal boxes are lightly reduced with a microfine diamond. Try-in the inlay again and repeat the process until the inlay completely seats.
13. Check interproximal contacts. If contact is light, roughen the proximal surface of the inlay, wash surface, place light-cured adhesive and resin composite, and light cure. Return inlay to the preparation, make necessary adjustments and polish the repaired proximal surface.
14. Air abrade the inner surface of the resin inlay with 50-µm aluminum oxide and wash or steam clean.

15. Place strips to protect the proximal surfaces of adjacent teeth, and place 37% phosphoric acid in the preparation for 20 seconds and rinse.
16. Place dentin primer on the prepared tooth according to the manufacturer's instructions.
17. Place silane on the inner surface of the inlay and air dry.
18. Mix dual-cured adhesive resin and place in a thin coat on the inner surface of the inlay and a thin layer into the preparation.
19. Mix dual-cured resin cement, and place into the preparation with a syringe.
20. Place inlay in the preparation, almost completely seat, and remove excess resin cement.
21. Completely seat the inlay, leaving a bead of resin cement at all accessible margins, and light cure for 5 seconds from the occlusal direction.
22. Completely clean out excess resin cement from the proximal surfaces with floss and interproximal instruments.
23. Light cure for 90 seconds from the occlusal aspect and 30 seconds from each interproximal direction.

Finishing

24. Finish occlusal margins with a 12-fluted pear-shaped finishing bur, and interproximal margins with a 12-fluted flame-shaped finishing bur and No. 12 or 12b scalpel blade.
25. Remove rubber dam and adjust occlusion.
26. Smooth and polish with a composite-finishing kit.
27. Etch with phosphoric acid for 5 to 10 seconds and rebond.

Direct/Indirect Resin Inlays

When the direct/indirect method is used, an impression is made of the prepared tooth and a cast is poured (Figs 9-8a to 9-8o). Because this technique can be done in one appointment, the master cast must be ready to use in a short period of time (5 minutes). Therefore the products used must be compatible with the technique. The master die can be made from a silicone material (Fig 9-8d); however, most clinicians prefer a master cast made from die stone (Snap Stone, Whip Mix) (Fig 9-8j). The restoration is fabricated on the die and usually undergoes a primary and secondary polymerization. This process may be performed in the dental office or at a commercial laboratory (see box for the direct/indirect resin inlay technique).

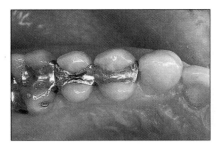

Fig 9-8a Preoperative view of the maxillary first and second premolars, which will be restored with direct/indirect resin composite inlays.

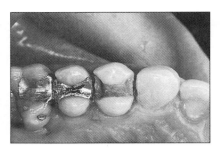

Fig 9-8b Preparation of the maxillary first premolar for a direct/indirect resin inlay.

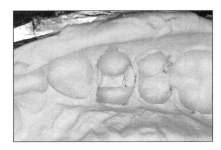

Fig 9-8c Impression of the inlay preparation.

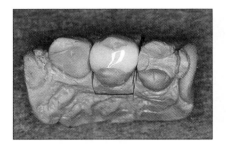

Fig 9-8d Indirect fabrication of the resin composite inlay on a silicone die that was made from the impression.

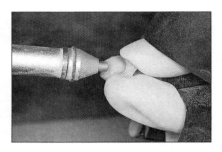

Fig 9-8e Air abrasion of the inner surface of the hybrid resin composite inlay with 50 µm aluminum oxide.

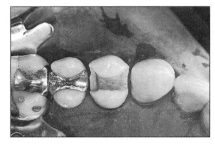

Fig 9-8f Preparation of the maxillary first premolar for cementation of the direct/indirect resin inlay.

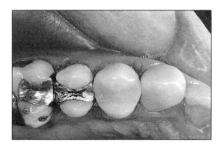

Fig 9-8g Indirect/direct resin composite inlay after cementation in the maxillary first premolar.

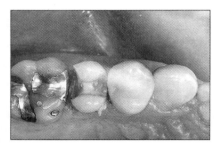

Fig 9-8h Preparation of the maxillary second premolar for direct/indirect resin composite inlay.

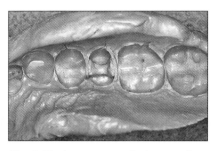

Fig 9-8i Impression of the maxillary second premolar for the resin composite inlay.

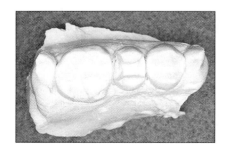

Fig 9-8j Stone die (Snap Stone) of the inlay preparation.

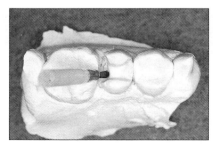

Fig 9-8k Painting the separator on the stone die prior to fabrication of the inlay.

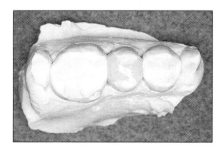

Fig 9-8l Fabrication of the direct/indirect resin composite inlay on the stone die.

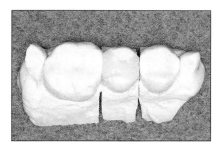

Fig 9-8m Stone die sawed and separated to allow for finishing of the inlay's margins.

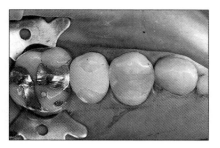

Fig 9-8n Try-in of the direct/indirect resin composite inlay in the maxillary second premolar.

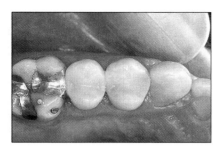

Fig 9-8o Direct/indirect resin composite inlays in the maxillary first and second premolars.

Indirect Resin Inlays and Onlays

Resin inlays and onlays are also available through commercial laboratories. They can be constructed from either hybrid resin composite or microfilled resin composite and exhibit the advantages and disadvantages inherent to each material (Figs 9-9a and 9-9b). However, the placement of an indirect inlay or onlay requires provisional restoration and two appointments, which increase the cost of the restoration. The technique for placement of the indirect resin inlay or onlay is the same as previously described in the direct/indirect resin inlay section.

Posterior Bonded Porcelain Restorations

The modern generation of bonded porcelain restorations was first described in 1983.[26,86] When it became clear that the technique had merit in anterior applications, interest developed in the use of bonded porcelain for posterior applications. In 1986, Redford and Jensen[59] described the strengthening effect of porcelain inlays on the fracture resistance of natural teeth. In 1988, Jensen[33] reported excellent clinical success in a 2-year in vivo study. During subsequent years, the technique has been refined to the point that porcelain inlays and onlays are now an accepted operative modality.

Ceramic inlays have been used since 1913,[57] but did not become popular because of difficulties in fabrication and a high failure rate.[2] In the 1980s, the development of compatible refractory materials made fabrication easier, and the development of adhesive resin cements greatly improved the clinical success rate.[11]

Indications

The indications for posterior bonded porcelain restorations clearly overlap the indications for direct and indirect posterior resin composite restorations, which have already been described. These restorations are indicated when there is an overriding desire for esthetics and all margins can be placed on enamel. Some clinicians recommend them instead of resin composite restorations for larger preparations.[11]

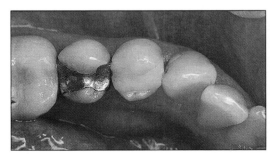

Fig 9-9a Mesio-occlusodistal resin composite restoration with recurrent caries in the mandibular first premolar.

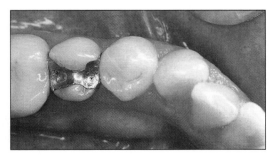

Fig 9-9b Indirect mesio-occlusodistal resin composite inlay (Concept, Williams) in the mandibular first premolar.

Ceramic Inlay Versus Resin Composite Inlay

Ceramic inlays are reported to leak less than resin composite inlays[35,69] and to fit better,[69] although marginal fidelity depends on technique and is laboratory dependent.[19] As previously described, adhesion of resin cement is more reliable and durable to etched ceramic inlays than to treated resin composite inlays.

The main advantage of resin composite inlays is that they tend to be more user friendly, both clinically and in the dental laboratory. The resin inlay can be placed into the preparation with moderate pressure to ensure complete seating without the fear of fracture. Also, if, during the process of adjustment, the interproximal contact is removed, it can be easily replaced with the addition of light-cured resin composite.

In contrast, the porcelain inlay is quite fragile and subject to fracture during the try-in phase. If the interproximal contact is inadvertently removed during adjustment, it can be replaced by the time-consuming procedure of adding porcelain and refiring it in a porcelain furnace.[63] Once it is removed from the porcelain furnace, the inlay must be re-etched with hydrofluoric acid. Alternatively, the contact can be replaced with resin composite after the proximal porcelain surface is etched with hydrofluoric acid and silanated.

Because, to date, no clinical studies have compared the success of these two treatment modalities, the resin composite inlay should be considered first for use in two- and three-surface inlay preparations of moderate width in premolar teeth.

Porcelain Onlay Versus Resin Composite Onlay

The porcelain onlay has the same disadvantages as the porcelain inlay. Although some ceramic materials cause wear of opposing enamel,[55] they also provide long-term occlusal stability, which resin composite may not provide in a complete coverage restoration. The stronger bond to porcelain is particularly important when cusps are covered. The stronger the bond, the more efficiently forces are transferred from the restoration through the cement and absorbed into the tooth.[17] For these reasons, when even one cusp of a posterior tooth is being covered with an esthetic bonded onlay, the porcelain onlay is preferred.

Porcelain onlays may be used routinely for the esthetic restoration of premolar teeth. They may also be used as cuspal-coverage restorations in molars, although the occlusal forces will be greater in the molar regions. An excellent indication for the porcelain onlay is for restoration of a molar with a short occlusogingival dimension. In this circumstance, it is difficult to gain axial retention and resistance with a conventional crown preparation.

However, the porcelain onlay preparation requires only 2 mm of occlusal reduction and requires no axial reduction for retention and resistance. The short molar tooth, which would have previously required crown-lengthening surgery prior to placement of a complete-coverage crown, can now be more conservatively restored with the porcelain onlay.

Selection of appropriate patients is paramount when placement of posterior bonded porcelain restorations is considered. Ideally, the patient should exhibit no signs of a parafunctional habit and should be provided with an occlusal guard to prevent wear of opposing teeth. In addition, the restoration should be fabricated so that it contacts in maximum intercuspation but has no contacts on the porcelain in eccentric mandibular positions.

Shade Selection

The shade used for a porcelain inlay or onlay is selected in the same way as for a ceramometal crown. Because of the thickness of the porcelain, the underlying tooth color and cement shade have a minimal effect on the shade of the final restoration except at the margins. As with porcelain veneers, use of a translucent resin cement is recommended to improve the esthetic blend at the margins.

Fabrication

The most common method of fabrication of porcelain inlays and onlays utilizes a refractory die. After a master die is poured in die stone, a refractory die is made by duplicating the master die or repouring the impression in a refractory material. The porcelain is baked on the refractory die, recovered, and fit to the master die. Variations in the fit of ceramic inlays and onlays is reported to be related more to the technician than the type of ceramic material used.[19] The use of refractory materials with ceramic restorations is discussed in more detail in chapter 15.

Isolation

It is universally acknowledged that strict isolation is necessary for bonding of posterior adhesive restorations. This unquestionably can be best accomplished with a well-placed rubber dam. If it is not possible to isolate the tooth from the oral environment with a rubber dam, then an adhesive restoration should not be placed (see box for the porcelain onlay technique).

Porcelain Onlay Technique

Preparation

1. Select a shade of porcelain prior to tooth dehydration.
2. Make a template if needed for the provisional restoration.
3. Remove the old restoration and proceed with tooth preparation.
4. After the preparation is completed, there should be room for at least a 2-mm thickness of porcelain in all areas. All internal line angles should be rounded and the walls should be quite divergent occlusally.
5. Make an impression using retraction cord if required.
6. Make a provisional restoration by one of the methods previously described in the text and cement with polycarboxylate cement.

Insertion

1. Check the restoration on the die for fit, and check for fracture lines with transillumination.
2. Place silane on the internal surface and allow to air dry.
3. Isolate the prepared tooth with a rubber dam.
4. Remove the provisional restoration and cement from the preparation. Clean the preparation with pumice and a brush.
5. Try-in the porcelain restoration. If it does not go completely to place, check proximal contacts with thin floss. If the contacts prevent seating, adjust with a coarse Sof-Lex disk (3M Dental) or a fine diamond bur, and then polish.
6. If the restoration still does not go to place, disclose inner surface of restoration that is binding. If a silicone disclosing material is used, the inner surface of the porcelain restoration must be re-etched with 9.5% hydrofluoric acid for 4 minutes and resilanated.[70]
7. It is preferable to adjust the tooth, rather than the inner surface of the porcelain, so that the etched surface is not disturbed.
8a. If color is important, try-in the restoration with base shade from a dual-cured composite. Either accept the color or use a different color of resin.
8b. Clean the restoration with acetone and then place it in an ultrasonic cleaner with clean acetone for 5 minutes.
8c. Place silane on the inner surface of the restoration and allow to air dry.
9. Place strips interproximally to ensure that the etchant is not in contact with adjacent teeth. Etch the preparation with 37% phosphoric acid for 20 seconds and then rinse for 5 seconds.
10. Place dentin primer on the tooth preparation according to the manufacturer's instructions. Mix and place a dual-cured adhesive. Do not light cure prior to placement of the restoration. Similarly, dual-cured adhesive must be placed on the inner surface of the restoration.
11. Mix a dual-cured composite luting resin and place into the preparation and on the inner surface of the restoration with a syringe.
12. Gently place the restoration into the preparation and vibrate with a hand instrument to ensure that it is almost fully seated.
13. Remove excess resin composite with a brush both occlusally and interproximally.
14. Gently seat the restoration completely with an instrument applied to the occlusal surface, making sure that a bead of composite is expressed at all margins.
15. Light cure for 10 seconds from the occlusal surface.
16. While continuing to hold the restoration with an instrument, remove the excess interproximal composite with floss and explorer or a No. 12 or 12b scalpel blade. The interproximal aspect must be completely finished before the composite polymerizes.
17. Complete light curing for 90 seconds from the occlusal direction and 30 seconds from each proximal surface.

Finishing

18. Finish all margins with carbide finishing burs, Sof-Lex disks, and/or porcelain polishing cups and points.
19. Remove the rubber dam and adjust the occlusion with articulating paper and a microfine diamond or 12-fluted, egg-shaped carbide finishing bur.
20. Polish adjusted areas with a rubber porcelain-polishing kit.
21. Etch with phosphoric acid for 5-10 seconds and rebond.

CAD/CAM Ceramic Restorations

A recent addition to the field of dental ceramics has been CAD/CAM technology. Several CAD/CAM systems are available, but by far the most widely used is the Cerec System (Siemens). The Cerec (ceramic reconstruction) System was initially developed by Dr. Werner Mörmann, a dentist, and Marco Brandestini, an engineer, in 1980. Siemens marketed the technology initially in Europe in 1985, and the first clinical trials took place in 1987.[49] It was introduced in the United States in 1989. With this system, a ceramic inlay, onlay, or veneer is created in a single appointment with the aid of an optical scanner, a computer, and a milling machine. The tooth is prepared, and the preparation is scanned into a computer. There the image is manipulated and output to a milling machine, where the restoration is milled from a ceramic block. After adjustments, the restoration is ready for cementation.[47-49]

Another CAD/CAM system, the CELAY system (Vident), is also available. A resin or wax pattern of the preparation is made and used as a model for the ceramic restoration. The external surface of the pattern is mechanically traced with a probe to input the dimensions into the computer, and a ceramic restoration is generated.[20]

Although CAD/CAM is not widely used at the present time, the accuracy to which the restorations can be milled has reached a clinically acceptable level. In both 3-year[29] and 5-year[51] clinical evaluations, CAD/CAM restorations have performed satisfactorily.

Advantages and Disadvantages

The main advantage of CAD/CAM technology is time savings. This technique affords the opportunity to prepare, design, and fabricate a ceramic restoration in a single appointment, without the need for conventional impressions, provisional restorations, or dental laboratory support.

The CAD/CAM technology also offers excellent esthetics, durability and, at least, short-term strengthening of the tooth. Roznowski et al[62] compared the fracture resistance of molars restored with various adhesive and nonadhesive restorations and reported that teeth restored with mesio-occlusodistal Cerec inlays were as strong as unprepared, unrestored teeth, while the nonadhesive restorations weakened the tooth.

The CAD/CAM systems are not without their disadvantages. The systems can fabricate inlays, onlays, and veneers, but there is, at present, no capability for making ceramic crowns. Occlusal anatomy must be created "free hand" with a high-speed handpiece after the restoration is bonded. This is generally not a problem with inlays, but presents a greater challenge for onlays.

A significant training period is required to achieve proficiency with the system. Participation in a 2- to 3-day initial training course is usually recommended, followed by laboratory practice on an additional 25 to 30 restorations. The cost of the systems is considerable, even if shared by several practitioners.

A major concern about CAD/CAM restorations is their marginal fit. Several studies have evaluated marginal openings in CAD/CAM restorations. Molin and Karlsson[46] reported that the marginal adaptation of CAD/CAM restorations is inferior to that of traditional ceramic or gold restorations. Krejci and others[39] reported precementation marginal openings to be in the range of 125 to 175 µm. After cementation, they found that more than 90% of enamel-ceramic interfaces had "continuous margins." They found that the quality of the marginal adaptation immediately after cementation does not seem to depend on precementation marginal fit.[39] Peters and Bieniek[56] reported on a clinical study of 22 Cerec inlays in which the average marginal fit was 121 µm with a range of 60 to 150 µm.

Wilder[79] reported the average film thickness of cement at the occlusal cavosurface margin to be 89 ± 65 µm. The average thickness at the gingival margin was 105 ± 81 µm. Inokoshi and others[28] evaluated the marginal gap of Cerec inlays with the initial COS 1.0 software (Siemens) and the updated software version, COS 2.0. They reported a mean occlusal marginal gap of 52 µm with the updated software, a significant improvement over that measured with the initial software program. Christensen,[15] by comparison, has reported that gold castings can be fabricated with marginal openings of less than 25 µm. Because of the relatively large precementation marginal gaps, the exposed resin cement may be the weak link in the CAD/CAM system.

Hardware and Software

The Cerec CAD/CAM system consists of an intraoral camera, a video monitor, a computer, and a milling chamber (Figs 9-10a and 9-10b). The computer utilizes software for design and construction of ceramic restorations. Currently available software packages allow fabrication of ceramic inlays, onlays, and veneers.

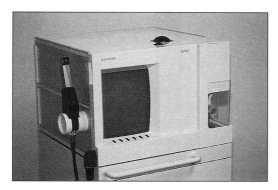

Fig 9-10a Cerec CAD/CAM unit, consisting of a computer and an intraoral camera hanging next to the video monitor.

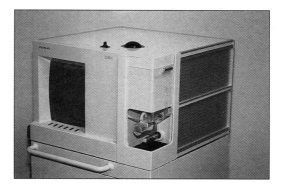

Fig 9-10b Milling chamber of the Cerec CAD/CAM unit.

Inlays

Preparation

How well the milled restoration fits depends, to a great extent, on the tooth preparation. The design of the cavity preparation is influenced by requirements dictated by the intraoral camera, design software, and the milling head.[30,50]

The cavity preparation for CAD/CAM inlays is similar to that for a conventional indirect ceramic inlay.[14,16] The occlusal aspect of the preparation should be at least 2 mm deep to provide adequate strength for the ceramic restoration. All cavosurface margins should be well defined and have a 90-degree butt joint. This will allow the camera head to record an accurate image of the cavosurface margin. Bevels and chamfer-style margins should not be utilized. The cavity walls of the proximal box should have 4 to 6 degrees of divergent taper[13] (Fig 9-11a). However, the occlusal aspect of the preparation should have parallel to slightly undercut walls to aid the camera in recording a sharp image of the cavosurface margin (Fig 9-11b). The axial wall should be prepared flat without convexity (Fig 9-11c). Any facial or lingual extensions of the occlusal portion of the preparation must follow the same angle as the axial wall of the box. The milling disk will not mill acute angles developed by extensions that are different from the axial wall direction (Fig 9-12). All preparation floors should be smooth and flat. Concavities created by removal of caries or prior restorations can be blocked out with a liner or base. In addition, a bump or convexity on the floor will prevent the restoration from seating completely.

Computer-assisted Design

A dry field is necessary to ensure that the preparation is optically scanned with precision and accuracy. It is also critical to clearly isolate the gingival extent of the preparation from the adjacent soft tissues. For these reasons, the use of a rubber dam is essential.

Following completion of the tooth preparation, an optical impression is recorded. The image is captured by way of the intraoral camera, which reflects an infrared beam off of the surface of the tooth[30] (Figs 9-13a and 9-13b). Because enamel, dentin, bases, and liners do not reflect the infrared beam equally well, the tooth must be coated with a uniform reflective material before imaging. The powder should also coat all adjacent structures that may be viewed in the optical scan (Figs 9-14a and 9-14b).

The electronic camera has a three-dimensional resolution that projects a two-dimensional image of the preparation on the monitor (Figs 9-15a and 9-15b). To ensure accurate scanning of the preparation, the camera head is aligned in the long axis of the tooth parallel to the path of insertion of the restoration. The image is viewed simultaneously on the video monitor. All portions of the preparation margins should be visible and distinct from adjacent structures. The camera head must be held motionless to record an accurate image without distortion of the preparation.

The design phase is initiated when the "bottom line" of the preparation is drawn on the computer image (Fig 9-15a). Then the proximal surface contour, the cavosurface margin, and the marginal ridge are drawn (Fig 9-15b). The image can be viewed both in profile and cross section, to aid in evaluating the accuracy of the tracing.

Computer-assisted Manufacture

When the milling function is activated, the software constructs a model of the restoration (Fig 9-16). Based on the calculated three-dimensional model of the restoration, the computer then requests the appropriately sized

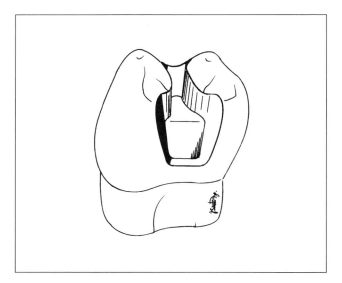

Fig 9-11a Preparation for a CAD/CAM inlay. The proximal box has a 4- to 6-degree occlusal taper.

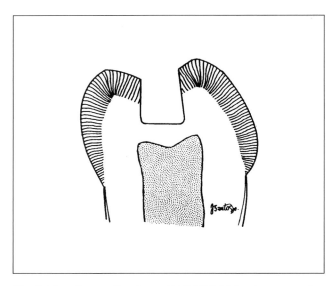

Fig 9-11b Preparation for a CAD/CAM inlay in a premolar. The opposing walls of the occlusal portion of the preparation should be parallel or slightly undercut.

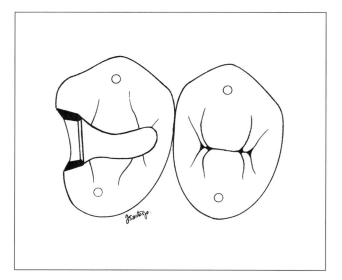

Fig 9-11c Preparation for a CAD/CAM inlay. The cavosurface margin should be sharp, without bevels, and the axial wall should be flat, rather than convex.

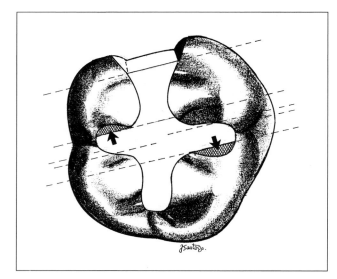

Fig 9-12 All walls must be parallel to or form obtuse angles with the axial wall of the proximal box. The CAD/CAM unit cannot mill walls at an acute angle to the axial wall.

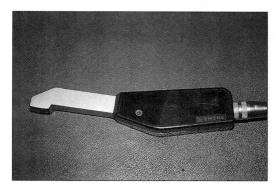

Fig 9-13a Electronic camera.

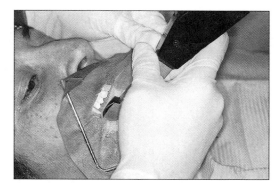

Fig 9-13b Electronic camera scanning the tooth and preparation onto the video monitor, making the electronic impression.

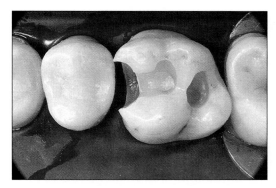

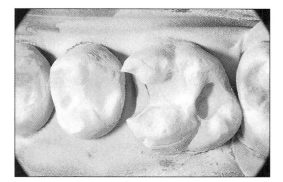

Figs 9-14a and 9-14b Since enamel, dentin, bases, and liners do not reflect the infrared beam equally well, the tooth and adjacent structures are coated with an adhesive and an imaging powder.

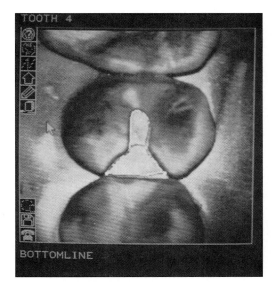

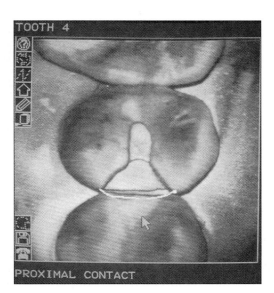

Figs 9-15a and 9-15b The margins of the restoration and the marginal ridge are drawn on the video screen.

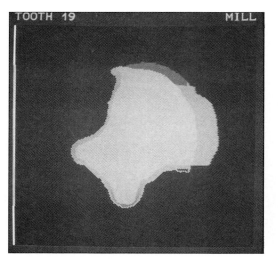

Fig 9-16 Computer software constructing a model of the restoration to use as a guide in milling.

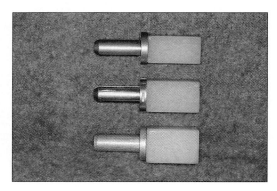

Fig 9-17 Ceramic blocks of three different sizes.

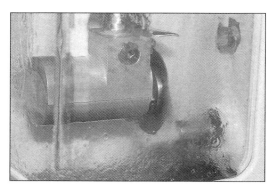

Fig 9-18 Ceramic block being milled with a diamond disk into an inlay based on the computer-constructed model.

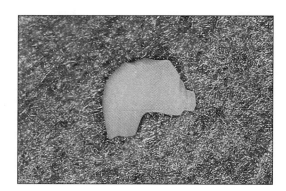

Fig 9-19 Completed inlay with the sprue still attached.

ceramic block to be inserted in the milling chamber (Fig 9-17).

The two ceramic materials most commonly used for machining are a fine-grained feldspathic porcelain (Vita Cerec Mark II, Vita Zahnfabrik) and a machinable glass ceramic (Dicor MGC, Dentsply). The fine grain of the Mark II porcelain is reported to increase hardness of the material but decrease wear of the opposing dentition[37]; the material comes in five Vita shades. Dicor MGC is a cast glass that is 70% mica and has a hardness value similar to that of enamel.[55] It comes in light and dark shades. Both materials have performed well in clinical studies.[29,50,54]

Once the ceramic block has been locked in the milling chamber, the unit is ready to mill the restoration. A diamond disk moves in contact with the metallic mounting

of the ceramic block, which calibrates the position of the milling head. The ceramic block, rotating as it goes, is fed uniformly across the milling disk (Fig 9-18). Milling occurs in three axes, from mesial to distal; the sprue of ceramic, where the restoration is separated from the ceramic block, ends up on the distal surface (Fig 9-19). Most restorations can be milled within 4 to 7 minutes.

Try-in and Cementation

Once the ceramic restoration is recovered from the milling chamber, the sprue is removed and the inlay is tried in (Fig 9-20a). Adjustments may have to be made for the restoration to fit accurately. The axiopulpal line angle and the gingival floor of the box are the places most likely to require adjustment.[79] Should the fit be unacceptable in some area, the design can be reloaded

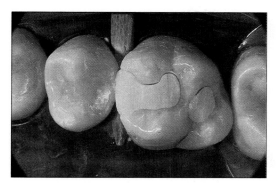

Fig 9-20a Trying the mesio-occlusal inlay in the maxillary first molar. Note that there is no occlusal anatomy in the inlay.

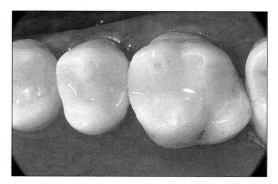

Fig 9-20b The mesio-occlusal inlay in the maxillary first molar after cementation, occlusal contouring, and polishing.

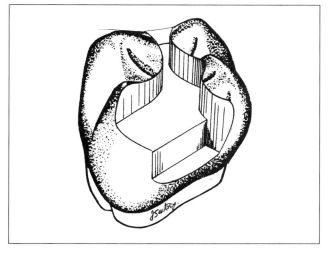

Fig 9-21a Preparation for a CAD/CAM onlay. The gingival shoulder must be extended to the buccal or lingual, adjacent to areas of cuspal coverage. The milling machine cannot produce both cuspal coverage and an adjacent proximal box.

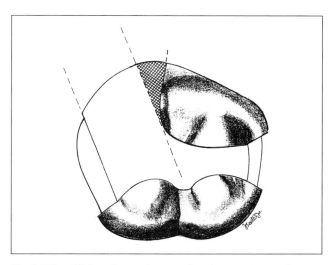

Fig 9-21b Walls adjacent to cuspal replacement must be parallel to the axial wall of the proximal box.

from the program disk and corrected, and a second restoration can be quickly milled.

There is no occlusal anatomy in the restoration when it is removed from the milling chamber. The surface is flat from the facial aspect of the cavosurface margin to the lingual aspect. The software program has no capacity to create occlusal anatomy. Although an attempt can be made to create some anatomy with a high-speed handpiece at this time, it is best done after cementation of the restoration.

The tissue surfaces of Vita Mark II restorations should be etched with hydrofluoric acid, and Dicor restorations should be etched with 10% ammonium bifluoride. Both materials should be treated with silane before cementation. Use of a conventional adhesive cementation technique and a dual-cured resin cement is recommended. Contouring and delineation of anatomy can be accom-

plished after cementation with various microfine diamonds or carbide burs.[66] Finishing and polishing are completed with abrasive rubber points, disks, and cups with diamond polishing paste as for other ceramic restorations (Fig 9-20b).

Onlays

The cavity design for an onlay differs significantly from that for a conventional ceramic onlay.[30] The principles of cavity design that apply to a CAD/CAM inlay also apply to an onlay. In addition, any cusp to be restored must be reduced to the level of the pulpal floor. The floor of the proximal box must also be extended to either the facial or lingual surface, in essence removing one wall of the box (Figs 9-21a and 9-21b). This is due to the fact that

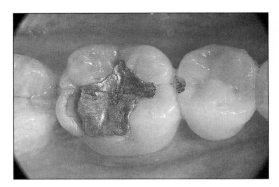

Fig 9-22a Mandibular first molar prior to preparation for a CAD/CAM onlay.

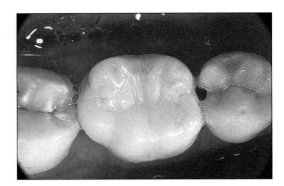

Fig 9-22b Disto-occlusobuccal CAD/CAM onlay on the mandibular first molar.

the milling disk cannot mill a design with "steps" in both the mesiodistal and faciolingual dimensions. Reducing the cusp to the level of the pulpal floor and modifying the adjacent proximal box will eliminate the presence of a faciolingual step in the preparation.

The computer design of an onlay is essentially the same as that for an inlay except that one or more cusps is being rebuilt. This is accomplished when the marginal ridge is drawn. The software program will draw in the marginal ridge as if the onlay were an inlay. This would result in a cuspal height equivalent to that of the marginal ridge. To create a cusp, the marginal ridge is edited in the profile view to elevate that portion of the marginal ridge over the area of the missing cusp. The milling of the restoration occurs in the same manner as for an inlay (Figs 9-22a and 9-22b).

References

1. Bailey L, Bennett R. Two year bond results of dicor ceramic/LA cement system [Abstract 1734]. J Dent Res 1989;68:398.

2. Banks RG. Conservative posterior ceramic restorations: A literature review. J Prosthet Dent 1990;63:619-626.

3. Bergmann P, Noack MJ, Roulet J-F. Marginal adaptation with glass ceramic inlays adhesively luted with glycerine gel. Quintessence Int 1991;22:739-744.

4. Bessing C, Lundqvist P. A one-year clinical examination of indirect resin composite inlays: A preliminary report. Quintessence Int 1991;22:153-157.

5. Bishop BM. A heat and pressure cured composite inlay system: A clinical evaluation. Aust Prosthodont J 1989;3:35-41.

6. Blair KF, Koeppen RG, Schwartz RS, Davis RD. Microleakage associated with resin composite-cemented, cast glass ceramic restorations. Int J Prosthodont 1993;6:579-584.

7. Brännström M. Infection beneath resin composite restorations: Can it be avoided? Oper Dent 1987;12:158-163.

8. Burgess JO, Haveman CW, Butzin C. Evaluation of resins for provisional restorations. Am J Dent 1992;5:137-139.

9. Burgoyne A, Nichols J, Brudvik J. In vitro two-body wear of inlay-onlay resin composite restorations. J Prosthet Dent 1991;65:206-214.

10. Burke FJT, Watts DC, Wilson MA. Current status and rationale for composite inlays and onlays. Br Dent J 1991;171:269-273.

11. Burke FJT, Qualtrough AJE. Aesthetic inlays: Composite or ceramic? Br Dent J 1994;176:53-60.

12. Burke FJT, Wilson NHF, Watts DC. The effect of cuspal coverage on the fracture resistance of teeth restored with indirect resin composite restorations. Quintessence Int 1993;4:875-880.

13. Burke FJT, Wilson NHF, Watts DC. The effect of cavity wall taper on fracture resistance of teeth restored with resin composite inlays. Oper Dent 1993;18:230-236.

14. Cerec Operator's Manual. Siemens, 1993.

15. Christensen GJ. Marginal fit of gold inlay castings. J Prosthet Dent 1966;16:297-305.

16. David SB, LoPresti JT. Tooth-colored posterior restorations using Cerec method CAD/CAM-generated ceramic inlays. Compend Cont Educ Dent 1994;15:802-810.

17. Derand T. Stress analysis of cemented or resin-bonded porcelain inlays. Dent Mater 1991;7:21-24.

18. DeSchepper EJ, Tate WH, Powers JM. Bond strength of resin cements to microfilled composites. Am J Dent 1993;6:235-238.

19. Dietschi D, Maeder M, Holz J. In vitro evaluation of marginal fit and morphology of fired ceramic inlays. Quintessence Int 1992;23:271-278.

20. Eidenbenz S, Lehner CR, Schärer P. Coping milling ceramic inlays from resin analogs: A practical approach with the CELAY System. Int J Prosthodont 1994;7:134-142.

21. Feilzer AJ, de Gee AJ, Davidson CL. Curing contraction of composites and glass ionomer cements. J Prosthet Dent 1988;59:297.

22. Gray W, Suzuki M, Jordan R, et al. Clinical evaluation of indirect composite restorations—3 year results [abstract 633]. J Dent Res 1991;70:344.

23. Hasegawa EA, Boyer DB, Chan DCN. Microleakage of indirect composite inlays. Dent Mater 1989;5:388-391.

24. Hasegawa EA, Boyer DB, Chan DCN. Hardening of dual-cure cements under resin composite inlays. J Prosthet Dent 1991;66:187-192.

25. Hilton TJ, Schwartz RS. The effect of air thinning on dentin adhesive bond strength [abstract 243]. J Dent Res 1994;73:132.

26. Horn HR. A new lamination: Porcelain bonded to enamel. NY State Dent J 1983;49:401-403.

27. Inokoshi S, Iwaku M, Fusayama T. Pulp response to a new adhesive restorative resin. J Dent Res 1982;61:1014-1019.

28. Inokoshi S, Van Meerbeek B, Willems G, et al. Marginal accuracy of CAD/CAM inlays made with the original and the updated software. J Dent 1992;20:171-177.

29. Isenberg BP, Essig ME, Leinfelder KF. Three year clinical evaluation of CAD/CAM restorations. J Esthet Dent 1992;4:173-176.

30. Jedynakiewicz NM, Martin N. CAD-CAM in Restorative Dentistry: The Cerec Method. Liverpool, England: University Press, 1993.

31. Jensen ME, Chan DCN. Polymerization, shrinkage and microleakage. In: Vanherle G, Smith DC (eds). Posterior Resin Composite Dental Restorative Materials. Utrecht, The Netherlands: Szulc, 1985:243-262.

32. Jensen ME, Redford DA, Williams BT, Gardner F. Posterior etched porcelain restorations; an in-vitro study. Compend Contin Educ Dent 1987;8:615-622.

33. Jensen ME. A two-year clinical study of posterior etched-porcelain resin-bonded restorations. Am J Dent 1988;1:27-33.

34. Kanca J. The effect of heat on the surface hardness of light-activated resin composites. Quintessence Int 1989;20:899-901.

35. Karaagaclioglu L, Zaimoglu A, Akoren AC. Microleakage of indirect inlays placed on different kinds of glass ionomer cement linings. J Oral Rehabil 1992;19:457-469.

36. Kawai K, Isenberg B, Leinfelder KF. Effect of gap dimension on resin composite cement wear. Quintessence Int 1994;25:53-58.

37. Krejci I. Wear of Cerec and other restorative materials. In: Mörmann WH (ed). Proceedings of an International Symposium on Computer Restorations. Chicago: Quintessence, 1991:245-251.

38. Krecji I, Krecji D, Lutz F. Clinical evaluation of a new pressed glass ceramic inlay material over 1.5 years. Quintessence Int 1992;23:181-186.

39. Krejci I, Lutz F, Reimer M. Marginal adaptation and fit of adhesive ceramic inlays. J Dent 1993;21:39-46.

40. Krejci I, Lutz F, Reimer M. Wear of CAD/CAM ceramic inlays: Restorations, opposing cusps, luting cements. Quintessence Int 1994;25:199-207.

41. Krejci I, Guntert A, Lutz F. Scanning electron microscopic and clinical examination of resin composite inlays/onlays up to 12 months in situ. Quintessence Int 1994;25:403-409.

42. Lambrechts P, Braem M, Vanherle G. In vivo wear of resin composites [abstract S23]. J Dent Res 1988;67:75.

43. Latta M, Barkmeier W. Bond strength of a resin cement and a cured composite inlay material. J Prosthet Dent 1993;72:189-93.

44. Lundin SA. Studies on posterior resin composites with special reference to class II restorations. Swed Dent J 1990;73 (suppl):6-33.

45. Meseros AJ, Evans DB, Schwartz RS. Influence of a dentin bonding agent on the fracture load of Dicor. Am J Dent 1994;7:137-140.

46. Molin M, Karlsson S. The fit of gold inlays and three ceramic inlay systems. Acta Odontol Scand 1993;51:201-206.

47. Mörmann WH, Brandestini M, Lutz F, Barbakow F. Chairside computer-aided direct ceramic inlays. Quintessence Int 1989; 20:329-339.

48. Mörmann WH, Symposium review. In: Mörmann WH (ed). Proceedings of an International Symposium on Computer Restorations. Chicago: Quintessence, 1991:17-21.

49. Mörmann WH, Gotsch T, Krejci I, Lutz F. Barbakow F. Clinical status of 94 Cerec ceramic inlays after 3 years in situ. In: Mörmann WH (ed). International Symposium on Computer Restorations. Chicago: Quintessence, 1991:355-363.

50. Mörmann WH. Chairside computer-generated ceramic restorations: The Cerec third generation improvements. Pract Periodont Aesthet Dent 1992;4(7):9-16.

51. Mörmann W, Krejci I. Computer-designed inlays after 5 years in situ: Clinical performance and scanning electron microscope evaluation. Quintessence Int 1992;23:109-115.

52. Nasedkin JN. Porcelain posterior resin-bonded restorations: Current perspectives on esthetic restorative dentistry. Part II. J Can Dent Assoc 1988;54:499-506.

53. O'Neal SJ, Miracle RL, Leinfelder LF. Evaluating interfacial gaps for esthetic inlays. J Am Dent Assoc 1993;124:48-54.

54. Pallesen U. Clinical performance of Cerec-restorations: Restorative procedure and preliminary results. In: Mörmann WH (ed). Proceedings of an International Symposium on Computer Restorations. Chicago: Quintessence, 1991:285-300.

55. Palmer DS, Barco MT, Pelleu GB. Wear of human enamel against a commercial castable ceramic restorative material. J Prosthet Dent 1991;65:192-195.

56. Peters A, Bieniek KW. SEM-examination of the marginal adaptation of computer machined ceramic restorations. In: Mörmann WH (ed). Proceedings of an International Symposium on Computer Restorations. Chicago: Quintessence, 1991:365-370.

57. Qualtrough AJE, Wilson NHF, Smith GA. The porcelain inlay: A historical review. Oper Dent 1990;15:61-70.

58. Qualtrough AJ, Cramer A, Wilson NH, Roulet J-F, Noack M. An in vitro evaluation of the marginal integrity of a porcelain inlay system. Int J Prosthodont 1991;4:517-523.

59. Redford DA, Jensen ME. Etched porcelain resin-bonded posterior restorations: Cuspal flexure, strength, and micro-leakage [abstract 1573]. J Dent Res 1986;65:334.

60. Retief DH. Do adhesives prevent microleakage? Int Dent J 1994;44:19-26.

61. Robinson PB, Moore BK, Swartz ML. Comparison of microleakage in direct and indirect resin composite restorations in vitro. Oper Dent 1987;12:113-116.

62. Roznowski M, Bremer B, Geurtsen W. Fracture resistance of human molars restored with various filling materials. In: Mörmann WH (ed). Proceedings of an International Symposium on Computer Restorations. Chicago: Quintessence, 1991:559-565.

63. Scherer W, Futter H, Cooper H. Clinical technique for an in-office porcelain modification. J Esthetic Dent 1991;3:23-26.

64. Schwartz RS, Davis RD, Mayhew R. The effect of ZOE on the bond strength of resin to enamel. Am J Dent 1990;3:28-30.

65. Schwartz RS, Davis RD, Hilton TJ. Effect of temporary cements on the bond strength of a resin cement. Am J Dent 1992;5:147-150.

66. Shearer AC, Kusy RP, Whitley JQ, Heymann HO, Wilson NHF. Finishing of MGC Dicor material. Int J Prosthodont 1994;7:167-173.

67. Shorthall AC, Baylis RL, Baylis MA, Grundy JR. Marginal seal comparisons between resin bonded Class 2 porcelain inlays, posterior composite restorations and direct resin composite inlays. Int J Prosthodont 1989;2:217-223.

68. Simonsen RJ, Calamia JR. Tensile bond strength of etched porcelain [abstract 1154]. J Dent Res 1983;62:297.

69. Thordrup M, Isidor F, Hørsted-Bindslev P. Comparison of marginal fit and microleakage of ceramic and composite inlays: An in vitro study. J Dent 1994;22:147-153.

70. Tjan AHL, Dunn JR, Grant BE. Effect of fitting paste on bond strength of composite/porcelain [abstract 714]. J Dent Res 1989;68:270.

71. Torstenson BC, Nordenvall KJ, Brännström M. Pulpal protection and microorganisms under clearfil resin composite in deep cavities with acid etched dentin. Swed Dent J 1982;6:167.

72. Van Meerbeek B, Inokoshi S, Willems G, Joack MJ, Braem M, Lambrechts P, et al. Marginal adaptation of four tooth-coloured inlay systems in vivo. J Dent 1992;20:18-26.

73. Walton JN. Esthetic alternatives for posterior teeth: Porcelain and laboratory-processed resin composites. J Can Dent Assoc 1992; 58:820-823.

74. Wendt SL. The effect of heat used as a secondary cure upon the physical properties of three resin composites. I. Diametral tensile strength, compressive strength and marginal dimensional stability. Quintessence Int 1987;18:265-271.

75. Wendt SL. The effect of heat used as a secondary cure upon the physical properties of three resin composites. II. Wear, hardness and color stability. Quintessence Int 1987;18:351-356.

76. Wendt SL, Leinfelder KF. The clinical evaluation of heat treated resin composite inlays. J Am Dent Assoc 1990;120:177-181.

77. Wendt SL. Microleakage and cusp fracture resistance of heat-treated resin composite inlays. Am J Dent 1991;4:10-414.

78. Wendt SL, Leinfelder KF. Clinical evaluation of a heat treated composite inlay: 3 year results. Am J Dent 1992;5:258-262.

79. Wilder AD. Clinical considerations of Cerec restorations. In: Mörmann WH (ed). Proceedings of an International Symposium on Computer Restorations. Chicago: Quintessence, 1991:141-149.

80. Wilson NHF, Wilson MA, Wastell DG, Smith GA. Performance of Occlusin in butt-joint and bevel-edged preparations: Five-year results. Dent Mater 1991;7:92-98.

Amalgam Restorations

James B. Summitt / J. William Robbins

The word amalgam means an alloy of mercury with another metal or metals.[114] This type of alloying is called amalgamation.[86] In dentistry, before these metals are combined with mercury to make dental amalgam, they are known as dental amalgam alloys. Before the development of high-copper amalgam alloys, dental amalgam alloys contained at least 65 wt% silver, 29 wt% tin, and less than 6 wt% copper. The high-copper amalgam alloys contain between 12 wt% and 30 wt% copper,[25] and this higher level of copper has resulted in the elimination of the highly corrodible and weak gamma 2 phase that existed in the low-copper amalgams.[82c]

Zinc is added to amalgam to enhance its physical properties and prolong the service of the amalgam restoration.[82c,86] However, when moisture is incorporated during condensation of a zinc-containing low-copper amalgam, a delayed expansion will occur. Although zinc-containing high-copper amalgams do not exhibit this delayed expansion, exclusion of moisture enhances other properties, as well as clinical performance, and isolation to prevent any moisture contamination is important.[80b]

Amalgam is made by mixing mercury with a powder of amalgam alloy. The powder may be of the lathe-cut variety (Fig 10-1a), which is made by milling an ingot of the alloy, or of the spherical type (Fig 10-1b), which is made by atomizing liquid alloy. The spherical particles usually are not true spheres but take on various rounded shapes. Amalgam alloy may also be composed of a mixture of lathe-cut and spherical particles; this type of amalgam is called an *admixed alloy*[25] (Fig 10-1c).

Dental amalgam constitutes approximately 75% of all restorative materials used by dentists.[64] It has served as a dental restorative for more than 165 years.[6,76] Its use has at times been controversial. The most recent controversy is related to amalgam's release of mercury during chewing. There is considerable evidence of the safety of dental amalgam. To date, there is no confirmed evidence to indicate that the mercury in dental amalgam is related to any disease.[76] The US Public Health Service in 1993 reaffirmed its position that there are no data to compel a change in the current use of dental amalgam.[6,23,110]

Any component of amalgam or any other restorative material can elicit an allergic reaction, but hypersensitivity to mercury is extremely rare. Of those who have a true allergy to mercury, fewer than 1% demonstrate clinically observable reactions to mercury in dental amalgam restorations.[76]

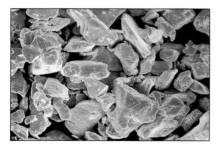

Fig 10-1a Lathe-cut amalgam alloy particles.

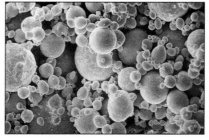

Fig 10-1b Spherical amalgam alloy particles.

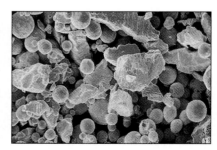

Fig 10-1c Admixed amalgam alloy particles.

Advantages and Disadvantages

In the United States, amalgam has been used since the middle of the 19th century.[6] Dental amalgam has many advantages as a restorative material. It is strong and relatively easy to use. It wears at a rate similar to that of tooth structure. It has the ability to corrode, resulting in a reduction in the amount of microleakage at its interface with tooth structure. Dental amalgam is the least expensive of the long-term restorative materials.

Dental amalgam also has some disadvantages. It is not tooth-colored. It does not bond to tooth structure, although there are some promising new agents that are designed to create a bond between amalgam and tooth structure. It contains mercury, which, if not handled properly, can cause a safety hazard for the dental staff. Nevertheless, because a tooth-colored dental material that has the advantages of dental amalgam has yet to be developed, it is still the primary posterior restorative material, with more than 100 million amalgam restorations placed in this country each year. In 1990, 94% of US dentists listed amalgam as their material of choice for Class 2 restorations.[111]

Amalgam, when inserted properly into well-designed tooth preparations, will serve well for long periods of time. Many studies have demonstrated the excellent longevity potential of dental amalgam.[77,94,100] This chapter will discuss Class 1 and 2 preparations and insertion techniques for dental amalgam. Also described will be complex restorations involving the replacement of cusps with dental amalgam.

Resistance Form

One of Black's steps in tooth preparation is obtaining resistance form. There are two considerations in resistance form when a tooth is being prepared to receive an amalgam restoration. First, resistance form should be developed for the restoration; the restoration must be of adequate thickness and have a marginal design that will allow it to bear the forces of mastication without fracture or deformation. In that regard, the restoration must have adequate occlusogingival depth to resist fracture in function or parafunction (bruxing or clenching). Second, the remaining tooth structure must be left in such a state that it, too, will resist the forces of mastication. As much sound tooth structure as possible must be maintained. If adequate resistance form cannot be maintained in the tooth to resist masticatory forces, the weak portion of

the occlusal surface should be reduced and restored with amalgam or another strong restorative material.

To maximize resistance form for tooth structure, minimum sound tooth structure should be removed when tooth preparations are cut for Class 1 or Class 2 amalgam restorations. Several studies[5,8,62,82a,112] have demonstrated that, as an amalgam restoration becomes wider faciolingually, the tooth is more subject to fracture and the integrity of the restoration is less likely to be maintained. An increase of the depth of the occlusal portion of an amalgam preparation has also been linked to a decrease in resistance to fracture of the tooth.[8] Class 2 restorations that are confined to the marginal ridge areas (proximal slot restorations) may minimize the severity of tooth fracture compared to Class 2 restorations that extend through occlusal grooves.[17,38] Based on this knowledge, the following goals should guide the preparation and restoration of teeth: (1) removal of pathosis (caries), (2) preservation of the integrity of the tooth and periodontium, and (3) maximization of the life of the restored tooth.

The Class 1 Preparation

Indications

Occlusal Caries

The indication for an initial Class 1 amalgam restoration is occlusal caries (and facial or lingual pit caries in posterior teeth) detected visually and with bitewing radiographs. The objectives of treatment are to eliminate the caries, to remove any enamel that has been undermined by the caries, to preserve as much sound tooth structure as possible, and to create a strong restoration that mimics the original sound tooth structure and allows little or no marginal leakage.

For the purpose of this chapter, it is necessary to review the definitions of the terms groove, fissure, and pit.[43] A groove, or a developmental groove, is a linear channel on the surface of a tooth, usually at the junction of dental lobes (cusps or ridges). A fissure is a developmental linear cleft, the result of the incomplete fusion of the enamel of adjoining dental lobes. A pit is a pinpoint fissure or is the junction of several fissures.

The presence of deep fissures alone does not justify the placement of a restoration. When there is concern that a deep fissure may develop caries at its base, it should be sealed with a resin pit and fissure sealant. In a tooth that has been diagnosed as having localized fissure caries, the caries should be removed and a restoration placed. Remaining fissures that are considered to be sus-

Figs 10-2a to 10-2f Amalgam should be used as a restorative material only in areas where actual caries has been removed; remaining noncarious fissures and amalgam restoration margins are etched and sealed with resin fissure sealant.

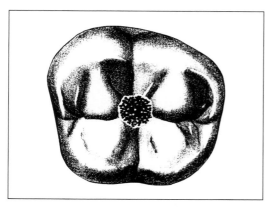

Fig 10-2a Caries is found only in the central fossa.

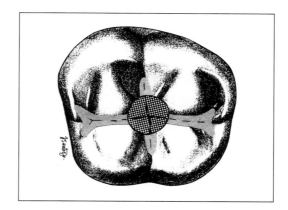

Fig 10-2b An amalgam restoration has been placed in the area where caries and unsupported enamel were removed; the remaining fissures are sealed.

Figs 10-2c and 10-2d Maxillary second molar preparation and sealed restoration.

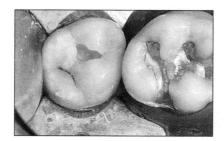

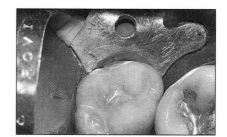

Figs 10-2e and 10-2f Mandibular first molar preparation and sealed restoration.

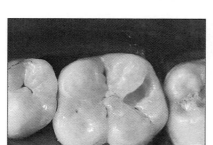

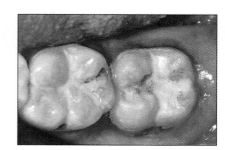

ceptible to caries should then be sealed with a resin sealant (Figs 10-2a to 10-2f).

Deep fissures that are to be sealed may benefit from being prepared with a small bur to a width and depth of approximately 0.5 mm before they are acid-etched and sealed with a resin fissure sealant[28,60,98] (Figs 10-3a to 10-3d). Alternatively, fissures may be opened or cleaned with an air-abrasive instrument or an air-polishing prophylaxis unit[9,41,47,113] (Figs 10-4a to 10-4d).

Traditionally, in a Class 1 amalgam preparation, occlusal fissures, or at least those in the developmental grooves, have been included in the preparation, even when caries has not extended throughout the fissures. The justification for this has been that occlusal caries, although not evident visually or radiographically, may be lurking at the base of one of those fissures. There is strong evidence that caries inadvertently left at the base of a sealed fissure does not progress[44,50,51,56,108] and that

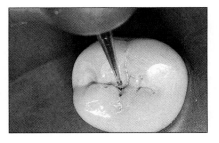

Fig 10-3a A No. ¼ bur (0.5 mm in diameter) is used to open the fissures.

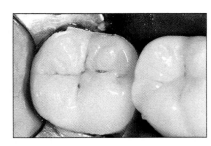

Fig 10-3b The fissure system of a mandibular second molar is shown pre-treatment.

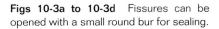

Figs 10-3a to 10-3d Fissures can be opened with a small round bur for sealing.

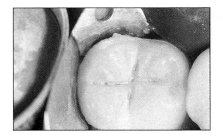

Fig 10-3c The fissures have been opened for sealing.

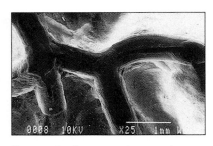

Fig 10-3d Scanning electron photomicrograph of fissures prepared with No. ¼ bur.

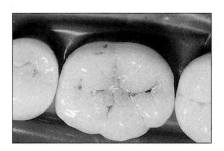

Fig 10-4a The fissure system of a mandibular molar is shown prior to air abrasion.

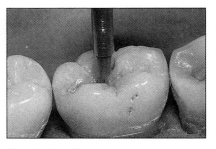

Fig 10-4b Fifty-micron alumina powder is projected into the fissure.

Figs 10-4a to 10-4d Fissures can be opened with an air-abrasion unit (KCP 2000).

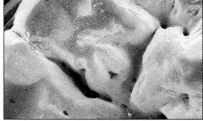

Fig 10-4c The fissures are shown after air abrasion.

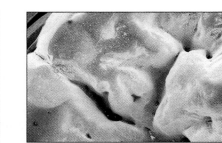

Fig 10-4d Scanning electron photomicrograph of fissures opened with air abrasion.

the sealing of fissures associated with occlusal amalgam restorations is an extremely effective treatment modality.[74,75] Therefore, the routine extension of cavity preparations through fissures not known to be carious can no longer be justified. Additionally, extension of cavity preparations through grooves in which there are no fissures is contraindicated.

Defective Restorations and Recurrent Caries

Another indication for a Class 1 restoration is the replacement of a restoration that is defective beyond repair or associated with recurrent caries. Recurrent caries is caries that occurs adjacent to an existing restoration. Optimally, the margins of a restoration are sealed or leakproof. In reality, most restorations exhibit some leakage at their margins, although it is minimal in most cases. When the leakage becomes greater, usually because of a defective restoration or flexure of tooth structure, plaque can form in the space between the tooth and the restoration and can lead to caries initiation. There is some evidence that cleaning, etching, and sealing leaky amalgam margins with a resin sealant can prolong the life of a restoration.[18]

Outline Form

When an occlusal restoration must be placed because of initial caries, two guidelines should be applied in establishing the outline form: *(1)* caries should be eliminated, and *(2)* margins should be placed on sound tooth structure. The enamel at the margin of the preparation should be supported by sound dentin. Any enamel prisms that have been undermined by the removal of caries should be removed. If a noncarious fissure is evident in the wall of a preparation, the preparation should not be extended solely to include the fissure; the fissure should, instead, be sealed after the amalgam has been inserted.

If there is no cavitation in the area of the caries, a bur such as a No. 56, 245, 329, or 330 is used to cut through enamel to gain access to the caries. The preparation is widened to give access to all dentinal caries and to remove any enamel that is not supported by sound dentin. The preparation should be widened only enough to obtain enamel margins supported by sound dentin.

Although the outline form should not contain sharp angles, sound tooth structure should not be removed simply to obtain wide, smooth curves in the outline form. The outline form should be smooth to facilitate the uncovering of the margins during carving of amalgam. That is, the margins of the preparation should not

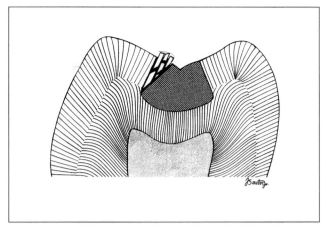

Fig 10-5 An acute cavosurface margin of enamel has the potential for fracture; a 90-degree enamel margin on the occlusal surface will withstand occlusion.

be jagged or rough, because it is difficult for the dentist to know whether a margin of the restoration appears to be irregular because the enamel margin is rough or because amalgam extends past the margins onto the surface of the tooth (overextended amalgam).

When replacing a defective restoration, or a restoration associated with recurrent caries, the outline form will be determined by several factors. First, the outline form of the old restoration will have a major influence. Also, the outline form may have to be extended because of additional pathosis. Finally, the resistance form for the tooth structure or restoration may have to be improved, and that will affect the outline form.

Resistance and Retention Form

To provide retention form for the amalgam, opposing walls of Class 1 occlusal restorations should be parallel to each other or should converge occlusally. Enamel prisms in most areas of the occlusal surface are directed roughly parallel to the long axis of the tooth,[39] and this factor should be considered when the angulation of the margin of the amalgam preparation is designed. To enhance their ability to resist fracture, enamel margins should be prepared at a 90-degree or more obtuse angle; enamel margins of less than 90 degrees are much more subject to fracture (Fig 10-5).

For resistance form in the amalgam restoration, amalgam margins should be approximately 90 degrees. Although many amalgam restorations will have amalgam margins that are significantly less than 90 degrees on the occlusal surface, very acute amalgam margins are much more subject to fracture (Fig 10-6). Marginal fracture will usually cause marginal gaps, or ditches, between the amalgam and the enamel.

If the faciolingual width of the preparation exceeds one third the distance between the tips of the facial and lingual cusps (intercuspal distance), the remaining cusps themselves should be carefully evaluated. Even in narrower preparations, cusps should be evaluated for cracks that could lead to fracture, and the functional loading to which they will be exposed should be assessed. If a cusp is too weak to withstand function (Figs 10-7a to 10-7c), it should be reduced for coverage with amalgam or attached in some way to the amalgam to provide cuspal reinforcement (described in the section on complex amalgam restorations).

Occlusal amalgam restorations should have an occlusogingival thickness of at least 1.5 mm, and preferably 2.0 mm to resist fracture during function (resistance form for the restoration). When dentinal caries and the overlying enamel are removed, the preparation will be at least that depth and will usually be deeper.

Figure 10-8a shows a diagram of a cross section of the crown of a posterior tooth with fissure caries. Figure 10-8b shows a cross section of the amalgam preparation that is indicated because of that carious lesion. Figure 10-9 shows the outline form of several occlusal amalgam restorations; the outline form was determined by the extent of dentinal caries at the base of the fissures. Again, fissures not known to be carious, in a surface receiving an amalgam restoration due to fissure caries, should be sealed with a resin fissure sealant.

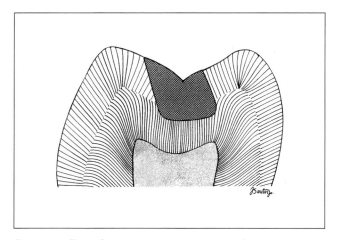

Fig 10-6 The left margin exhibits an acute "fin" of amalgam, which has a greater propensity for fracture, depending on the load applied to it during mastication. The right marginal configuration allows nearly a 90-degree angle for amalgam, imparting greater strength.

If occlusal caries encroaches on the enamel of the proximal surface, so that, when the caries is removed, the proximal enamel has no dentinal support, consideration should be given to converting the Class 1 preparation to a Class 2 preparation. An important part of this consideration should be the determination of the forces to which the marginal ridge will be exposed. If there is direct occlusal contact between the opposing tooth and the weakened marginal ridge, the marginal ridge should be removed and restored with amalgam.

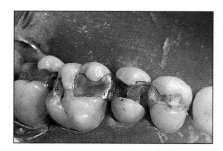

Fig 10-7a The mesio-occlusodistal preparation in the premolar, after removal of a defective restoration, is greater than one third the intercuspal distance; therefore, the cusps should be protected by reduction and coverage with a restoration, or they should be cross splinted (Fig 10-40).

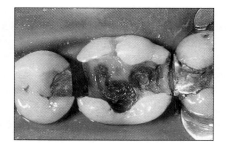

Fig 10-7b The mesio-occlusodistal preparation in the molar leaves cusps much too thin to resist occlusal loading; they must be reduced and protected with a complete–occlusal coverage restoration.

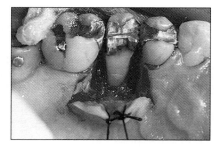

Fig 10-7c The lingual cusp of the maxillary premolar, which was not protected or reinforced during restoration, has fractured.

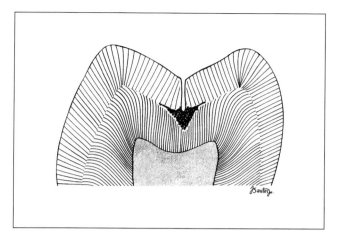

Fig 10-8a Fissure caries in this tooth involves demineralization of the enamel at the depth of the fissure, spread of caries along the dentinoenamel junction, and the penetration of caries into dentin.

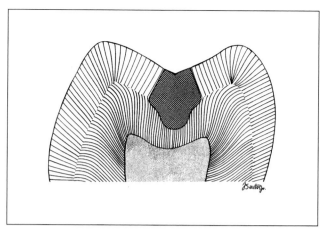

Fig 10-8b Tooth preparation involves the removal of the caries and of the enamel not supported by sound dentin. Only the diseased dentin is removed; additional dentin is not removed simply to create a flat pulpal floor for the preparation.

Fig 10-9 Outline form of various Class 1 preparations. The extent of caries is the determinant of outline form, so outline form will vary in every situation involving caries. Fissures not known to be carious may be sealed with a resin fissure sealant; fissures may be opened with a small bur to a depth of approximately 0.5 mm for inspection prior to sealing.

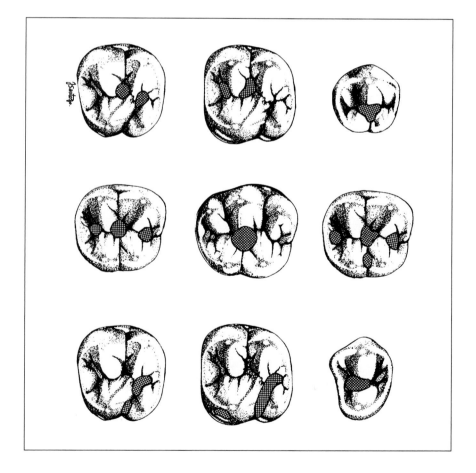

The Class 2 Preparation

Indications

An initial Class 2 restoration is usually placed because caries is present in a proximal surface of a molar or premolar. Proximal caries can sometimes be diagnosed visually during a clinical examination, but it is usually diagnosed with bitewing radiographs. The depth of the penetration of caries in enamel and dentin is actually greater than it appears to be in a bitewing radiograph. A carious lesion that appears radiographically to have penetrated about two thirds of the way through the proximal enamel has actually penetrated the dentinoenamel junction (DEJ). However, even if caries has slightly penetrated the DEJ, the tooth still has the potential for remineralization if the etiologic conditions are changed.[1] Each patient must be individually evaluated for improved oral hygiene, alteration of diet, and reduction in cariogenic bacteria before it is decided to surgically remove a minimally deep carious lesion. In most cases, restorative procedures should not be undertaken to treat proximal caries unless there is radiographic evidence of spread of the caries at the DEJ and at least slight penetration in dentin toward the pulp.[1]

If minimal dentinal caries initiated through demineralization of enamel in a proximal surface necessitates a restoration, it can possibly be treated by what is referred to as a tunnel restoration. Because this restoration does not usually involve the use of dental amalgam, it is discussed in the chapter on esthetic posterior restorations (chapter 8).

Outline Form

As with Class 1 restorations, Class 2 restorations that leave as much sound tooth structure as possible will contribute to resistance form for the tooth. Tooth preparation necessitated by a carious lesion on a proximal surface should, when possible, avoid extension of the occlusal outline more than is necessary to allow access to the proximal caries, to remove demineralized enamel, and to remove enamel not supported by sound dentin. If occlusal caries is present, it should be treated with a separate occlusal restoration. If occlusal caries is in close proximity to the occlusal outline of the proximal restoration, so that there is minimal or no sound tooth structure separating the two preparations, they should be joined. As when Class 1 occlusal restorations are placed, fissures not known to be carious but believed to be susceptible

to caries should be sealed with a resin fissure sealant.[75] Fissures that contact the outline of a Class 1 or Class 2 preparation should be sealed. Retention form for the proximal restoration should be attained within the proximal preparation; the preparation should not be extended further into the occlusal grooves to provide retention of the proximal restoration, because this will weaken the tooth's resistance to fracture.

Access to the caries is usually made by preparation through the marginal ridge. The proximal preparation is begun by creating a slot, cut with a small bur in the center (mesiodistally) of the crest of the marginal ridge and occlusal to the carious lesion (Fig 10-10a). The slot is deepened gingivally until the bur "falls" into the carious lesion. The preparation is widened facially and lingually to eliminate all caries at the DEJ and to remove enamel that is not supported by sound dentin. All enamel demineralization should usually also be removed. However, if demineralization is superficial (less than half way through the enamel), consideration should be given to using an acid etchant and coating the white-spot demineralization with resin.[42] Alternatively, the demineralized enamel can be removed with a round bur or hand instrument; then the sound enamel walls of the dished-out area can be etched and the area can be restored to contour with bonded resin composite.

The Class 2 restoration necessitated only because of proximal caries and having an occlusal outline limited to the marginal ridge area will be referred to in this chapter as a *slot restoration*. If it involves the distal surface with access from the occlusal surface, it will be called a disto-occlusal (DO) slot restoration (Fig 10-11).

When the proximal slot restoration is prepared, a shell of enamel should be left between the preparation and the adjacent tooth as long as a high-speed dental bur is being used (Figs 10-10b and 10-12a to 10-12c). This will prevent accidental nicking and scarring of the adjacent tooth. One study[92] found unfilled proximal surfaces were damaged during Class 2 preparation in adjacent teeth 69% of the time, and that damaged surfaces were almost three times as likely to become carious as were undamaged surfaces. Special care to avoid damage to the adjacent tooth is warranted. Any nicking or scarring of an adjacent tooth should be polished before the restoration is placed.

The proximal surface margins of a Class 2 amalgam preparation should not be in contact with the adjacent tooth (Fig 10-10c). Breaking contact slightly will allow the amalgam at those margins to be carved and burnished (with a very thin carver, such as the interproximal carver) during the restoration placement procedure. If, to eliminate contact with the adjacent tooth, a significant

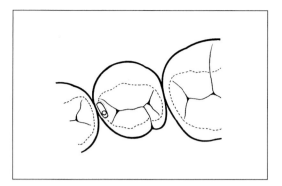

Fig 10-10a For a Class 2 preparation to treat initial proximal-surface caries, an initial cut is made through the marginal ridge with a narrow bur to penetrate to caries; then the slot is widened faciolingually.

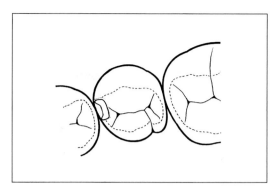

Fig 10-10b The mesial and distal aspects of the proximal enamel plate are thinned to facilitate its fracture and removal.

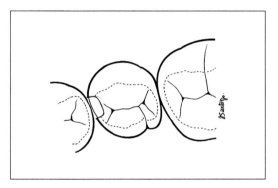

Fig 10-10c The final preparation outline will be determined after all caries is removed. It should provide for at least minimal separation of margins from the adjacent tooth.

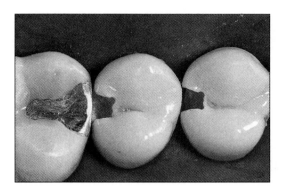

Fig 10-11 In the disto-occlusal slot preparations in the maxillary first and second premolars, the preparations have been opened facially and lingually so that contact is just broken to allow for carving and burnishing.

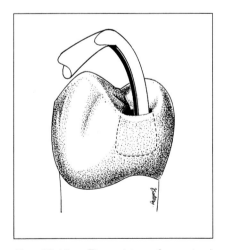

Fig 10-12a The plate of proximal enamel is often fractured with hand instruments to prevent damage to the adjacent tooth by a bur. The instrument is placed in the slot.

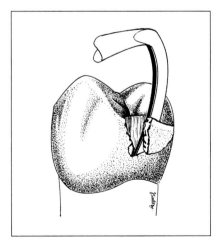

Fig 10-12b The instrument is rotated to fracture the plate.

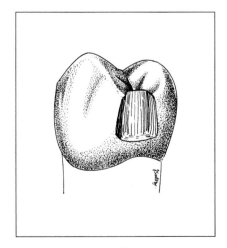

Fig 10-12c The fractured margins have been planed with a gingival margin trimmer or hatchet.

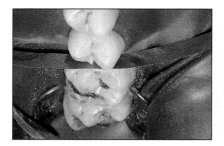
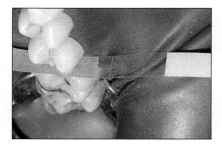
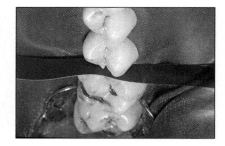

Fig 10-13a A metal-backed abrasive strip is used to provide minimal separation between the proximal cavosurface margins of a Class 2 preparation and the adjacent tooth. The tooth with the preparation or (as in this case) the adjacent tooth surface may be stripped in this way.

Figs 10-13b and 10-13c Strips with successively finer abrasives should be used to polish the abraded surface after separation is obtained.

amount of sound enamel that is supported by sound dentin would have to be cut away, consideration should be given to allowing contact to remain or to using proximal surface stripping with abrasive strips (Figs 10-13a to 10-13c) to avoid widening the preparation simply to break contact with the adjacent tooth.

During removal of dentinal caries, the demineralized dentin in the periphery of the preparation (at or near the DEJ) should be removed and the outline form should be extended to assure that the enamel at the margins of the preparation is supported by sound dentin. Dentinal caries should be removed with the largest round bur that will fit into the area. After the caries in the periphery of the preparation is removed, the caries in the dentin overlying the pulp should be removed. The bur should be rotated very slowly in a low-speed handpiece; the rotation should be so slow that the blades of the bur can be seen as it rotates. The blades of the slowly rotating bur are like multiple spoon blades, but the depth that a blade can penetrate into the carious dentin is limited by the edge angle of the bur and by the depth of each bur blade toward the center of the bur, so the bur will only remove a limited depth of caries during each rotation. During removal of deep caries, this procedure is less likely to result in a pulpal exposure than the use of a spoon excavator.

Resistance and Retention Form

After the shape of the preparation is roughed out with a bur, hand instruments, such as a gingival margin trimmer (10-80-8-14 or 10-95-8-14), may be used to fracture away the shell of enamel, to shape the facial, lingual, and gingival walls and margins, and to scrape away any fragile enamel from the margins (Figs 10-14a to 10-14e). The facial and lingual walls of a Class 2 slot preparation should converge slightly toward the occlusal surface to provide retention form for the restoration (Fig 10-15).

To provide resistance form for the Class 2 amalgam restoration, the proximal preparation should have a mesiodistal dimension of about 1.5 mm or more. If there is sound dentin supporting occlusal enamel in the fossa adjacent to the marginal ridge, that dentin and enamel should be left intact. If caries extends from the proximal DEJ deeper into dentin, the demineralized dentin should be removed completely, especially in the areas near the DEJ, and sound dentin should be left in place.

The gingival floor of the proximal preparation may be flat and approximately perpendicular to the long axis of the tooth, or it may be curved faciolingually, as determined by the extent and configuration of the caries that necessitated the restoration. The location of the gingival floor, therefore, should be determined by the gingival extent of the carious lesion and/or by the level necessary to provide separation of the gingival margin from the adjacent tooth. The gingival wall, like the facial and lingual walls of the proximal preparation, should form an angle of approximately 90 degrees with the surface of

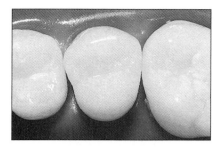

Fig 10-14a An amalgam preparation will be made because initial caries is present.

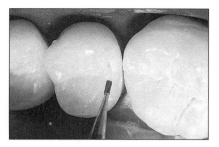

Fig 10-14b A small bur is used to cut a slot, beginning at crest of marginal ridge and extending gingivally to "fall" into caries. A thin plate of enamel separates the bur from the adjacent tooth to prevent damage to the adjacent tooth.

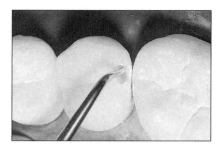

Fig 10-14c A gingival margin trimmer is placed into the slot created by the bur and rotated to apply pressure to the thin plate of proximal enamel.

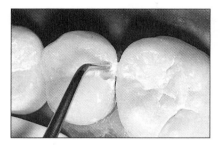

Fig 10-14d The thin plate is fractured.

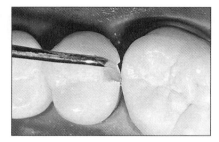

Fig 10-14e The walls and margins are planed with the margin trimmer to smooth them and to eliminate any remaining fragile enamel.

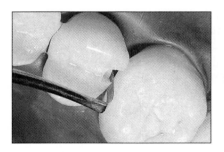

Fig 10-14f There is enough separation of margins from the adjacent tooth to allow access to a thin carver (IPC) to carve and burnish margins.

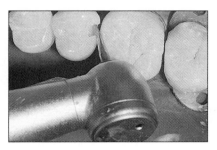

Fig 10-14g Retention grooves are placed with No. ¼ bur.

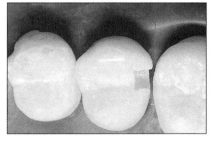

Fig 10-14h The preparation is completed.

the tooth; this is to give strength to both the amalgam and enamel and to prevent enamel prisms that are not supported by sound dentin from being left at the margins of the restoration.

Convergence toward the occlusal surface of the facial and lingual walls of the proximal slot preparation gives retention form to the restoration to keep it from dislodging occlusally. Although, with initial proximal-surface caries, it is not often necessary to extend the Class 2 preparation into occlusal grooves, the operator will frequently need to replace an existing restoration that was prepared with an occlusal extension. If the restoration is extended into occlusal grooves, this extension will provide resistance to displacement of the restoration proximally (that is, toward the adjacent tooth). To provide enough resistance, however, the extension into the

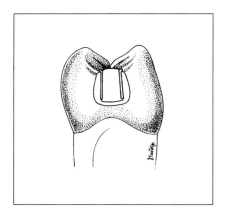

Fig 10-15 The proximal slot preparation, or the proximal box of a Class 2 preparation, should have walls that meet the proximal surface of the tooth at 90 degrees and converge occlusally to provide resistance and retention form.

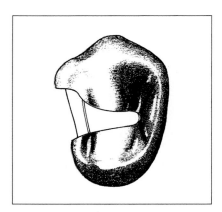

Fig 10-16a Although extension of a Class 2 preparation into occlusal grooves is not usually necessitated by caries, if such an extension is already present from a previous restoration of the tooth, it will provide some resistance form for the proximal portion.

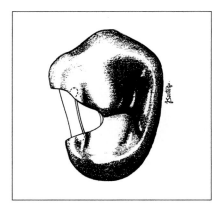

Fig 10-16b An extension without parallel cavosurface margins, however, will not provide the resistance form needed to prevent displacement of the proximal amalgam during mastication, so retention grooves *(dotted lines)* should be added.

occlusal surface must have a faciolingual dimension of at least one fourth the distance between the facial and lingual cusp tips[105] (intercuspal distance), and the facial and lingual margins of the occlusal extension must be approximately parallel to each other in a mesiodistal direction (Fig 10-16a).

Retentive Undercuts

If the extension into the occlusal surface is narrower, or if there is no extension into the occlusal grooves, as with the proximal slot restoration, retentive undercuts (retention grooves or points) must be cut into the dentin of the facial and lingual walls of the proximal box (Fig 10-16b). Use of a No. ¼ round bur, with a head diameter of 0.5 mm, is recommended for preparation of retention grooves and points for Class 2 amalgam restorations[104] (Figs 10-14g). For a proximal slot restoration, retentive undercuts should be very distinct (at least 0.5 mm deep) and should oppose each other to form a dovetail effect in the dentin. Long grooves, extending from the gingival floor to the occlusal surface are recommended for a proximal slot restoration[102,106] (Fig 10-17a). If the occlusal extension is narrow, short retention grooves, or retentive points, should be prepared in the facial and lingual walls to supplement the resistance form provided by the occlusal extension[104] (Fig 10-17b). If there is a bulky extension of amalgam into the occlusal surface of the tooth, retentive undercuts should not be necessary[105] (Fig 10-17c). For preparing any retentive undercuts with

a bur, it is advisable to use a handpiece at low speed and to use magnification to enable visualization, because the location and direction of the undercuts are critical to the success of the restoration.

Retentive undercuts in the dentin of the facial and lingual walls should be completely in dentin and not at the DEJ; this avoids the removal of the dentinal support for the proximal enamel adjacent to the restoration. The undercuts should not, however, be inserted so far away from the DEJ that the pulp chamber could be penetrated. A good rule of thumb is to place retentive undercuts so that there is approximately 0.25 to 0.5 mm of dentin between the groove and the DEJ and so that the groove is approximately 0.5 mm deep and 0.5 mm wide. Again, the 0.5-mm diameter of the No. ¼ round bur is ideal as a gauge of dimension. So that retentive undercuts do not penetrate through the dentin to the DEJ when they are placed in the facial and lingual walls, they should be cut to be parallel faciolingually to the DEJ and to the external surface of the tooth (Fig 10-18).

When retentive undercuts are necessary, they must be actual undercuts in the facial and lingual dentin that oppose each other (Fig 10-18). This is especially important in proximal slot restorations, in which the undercuts are the only feature that will prevent dislodgment of the restoration proximally. Without correctly located, distinct retention grooves, a proximal slot restoration is doomed to failure. When well designed, the proximal slot restoration can last indefinitely. Figures 10-19a and

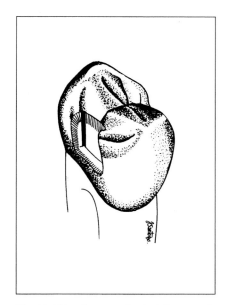

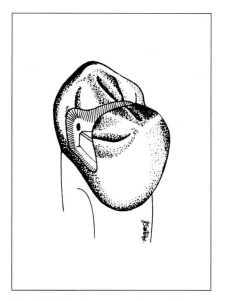

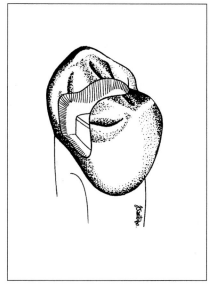

Fig 10-17a In a proximal slot or proximal box–only preparation, retention grooves should be long and very distinct.

Fig 10-17b In preparations with narrow occlusal extensions, a short (0.5- to 1.0-mm) retention groove or point is placed just gingivally to the occlusal DEJ.

Fig 10-17c When the occlusal extension is wide (1.5 mm or more faciolingually) and has parallel walls, retention points or grooves are not necessary.

Fig 10-18 Location and direction of retentive undercuts (retention grooves) for the proximal portion of a Class 2 restoration. The illustrated grooves are approximately 0.5 mm wide and 0.5 mm deep (No. ¼ bur head is shown) and are directed approximately parallel to the DEJ (and the external surface of the tooth). *(left)* For a fairly flat surface, such as the proximal surface of a maxillary premolar, the grooves are directed almost in the facial and lingual directions. *(right)* For a convex proximal surface, such as in a mandibular premolar, their direction is considerably vectored.

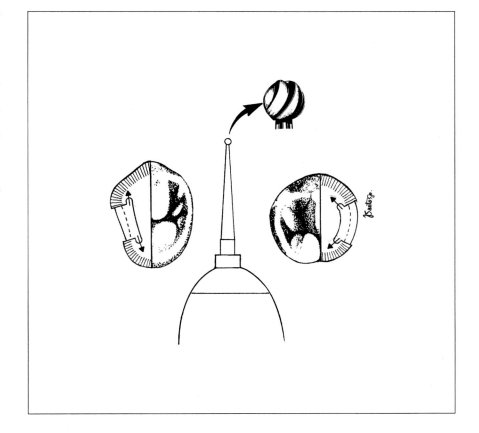

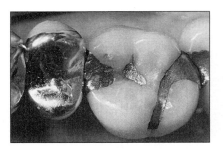

Fig 10-19a This restoration has served for more than 58 years.

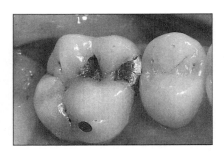

Fig 10-19b This restoration is more than 20 years old.

Figs 10-19a and 10-19b Proximal slot restorations placed by Dr Miles Markley in his practice in Denver, Colorado, were photographed in 1992.

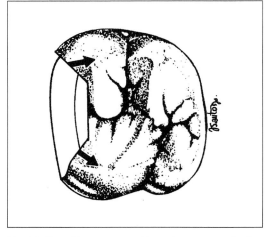

Fig 10-20a For a proximal box that is so wide that retentive undercuts, if placed parallel to the adjacent DEJ, would not oppose each other to provide any undercut retention, undercuts (retention grooves) should not be placed.

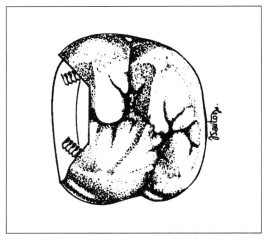

Fig 10-20b Instead, other types of resistance and retention, such as these horizontal self-threading pins, should be employed.

10-19b show two Class 2 slot amalgam restorations, both placed by Dr Miles Markley; one has been in function for more than 58 years and the other for more than 20 years.

Mechanical Retention

If a proximal box or slot is so wide that retentive undercuts will not oppose each other (Fig 10-20a), another type of retention and resistance feature, such as a self-threading pin, placed horizontally or vertically, should be used (Fig 10-20b). (Pins are discussed in a later section.) The need for pins and other forms of mechanical resistance features may one day be negated by the ability to bond amalgam restorations to tooth structure,[16,54,55] but the consistency and longevity of bonded amalgam restorations have yet to be confirmed.

The outline form of Class 2 amalgam restorations is always determined by the pathologic problem they are treating, so there will be an infinite number of variations in occlusal outline form. Figure 10-21 illustrates the outline form of some typical Class 2 restorations that would be placed to treat initial caries.

Facial and Lingual Access

Most Class 2 amalgam restorations have occlusal access, as already discussed. If proximal caries is at or apical to the cementoenamel junction, however, it is often more conservative to use facial, and occasionally lingual, access.[2] The preparation for a Class 2 amalgam restoration with facial or lingual access, sometimes referred to as a *keyhole preparation* or *facial or lingual slot preparation*, is similar to a slot preparation with occlusal access. The entire preparation is apical to the proximal contact. The location and configuration of the caries and the

Fig 10-21 Typical outline forms of Class 2 restorations placed to treat initial caries. Because outline form is determined by the pathosis present and the morphology and position of the tooth, there are an infinite number of variations. The bottom right-hand restoration represents a facial slot or keyhole restoration to treat root caries, or caries at the cervical line.

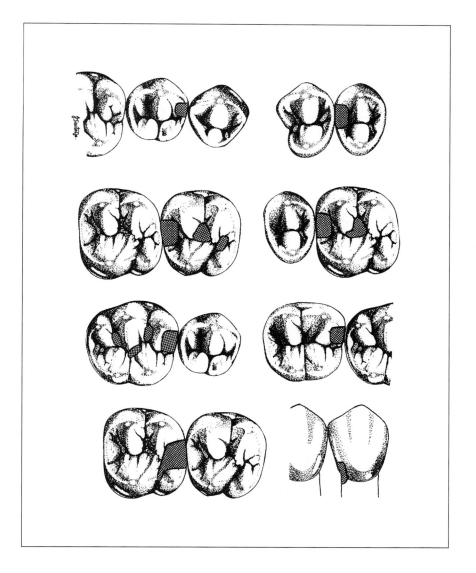

access preparation determine the outline form of the keyhole preparation (Fig 10-21, bottom right). Its margins, which are usually on cementum or dentin, should be at approximately 90 degrees to the external surface of the tooth. Groove retention, similar to that recommended for a proximal slot preparation with occlusal access, is indicated and can usually be placed with a No. 1/4 bur; occasionally grooves must be placed with a hand instrument, such as a gingival margin trimmer.

Replacement of Restorations with Occlusal Extensions

Patients commonly will have existing Class 2 amalgam restorations that have extensions of the preparation through occlusal fissures and even through nonfissured grooves. Although this preparation outline form should not currently be advocated, existing restorations of this type will need to be replaced from time to time. Therefore, some aspects to promote their longevity must be discussed. First, the narrower the extension through the occlusal surface is faciolingually, the less marginal breakdown will occur[5,81,82a] (Fig 10-22). Second, the junction of the proximal portion and the occlusal extension of the Class 2 amalgam preparation must have adequate depth occlusogingivally (1.5 to 2.0 mm) or the proximal portion must have distinct and effective undercuts in the dentin of the facial and lingual walls.[106] The occlusal outline form at the junction of the proximal and occlusal components should not be sharp or jagged, but sound cuspal enamel should not be sacrificed to make the junction smooth and flowing.

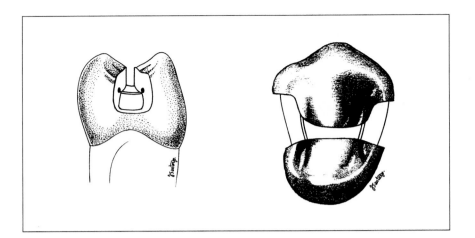

Fig 10-22 When extension through occlusal fissures or grooves cannot be avoided, such as when an old, defective amalgam restoration is being replaced, the faciolingual width of the occlusal portion of the preparation should be kept as narrow as possible to maintain tooth strength. *(left)* Proximal view; *(right)* occlusal view of mesio-occlusodistal preparation.

Complex Preparations

Historically, the term *complex amalgam restoration* referred to one that involved three or more surfaces of a tooth. The term has been redefined in recent years[94] to refer to an amalgam restoration that replaces one or more cusps.

When a metal cuspal-coverage restoration is indicated, a gold casting is considered the restoration of choice. Gold has wear characteristics similar to those of enamel and has the ability to maintain a stable occlusion. However, for various reasons, a gold casting cannot always be chosen as the definitive restoration. In these situations, amalgam is an excellent alternative restorative material.

The efficacy of the amalgam cuspal-coverage restoration has been shown in both clinical and laboratory studies.[65,94,100] The key to the successful placement of cuspal-coverage restorations is a thorough understanding of the underlying engineering principles. Preparations for amalgam restorations have traditionally been designed to provide adequate retention form. *Retention* has been defined as prevention of dislodgment of the restoration along the path of insertion (with tensile forces). *Resistance* is defined as prevention of dislodgment or fracture by oblique or compressive forces. Although retention form is important in the complex amalgam restoration, more emphasis should be placed on the resistance of both the restoration and the remaining tooth structure. Retention and resistance form can be obtained through the use of both metal threaded pins and non-pin features, which will be described.

Cuspal Coverage Preparations

Often, individuals seek treatment because of a fractured cusp or cusps in posterior teeth. If the treatment option agreed on for the tooth is a complex amalgam restoration, the tooth preparation will usually include removal of any existing amalgam restoration, removal of any caries and fragile enamel and/or dentin, and preparation of margins to provide a cavosurface angle of approximately 90 degrees in all areas. But in addition weak cusps that have not fractured should be reduced for coverage and protection with amalgam.

The thickness of amalgam needed for cuspal protection will vary, depending on the functional load to which the cusp will be exposed. A good rule of thumb for amalgam thickness in centric holding cusps (stamp cusps) of molars and premolars is 2.5 mm. In a facial cusp of a maxillary premolar, occasionally a reduced thickness of amalgam is acceptable to allow a maximum amount of facial enamel to remain for esthetics (Figs 10-23a to 10-23c).

When cusps are reduced for coverage, the occlusal tooth structure should be reduced anatomically to provide for an adequate and consistent occlusal amalgam thickness. To facilitate consistent reduction, depth cuts are recommended. Figure 10-24 illustrates the use of depth cuts to assure consistent reduction of occlusal tooth structure for coverage. Figures 10-25a to 10-25i show a clinical case in which depth cuts provided consistent reduction. The length of the head of the bur that is used for depth cuts must be known. Because head lengths vary from manufacturer to manufacturer, and even among burs of a single manufacturer, it is good

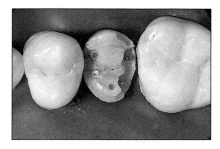

Fig 10-23a Because of a diagnosis of incomplete tooth fracture, the maxillary premolar has been prepared for a complex amalgam restoration.

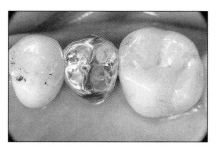

Fig 10-23b The tooth has been restored with a complex amalgam restoration that protects the entire occlusal surface.

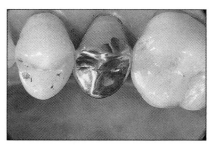

Fig 10-23c The occlusal height of the mesial aspect of the nonfunctioning facial cusp was only reduced 1.5 mm to preserve facial enamel for esthetics.

Fig 10-24 Depth cuts are used to provide for even reduction of occlusal tooth structure of a mandibular molar and consistent thickness of amalgam. (a) Depth cuts 2.5 mm deep; (b) cuspal reduction viewed from the facial aspect; (c) cuspal reduction viewed from the mesial aspect.

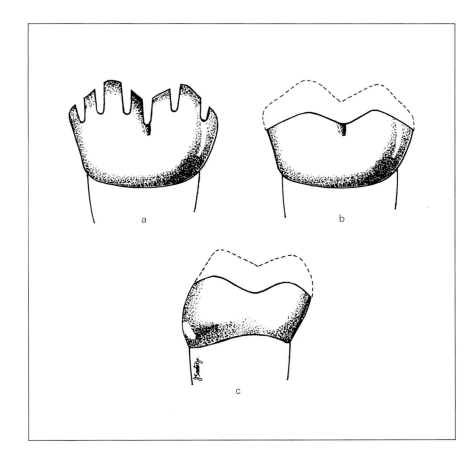

Figs 10-25a to 10-25i   Reduction of weak cusps of a mandibular molar for coverage.

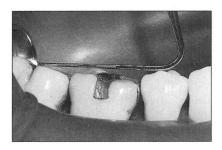

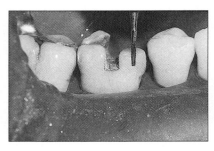

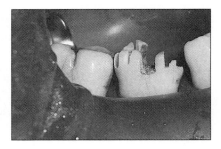

Fig 10-25a   An instrument is placed so that it touches the cusp tips of the adjacent teeth. This way the cusps to be reduced and rebuilt in amalgam may be carved to approximately the correct height before the rubber dam is removed.

Fig 10-25b   Half the 5.5-mm length of a No. 169L bur is used to make depth cuts approximately 2.5 mm deep in the cusps.

Fig 10-25c   The depth cuts are completed.

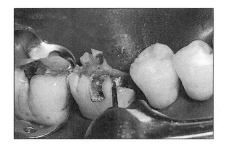

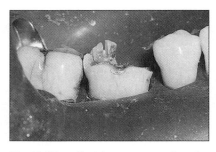

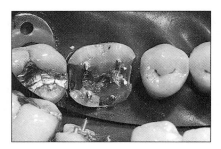

Fig 10-25d   The head of the handpiece is rotated so that the 169L bur can be used to reduce the cuspal structure between the depth cuts.

Fig 10-25e   Facial cusps are reduced.

Fig 10-25f   All cusps are reduced, and resistance features are placed.

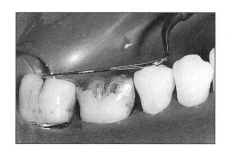

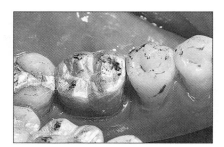

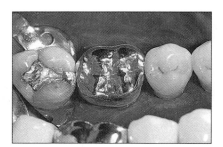

Fig 10-25g   Amalgam is placed, carved, and smoothed. An instrument is placed to ensure that cuspal height is similar to preoperative cuspal height.

Fig 10-25h   Completed restoration.

Fig 10-25i   Polished restoration.

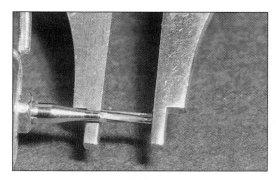

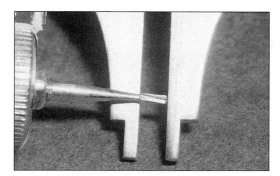

Fig 10-26a A Boley gauge is used to measure a No. 56 bur head (4.0 mm in this case).

Fig 10-26b A Boley gauge is used to measure a No. 330 bur head (2.0 mm in this case). A handy instrument for measuring bur head length is the periodontal probe.

Figs 10-27a to 10-27c Preoperative registration of the height of cusps to be reduced and restored with amalgam.

Fig 10-27a The midfacial and distofacial cusps are to be reduced for coverage. A periodontal probe is placed along the facial cusp tips of the tooth to be restored and the adjacent teeth, and the relationships of the cusp tips to the probe is remembered or drawn.

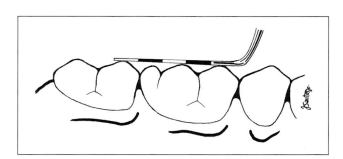

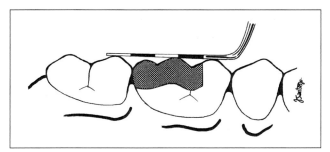

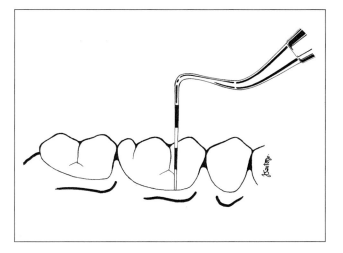

Fig 10-27b The amalgam cusp tips of the carved restoration are seen to have a similar relationship to the probe.

Fig 10-27c If there are no adjacent teeth or cusp tips to guide the height of amalgam cusp tips, the distance from a landmark (such as the cervical line) may be measured with a periodontal probe.

practice to measure the length of a bur head prior to preparation of depth cuts (Figs 10-26a and 10-26b). A periodontal probe should be available for measuring the length of bur heads.

Consistent reduction of cusps provides anatomic reduction rather than flat reduction. Anatomic reduction imparts adequate strength to the amalgam while preserving and protecting as much natural tooth structure as possible. Some operators reduce to a flat surface that is perpendicular to the long axis of the tooth; no scientific justification for this practice can be found in the literature. The authors have been using anatomic reduction for many years with excellent results.

A time-saver in practice is to take note of cuspal height and cusp tip location, or even to make a drawing, prior to cuspal reduction so that cusps may be built and carved back to their original height prior to removal of the rubber dam (Figs 10-27a to 10-27c).

Figs 10-28a and 10-28b Scanning electron micrographs of self-threading pins. (Courtesy of Dr. John O. Burgess.)

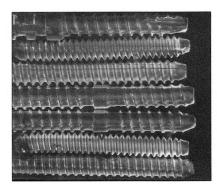

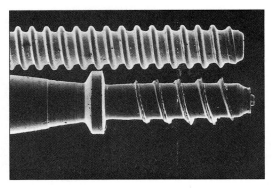

Fig 10-28a *(top to bottom)* Brasseler PPS (titanium alloy); Denovo Denlok (stainless steel); Vivadent Filpin (titanium); Coltene/Whaledent TMS Link Plus (titanium alloy); Coltene/Whaledent TMS Link Plus (stainless steel); Coltene/Whaledent TMS Minim (stainless steel); Fairfax Dental Stabilok (stainless steel).

Fig 10-28b *(top)* Coltene/Whaledent TMS Minim pin and *(bottom)* Max pin (with threads more widely separated to allow for greater thickness of dentinal threads).

Resistance and Retention Features

For amalgam restorations that do not replace cusps, or at least large portions of cusps, the walls of the preparation provide retention and resistance form. Retention form is provided by convergent walls and undercuts placed in dentin. When a large amount of cuspal tooth structure is lost or removed, the walls, or portions of them, that provide resistance and retention for the amalgam are lost. For this reason, it is necessary to add features to the preparation that will provide adequate resistance and retention for the restoration. Several methods of obtaining resistance and retention for complex amalgam restorations will be discussed below.

Pins

Although pins were first described in the 19th century,[33,53] Markley[67–69] popularized the concept of cemented stainless steel pins in his lectures and articles. Later, stainless steel pins, which were malleted into slightly undersized channels in dentin (friction-locked pins),[46] and threaded stainless steel pins, which were screwed into channels in dentin,[45] were developed. Laboratory studies have since investigated the properties of these three types of pins (cemented, friction-locked, and self-threading), and, because of these studies, the self-threading pins are the only ones that are currently popular (Figs 10-28a and 10-28b). In a study by Dilts and coworkers,[30] self-threading pins were found to be more retentive in dentin than cemented or friction-locked pins. They also recommended a depth in dentin of 2.0 to

3.0 mm as optimum for self-threading pins. Moffa and others[78] found that a pin length of approximately 2.0 mm into amalgam provides optimum retention. The relationship between retention and the diameter of the pin has also been investigated. As would be expected, larger-diameter pins are more retentive.[30,31,78]

Self-threading pins are manufactured in a variety of configurations. Some are self-shearing and some have heads. Figure 10-28a shows several pins from various manufacturers. In one study of self-threading pins,[15] pins manufactured by Coltene/Whaledent and Brasseler demonstrated superior resistance and retention.

An innovation in pin thread design has been to place the metal threads further apart so that, once the pin is threaded into dentin, the dentinal threads are thicker. When a pin is pulled from a pin channel, it is the dentinal threads that shear, and not the metal threads. The pin design with wider dentinal threads retains well in dentin (Fig 10-28b). Another innovation has been the addition of a shoulder stop to prevent the end of the pin from putting stress on the dentin at the end of the pin channel; the PPS pin (Brasseler) and the Max pins (Coltene/Whaledent) have an effective shoulder stop incorporated into their design. A shoulder is a part of the design of the Link Plus pins (Coltene/Whaledent), but its diameter is similar to that of the threads, so it does not provide an effective stop.[70] Although a definite shoulder stop is theoretically beneficial, there is no evidence that problems are associated with pins that lack effective shoulder stops.

Figs 10-29a and 10-29b Color-coded pin channel (twist) drills and pins of various diameters and lengths (Coltene/Whaledent TMS [Thread Mate System]).

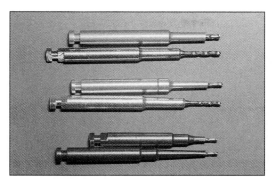

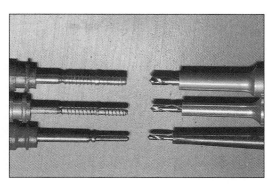

Fig 10-29a Pin channel (Kodex) drills: *(top to bottom)* Regular (gold, 0.027-inch [0.675-mm] diameter, 2.0- and 5.0-mm lengths); Minim (silver, 0.021-inch [0.525-mm] diameter, 2.0- and 5.0-mm lengths); Minikin [red, 0.017-inch [0.425-mm] diameter, 1.5-mm length).

Fig 10-29b Pins with corresponding pin channel drills: *(top to bottom)* Regular (0.031-inch diameter) gold-plated stainless steel Link Plus pin with Regular (0.027-inch diameter) pin channel drill (2.0-mm depth-limiting); Minim (0.024-inch diameter) titanium alloy Link Plus pin with Minim (0.021-inch diameter) pin channel drill (2.0-mm depth-limiting); Minikin (0.019-inch diameter) titanium alloy Link Series pin with Minikin (0.017-inch diameter) pin channel drill (1.5-mm depth-limiting).

Coltene/Whaledent pins and pin channel drills in Regular, Minim, and Minikin sizes are shown in Figs 10-29a and 10-29b; a smaller size (Minuta, 0.0135-mm diameter twist drill; 0.015-mm diameter pin) is available, but the authors have been unable to find a practical use for it. The gold-plated stainless steel TMS Regular and Minim pins (see Figs 10-34b and 10-34c) are also available as self-shearing pins, and in double-shear (two pins in one) form as well as single-shear form. All TMS Link and Link Plus (with shoulder) pins are self-shearing; Link Plus Regular and Minim pins are also available in the two-in-one form. Selection among these pins should be based on operator preference because they all have performed well in laboratory studies.

Number to use. A commonly stated rule for deciding the number of pins required to retain a restoration is one pin for each missing cusp and one pin for each missing proximal surface. However, it is difficult to make a rule that is appropriate for all situations. Although it has been demonstrated that, as the size and number of pins increase, the amount of resistance form imparted by the pins increases,[12] the number of pins used will vary with the size of pin, the amount of remaining tooth structure, other resistance features used, and the functional requirements of the final restoration.

Channel preparation. A rubber dam should be in place when pin channels are prepared and when pins are placed to protect the patient from aspiration and to prevent contamination by saliva in case there is pulpal perforation during pin channel preparation.

Because the tips of pin channel drills tend to "walk around" when the rotating tip is placed against dentin, it is often useful to place an indentation or starting point in the dentin at the desired location for the initiation of the pin channel. The starting point may be placed with a small bur, such as a No. 1/4 or No. 1/2 bur.

Various lengths and diameters of twist drills are available for preparation of pin channels (Figs 10-29a and 10-29b). The most popular twist drills have depth-limiting shoulders, which assure that the optimum pin channel depth is not exceeded. To avoid perforation of either the pulp or the external surface of the tooth, location of the pin channel is critical. The channel should usually be prepared parallel to the nearest external tooth surface. Before channel preparation is initiated, approximately 2.0 mm of the end of the twist drill should be placed against the external surface of the tooth. If that much of the side of the tooth is exposed above the rubber dam, alignment is facilitated. Frequently, however, adjacent soft tissue under the dam obscures visualization of the tooth surface in the area adjacent to the desired pin

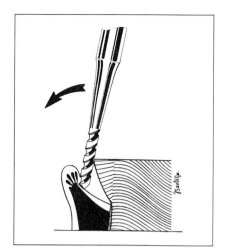

Fig 10-30a To align the twist drill with the side of the tooth when the external tooth surface is obscured, the drill is placed in the sulcus so that the drill is touching the preparation margin; the drill is then rotated *(arrow).*

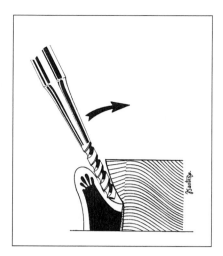

Fig 10-30b With that movement, the tip contacts the external surface and the portion of the drill that was in contact with the margin is rotated slightly away from it; then the length of the drill is rotated *(arrow).*

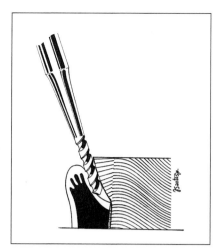

Fig 10-30c With that rotation, the drill returns just to touch the margin. It is now aligned parallel to the external surface.

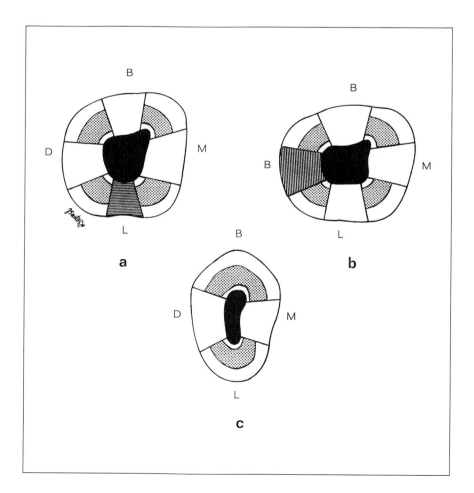

Fig 10-31 Preferred locations for pin placement in a (a) maxillary molar, (b) mandibular molar, and (c) maxillary premolar. *(dotted areas)* The most preferred locations at the line angles; *(white areas)* areas to avoid because of concavities, furcations, or thin dentin; *(lined areas on the molars)* areas where pins may be placed with added caution because the angulation of the root in relation to the crown is frequently severe.[48]

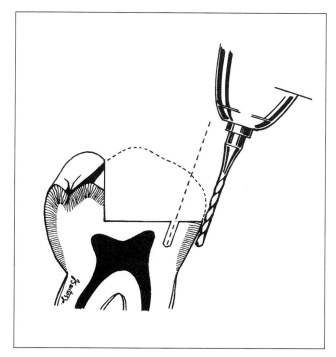

Fig 10-32a To align a pin channel drill, a non–depth-limiting pin channel drill is aligned parallel to the external surface.

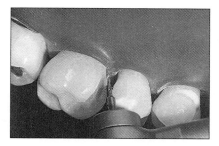

Fig 10-32b A pin channel drill is aligned with the mesial surface of the maxillary molar before it is carried into the preparation.

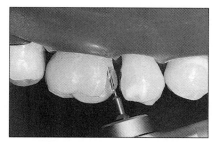

Fig 10-32c The drill is used to cut the pin channel to the same alignment.

location. For alignment, the twist drill is placed against the external tooth surface, the angulation of the drill is changed until the drill separates from the margin of the preparation; it is then rotated back until it just contacts the margin (Figs 10-30a to 10-30c).

Pin channels should be initiated at least 0.5 mm from the DEJ if the entrance to the pin channel is coronal to the cementoenamel junction; a 1.0-mm distance from the DEJ is preferable.[30] If the pin channel entrance is apical to the cementoenamel junction, there should be at least 1.0 mm of dentin between the channel and the external surface of the tooth.

The most common location for pins is at the line angles of the tooth because of the greater thickness of dentin between the external surface and the pulp and the decreased risk of perforation. The risk of perforation is especially increased in furcation areas. Figure 10-31 illustrates the preferable locations for pins.[48] Areas to be avoided in posterior teeth include interproximal areas and tooth structure that lies over furcations or concavities in the root. Wherever the pin is to be located, the external surface of the tooth should be assessed and the pin channel drill aligned parallel to it (Figs 10-32a to 10-32c).

Pins should be located so that the channels enter the dentin at approximately 90 degrees to the prepared dentinal surface. If a depth-limiting twist drill is used, the drill will not be able to achieve optimum pin channel depth if the surface of dentin adjacent to the entrance to the channel is at an angle to the drill. In addition, a pin should not be located immediately adjacent to a wall of the preparation; there should be access to condense amalgam around the full circumference of the pin. If a pin is located an optimal distance from the DEJ and a dentinal wall is adjacent to the pin, a "cove" may be cut in the dentin to provide adequate space for amalgam (Fig 10-33).

To provide maximum cutting efficiency, the twist drill must be sharp so that it will be efficient at low speeds. A twist drill loses cutting efficiency with extended use and steam autoclaving.[22,109] Twist drills should be sterilized with dry heat, chemical vapor, or immersion in glutaraldehyde rather than steam autoclave. Drills should be discarded when a diminished cutting efficiency is sensed by the operator.[71,80a] If preparation of a pin channel is difficult, it is likely that the flutes of the twist drill are obstructed by debris, the drill is dull, the handpiece is running in reverse, or the tip of the drill is in contact with enamel rather than dentin.

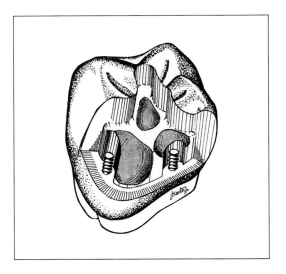

Fig 10-33 There should be adequate space around the full circumference of a pin for amalgam. If a pin is located adjacent to a dentinal wall, a small cove may be cut in the wall to provide adequate space for condensation of amalgam.

The correctly prepared pin channel will be slightly smaller in diameter than the pin; this size difference is called the pin-to–pin channel mismatch. The mismatch must be small to ensure that excessive stresses are not exerted on the dentin during insertion of the pin and that the pin will be retained by the dentin.

During preparation of a pin channel to a depth of 2.0 mm or more, it is advisable to withdraw the twist drill from the channel at least once to allow dentinal cuttings to be cleared from the flutes of the drill; this allows more efficient pin channel preparation and less heat generation. Care must be taken, however, to avoid overenlargement of the channel with multiple entries and withdrawals.

If a cavity varnish is used, it is best applied prior to insertion of the pin so that it thinly coats the channel and so that it does not coat the pin. When a dentin bonding agent is used, if it is applied prior to placement of the pin, the adhesive will occlude the channels, and they will have to be redrilled; so it is best to apply the dentin bonding agent after the pin is placed. If amalgam bonding materials are used, they are applied after the pin so that amalgam can be condensed immediately after placement of the bonding material.

Insertion. The insertion of self-threading pins may be accomplished in several ways. Placement by hand with a small pin wrench (Figs 10-34a to 10-34c) or a hand-operated handpiece[89] (Figs 10-35a and 10-35b), is preferred by some dentists because (1) it allows the operator to feel the insertion and to reverse the pin one-quarter turn once the tip has contacted the end of the channel, thus avoiding excessive stresses in the dentin; and (2) stripping of the dentinal threads created by the self-threading pin is less likely. Insertion of pins with a low-speed handpiece is preferred by many because it is much more time efficient (Fig 10-36). The thread design of some pins (such as the Link-Plus series) provides for wider dentinal threads; dentinal stripping is less frequent when such designs are used.

Because the portion of a pin that will extend into the amalgam usually is only 2.0 mm long or less, the pin is aligned parallel to the external surface of the tooth, and the channel entrance is about 1.0 mm inside the DEJ, a pin rarely needs to be bent. The only reason for bending a pin is to keep it within the bulk of the planned amalgam restoration. If bending should be needed, it may be accomplished with a small, fork-shaped pin bender (Fig 10-37a) or a small hemostat (Fig 10-37b) before the pin is shortened.

Figs 10-34a to 10-34c   Pins and pin drivers (or wrenches) (TMS system).

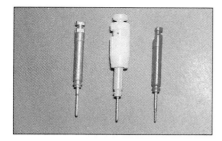

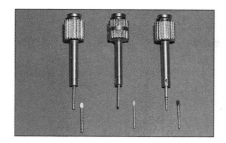

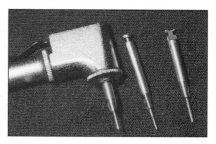

Fig 10-34a *(right to left)* Link Plus Regular pin, Link Plus Minim pin, and Link Series Minikin pin. A plastic Universal Hand Driver (for Link Plus and Link Series pins) is shown on the Link Plus Minim pin.

Fig 10-34b Metal hand wrenches or drivers with individual TMS gold-plated stainless steel pins: *(left to right)* Regular, Minim, and Minikin. The hand driver with the band around the handle is for Minim pins; the nonbanded hand driver is for Regular and Minikin pins.

Fig 10-34c Pin drivers for insertion into a motorized or hand-operated handpiece to place individual gold-plated stainless steel pins (shown installed in drivers).

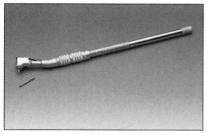

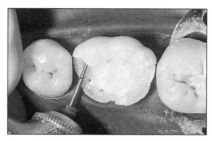

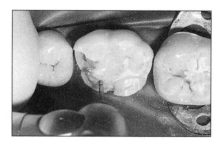

Fig 10-35a Hand-operated handpiece (E-Z Place Driver, Whip Mix) for hand insertion of pins in areas that are difficult to access with a hand wrench.

Fig 10-35b Insertion of a horizontal Link Series Minikin pin in a facial cusp of a mandibular molar, using an E-Z Place Driver.

Fig 10-36 Low-speed handpiece is used to insert a vertical Link Plus Minim pin.

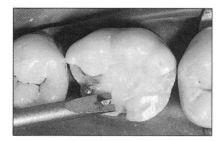

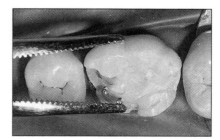

Fig 10-37a To bend pins, a Coltene/Whaledent pin bender can be used.

Fig 10-37b If a hemostat is used to bend a pin, the jaw of the hemostat should contact the pin at its tip, and very controlled pressure should be used in bending the pin.

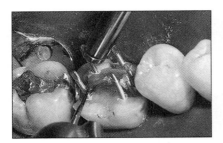

Fig 10-38a   When a No. 169L tapered fissure bur is used to approach the pin at approximately 90 degrees, no stabilization is necessary.

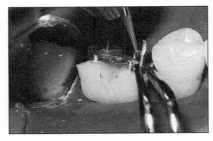

Fig 10-38b   When a No. 35 inverted cone bur is approaching the pin obliquely, the pin is stabilized to prevent it from being unscrewed from the pin channel.

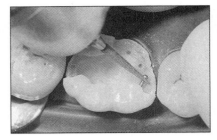

Fig 10-38c   This needle-shaped diamond is approaching the pin at approximately 90 degrees.

Shortening. The portion of a pin extending from the pin channel is usually longer than desired, so it will need to be shortened after insertion. The pin may be efficiently and safely cut by gently brushing the pin with either a fissure bur or a diamond in a high-speed handpiece. Both the bur and the diamond should be used with air or water coolant to prevent the pin, and therefore the surrounding tooth structure, from being overheated during the operation. If a bur is used, it must be sharp (Fig 10-38a). If the bur can approach perpendicularly to the pin, the pin does not require stabilization during the cutting process. If the bur approaches from an oblique angle, the clockwise rotation of the bur can cause counterclockwise rotation of the pin so that it is unscrewed. Therefore, if the pin cannot be approached perpendicularly by the bur, it should be grasped with cotton forceps or a hemostat to stabilize it during the cutting process (Fig 10-38b), or, minimally, an instrument should be pressed against the pin during the process to dampen vibration from the bur, which tends to initiate the unscrewing. A long, narrow diamond is preferred by many operators for cutting pins, because it causes less vibration and it is less likely to "catch" in the metal of the pin to initiate reverse rotation (Fig 10-38c).

Horizontal Pins

Until a decade or so ago pins had been, for the most part, oriented vertically, approximately in line with the long axis of the tooth. Studies[13,61] have also demonstrated the efficacy of using pins oriented horizontally, that is, inserted into the dentin of a vertical wall of a preparation (Figs 10-39a and 10-39b). Burgess[13] found two horizontal self-threading pins (Whaledent TMS Minim and Minikin) placed into a free-standing facial cusp of a maxillary premolar to be effective in reinforcing the cusp (Fig 10-39a). Other investigators[61] have found that hori-

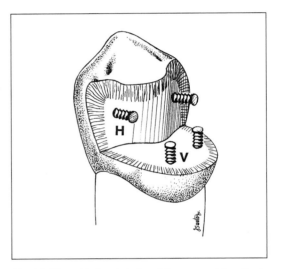

Fig 10-39a   Horizontal pins (H) are used to attach the wall of a cusp to the amalgam restoration. Vertical pins (V) attach the restoration to the radicular portion of the tooth.

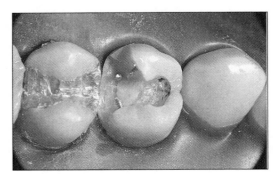

Fig 10-39b Horizontal pins can be used in conjunction with vertical pins. In this clinical situation, a proximal box had to be extended significantly facially to eliminate caries and unsupported enamel.

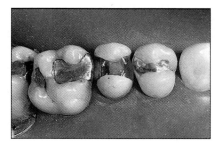

Fig 10-40 Horizontal pins are used to cross splint the cusps of a maxillary premolar.

Fig 10-41 A circumferential slot is prepared with a small, inverted cone bur, such as a No. 33½.

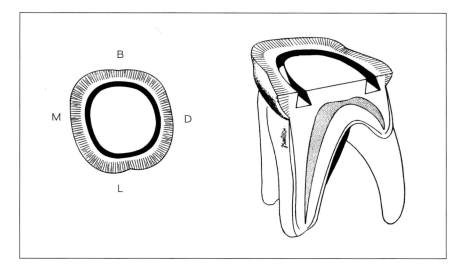

zontal pins used to cross-splint cusps of maxillary premolars reinforce and strengthen the cusps (Fig 10-40).

Adequate dentin must be present for horizontal pins to be employed. When the channels for horizontal pins are prepared, they should be initiated in dentin 0.5 to 1.0 mm from the DEJ. They should be directed approximately parallel to the adjacent DEJ (and external surface of the tooth). But, because of their horizontal orientation, such pin channels, prepared only 1.5 to 2.0 mm deep, will often contact enamel. When the twist drill, in its progress through dentin, seems to stop its penetration short of reaching its depth-limiting shoulder, it is probably because it has reached enamel. Further deepening of the channel should not be attempted; even 1.0 mm of depth will impart some retention for a pin, and attempts to deepen the channel into enamel will result in an enlarged dentinal channel and the increased potential for enamel fracture.

Horizontal pins should be positioned fairly near to the occlusal surface in the dentin of a vertical wall, 0.5 mm to 1.0 mm gingival to the occlusal DEJ, so that their mechanical advantage is enhanced for reinforcement of the cusp. A horizontal pin should be oriented so that it will not be near the anticipated surface of the amalgam and so that amalgam may be condensed around the entire circumference of the pin.

Perforation During Pin Channel Preparation

Perforations during pin channel preparation should be avoided through careful design and placement of the channel. However, if a perforation does occur, it is important to determine what has been perforated, the external surface of the tooth or the pulp chamber. When the pulp chamber has been perforated, the channel should be covered with calcium hydroxide, and the pin

channel should be placed in another location, or a different type of resistance feature should be used. A perforation of the external surface of the tooth may be more problematic. If the perforation is located above the epithelial attachment, the channel should be filled with amalgam. If the pin is inserted and the tip protruding on the external surface is cut even with the surface and polished, the pin will not totally obturate the perforation, and leakage will occur.[21] If the perforation occurs below the epithelial attachment, the channel may be obturated with gutta-percha and zinc oxide–eugenol sealer or with amalgam.

Non-Pin Resistance and Retention Features

Birtcil and Venton[7] suggested that more attention be directed toward using the available tooth structure to provide retention and resistance form in complex amalgam restorations. They recommended parallelism in all walls of the preparation, proximal box form, retention grooves in the proximal line angles, box form in buccal and lingual groove areas of molars, dovetails, rectangular boxes in areas other than interproximal surfaces, and reduction of undermined cusps for coverage with amalgam. In recent years, several additional non-pin resistance and retention features have been described and investigated. These include the circumferential slot, the amalgapin, and the peripheral shelf.

Circumferential slots. Outhwaite and others,[83] who introduced the circumferential slot prepared with a No. 33½ inverted cone bur (Fig 10-41), compared it with four pins (TMS Minim) and found no significant differences between the resistance provided by the two techniques. They also reported that the pin restorations had a greater tendency to slip on their bases before failure,

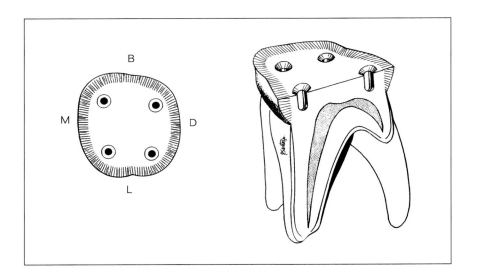

Fig 10-42a The entrances to amalgapin channels are beveled.

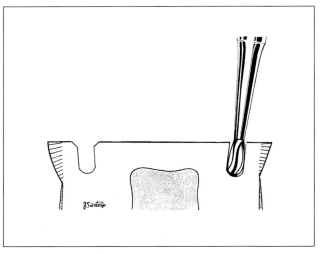

Fig 10-42b A variety of burs may be used to prepare amalgapin channels. A bur with a diameter of 0.8 to 1.0 mm, for example, the No. 330 bur, is desirable.

whereas slippage did not occur with circumferential slots. However, slot-retained restorations are more sensitive to displacement during matrix removal than are pin-retained restorations.

Amalgapins. Seng and others[97] tested circular chambers that they cut vertically into dentin to provide resistance and retention form for the restoration; they called these features *amalgam inserts*. Preparations for the inserts were made with a No. 35 inverted cone bur and were approximately 1.4 mm in diameter and depth. In their study, amalgam inserts provided resistance to displacement similar to that provided by self-threading pins. Shavell[99] described a variation of the amalgam

insert, which he termed the amalgapin (Figs 10-42a and 10-42b). The amalgapin channel described by Shavell was prepared with a No. 1157 or No. 1156 bur and had a depth of 3.0 mm. The margin of the channel entrance was beveled to decrease stress concentration in the amalgam. Laboratory studies of the amalgapin[27,95] have demonstrated that the resistance to displacement provided by amalgapins is similar to that provided by pins. It has been demonstrated[95] that a depth of 1.5 to 2.0 mm is adequate for amalgapins, and that an amalgapin with a diameter of 0.8 mm provides resistance similar to that of an amalgapin with a diameter of 1.0 mm. In addition to the burs advocated by Shavell (No. 1156 & No. 1157), others with similar diameters (such as the No. 330 and No. 56) also function well in creating amalgapin channels.[95]

Peripheral shelves. Peripheral shelves provide another form of resistance for complex amalgam restorations (Figs 10-43 and 10-44). A narrow (1.0 mm axially and 1.0 mm cervically) shelf did not perform well in tests for resistance form.[93,103] A wider shelf (2.0 mm axially and 1.0 mm cervically) (Fig 10-43) provided significantly more resistance form. Typically, peripheral shelves, like circumferential slots, are not used circumferentially, but are used only in areas of the preparation where they are needed (Fig 10-44).

Efficacy of Resistance and Retention Features

For the most part, the resistance form provided by various resistance and retention features has been tested in flattened molars, as described by Buikema and others,[12] with 4.0-mm high restorations retained by a given resistance feature. These teeth were mounted at a 45-degree

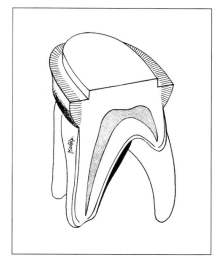

Fig 10-43 The circumferential peripheral shelf has been prepared with a 2.0-mm axial depth and a 1.0-mm cervical depth. For a flat preparation such as this, a peripheral shelf would not be adequate without other forms of resistance.

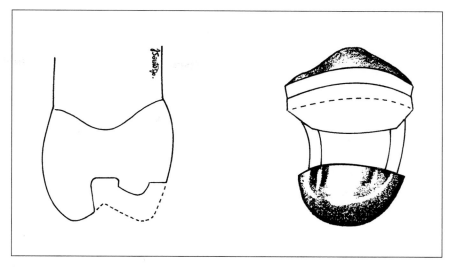

Fig 10-44 A more typical clinical use of a peripheral shelf is for resistance form for the amalgam-covered facial cusp of a premolar. *(left)* Cross-sectional view; *(right)* occlusal view.

angle and were loaded in compression; the mean loads at the time of failure have been calculated. Although this method of testing is not as enlightening as long-term clinical tests, it probably provides a good indicator of how well a resistance feature will perform in a clinical situation. It has been shown, however, that if these standard resistance-test restorations are loaded at a 90-degree angle instead of a 45-degree angle, the stainless steel pins provide significantly more resistance than amalgam inserts.[63,107] Few forces in the mouth are directed at a 90-degree angle to the long axis of the tooth, however, and few restorations are placed on preparations that are totally flat, without any walls or irregularities in the dentin.

One of the most telling studies pertaining to resistance form for complex amalgam restorations was reported by Plasmans and coworkers.[88] This group created preparations for complex amalgam restorations that combined the use of boxes, shelves, and amalgapins as resistance and retention features. They then loaded specimens at 45 degrees, as in most previous studies of resistance form, but they loaded half of the restorations from one side and half from the other. Their finding was, generally, that more load was required to cause failure of a restoration when the resistance and retention features (walls of shelves, boxes, and amalgapin channels) that opposed the direction of the load were increased.

It is important to distribute resistance features into all areas of the preparation and not to cluster them in any area.[19,88,107] Figures 10-45a to 10-45g show a restoration that originally replaced two missing cusps of a mandibular molar. The probable cause of failure was that the resistance features (pins) were clustered on the lingual aspect of the cavity preparation. In function, there was nothing to attach the facial aspect of the restoration to the tooth. If two of the four vertical pins had been placed in the facial portion of the preparation, or if two horizontal pins had been placed in the facial cusps, the restoration would, in all likelihood, have had adequate resistance to withstand its load in function.

When the technical requirements for placement of vertical pins can be met, vertical pins provide excellent retention and resistance form. However, risks are involved with pin placement: crazing of tooth structure, perforation into the pulp or periodontium, and weakening of the amalgam restoration over pins.[14] Additionally, the use of both vertical and horizontal pins may be limited by inadequate access; in these cases, alternative resistance and retention features should be employed. When a cusp has been reduced, and increased resistance form is needed, an amalgapin or a segment of a peripheral shelf or circumferential slot may be indicated.

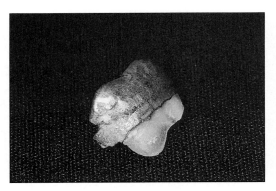 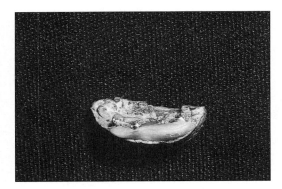

Figs 10-45a and 10-45b Failed complex amalgam restoration that replaced the lingual cusps of a mandibular molar. Note the fin of cervical tooth structure that fractured.

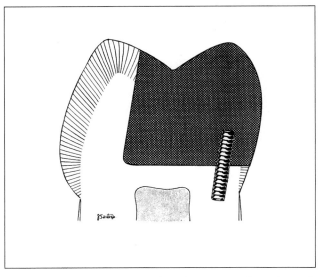 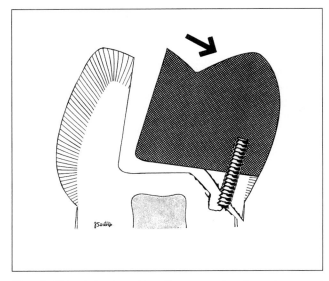

Fig 10-45c The dentin lingual to the pin was the only tooth structure that was opposing a lingually directed load on the restoration.

Fig 10-45d A load pushing the restoration lingually caused failure. Failure can be attributed to a lack of distribution of resistance and retention features.

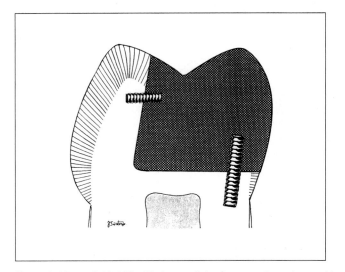 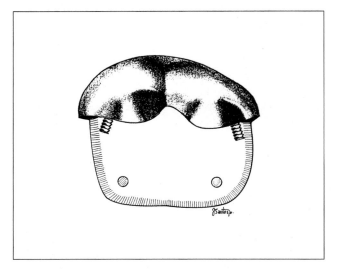

Figs 10-45e and 10-45f Had two of the four pins been located horizontally, failure would likely have been averted.

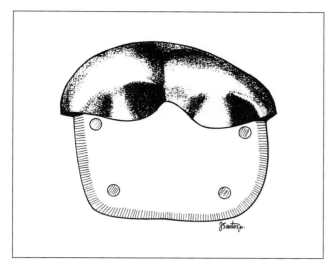

Fig 10-45g Alternatively, had two of the pins been placed vertically in the facial aspect of the preparation, this could have reduced the likelihood of failure.

Bonded Amalgam Restorations

In recent years, the use of adhesive resins to increase the retention and resistance of amalgam restorations has gained much attention. Although some researchers have found products such as Amalgambond (Parkell) and Allbond (Bisco) to be quite effective,[16,29,59] others have not been able to confirm these findings.[96] Based on laboratory studies,[79,101] it is widely held that resin composite restorations can strengthen remaining tooth structure. However, it has also been shown that thermal stressing and the moisture of the oral environment can decrease this reinforcing effect with time.[34,49] This same decrease in reinforcement may occur in bonded amalgam restorations placed with the current generation of amalgam bonding materials, but there is evidence that at least some of the reinforcement may be sustained.[35] Although there is great promise for future amalgam bonding materials, dentists should be cautious about abandoning proven resistance and retention features in favor of amalgam bonding. Until clinical research data are available to support the efficacy of bonding as the sole provider of resistance and retention, resin bonding agents should be used only in conjunction with proven mechanical forms of resistance and retention.

Cavity Sealers

Traditionally, in amalgam restorations, a base material was used whenever the restoration extended further pulpally than was considered to be "ideal." The cavity preparation was built up with the base so that the "ideal" cavity preparation could be made; a portion of the walls of the cavity preparation were composed of the base material. The rationale was that amalgam, as a metal, conducts temperature changes rapidly and does not have the thermal insulation qualities of tooth structure. It was believed that replacement of deeper carious dentin with amalgam would lead to permanent thermal sensitivity in the tooth or possibly to loss of pulpal vitality.

This belief in the need for thick bases for thermal insulation has not been borne out in research.[26,87] There is strong evidence[24,52,84] that long-term thermal sensitivity is the result of leakage of bacteria-produced irritants through dentinal tubules to the pulp, causing inflammation and hyperreactivity or sensitivity.

The use of bases in amalgam preparations is not indicated. The use of a bacteriostatic, bactericidal, or fluoride-leaching liner in areas of a preparation that are very deep pulpally, may be of some benefit, especially when a small pulpal exposure is detected or an undetected microexposure of the pulp could be present. But, of primary importance in protecting the pulp and preventing tooth sensitivity after amalgam restorations are placed is the sealing of the dentinal tubules against the ingress of oral fluids or of toxins generated by bacteria.[24]

For several decades, the use of a copal resin cavity varnish under amalgam restorations has been recommended by many teachers and researchers. Numerous laboratory and clinical studies have been carried out to determine the performance of various cavity varnishes.[40,58,66,85,116] Varnishes have been at least partially successful in preventing or slowing microleakage at the amalgam-tooth interface,[40,58,73] and they have decreased the penetration of fluids and irritants into dentinal tubules, but their success has been limited. In recent years, several investigators have advocated the use of resin adhesive systems under amalgam. Many of the bonding agent systems incorporate superficial etching of dentin and the application of a soluble hydrophilic resin to penetrate the etched dentinal surface and encapsulate the network of collagen fibers exposed by the etching process.[4,20,32,37] Some investigators have recommended the use of a primer only[32]; others have recommended the addition of the adhesive, which is then polymerized. The long-term clinical implications of use of dentin adhesive systems under amalgam are still unknown. A thorough discussion of dentin adhesive systems can be found in chapter 6.

Most of the dentin bonding systems that have been advocated for sealing the walls of amalgam preparations were designed for use with resin composite materials, and their use was simply expanded to include sealing the walls of amalgam restorations. Recently, several products specifically manufactured for use with amalgam have been used and tested. In the laboratory setting, these products provide an effective seal of the cavity walls and also some attachment of the amalgam to the tooth structure.[16,20,37] Although these so-called amalgam-bonding systems have not yet been clinically tested over a long period of time, their use for both sealing cavity walls of amalgam preparations and bonding amalgam to tooth structure is promising.

Based on current research findings, the following recommendations are made concerning sealing, lining, and basing amalgam restorations:

1. It is unnecessary to use bases in amalgam preparations to achieve "ideal internal form."
2. Near or suspected pulpal exposures should receive a calcium hydroxide–containing liner confined to the area overlying the pulp.
3. Neither liners nor bases should routinely be used for "insulation." Rather than relying on insulation, the dentist should look for a reason for tooth hyperreactivity (sensitivity), such as incomplete tooth fracture, caries, hyperocclusion, or erosion, and treat the problem.
4. The anticariogenic effect of fluoride-containing bases and liners is still being researched. Their use should be considered when the risk of caries is high.
5. A copal varnish or resin dentin bonding agent should be used on amalgam cavity walls.

Matrices

To confine the amalgam and allow adequate pressure for optimum condensation, the preparation must have a floor (or floors) plus walls completely surrounding the floor(s). A Class 1 occlusal preparation provides these by virtue of its location and definition. Whenever an amalgam preparation extends from one surface of the tooth to another, some form of matrix is needed to confine the amalgam for condensation. If a matrix is not used, condensation force will tend to push the amalgam out of the preparation rather than condensing the amalgam.

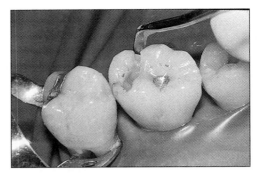

Fig 10-46　An instrument is held in place to act as a matrix for a small occlusolingual Class 1 restoration in a maxillary molar.

The simplest and fastest method of adequately providing a matrix should be used. Occasionally, as with the occlusolingual restoration of the maxillary molar, the blade of a hand instrument placed on the lingual surface of the molar and held in place during condensation may be adequate (Fig 10-46). In most cases, a matrix system, such as a Tofflemire matrix, is indicated. Rarely, a customized matrix will be necessary for a particular situation. A matrix system is needed in almost every case for Class 2 amalgam restorations.

There are myriad types of matrix systems; most involve a thin piece of stainless steel that is contoured and placed adjacent to the proximal portions of Class 2 preparations. The purpose of the matrix is to:

1. Substitute for missing walls so that adequate condensation forces can be applied.
2. Allow reestablishment of contact with the adjacent tooth.
3. Restrict extrusion of the amalgam and the formation of an overhang at a hidden margin, such as the interproximal gingival margin.
4. Provide for adequate physiologic contour for the proximal surface of the restoration.
5. Impart an acceptable surface texture to the proximal surface, especially in the area of the contact that cannot be carved and burnished.

Tofflemire Matrix

Probably the most commonly used type of matrix system in the United States is the Tofflemire system. The system consists of a matrix band and retainer (Figs 10-47a to 10-47j). The Tofflemire retainer consists of four parts (Fig 10-47b).

Figs 10-47a to 10-47j Tofflemire matrix system.

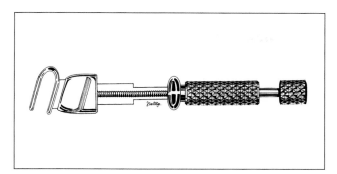

Fig 10-47a Matrix retainer.

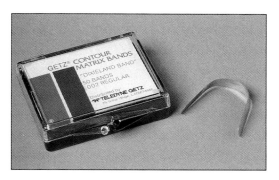

Fig 10-47d Precontoured Dixieland bands.

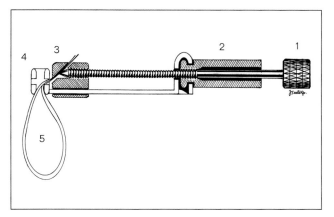

Fig 10-47b Parts of the assembly: (1) set-screw; (2) rotating spindle; (3) slide; (4) head; (5) band.

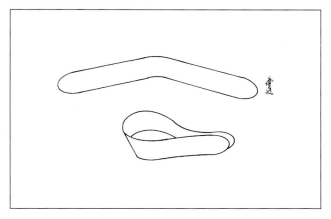

Fig 10-47e The matrix band is folded for insertion into retainer.

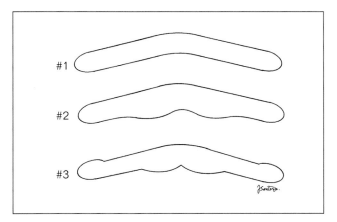

Fig 10-47c Three common shapes of Tofflemire matrix flat bands (Number 1 is also called a *Universal band;* numbers 2 and 3 are also called MOD bands).

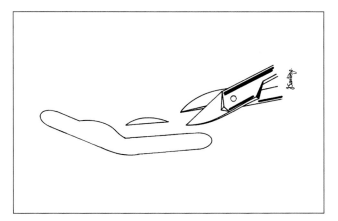

Fig 10-47f One of the projections of a No. 2 or 3 band may be cut if there is only one deep proximal area of the preparation.

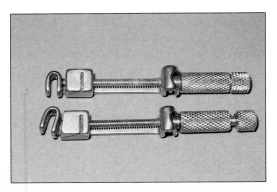

Fig 10-47g Two types of Tofflemire retainer: *(top)* straight; *(bottom)* contra-angled.

Parts

Head. This is the part that has the open side. In the U-shaped head, there are two slots in the open side. These slots are used to position the matrix band. The open side of the head should be held facing upward while the band is installed. The open side of the head faces gingivally when the band is placed around the tooth. There are two types of Tofflemire retainers based on the angulation of the head (Fig 10-47g).

Slide. This element has a diagonal slot; it is brought close to the head for band installation. The round ends

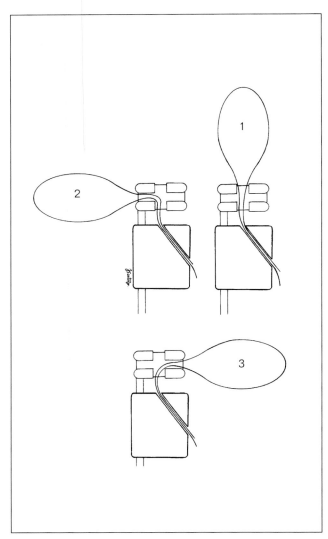

Fig 10-47h The loop of the band may extend from the head of the retainer in one of three directions: (1) straight; (2) left; (3) right.

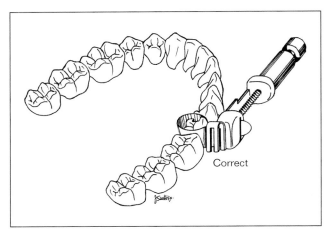

Fig 10-47i The matrix must be assembled with the slots in the head directed gingivally.

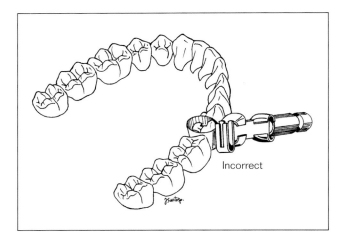

Fig 10-47j The slots in the head of the matrix should not be directed occlusally.

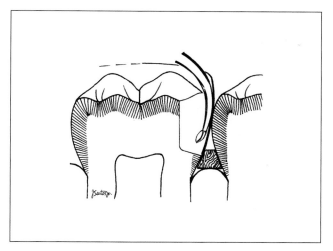

Fig 10-48a The convex side of a spoon excavator is used to impart a convex contour to the matrix band.

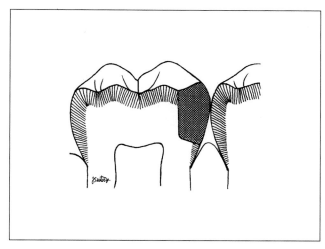

Fig 10-48b This will help to achieve a contact area, as opposed to a pinpoint contact, with the adjacent tooth.

of the band, when installed, extend at least 1.0 or 2.0 mm beyond the slot in the side of the slide. The amount of the band extending beyond the slot in the side of the slide will depend on the size of the tooth being treated. More band should extend from the slide for premolar teeth than for molar teeth. The slide is positioned near the head for installation of the band in the retainer and for placement of the band around the tooth.

Rotating spindle. This is used to adjust the distance between the slide and the head. The retainer is held with the thumb and forefinger of one hand (contacting both the head and slide) while the rotating spindle is turned with the other hand, clockwise and counterclockwise, to advance and retract the slide. This movement adjusts the size of the loop of the matrix band.

Set-screw. This threaded shaft of the set screw locks and unlocks the matrix band in the slide.

Types

The types of Tofflemire bands include flat bands of multiple shapes, precontoured bands, and bands with and without memory (dead-soft metal).

Flat bands. Bands for the Tofflemire system come in several shapes (Fig 10-47c) and three thicknesses. The thicknesses available are 0.010, 0.015 and 0.020 inch. The thicker band is stiffer to resist deformation during condensation; the thinner bands are often used to help

assure a tight contact in Class 2 restorations. Either thickness can be used to achieve excellent results, and selection is primarily a matter of operator preference.

By far the most frequently used shape is the No. 1, or Universal, band. The No. 2 band (so-called MOD band) has two extensions projecting at its gingival edge to allow matrix application in teeth with very deep gingival margins. In most cases, there will be only one deep area, so one of the extensions is usually cut off with curved scissors (Fig 10-47f). The No. 3 band also has projections for deeper gingival margins, but the band is narrower than the No. 2 band. The No. 3 band is ordinarily thought of as being for premolars and the No. 2 band for molars, but the size that best suits the situation should be used.

Because these bands are flat, they should be contoured so that they will impart physiologic contours to the restorations. A flat band may be contoured before it is inserted in the retainer. The band is laid on a paper pad, or other compressible surface, and the area to be contoured is heavily rubbed with an ovoid burnisher, a beavertail burnisher, the convex back of the blade of a spoon excavator, or a convex side of the cotton forceps. A band may also be contoured after it has been applied to the tooth. The area to be contoured is rubbed with the back of the blade of the spoon excavator or other thin, convex instrument (Fig 10-48a). The contact with the adjacent tooth should have some area and not have only a pinpoint touch (Fig 10-48b).

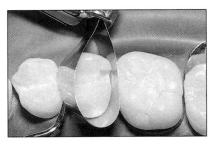 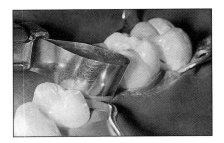

Figs 10-49a and 10-49b The blade of a plastic filling instrument has been placed into the gingival embrasure and is being slightly rotated (torqued) to provide enough separation to allow the matrix band to slip through the contact.

Pre-contoured bands. Precontoured Tofflemire matrix bands are also available. One such band is the Dixieland Band, developed by Dr Wilmer Eames (Fig 10-47d). When these bands are removed from interproximal contacts, the contour must be considered, and the band must be rotated in such a way that the trailing edge does not break or alter the shape of the marginal ridge as the band is being removed.

Insertion

Assembly. When the matrix retainer and band are assembled, the two ends of the matrix band must be even as they protrude from the diagonal slot of the slide. The loop can extend from the retainer in three different ways: straight, to the left, or to the right (Fig 10-47h). The straight assembly is for restorations near the front of the mouth where the rubber dam–covered cheek will not get in the way if the retainer protrudes perpendicularly from the line of teeth. The right and left assemblies are to allow the retainer to be aligned parallel or tangent to the line of teeth in more posterior areas. The band should be inserted into the retainer so that the loop extends from the appropriate side of the retainer and the set-screw knob is directed toward the front of the mouth. Because of the shape of the Tofflemire matrix band, when it is inserted into the retainer, one opening of the loop has a greater diameter than the other (Fig 10-47e). In other words, the loop will be shaped somewhat like a funnel. The wider opening goes toward the occlusal. The short knob of the set-screw is tightened so that the matrix band is held securely.

Application. The matrix is applied to the tooth to be restored. The matrix band will slide easily through the proximal contact area when the preparation has opened the contact. It will often slide through an intact contact as well (for example the mesial contact when a disto-occlusal restoration is being accomplished). If it will not slide through the intact contact, a bladed plastic filling instrument (such as the No. 1-2, Figs 10-49a and 10-49b) may be used to open the contact slightly to allow the band through. For this slight tooth separation, the blade of the instrument is placed in the gingival embrasure (gingival to the contact), moved occlusally until it is stopped by the contact, and torqued very slightly. At the same time, the matrix band is slipped through the contact. When the matrix is around the tooth, it should be tightened snugly, but not too tightly because a very tight matrix will deform the tooth.[3,90,91]

Wedging. Wooden wedges may be placed from either the facial or the lingual aspect. A wedge should usually be inserted from the side with the widest embrasure. For example, between the first and second premolars, the largest embrasure is usually the lingual embrasure. The wedge should be tightly inserted to enable development of an adequate contact despite the thickness of the matrix material.

Wedges are available in a variety of shapes and sizes. Figure 10-50a shows Wizard Wedges (Teledyne-Water Pik), which are triangular and available in four sizes. Figures 10-50b and 10-50c show Sycamore wedges (Premier), which are shaped to aid in the establishment of physiologic proximal contours. The Premier wedges, with seven color-coded sizes, are recommended for amalgam restorations.

It is necessary that the matrix band extend gingival to the gingival margin of the proximal box of a Class 2 restoration and that the wedge be positioned so that its base is also gingival to the gingival margin. If the wedge cannot be placed so that its base is gingival to the preparation margin, a concavity will be created in the matrix just occlusal to the gingival margin, and this concavity

Figs 10-50a to 10-50d Wooden inter-proximal wedges.

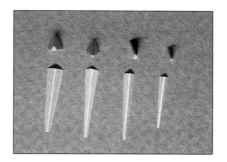

Fig 10-50a Wizard Wedges have a triangular shape.

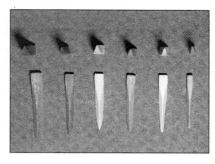

Fig 10-50b Premier Sycamore Wedges are shaped to impart a more physiologic contour to the matrix. There is a larger selection of sizes, and they are color coded for easy selection.

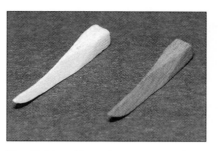

Fig 10-50c Note the anatomic shape of the Premier Sycamore wedges. The snow sled point helps to prevent catching of the rubber dam during insertion.

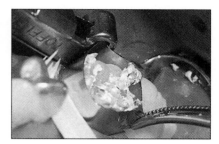

Fig 10-50d A custom-made wooden wedge may also be used, such as this one, which was made from a tongue blade.

will be transferred to the amalgam. Occasionally the gingival papilla will need to be surgically reflected from the interproximal area to allow the wedge to be positioned apical to the gingival margin. Another option might be to use a rigid bladed instrument to hold the matrix against the gingival margin during condensation. Custom wedges may be made for special situations; the wedge in Fig 10-50d was fabricated from a wooden tongue blade.

Contouring. The band should be burnished and contoured to impart desired proximal contours to the restoration. This can be accomplished with the back (convex side) of a spoon excavator (Fig 10-48a). The wedged matrix should be in solid contact with the adjacent tooth in the desired contact area. It should be pos-

sible to feel the convexity of the proximal surface of the adjacent tooth with an instrument through the matrix as the matrix is burnished.

Removal

In a multiple surface restoration, amalgam is condensed in the preparation after matrix placement. Amalgam condensation will be discussed in the next section.

When restoration with a Tofflemire matrix has been completed, first the slide, and then the set-screw is loosened. A finger or thumb is placed on the loop of the matrix band to keep it in place and the retainer is pulled occlusally to remove it. The distal end of the matrix is grasped and pulled occlusally and lingually (if the free ends are on the facial aspect) and out of the distal contact of the tooth. The mesial end is then grasped and pulled facially and occlusally until it is out of the contact. The matrix band can be grasped with fingers, the cotton forceps, or a hemostat. There are a few tricks that may help the dentist remove the Tofflemire matrix without breaking the marginal ridge:

1. As the matrix edge is coming out of the contact, the matrix can be tipped so that the edge will not "flip" the newly carved marginal ridge and break it.
2. Some dentists like to hold a condenser against the marginal ridge to support it and prevent it from breaking as the matrix is removed.
3. The movement of the band should be primarily to the facial or the lingual aspect as the band slips occlusally out of the contact.
4. Some dentists like to cut the band close to the teeth on the lingual aspect and then pull it facially from the contact.

The matrix band should be used once only and then discarded.

If a cavity varnish or bonding agent is used to coat the walls of the preparation, the material should be applied before the matrix is placed, otherwise, the material may cause the matrix to stick to the amalgam. This sticking can lead to fracture of the amalgam during removal of the matrix. Attachment of the matrix to the amalgam is a significant problem when amalgam-bonding materials are used. Because amalgam must be inserted immediately after placement of the adhesive, the bonding material cannot be placed prior to matrix application; the best solution at present is to avoid, as much as possible, getting the bonding material on the matrix. It is hoped that, as amalgam bonding evolves, matrices that resist the bonding materials will be made available. Until that time, a thin coat of wax, applied to the matrix with a wax pencil or crayon, may be helpful.

Other Matrix Systems

Many systems other than Tofflemire matrices are available (Figs 10-51 to 10-55). Each has its own advantages and disadvantages. In addition, stainless steel matrix material may be spot welded to provide a custom matrix for any situation. One commercial system (Denovo) has prewelded bands in various sizes (Figs 10-51a and 10-51b). To remove spot-welded matrices, a small bur in a high-speed handpiece is used to cut through the weld and allow the two ends of the matrix to separate for removal. The absence of a matrix retainer in the Denovo system is a distinct advantage.

T-bands have long been used in dentistry and provide a very simple and inexpensive matrix system (Figs 10-52a and 10-52b). The AutoMatrix system (Caulk/Dentsply) has a built-in matrix retainer that is much smaller than the Tofflemire matrix retainer, and this is an advantage (Figs 10-53a and 10-53b). The Palodent matrix (Darway) system provides small, precontoured matrices that are placed, wedged, and held in place by a flexible metal Bitine ring. A major advantage of this system is that, for a restoration involving only one proximal surface, there is no need for the matrix to be placed in the other contact (Figs 10-54a to 10-54c). The Omni-Matrix (Innovadent) is basically a disposable Tofflemire retainer and band that is preassembled and has a head that moves from side to side (Fig 10-55). This system takes less time to use than a Tofflemire matrix because there is no assembly time, but it is more expensive.

Reinforcing Matrices with Modeling Compound

Among the desirable qualities of a matrix are rigidity and maintenance of the shape established by the operator. When a Class 2 preparation has only proximal boxes that are adjacent to other teeth, and when the preparation does not, to any significant degree, extend to facial and lingual surfaces, the stainless steel matrix is usually well supported by the adjacent tooth or teeth. In these cases, no reinforcement is necessary. In larger restorations that involve surfaces not supported by adjacent teeth, it is often desirable to reinforce or support the matrix in some way in these areas to maintain the rigidity and shape of the matrix.

Occasionally, a single unsupported area of a matrix may be reinforced during condensation by the operator, who places a finger or holds an instrument against the matrix in a facial or lingual area. For large unsupported areas, however, modeling compound may be used (Figs 10-56a to 10-56j).

There are various ways of applying compound to support a metal matrix. Probably the most simple is to employ a stick of compound (Fig 10-56a). Approximately 1.0 inch of one end of the compound stick is heated over an alcohol burner. The stick is moved back and forth over the tip of the flame, while at the same time, the stick is rotated in the fingers (Fig 10-56b). After 5 to 10 seconds, the stick is removed from the flame and held for a few seconds until the heat has diffused to the center of the stick, as indicated by its starting to droop or sag (Fig 10-56c). At that point, the 1.0-inch end is soft enough to carry to the matrix and press into place with a dampened, gloved finger (Fig 10-56d). If adhesion of the

Figs 10-51a and 10-51b Denovo matrix system.

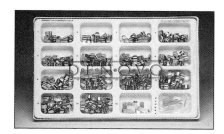

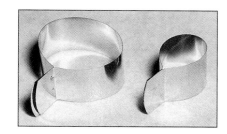

Figs 10-52a and 10-52b T-band matrix.

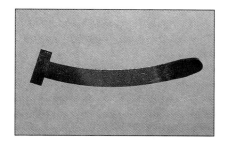

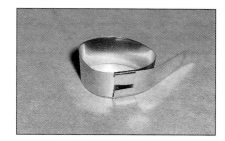

Figs 10-53a and 10-53b AutoMatrix system. Note the cable-drive wrench for adjusting the size of the loop.

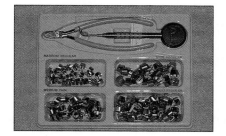

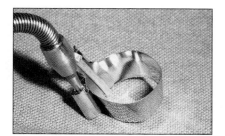

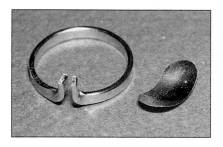

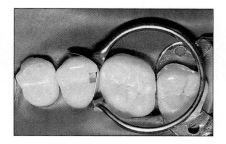

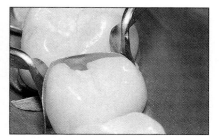

Figs 10-54a to 10-54c Palodent matrix system. Note the metal ring for holding the ends of the matrix snugly against the facial and lingual enamel. It will also provide some tooth separation.

Fig 10-55 The Omni-Matrix is basically a preassembled Tofflemire retainer and band that is intended for one-time use and then disposal.

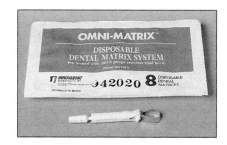

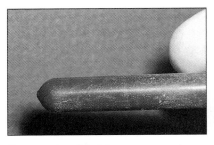

Fig 10-56a Modeling compound can be used to support a matrix.

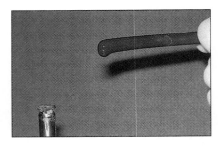

Fig 10-56b The compound stick is heated over an alcohol flame, then removed from the flame to allow warmth to diffuse to the core of the stick.

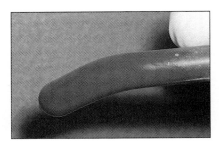

Fig 10-56c When the warmed tip of compound stick begins to droop, softness is through and through, and the compound is ready for use.

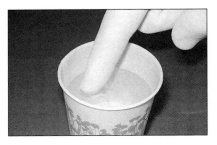

Fig 10-56d A finger is dampened in water to prevent the glove from sticking to the softened compound.

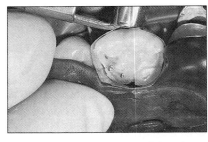

Fig 10-56e The compound has been pressed into place. It will be cooled with air to reharden it.

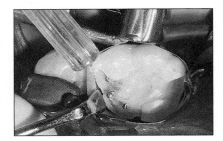

Fig 10-56f The matrix may be recontoured after application of the compound. A warmed instrument is used to soften the compound and reshape the matrix.

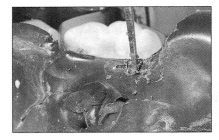

Fig 10-56g Any compound extending past the edge of the matrix should be trimmed to prevent chipping during amalgam condensation.

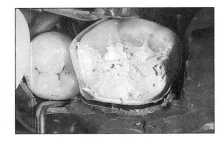

Fig 10-56h The compound is removed after amalgam condensation and initial carving.

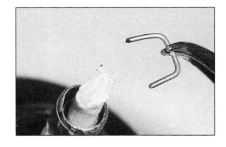

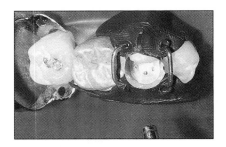

Figs 10-56i and 10-56j A staple can be used to hold compound segments in place.

compound to the matrix and adjacent teeth is desired, the softened end of the stick should be passed through the flame again before it is carried to the mouth; this will provide a tacky surface that will impart some adhesion.

After the compound is pressed into place (Fig 10-56e), it is cooled and hardened with air from the three-way syringe. The matrix may be recontoured after compound application. A warmed instrument is used inside the matrix to soften the compound and exert pressure on the matrix to give it the shape that will allow the restoration contours and shape to be similar to the original shape of the tooth (Fig 10-56f). Again, the compound should be cooled with air after reshaping with a warmed instrument. If modeling compound extends occlusal to the occlusal edge of the matrix band, it should be trimmed back with a sharp instrument (Fig 10-56g), or pieces of compound could chip off during amalgam condensation and contaminate the amalgam.

If compound is dislodged by condensation forces, the reinforcement will be lost; steps should be taken, therefore, to assure that the compound does not dislodge. While it is soft, a portion of it may be pushed onto the cusps of an adjacent tooth to provide retention, or, when compound is present on both the facial and lingual aspects, a staple-shaped piece of metal, made from a paper clip or other wire, may be warmed in the flame (Fig 10-56i) and placed to hold the facial and lingual segments of compound together (Fig 10-56j). When it is time to remove the staple, the tips of a hemostat are warmed in the flame, the staple is grasped, and the heat is allowed to diffuse into the compound surrounding the staple so that it is softened. The compound can usually be pried away from the adjacent teeth and matrix with an instrument such as a Hollenback carver or enamel hatchet (Fig 10-56h). After the compound is removed, the matrix may be removed as previously described.

Insertion of Amalgam

The technique for insertion of amalgam is basically the same no matter the type or classification of the preparation. Amalgam is mixed (triturated), carried to the cavity preparation, condensed into the preparation so that voids are eliminated and all areas of the preparation are obturated, and then carved to shape to reproduce the portion of the tooth that is missing.

As stated earlier in this chapter, the particles in amalgam alloys are either filings, produced by milling an ingot of the alloy, or spheres, produced by solidifying a spray of molten alloy. Some dental amalgam alloys contain only filings, others contain only spheres, and some contain both spheres and filings. Those containing only filings are called *conventional* or *lathe-cut amalgam alloys*, those containing only spheres are called *spherical alloys*, and those containing both filings and spheres are called *admixtures*.[25]

Spherical alloys produce an amalgam that requires a lower mercury-alloy ratio and less condensation force; they are said to be less condensable than conventional alloy amalgams or admixtures, and it is somewhat more difficult to obtain good interproximal contacts in Class 2 amalgam restorations with spherical amalgams than with lathe-cut alloys or admixtures. It has been demonstrated, however, that spherical amalgams are less sensitive to variations in condensation pressure than the alloys containing nonspherical particles.[10] In addition, the spherical alloys generally have a shorter working time than the admixed alloys.

Trituration

The trituration process includes the combining or mixing of liquid mercury with dry amalgam alloy powder. Electric amalgam mixers (also called *amalgamators* and *amalgam triturators*) are used for the trituration process (Figs 10-57a and 10-57b). The objective is to coat each particle of alloy with mercury and to begin the reaction that will produce a solid mass. Although amalgam alloy pellets and bottled mercury are available separately, use of precapsulated amalgam alloy, that is, a weighed, standardized amount of amalgam powder and mercury sealed into a capsule, ready for trituration, is recommended. The precapsulated products provide more consistent mixes of amalgam and are safer for those working in the dental office.

Amalgam must be condensed into the preparation as soon as trituration is completed. The duration and speed of trituration should be just enough to coat all alloy particles with mercury and to produce a plastic mix. Excessive trituration should be avoided. In general, the instructions that come with the amalgam regarding the duration and speed of trituration should be followed. An overtriturated mix of amalgam will set prematurely during or soon after trituration, and this will prevent adequate condensation and result in a weakened product. A mix of amalgam that is difficult to manipulate, that is too plastic, or, as is more frequently the case, not plastic enough, must be discarded. A good mix of amalgam does not fall apart but is plastic enough to condense well; if the mix is too hard, brittle, or hot, reduction of the mixing time and/or the mixing speed is indicated.

Condensation

Condensation is the process of compressing and directing the dental amalgam into the tooth preparation with amalgam-condensing instruments (called *condensers* or *pluggers*) until the preparation is completely filled, and then overfilled, with a dense mass of amalgam. Proper condensation of the amalgam promotes adaptation of the amalgam to the walls of the preparation, and it compacts the material, eliminating voids and reducing the amount of residual mercury in the restoration. Both voids and increased residual mercury have been associated with a weakened amalgam product, so effective condensation increases the strength of the restoration.[86]

Adequate condensation technique requires that a significant amount of force be applied to the condenser.[10] The force should be 2 to 5 kg (5 to 10 lbs) for a condensible amalgam (admixture or conventional); the condensation force required for spherical amalgams will be considerably less,[10] because heavy forces tend to push the spherical particles to the side and "punch through" the amalgam mass. The size of the condenser nib (end) determines the amount of pressure actually transferred from the operator's hand to the amalgam mass; the larger the nib, the less force per unit area (pressure) is applied to the mass for a given force from the operator's hand. In other words, when a larger-faced condenser is used, the operator must exert more force on the condenser to deliver adequate condensation pressure. Larger condensers should be used for spherical amalgam than for admixtures to allow adequate force to be applied without displacement of the spherical amalgam to the side.

Adequate condensation force will cause a slight movement of the patient's mandible or head, and often this movement will need to be stabilized by the dentist or assistant. A secure finger rest will enable the operator to perform more controlled, forceful strokes, using arm as well as finger pressure. The condensers are held with the pen grasp or a modification. Many operators use a finger or thumb of the hand that is not holding the condenser to apply additional condensation force. It has been demonstrated that dentists tend to use less condensation pressure during the later stages of insertion of amalgam; investigators[11] have emphasized the need for maintaining condensation pressures for both admixed and spherical amalgams throughout the condensation process.

After the preparation has been made ready to receive the amalgam, the amalgam alloy and mercury should be mixed or triturated to give a plastic and moldable mass of amalgam. For most restorations, an amalgam carrier is valuable for carrying the amalgam to the preparation (see Fig 4-35). For very large complex amalgam preparations, the entire mix may be carried to the preparation, or the mix may be divided in half and one half at a time carried to the preparation with cotton forceps. No matter how the amalgam is carried, it should be spread in the preparation so that the increment is thin for optimum condensation. Each portion of amalgam carried to the preparation should result in an increment thickness of 1.0 mm or thinner to ensure maximum condensation effectiveness.

Condensers that fit into all areas of the preparation should be used. Flat-faced, round condensers are generally considered to allow maximum condensation pressure. Convex-ended condensers are also available, as are flat-ended condensers with diamond, rectangular, and triangular shapes. A large condenser should be used for the overfilling of the preparation.

One increment of amalgam should not be allowed to set significantly before the next increment is added. Amalgam should be condensed both vertically and horizontally or laterally (toward the walls of the preparation). This will ensure a close adaptation of the amalgam to the walls as well as to the floor of the preparation. Lateral condensation can be achieved in more than one way; the direction of the face (end) of the condenser can be altered so that the face is pushed toward the walls, or the condenser can be inserted into the preparation vertically then moved laterally toward the walls so that the side of the condenser condenses the amalgam toward the walls (Fig 10-58a). Lateral condensation is especially important for spherical amalgams because, paradoxically, it is more difficult to adapt these materials to cavity walls.

When amalgam is condensed, mercury tends to be brought to the surface, creating a mercury-rich amalgam on the surface. To reduce the amount of mercury left in the restoration (residual mercury), the preparation is overfilled (Fig 10-58b), and the mercury-rich excess is carved off. The lower the residual mercury in the carved restoration, the higher its strength.

Precarve Burnishing

After it is condensed with amalgam condensers, the amalgam should be further condensed with a large burnisher, such as an ovoid (football) burnisher (see Fig 10-66h). This is called precarve burnishing, and it should take place immediately after completion of condensation. The burnisher should be used with heavy strokes, made in the mesiodistal and faciolingual directions, that pinch much of the amalgam off as the burnisher contacts the cusp inclines and, in some places, the margins of the preparation. It has been shown that precarve burnishing

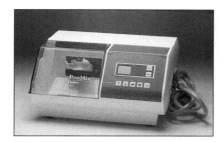

Fig 10-57a Pro-Mix amalgamator (Caulk/Dentsply).

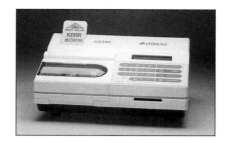

Fig 10-57b Automix amalgamator (Kerr/Sybron). Both the Automix and the Pro-Mix represent advanced technology in control of time, speed, and energy.

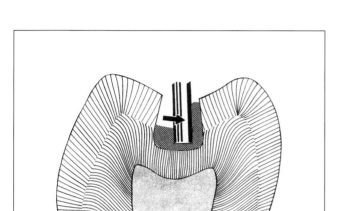

Fig 10-58a Lateral condensation, toward all walls, and toward the adjacent tooth in a Class 2 restoration, will improve adaptation to walls and ensure a contact area with the adjacent tooth.

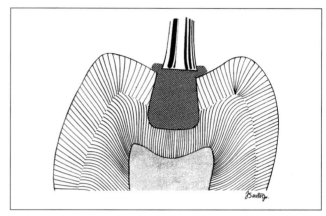

Fig 10-58b Overfill should be condensed with a large condenser.

produces denser amalgam at the margins of restorations.[57] In addition to aiding condensation, precarve burnishing is the first step in shaping the occlusal surface of the restoration.

Carving

Amalgam may be carved with any bladed dental instrument that has a sharp edge. Numerous carvers are available, and each has its own merit. Recommended amalgam carvers that satisfy most amalgam carving needs are a small cleoid-discoid carver; a Walls No. 3 (or Tanner No. 5) carver: a Hollenback No. ½ carver; an interproximal carver (developed by Baum); and a No. 14L sickle-shaped carver (see Fig 4-38). In addition some cutting instruments, such as a small spoon excavator and hoe, make excellent amalgam carvers, especially for carving occlusal anatomy in large restorations. The carving instruments that are selected should allow the operator

to create contours and occlusion that reproduce, or occasionally improve upon, the missing tooth structure.

Carving may begin immediately after condensation and precarve burnishing. Before the setting of the amalgam is very advanced, it carves very easily, but it is also easy to miscarve or overcarve, so care must be taken. As the setting of the amalgam advances, it does not carve as easily, but it remains carvable with sharp carvers for a long time. In fact, amalgam that has been in the mouth for many years can still be carved with sharp carvers.

The need for sharp carvers cannot be overemphasized, and it is advisable to have a sterilized sharpening stone available during placement of a large amalgam restoration. Amalgam seems to cause rapid dulling of carvers, possibly because of the effect of the mercury in penetrating and imparting brittleness to the steel.

Most occlusal carving is performed with pulling strokes, but the pushing stroke can also be advantageous in developing occlusal anatomy (grooves). Smaller occlusal and Class 2 restorations should be carved with

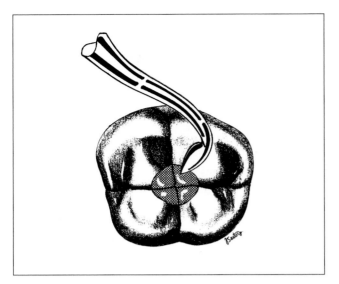

Fig 10-59a Cleoid carver viewed from the occlusal aspect.

Figs 10-59a and 10-59b The enamel margin is used as a guide for carving smaller restorations.

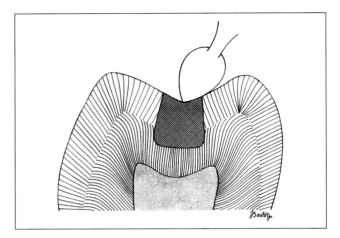

Fig 10-59b Cleoid carver viewed in cross section.

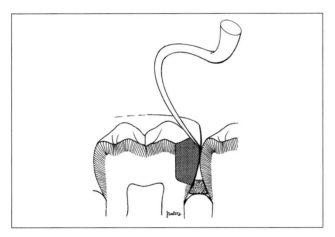

Fig 10-60 The tip of the No. 23 explorer is used at a 45-degree angle to the matrix to begin shaping the occlusal embrasure.

the enamel tooth surface as a guide (Figs 10-59a and 10-59b). The carver should rest on the enamel adjacent to the preparation and be pulled in a direction parallel to the margin of the preparation. When a stroke that is perpendicular to the margin of the preparation is needed, the carver should be pulled from enamel to amalgam. If it is pulled from amalgam to enamel, it will be more likely to carve the surface of the amalgam to a level that is below the surface of the enamel. It is desirable that the two surfaces be even (at the same level) so that there is no step down from the enamel to the amalgam.

It is good to register a mental picture of the outline of the preparation before the amalgam is inserted so that

the same outline can be visualized after carving. Because amalgam preparations should have enamel margins that are not jagged or rough, if the margins of a carved restoration appear ragged, it will be due to thin amalgam flash that extends outside of the preparation onto the adjacent enamel surface.

Amalgam should not be overcarved so that groove anatomy is deep, leaving thin fins of amalgam adjacent to the preparation margins. The operator should try to develop margins of amalgam that will leave a 75- to 90-degree angle at the margin of occlusal amalgam. Acute angles (fins) of amalgam at the margins on an occlusal surface are subject to fracture during function.

For Class 2 restorations, while the matrix is in place (Fig 10-60), the marginal ridge should be carved very nearly to the height of the adjacent marginal ridge (see Fig 10-66i). The occlusal embrasure of the marginal ridge is shaped with the tip of an explorer angled at approximately a 45-degree angle to the long axis of the tooth and touching the matrix band (Fig 10-60; also see Fig 10-66j). The explorer tip should be moved from the facial margin of the box to the center of the marginal ridge, and then from the lingual margin of the box to the center. The explorer should not be moved from the amalgam toward the margin, because this movement could easily result in overcarving, leaving the marginal ridge with a deficient contour.

Most carving will be accomplished while the rubber dam is in place. For Class 2 restorations, after the matrix is removed, amalgam flash on proximal surfaces should be removed and the proximal contours should be refined. A thin carver, such as the interproximal carver,

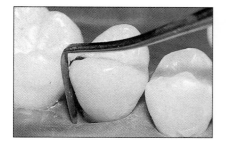
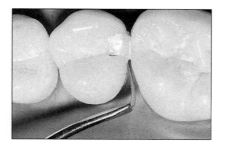
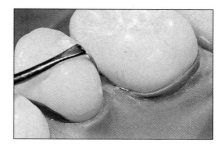

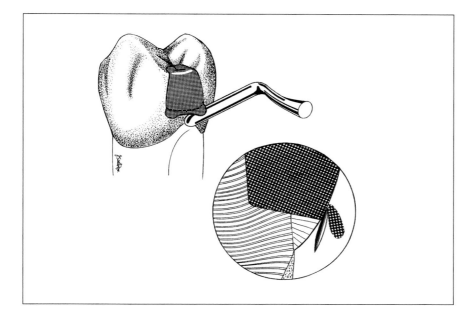

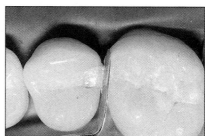

Figs 10-61a to 10-61e An interproximal carver is used to remove flash and to contour and burnish the amalgam in interproximal areas.

is useful for both removing flash and refining proximal contours (Figs 10-61a to 10-61e; also see Figs 10-66w to 10-66y).

Adjusting the Occlusion

When the carving appears to be correct, the dam is removed, and the occlusion is checked. This is accomplished with articulating ribbon, which marks the points of contact when the mandibular and maxillary teeth are brought together (Figs 10-62a and 10-62b). It is wise not to ask the patient to close, because, if the amalgam has not been carved adequately, it will be "high" in occlusion so that it contacts first, prior to any other tooth contact. The masseter muscles are very strong, and when the proprioceptive innervation relates to the patient's brain that there is something between the maxillary and mandibular teeth, it is reflex action for the patient to attempt to masticate it. If the patient senses that there is

something between the teeth, but it is actually a high amalgam restoration, disaster will result; the amalgam will usually be fractured, and the operator will have to remove the remaining amalgam and begin again with amalgam insertion.

It is best, therefore, for the dentist to perform the tapping of the teeth by grasping the patient's chin, having the patient close to very near contact, and then, by hand, manipulating the mandible so that mandibular and maxillary teeth are tapped together in centric occlusion (maximum intercuspation). The dentist's arm, no matter how strong, will be unable to impart nearly as much force in mandibular closure as the masseter muscle is capable of achieving. An alternative to this tapping by the dentist is to instruct the patient to "very, very gently, tap the back teeth together."

The amalgam must be carved until contacts on the restoration occur simultaneously with other centric contacts on that tooth and adjacent teeth. These can be seen as marks made by articulating ribbon, but they should

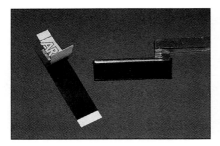

Fig 10-62a For initial gross adjustment, a piece of articulating paper with a thickness of 20 µm (0.0008-inch) or more is useful. When articulating paper forceps are used, the total length of the piece of articulating tape or paper should be supported by the forceps.

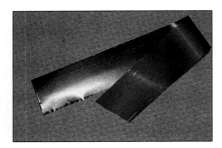

Fig 10-62b For refining occlusion, especially in complex amalgam restorations, an articulating tape with a thickness of 15 µm (0.0006-inch) or less is advantageous

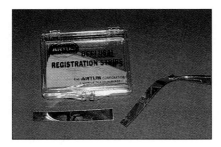

Fig 10-63a Shimstock (0.0005-inch thick Mylar) is supplied in books with paper separators between pieces of silver-colored shimstock. It may be held in the fingers or with a hemostat (as shown at lower right).

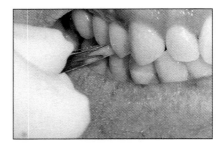

Fig 10-63b Shimstock is used to "feel" contacts between maxillary and mandibular teeth.

also be felt by the dentist with 0.0005-inch (12 µm) thick shimstock (Artus) (Figs 10-63a and 10-63b). To do this, the patient should be instructed to close in centric occlusion ("bite the back teeth together") while shimstock is in place on the tooth being restored. With the teeth in centric occlusion, the shimstock should be held securely in place. The same test should be performed with the shimstock on adjacent teeth, and it should again be held securely (assuming that those teeth held shimstock prior to the restorative procedure). If the adjacent teeth do not hold the shimstock, the newly placed restoration is probably in hyperocclusion and needs additional carving.

When the restoration is correct in centric occlusion, it must be checked to ensure that no interferences are caused by the restoration in eccentric movements. This may also be evaluated with the use of the shimstock. Two colors of articulating ribbon (preferably ribbons that do not easily cause smudge marks), one color for lateral and protrusive excursions, and the other to mark centric occlusion, are used. To eliminate eccentric con-

tacts in the amalgam, the amalgam marked with the color used to register the excursions should be carved, and the amalgam marked with the centric marks should be left alone. For complex amalgam restorations, it should be ensured that the restoration does not cause interference in the slide between centric relation and centric occlusion (or maximum intercuspation).

Postcarve Burnishing

Postcarve burnishing is the light rubbing of the surface of a carved amalgam restoration with a burnisher, such as the PKT3. Heavy forces should not be used, and postcarve burnishing should be avoided near the margins of restorations of fast-setting amalgam.[115] The purpose of postcarve burnishing is to smooth the surface of the restoration.

After completion of carving and postcarve burnishing, if the carving time was short and the amalgam is still fairly soft, the surface may be wiped over with a cotton

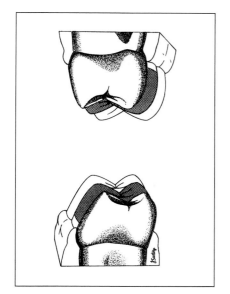

Fig 10-64 Facial and lingual contours are sighted in by looking down the line of teeth in a quadrant. The contour of the restoration must harmonize with natural tooth contours in the quadrant.

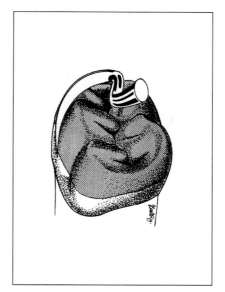

Fig 10-65a A No. 14L sickle-shaped carver will carve a very convex surface if it approaches the surface to be carved at just less than a 90-degree angle.

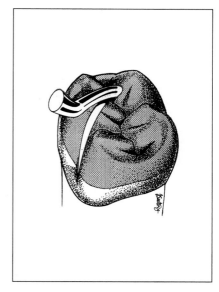

Fig 10-65b The No. 14L sickle-shaped carver will carve a surface with less convexity if it is rotated so that it approaches the surface at an angle of much less than 90 degrees.

ball or cotton roll saturated with water to provide additional smoothing. If the set of the amalgam is advanced, so that the saturated cotton will not smooth the surface, a rubber prophylaxis cup with damp flour of pumice or prophylaxis paste will smooth the amalgam (see the section on finishing and polishing). If the cup is used, it should be rotating at very low speed and should be kept moving at all times; if the cup is allowed to rotate in one place, it will groove the recently carved amalgam.

Insertion of Amalgam in Complex Preparations

Several special considerations for placing complex amalgam restorations have already been discussed, such as the need for reinforcement of matrices with compound. Following are some other considerations that may help the operator place successful complex amalgam restorations:

1. Visualize the finished product, and shape the matrix to allow for that product.
2. In addition to visualizing the height of the cusp tip prior to making the tooth preparation and then building cusps back to that height, make a mental picture of facial and lingual contours prior to cutting away natural tooth structure so that you can repro-

duce the natural contours in amalgam as closely as possible. Sight in contours by viewing down the line of teeth from the facial and/or lingual aspect. Make sure that the final contours harmonize with the contours of other teeth in the quadrant (Fig 10-64; also see 10-66ee).
3. Insert larger increments of amalgam (for instance, the entire two-spill mix when replacing the entire occlusal surface of a molar, or a half mix for smaller restorations).
4. Consider the use of carvers that contribute to proper contours, such as the No. 14L carver, which simplifies the carving of convex axial contours (Figs 10-65a and 10-65b).
5. Because carving large amalgam restorations involves the carving of more surface area, consider sharpening the carvers during the procedure to allow more efficient carving.
6. Smooth the carved amalgam with a slurry of flour pumice or with a prophylaxis paste.

A series showing the insertion of a complex amalgam restoration, beginning with matrix application and ending just before rubber dam removal, is shown in Figs 10-66a to 10-66ee. Several amalgam preparations and restorations are shown in Figs 10-67 to 10-79.

Figs 10-66a to 10-66ee Condensation and carving of a complex amalgam restoration.

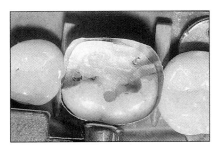

Fig 10-66a A Tofflemire matrix is placed and shaped to provide desired contours.

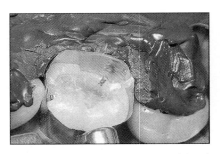

Fig 10-66b The matrix is stabilized with modeling compound.

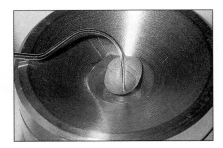

Fig 10-66c A two-spill mix of amalgam is halved.

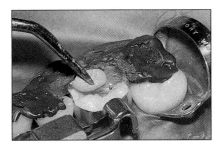

Fig 10-66d Half of the mix of amalgam is carried to the mouth.

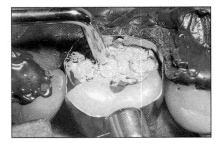

Fig 10-66e Amalgam is spread over the entire preparation floor and condensed.

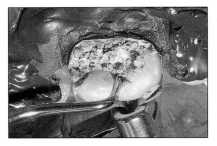

Fig 10-66f A small condenser is used to condense amalgam into the amalgapin channel.

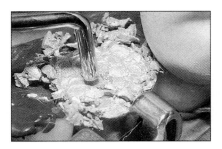

Fig 10-66g Amalgam increments are added in 1.0-mm thicknesses until the preparation is overfilled.

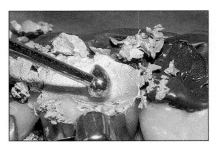

Fig 10-66h Amalgam shaping is begun with a large ovoid burnisher used to pinch excess amalgam off against the enamel.

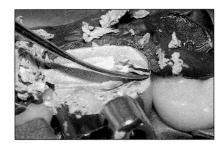

Fig 10-66i Marginal ridge shaping is begun by reducing amalgam in the area to the approximate desired height of the marginal ridge.

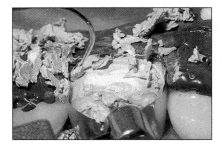

Fig 10-66j The occlusal embrasure is formed with an explorer tip.

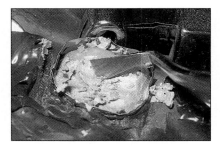

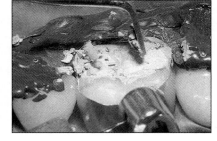

Figs 10-66k and 10-66l A chisel-shaped carver (Walls No. 3) is used to begin shaping cusps and grooves while the matrix is still in place.

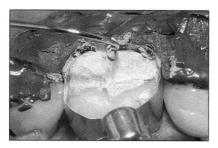

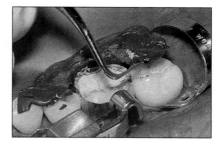

Fig 10-66m An explorer tip is used to begin shaping the lingual contour inside the matrix.

Fig 10-66n The compound and matrix are removed.

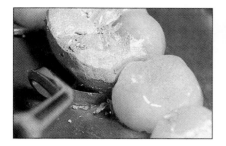

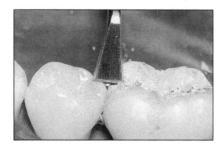

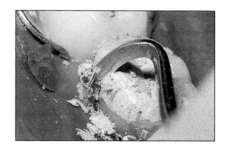

Figs 10-66o to 10-66q A sickle-shaped carver (No.14L) is used to remove gingival flash, shape proximal surfaces, and shape lingual contour.

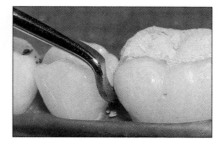

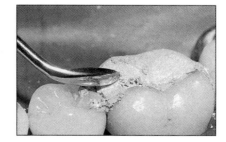

Figs 10-66r and 10-66s The marginal ridges are adjusted to height by resting the carver (Walls No. 3) on the adjacent marginal ridges.

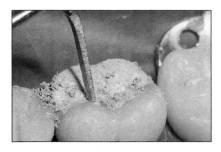

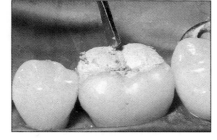

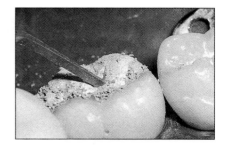

Figs 10-66t to 10-66v The occlusal anatomy is refined with a hoe.

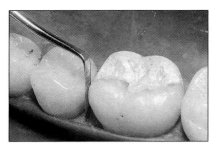

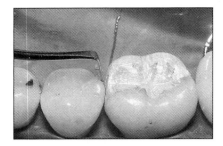

Figs 10-66w and 10-66x The proximal contours and contact position are refined with a very thin interproximal carver.

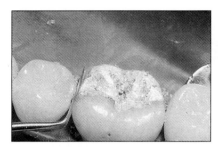

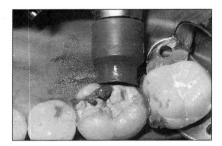

Fig 10-66y The occlusal embrasure is refined with an interproximal carver, which is rested on the adjacent enamel to guide the marginal ridge contour.

Fig 10-66z The surface is smoothed with a medium-grit prophylaxis paste in a rubber cup.

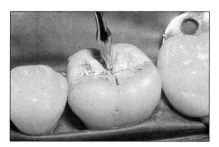

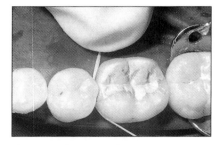

Fig 10-66aa The bases of the grooves are smoothed with a burnisher (PKT 3).

Fig 10-66bb The proximal contours are "felt" with floss to assure smoothness and to clear any amalgam carvings from the contact.

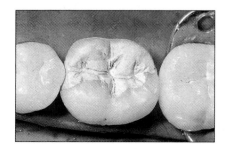

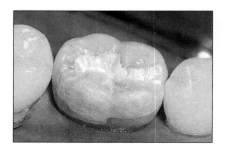

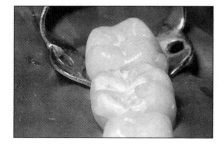

Figs 10-66cc to 10-66ee Carving is completed. Note that the lingual contour harmonizes with the contours of the adjacent teeth. The rubber dam is then removed, the occlusion is refined, and the surface is resmoothed with pumice or a prophylaxis paste.

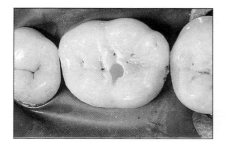

Fig 10-67a A small area of occlusal caries has been removed.

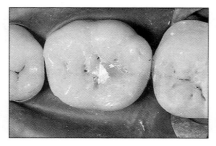

Fig 10-67b The preparation is filled with amalgam.

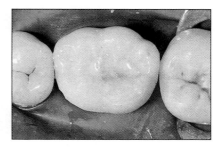

Fig 10-67c The remaining occlusal fissures were opened with a No. ¼ bur to a depth of 0.5 mm, etched, and sealed with resin fissure sealant.

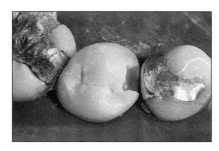

Fig 10-68a Mesio-occlusal slot preparation.

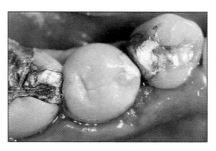

Fig 10-68b Slot restoration. There was no treatment of occlusal fissures.

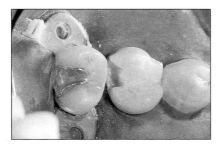

Fig 10-69a Disto-occlusal slot preparation.

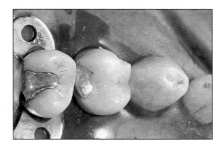

Fig 10-69b Slot restoration. There was no treatment of occlusal fissures.

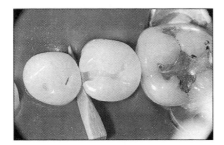

Fig 10-70a Mesio-occlusal preparation.

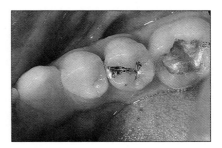

Fig 10-70b Restoration with conservative extension through the occlusal fissures in lieu of using a fissure sealant.

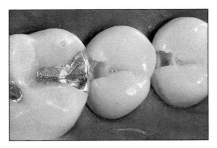

Fig 10-71a Disto-occlusal slot preparations.

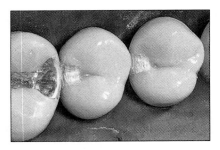

Fig 10-71b Slot restorations. The occlusal fissures were sealed without being opened.

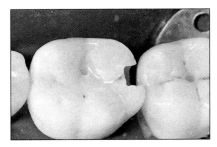

Fig 10-72a Small occlusal and disto-occlusal slot amalgam preparations.

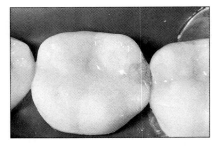

Fig 10-72b Restorations with sealed occlusal fissures.

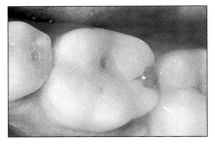

Fig 10-72c Restorations at 2 years.

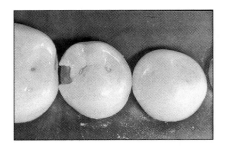

Fig 10-73a Disto-occlusal slot preparation.

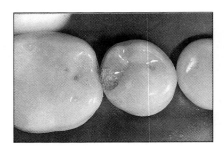

Fig 10-73b Restoration with sealed occlusal fissures.

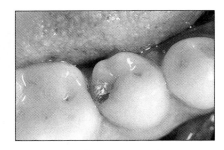

Fig 10-73c Restoration at 2 years.

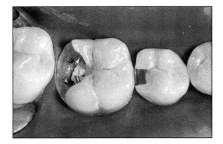

Fig 10-74a Complex amalgam preparation with vertical and horizontal pins in the molar and a disto-occlusal slot preparation in the premolar.

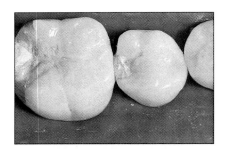

Fig 10-74b Restorations with sealed occlusal fissures.

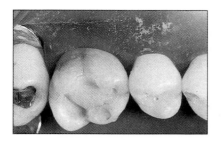

Fig 10-75a Old resin composite restoration with recurrent caries.

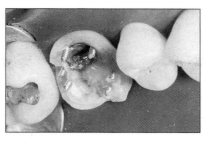

Fig 10-75b Complex amalgam preparation with six vertical pins.

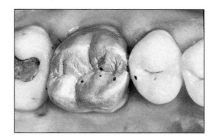

Fig 10-75c Complex amalgam restoration.

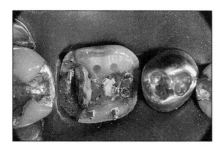

Fig 10-76a Complex amalgam preparation with pins, boxes, amalgapins, and a shelf.

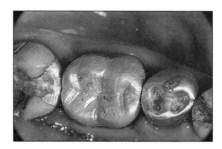

Fig 10-76b Complex amalgam restoration.

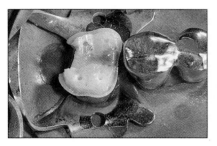

Fig 10-77a Complex amalgam preparation with boxes, amalgapins, and a shelf.

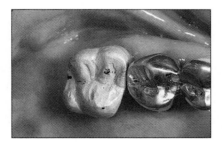

Fig 10-77b Complex amalgam restoration.

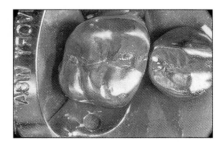

Fig 10-77c Restoration at 3 years.

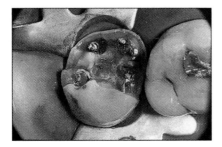

Fig 10-78a Complex amalgam preparation, which used horizontal and vertical pins.

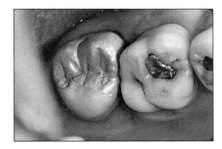

Fig 10-78b Complex amalgam restoration.

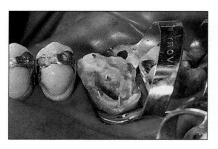

Fig 10-79a Complex amalgam preparation for a severely broken-down, endodontically treated molar, utilizing the chamber plus horizontal and vertical pins.

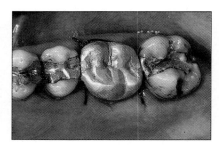

Fig 10-79b Complex amalgam restoration.

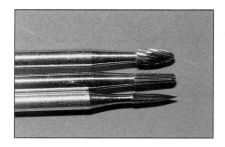

Fig 10-80 Finishing burs for a friction-grip handpiece: *(top to bottom)* No. 7404 (bud or egg shaped), No. 7803 (bullet shaped), No. 7901 (needle shaped).

Finishing and Polishing Amalgam Restorations

Finishing of an amalgam restoration includes evaluating the restoration for problems and correcting those, assuring that the margins are even and that the contours and occlusion are correct, and smoothing the restoration. *Polishing* is defined as smoothing the surface to a point of high gloss or luster. It has been demonstrated that polishing a high-copper amalgam restoration does not enhance its clinical performance,[72] but finishing is an important part of restoration placement. Finishing is usually accomplished at the placement appointment, but the finish may be refined at succeeding appointments.

Despite the lack of evidence that longevity is increased or performance is improved when an amalgam restoration is polished, a high luster is often more comfortable to the patient's tongue than a rough surface, so polishing is sometimes desirable. There are no contraindications to polishing a restoration, but care should be taken not to create excessive heat during the polishing procedure.

After placement of a restoration, its surface should be rubbed with a burnisher or with a damp cotton pellet until it is smooth. For amalgam with a more advanced set, a rubber cup with wet pumice or a prophylaxis paste may be used to smooth the restoration. Polishing of an amalgam restoration should be accomplished at a succeeding appointment, or at least several hours after placement of the restoration. If an amalgam is adequately smoothed at the placement appointment, imparting a high luster is usually a very simple and quick procedure.[36] If the restoration is not made smooth at placement, more time is required for polishing.

If, at the time of polishing, the restoration surface is not smooth, it should be smoothed. Gross smoothing of set amalgam can be accomplished with sharp amalgam carvers and finishing burs (Fig 10-80). For polishing convex surfaces (facial, lingual, and proximal), a series of progressively finer disks may be used (Figs 10-81a and 10-81b). Alternatives for smoothing and polishing convex surfaces are the abrasive-impregnated rubber cups, first the coarser cups, and then the finer cups (Figs 10-82a and 10-82b). Abrasive-impregnated rubber points are useful for smoothing and polishing concave surfaces such as the occlusal surface. It is especially important when rubber polishers and abrasive disks are used to use an abundance of air coolant and intermittent contact with the amalgam to prevent excessive generation of heat.

Although the disks and rubber polishers are more convenient, a less expensive, time-tested alternative method is the use of a prophylaxis cup, first with pumice in a water carrier as the "prepolishing" step, and then with tin oxide in a water or alcohol carrier for a high shine. One study[36] showed the pumice and tin oxide polishing procedure to be faster, but the investigator concluded that the impregnated points and cups are more desirable because they do not produce splatter.

A highly polished amalgam restoration is often more pleasing to the dentist than to the patient. A high polish can make a posterior amalgam restoration more noticeable, and this can be esthetically unpleasing to the patient. If this should occur, air abrasion with 50-μm aluminum oxide (Microetcher, Danville Engineering) or abrasion with pumice and a prophylaxis cup may be used to take away the high shine without making the restoration noticeably rough to the patient's tongue.

Figs 10-81a and 10-81b Abrasive disks, manufactured for polishing resin composite restorations, are also useful for polishing amalgam.

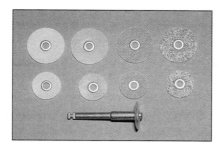

Fig 10-81a Brown-yellow series of Sof-Lex disks and the pop-on mandrel (3M Dental). Also available is the thicker, but more flexible, black-blue series of Sof-Lex disks.

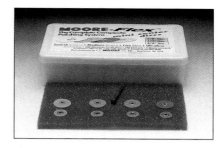

Fig 10-81b Moore-Flex disks (EC Moore) are similar to the Sof-Lex disks.

Figs 10-82a and 10-82b Abrasive-impregnated rubber cups and points.

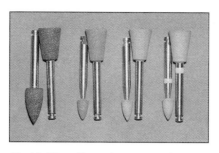

Fig 10-82a Brasseler cups and points: *(left to right)* coarsest (black), pre-polish (brown), high shine (gray), and super high shine (yellow band).

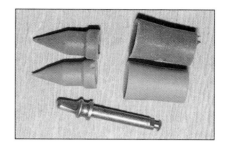

Fig 10-82b Min-Identoflex polishers (Centrix): brown (prepolish) point and cup; green (final polish) point and cup. These polishers snap onto the mandrel shown.

References

1. Anusavice KJ. Treatment regimens in preventive and restorative dentistry. J Am Dent Assoc 1995;126:727-743.

2. Battock RD, Rhoades J, Lund MR. Management of proximal caries on the roots of posterior teeth. Oper Dent 1979;4:108-112.

3. Bell JG. An elementary study of deformation of molar teeth during amalgam restorative procedures. Aust Dent J 1977;22:177-181.

4. Ben-Amar A, Liberman R, Judes H, Nordenberg D. Long-term use of dentine adhesive as an interfacial sealer under Class II amalgam restorations. J Oral Rehabil 1990;17:37-42.

5. Berry TG, Laswell HR, Osborne JW, Gale EN. Width of isthmus and marginal failure of restorations of amalgam. Oper Dent 1981;6:55-58.

6. Berry TG, Nicholson J, Troendle K. Almost two centuries with amalgam: Where are we today? J Am Dent Assoc 1994;125:392-399.

7. Birtcil RF, Venton EA. Extracoronal amalgam restorations utilizing available tooth structure for retention. J Prosthet Dent 1976;35:171-178.

8. Blaser PK, Lund MR, Cochran MA, Potter RH. Effects of designs of Class 2 preparations on resistance of teeth to fracture. Oper Dent 1983;8:6-10.

9. Brocklehurst PR, Joshi RI, Northeast SE. The effect of air-polishing occlusal surfaces on the penetration of fissures by a sealant. Int J Paediatr Dent 1992;2:157-162.

10. Brown IH, Miller DR. Alloy particle shape and sensitivity of high-copper amalgams to manipulative variables. Am J Dent 1993;6:248-254.

11. Brown IH, Maiolo C, Miller DR. Variation in condensation pressure during clinical packing of amalgam restorations. Am J Dent 1993;6:255-259.

12. Buikema DJ, Mayhew RB, Voss JE, Bales DJ. Pins and their relation to cavity resistance form for amalgam. Quintessence Int 1985;16:187-190.

13. Burgess JO. Horizontal pins: A study of tooth reinforcement. J Prosthet Dent 1985;53:317-322.

14. Burgess JO, Hartsfield C, Jordan T. Strength of amalgam with varying amalgam thickness covering the pins [abstract 549]. J Dent Res 1990;69:177.

15. Burgess JO, Summitt JB. Retention and resistance provided by nine self-threading pins. Oper Dent 1991;16:55-60.

16. Burgess JO, Alvarez AN, Summitt JB. Fracture resistance of complex amalgams [abstract 228]. J Dent Res 1993;72:132.

17. Caron GA, Murchison DF, Broom JC, Cohen RB. Resistance to fracture of teeth with various preparations for amalgam [abstract 208]. J Dent Res 1994;73:127.

18. Cassin AM, Pearson GJ, Picton DCA. Fissure sealants as a means of prolonging longevity of amalgam restorations—an in-vitro feasibility study. Clin Mater 1991;7:203-207.

19. Certosimo AJ, House RC, Anderson MH. The effect of cross-sectional area on transverse strength of amalgapin-retained restorations. Oper Dent 1991;18:70-76.

20. Charlton DG, Moore BK, Swartz ML. In vitro evaluation of the use of resin liners to reduce microleakage and improve retention of amalgam restorations. Oper Dent 1992;17:112-119.

21. Collins JF, Antonson DE. Treatment of external pin perforations. J Acad Gen Dent 1987;35:200-202.

22. Cooley RL, Marshall TD, Young JM, Huddleston AM. Effect of sterilization on the strength and cutting efficiency of twist drills. Quintessence Int 1990;21:919-923.

23. Corbin SB, Kohn WG. The benefits and risks of dental amalgam: Current findings reviewed. J Am Dent Assoc 1994;125:381-388.

24. Cox CF, Suzuki S. Re-evaluating pulp protection: Calcium hydroxide liners vs. cohesive hybridization. J Am Dent Assoc 1994;125:823-830.

25. Craig RG. Restorative Dental Materials, ed 9. St Louis: Mosby-Year Book, 1993.

26. Dachi SF, Stigers RW. Reduction of pulpal inflammation and thermal sensitivity in amalgam-restored teeth treated with copal varnish. J Am Dent Assoc 1967;74:1281-1285.

27. Davis SP, Summitt JB, Mayhew RB, Hawley RJ. Self-threading pins and amalgapins compared in resistance form for complex amalgam restorations. Oper Dent 1983;8:88-93.

28. DeCraene LGP, Martens LC, Dermaut LR, Surmont PAS. A clinical evaluation of a light-cured fissure sealant (Helioseal). J Dent Child 1989;56:97-102.

29. Diefenderfer KE, Reinhardt JW. Shear bond strengths of ten adhesive resin/amalgam combinations [abstract 740]. J Dent Res 1995;74:104.

30. Dilts WE, Welk DA, Stovall J. Retentive properties of pin materials in pin-retained silver amalgam restorations. J Am Dent Assoc 1968;77:1085.

31. Dilts WE, Duncanson MG, Collard EW, Parmley LE. Retention of self-threading pins. J Can Dent Assoc 1981;47:119-120.

32. Dutton FB, Summitt JB, Chan DCN, Garcia-Godoy F. Effect of a resin lining and rebonding on the marginal leakage of amalgam restorations. J Dent 1993;21:52-56.

33. Dwinelle WH. Crystalline gold, its varieties, properties, and use. Am J Dent Sci 1855;5:249-297.

34. Eakle WS. Effect of thermal cycling on fracture strength and microleakage in teeth restored with a bonded composite resin. Dent Mater 1986;2:114-117.

35. Eakle WS, Staninec M, Lacy AM. Effect of bonded amalgam on the fracture resistance of teeth. J Prosthet Dent 1992;68:257-260.

36. Eames WB. A comparison of amalgam polishing procedures. Quintessence J 1981;9:467-473.

37. Edgren BN, Denehy GE. Microleakage of amalgam restorations using Amalgambond and Copalite. Am J Dent 1992;5:296-298.

38. El-Mowafy OM. Fracture strength and fracture patterns of maxillary premolars with approximal slot cavities. Oper Dent 1993;18:160-166.

39. Fernandes DP, Chevitarese O. The orientation and direction of rods in dental enamel. J Prosthet Dent 1991;65:793-800.

40. Fitchie JG, Reeves GW, Scarbrough AR, Hembree JH. Microleakage of a new cavity varnish with a high-copper spherical amalgam alloy. Oper Dent 1990;15:136-140.

41. Garcia-Godoy F, Medlock JW. An SEM study of the effects of air-polishing on fissure surfaces. Quintessence Int 1988;19:465-467.

42. Garcia-Godoy F, Summitt J, Donly K, Buikema D. Resistance to further demineralization of white spot lesions by sealing [abstract 1643]. J Dent Res 1993;72:309.

43. Glossary of Operative Dentistry Terms, ed 1. Washington DC: Academy of Operative Dentistry, 1983.

44. Going RE. Pin-retained amalgam. J Am Dent Assoc 1966;73:619-624.

45. Going RE, Loesche WJ, Grainger DA, Syed SA. The viability of microorganisms in carious lesions five years after covering with a fissure sealant. J Am Dent Assoc 1978;97:455-462.

46. Goldstein PM. Retention pins are friction-locked without use of cement. J Am Dent Assoc 1966;73:1103-1106.

47. Goldstein RE, Parkins FM. Using air-abrasive technology to diagnose and restore pit and fissure caries. J Am Dent Assoc 1995;126:761-766.

48. Gourley JW. Favorable locations for pins in molars. Oper Dent 1980;5:2.

49. Gwinnett AJ, Yu S. Effect of long-term water storage on dentin bonding. Am J Dent 1995;8:109-111.

50. Handelman SL, Washburn F, Wopperer P. Two-year report of sealant effect on bacteria in dental caries. J Am Dent Assoc 1976;93:967-970.

51. Handelman SL, Leverett DH, Iker HP. Longitudinal radiographic evaluation of the progress of caries under sealants. J Pedod 1985;9:119-126.

52. Hovgaard O, Larsen MJ, Fejerskov O. Tooth hypersensitivity in relation to the quality of restorations [abstract 1667]. J Dent Res 1991;70:474.

53. How WS. Bright metal screw posts and copper amalgam. Dent Cosmos 1839;31:237-238.

54. Imbery TA, Burgess JO, Batzer RC. Comparing the resistance of dentin bonding agents and pins in amalgam restorations. J Am Dent Assoc 1995;126:753-758.

55. Imbery TA, Hilton TJ, Reagan SE. Retention of complex amalgam restorations using self-threading pins, amalgapins, and Amalgambond. Am J Dent 1995;8:117-121.

56. Jensen ME, Handelman SL. Effect of an autopolymerizing sealant on viability of microflora in occlusal dental caries. Scand J Dent Res 1980;88:382-388.

57. Kanai S. Structure studies of amalgam. II. Effect of burnishing on the margins of occlusal amalgam fillings. Acta Odontol Scand 1966;24:47-53.

58. Karamursel-Ulukapi I, Lussi A, Stich H, Hotz P. Comparison of the sealing ability of four cavity varnishes: An in vitro study. Dent Mater 1991;7:84-87.

59. Kline J, Boyer D. Comparison of bonding amalgam and composite to enamel and dentin [abstract 741]. J Dent Res 1995;74:104.

60. Kramer PF, Zelante F, Simionato MRL. The immediate and long-term effects of invasive and noninvasive pit and fissure sealing techniques on the microflora in occlusal fissures of human dentin. Pediatr Dent 1993;16:108-112.

61. Lambert RL, Robinson FB, Lindemuth JS. Coronal reinforcement with cross-splinted pin-amalgam restorations. J Prosthet Dent 1985;54:346-349.

62. Larson TD, Douglas WH, Geisfeld RE. Effect of prepared cavities on the strength of teeth. Oper Dent 1981;6:2-5.

63. Leach CD, Martinoff JT, Lee CV. A second look at the amalgapin technique. J Calif Dent Assoc 1983;11:43-49.

64. Leinfelder KF. Dental amalgam alloys. Curr Opin Dent 1991;1:214-217.

65. Liberman R, Judes H, Cohen E, Eli I. Restoration of posterior pulpless teeth: Amalgam overlay versus cast gold onlay restorations. J Prosthet Dent 1987;57:540-543.

66. Manders CA, Garcia-Godoy F, Barnwell GM. Effect of a copal varnish, ZOE or glass ionomer cement bases on microleakage of amalgam restorations. Am J Dent 1990;3:63-66.

67. Markley MR. Pin reinforcement and retention of amalgam foundations. J Am Dent Assoc 1958;56:675-679.

68. Markley MR. Pin-retained and pin-reinforced amalgam. J Am Dent Assoc 1966;73:1295-1300.

69. Markley MR. Pin retained and reinforced restorations and foundations. Dent Clin North Am 1967;3:229-244.

70. Marshall TD, Porter KH, Re GJ. In vitro evaluation of the shoulder stop in a self-threading pin. J Prosthet Dent 1986;56:428-430.

71. Marshall TD, Cooley RL. Evaluation of the Max titanium alloy retentive pins. Am J Dent 1989;2:349-353.

72. Mayhew RB, Schmeltzer LD, Pierson WP. Effect of polishing on the marginal integrity of high-copper amalgams. Oper Dent 1986;11:8-13.

73. McComb D, Ben-Amar A, Brown J. Sealing efficacy of therapeutic varnishes used with silver amalgam restorations. Oper Dent 1990;15:122-128.

74. Mertz-Fairhurst E, Smith CD, Williams JE, et al. Cariostatic and ultraconservative sealed restorations: Six-year results. Quintessence Int 1992;23:827-838.

75. Mertz-Fairhurst E, Ergle JW. Cariostatic and ultraconservative sealed Class I restorations: Nine year results [abstract 2513]. J Dent Res 1994;73:416.

76. Miller A, Okabe T, DePaola DP, Cole JS. Amalgam and mercury toxicity: An update. Tex Dent J 1991;108:25-29.

77. Mjör IA, Jokstad A, Qvist V. Longevity of posterior restorations. Int Dent J 1990;40:11-17.

78. Moffa JP, Razzano MR, Doyle MG. Pins—A comparison of their retentive properties. J Am Dent Assoc 1969;78:529.

79. Morin D, DeLong R, Douglas WH. Cusp reinforcement by the acid-etch technique. J Dent Res 1984;63:1075-1078.

80a. Newitter DA, Gwinnett AJ, Caputo L. The dulling of twist drills during pin channel placement. Am J Dent 1989;2:81-85.

80b. Osborne JW, Berry TG. Zinc containing high copper amalgam: a three-year clinical evaluation. Am J Dent 1992;5:43-45.

81. Osborne JW, Gale EN. Failure at the margin of amalgams as affected by cavity width, tooth position, and alloy selection. J Dent Res 1981;60:682-685.

82a. Osborne JW, Gale EN. Relationship of restoration width, tooth position, and alloy to fracture at the margins of 13- to 14-year old amalgams. J Dent Res 1990;69:1599-1601.

82b. Osborne JW, Howell ML. Effects of water contamination on certain properties of high copper amalgams. Am J Dent 1994;7:337-341.

82c. Osborne JW, Norman RD. 13-year clinical assessment of 10 amalgam alloys. Dent Mater 1990;6:189-194.

83. Outhwaite WC, Garman TA, Pashley DH. Pin vs. slot retention in extensive amalgam restorations. J Prosthet Dent 1979;41:396-400.

84. Panopoulos P, Mejare B, Edwall L. Effects of ammonia and organic acids on the intradental sensory nerve activity. Acta Odontol Scand 1983;41:209-215.

85. Pashley EL, Galloway SE, Pashley DH. Protective effects of cavity liners on dentin. Oper Dent 1990;15:10-17.

86. Phillips RW. Skinner's Science of Dental Materials, ed 9. Philadelphia: Saunders, 1991.

87. Piperno S, Barouch E, Hirsch SM, Kaim JM. Thermal discomfort of teeth related to presence or absence of cement bases under amalgam restorations. Oper Dent 1982;7:92-96.

88. Plasmans PJJM, Kusters ST, Thissen AMG, Van't Hof MA, Vrijhoef MMA. Effects of preparation design on the resistance for extensive amalgam restorations. Oper Dent 1987;12:42-47.

89. Podshadley AG, Chambers MS. A new instrument for placement of self-threading retention pins. J Prosthet Dent 1994;71:429.

90. Powell GL, Nicholls JI, Shurtz DE. Deformation of human teeth under the action of an amalgam matrix band. Oper Dent 1977;2:64-69.

91. Powell GL, Nicholls JI, Molvar MP. Influence of matrix bands, dehydration, and amalgam condensation on deformation of teeth. Oper Dent 1980;5:95-101.

92. Qvist V, Johannessen L, Bruun M. Progression of approximal caries in relation of iatrogenic preparation damage. J Dent Res 1992;71:1370-1373.

93. Reagan SE, Gray SE, Hilton TJ. Fracture resistance of complex amalgam restorations with peripheral shelves used as resistance features. Am J Dent 1993;6:225-228.

94. Robbins JW, Summitt JB. Longevity of complex amalgam restorations. Oper Dent 1988;13:54-57.

95. Roddy WC, Blank LW, Rupp NW, Pelleu GB. Channel depth and diameter effects on transverse strength of amalgapin-retained restorations. Oper Dent 1987;12:2-9.

96. Santos AC, Meiers JC. Fracture resistance of premolars with MOD amalgam restorations lined with Amalgambond. Oper Dent 1994;19:2-6.

97. Seng GF, Rupell OL, Nance GL, Pompura JP. Placement of retentive amalgam inserts in tooth structure for supplemental retention. J Acad Gen Dent 1980;28:62-66.

98. Shapira J, Eidelman E. The influence of mechanical preparation of enamel prior to etching on the retention of sealants: Three-year follow-up. J Pedod 1984;8:272-277.

99. Shavell HM. The amalgapin technique for complex amalgam restorations. J Calif Dent Assoc 1980;8:48-55.

100. Smales RJ. Longevity of cusp-covered amalgams: Survivals after 15 years. Oper Dent 1991;16:17-20.

101. Stampalia LL, Nicholls JI, Burdvik JS, Jones DW. Fracture resistance of teeth with resin-bonded restorations. J Prosthet Dent 1986;55:694-698.

102. Sturdevant JR, Taylor DF, Leonard RH, Straka WF, Roberson TM, Wilder AD. Conservative preparation designs for Class II amalgam restorations. Dent Mater 1987;3:144-148.

103. Summitt JB, Burgess JO, Kaiser DA, Rux HW, Dutton FB. Resistance form provided to complex amalgam restorations by pins, amalgapins, peripheral shelves, and combinations. Am J Dent 1991;4:268-272.

104. Summitt JB, Howell ML, Burgess JO, Dutton FB, Osborne JW. Effect of grooves on resistance form of conservative Class 2 amalgams. Oper Dent 1992;17:50-56.

105. Summitt JB, Osborne JW, Burgess JO, Howell ML. Effect of grooves on resistance form of Class 2 amalgams with wide occlusal preparations. Oper Dent 1993;18:42-27.

106. Summitt JB, Osborne JW, Burgess JO. Effect of grooves on resistance/retention form of Class 2 approximal slot amalgam restorations. Oper Dent 1993;18:209-213.

107. Summitt JB, Rindler EA, Robbins JW, Burgess JO. Effect of distribution of resistance features in complex amalgam restorations. Oper Dent 1994;19:53-58.

108. Swift EJ. The effect of sealants on dental caries: A review. J Am Dent Assoc 1988;116:700-704.

109. Ulusoy N, Denli N, Atakul F, Nayyar A. Thermal response to multiple use of a twist drill. J Prosthet Dent 1992;67:450-453.

110. US Department of Health and Human Services, Public Health Service. Dental Amalgam: A Scientific Review and Recommended Public Health Service Strategy for Research, Education, And Regulation. Washington, DC: US Dept. of Health and Human Services, Public Health Service, Jan 1993.

111. Use survey—1990. Clin Res Assoc Newsletter 1990;14(12):1.

112. Vale WA. Cavity preparation. Ir Dent Rev 1956;2:33-41.

113. Vesterhus Strand G, Raadal M. The efficiency of cleaning fissures with an air-polishing instrument. Acta Odontol Scand 1988;46:113-117.

114. Webster's Unabridged Dictionary of the English Language. New York: Portland House, 1989.

115. Woods PW, Marker VA, McKinney TW, Miller BH, Okabe T. Determining amalgam marginal quality: Effect of occlusal surface condition. J Am Dent Assoc 1993;124:60-65.

116. Wright W, Mazer RB, Teixeira LC, Leinfelder KF. Clinical microleakage evaluation of a cavity varnish. Am J Dent 1992;5:273-265.

Class 5 Restorations

Richard S. Schwartz

In the United States, the average age of the population is increasing. This fact, combined with systemic administration of fluorides, improved nutrition, and better access to dental care, has led to an older population that retains its teeth longer.[33] These patients have an increasing prevalence of root caries and cervical erosion/abrasion lesions[33] that require restorations. This chapter will address the restoration of teeth with Class 5 lesions, including isolation and soft tissue management.

Indications

Caries is the most clear-cut indication for Class 5 restorations. Root caries is common among older patients with high sucrose intake or low salivary flow and among patients who have received head and neck radiation.[33]

Another common indication for Class 5 restorations is cervical erosion/abrasion lesions (Figs 11-1a and 11-1b). In many instances, no treatment is necessary, but restorations may be indicated when sensitivity is present, the lesions are esthetically objectionable, or a progressive loss of tooth structure is observed. The etiology of these lesions is somewhat controversial. It was traditionally thought that they resulted from toothbrush abrasion. In recent years, it has been postulated that flexure of the tooth from occlusal trauma causes stress concentration at the cervical portion of the tooth, resulting in loosening and gradual loss of enamel rods (Fig 11-2). This process is referred to as *abfraction*.[8,14] The abfraction theory is hard to support as the sole source of cervical lesions, however, because the lesions rarely occur on the lingual surfaces of teeth, and because existing Class 5 restorations sometimes exhibit V-shaped wear patterns (Fig 11-3). Cervical erosion/abrasion lesions probably have a multifactorial etiology, which includes chemical softening, as well as mechanical abrasion.

A variety of restorative materials may be used for Class 5 restorations, depending on the clinical situation. Amalgam may be used in situations in which esthetics is not a concern and mechanical retention can be easily obtained, and in patients with a low caries index.[6,33] Glass-ionomer restorative materials are often recommended for patients with a high caries index (although there is little clinical proof of anticaries effects). Resin composite is recommended when esthetics is of prime importance and may be used with or without a glass-ionomer liner.[33]

Restorative Materials

Silver Amalgam

Amalgam has several advantages for Class 5 restorations. It has excellent wear characteristics and is resistant to toothbrush abrasion. Because of corrosion products that form between the restoration and tooth preparation, amalgam is self-sealing. It is easy to place (in most cases), and natural contours can usually be obtained. Because of improvements in resin composites and glass-ionomer cements, amalgam is no longer commonly used in Class 5 restorations. When isolation is a problem, however, amalgam is probably the material of choice. The physical properties and characteristics of amalgam are discussed in chapter 10.

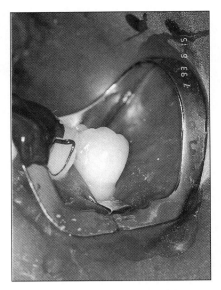

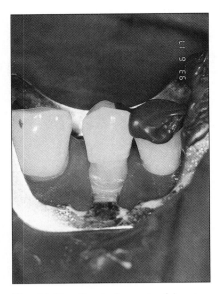

Fig 11-1a Cervical erosion/abrasion lesions may be V shaped.

Fig 11-1b Cervical erosion/abrasion lesions may be saucer shaped.

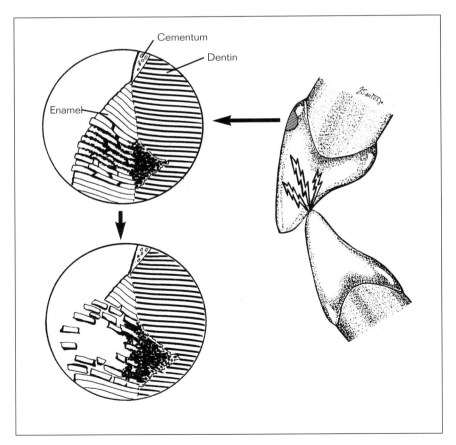

Fig 11-2 The abfraction theory holds that tooth flexure causes loosening of enamel rods, which initiates the cervical lesions.

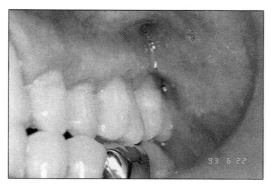

Fig 11-3 The notchlike wear pattern in the Class 5 resin composite restoration in the maxillary left second premolar suggests that toothbrush abrasion is a major contributor to cervical lesions.

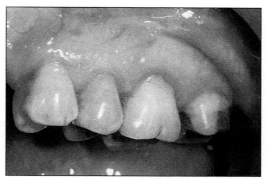

Fig 11-4 Traditional glass-ionomer restorations in the maxillary left second premolar and first molar.

Resin Composite

Continual improvements in dental adhesives have made resin composites very popular for Class 5 restorations. Resin composite is the most esthetic of the materials available for this application and has good wear resistance and longevity. Current adhesive systems provide relatively good retention, marginal seal, and resistance to polymerization shrinkage. In Class 5 composite restorations, as in other applications, the composite material tends to pull away from the gingival margin during polymerization, particularly when the margin is on cementum or dentin. The physical characteristics of composites and the problems associated with polymerization shrinkage are discussed in chapters 7 and 8. Because of their polishability and relative flexibility, microfilled composites are often used for Class 5 restorations.

Glass-Ionomer Restorative Materials

Glass-ionomer cement was introduced as a restorative material in the 1970s. It was dispensed as a powder and liquid, which were hand mixed. It was the first restorative material that offered true chemical adhesion to tooth structure and had the additional benefit of fluoride release.

Glass-ionomer cements consist of an alumina-silica glass that interacts with a polyalkenoic acid (usually polyacrylic or polymaleic acid). The resulting chemical reaction produces partially dissolved glass particles surrounded by a matrix of aluminum polyacrylate chains.

Fluoride is released from the glass particles rather than the matrix, so no breakdown of the cement results from the loss of fluoride.[20] Glass-ionomer cements have gradual polymerization shrinkage. Their coefficient of thermal expansion is similar to that of tooth structure.[18] This means that, once polymerized, glass-ionomer cement expands and contracts about the same amount as tooth structure during temperature changes (caused by coffee or ice cream, for example). The compatibility of thermal expansion between tooth structure and glass-ionomer cement is thought to account for the high rates of retention of glass-ionomer restorations in clinical studies,[16,24,31] despite having relatively low bond strengths to tooth structure.

The original restorative materials were extremely moisture sensitive, requiring 24-hour protection from moisture before finishing,[18] and were quite opaque. Throughout the 1980s, glass-ionomer cements were improved to the point that finishing could be accomplished in as little as 7 minutes. They are now encapsulated and are triturated, rather than hand mixed, prior to placement. Esthetics are somewhat improved (Fig 11-4).

Most current glass-ionomer restorative materials, called resin-modified glass ionomers, contain a small amount of light-cured and/or autocured resin, which allows immediate finishing after light polymerization. The original light-cured materials had properties similar to those of glass-ionomer cement, whereas most of the current products are more like resins.[33] The addition of resin resulted in improved bond strengths, esthetics, smoothness, and wear characteristics.[12] Microleakage is minimal,[4] and pulpal compatibility is excellent.[7] They

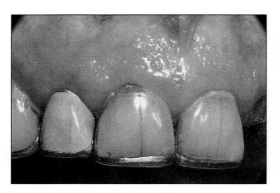

Fig 11-5a A Class 5 lesion is present in the maxillary right central incisor.

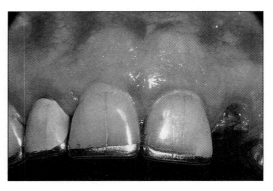

Fig 11-5b A resin-modified glass-ionomer restoration has been placed.

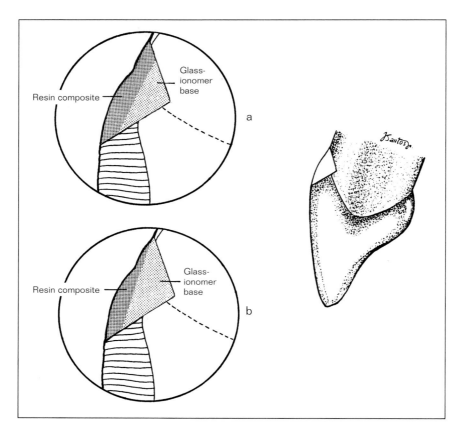

Fig 11-6 (a) The sandwich technique combines a glass-ionomer base with a veneer of resin composite. (b) Some clinicians advocate extension of the glass-ionomer cement material to the gingival margin if the restoration extends to the root surface.

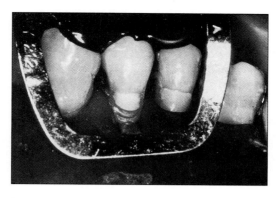

Fig 11-7 The rubber dam and No. 212 clamp provide retraction and isolation.

are hand mixed or mechanically triturated prior to insertion and can be placed in bulk because they have dual-curing characteristics. The addition of resin increases the coefficient of thermal expansion and the polymerization shrinkage, however. Some resin-modified glass-ionomer materials utilize a dentin adhesive system for retention and some utilize only an acid conditioner. The long-term clinical performance of these materials is not yet known. A resin-modified glass-ionomer restoration is shown in Figs 11-5a and 11-5b.

Sandwich Technique

The so-called sandwich technique was introduced to combine the fluoride release of glass-ionomer cements with the excellent esthetics of resin composites.[12,19,23,24,33] The sandwich technique is thought to lessen the amount of polymerization shrinkage of resin composites by lessening the bulk of material.[33] In the sandwich technique, the dentin is covered with a glass-ionomer liner or base. Some advocate that the glass-ionomer liner be carried to the gingival margin if it is on cementum or dentin. The enamel margins are then etched and the restoration is completed with a dentin adhesive and resin composite (Fig 11-6).

Restorations placed using the sandwich technique had the highest retention rate in a clinical study that compared them to resin composite and traditional glass-ionomer restorations,[24] and had the greatest reduction in sensitivity after 6 months.[23] With the introduction of the resin-modified glass-ionomer materials and the improvements in dentin adhesives, use of the sandwich technique has declined.

Other Materials

Several other materials are used by a small number of clinicians to restore Class 5 lesions. These materials include gold foil and gold or porcelain inlays.

Isolation

Rubber Dam

As discussed in chapter 5, adequate isolation of the operative field is essential for most restorative materials. Class 5 restorations often present a special challenge, because the gingival margin may extend into the sulcus. Rubber dam isolation should include at least two teeth on either side of the tooth to be restored. In most cases, it is necessary to place a second retainer on the tooth being restored to displace the gingiva and allow access for preparation and restoration. A No. 212 is the retainer most commonly used for Class 5 restorations (Fig 11-7). The lingual beak of the No. 212 retainer may be bent to accommodate the difference in height between the facial and lingual soft tissue margins. The rubber dam should be retracted 1 mm below the anticipated margin of the preparation so that it does not interfere with preparation and finishing. Compound should be used to provide stabilization for the No. 212 retainer (Fig 11-7).

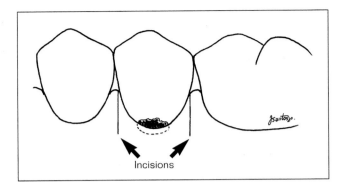

Fig 11-8a Short vertical incisions are made within the keratinized tissue at the line angles of the tooth. This allows additional tissue retraction with minimal trauma to the tissue or attachment apparatus.

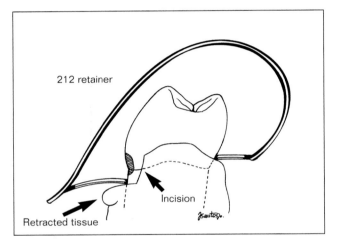
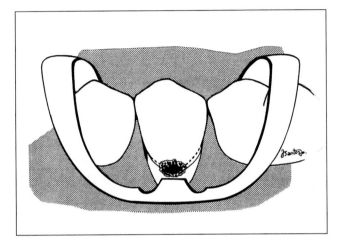

Figs 11-8b and 11-8c The No. 212 retainer and rubber dam are in place.

Miniflap

Occasionally, a Class 5 restoration will extend deep into the sulcus, and a miniflap procedure will be necessary to obtain adequate tissue retraction and isolation. A miniflap allows additional reflection of the gingival tissue with minimal trauma to the free gingival crest or attachment apparatus.[25,26] The simplest miniflap procedure utilizes two short vertical incisions at the line angles of the tooth (Fig 11-8a and Fig 5-46). The free gingiva can then be reflected, and the rubber dam can be placed as previously described (Figs 11-8b and 11-8c). If additional retraction is needed, a sulcular incision is made or a full mucoperiosteal flap is reflected.

Care must be taken that the completed restoration does not impinge on the biologic width. As discussed in chapter 1, the biologic width is the 2 mm of root surface coronal to the crestal bone that is occupied by the connective tissue and epithelial attachments. If a restoration extends into this area, chronic inflammation is often the result. See chapter 5 for additional information.

Crown Lengthening

If the depth of the sulcus is minimal, and encroachment on the biologic width is a possibility, bone levels can be determined by a method sometimes referred to

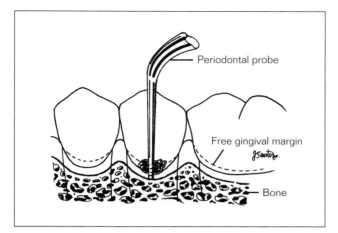

Fig 11-9a Occasionally a carious lesion extends to the base of the sulcus, making restoration difficult. Sounding with the periodontal probe shows that the restoration is likely to encroach on the biologic width. Therefore, crown lengthening is indicated.

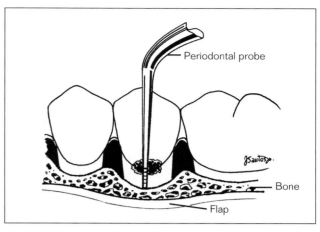

Fig 11-9b A full-thickness mucogingival flap is reflected and bone is removed so that 3 mm of root surface separate the bone and the carious lesion. The restoration can be placed prior to suturing, or restorative procedures can be delayed while the tissue heals.

as *sounding*. After anesthesia is administered, a thin periodontal probe is pushed through the base of the sulcus at several locations, to measure the distance to the crestal bone. If it is determined that the restoration will extend to within 2 mm of the bone, crown-lengthening procedures should be performed to adjust the bone level to at least 3 mm from the margin of the restoration (Figs 11-9a and 11-9b). Crown lengthening can be performed prior to or at the time of restoration. The gingival margin of the restoration should be at least 1 mm coronal to the base of the sulcus.

Preparations for Root Caries

Amalgam

The traditional amalgam preparation necessitated by facial root caries was extended beyond the caries to form a trapezoid with flat walls and sharp corners (Fig 11-10a). Currently, more conservative preparations are recommended that extend only far enough to allow removal of caries and unsupported enamel (Figs 11-10b and 11-10c). Internal angles should be rounded, and the cavo-surface margins should be as close to 90 degrees as possible. Cavosurface bevels are contraindicated with amalgam because of its low edge strength. Because of the curvature of the tooth, walls of the Class 5 preparation often diverge, so retentive points or grooves should be placed in the dentin of occlusal and gingival walls with a small round bur. If the preparation is very large, pins may be indicated to increase retention and resistance form. They should be placed in proximal areas to avoid the pulp. An example of pin placement is shown in Fig 11-11.

Glass-Ionomer Restorative Materials

The preparation for glass-ionomer restorations is essentially the same as that for amalgam. Tooth structure should be conserved as much as possible. The need for mechanical retention is somewhat controversial. Theoretically, the compatibility between coefficients of thermal expansion of tooth structure and glass-ionomer cement should obviate the need for mechanical retention. However, because of tooth flexure and other factors, mechanical retention is advisable.[33] Cavosurface bevels are not recommended for the preparation because glass ionomer is a brittle material that requires bulk.

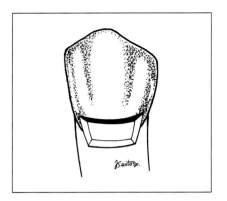
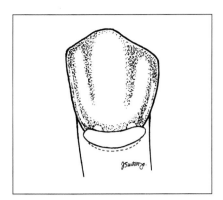
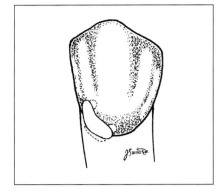

Fig 11-10a The traditional preparations for Class 5 restorations had a trapezoidal outline form.

Figs 11-10b and 11-10c The outline form currently recommended for all restorative materials includes removal of caries and unsupported enamel and the addition of undercuts.

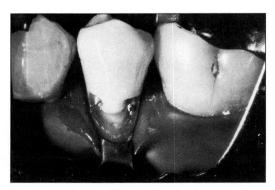

Fig 11-11 Large Class 5 amalgam restorations may require additional retention and resistance. In this case, proximal pins were used.

Resin Composite

Once again, the preparation should extend only far enough to include caries. Although high rates of retention are reported for Class 5 resin composite restorations without undercuts,[5,24] mechanical retention is recommended. In addition, a groove at the gingivoaxial line angle has been shown to lessen gap formation at the gingival margin when the preparation extends to the root surface.[33] Unless a bevel would remove thin enamel, all enamel margins should be beveled to maximize enamel bonding.

Preparations for Cervical Erosion/Abrasion Lesions

Minimal tooth preparation is necessary for restoration of teeth with cervical erosion/abrasion lesions. Enamel margins should be beveled for resin composite restorations only, and mechanical retention is recommended. Some clinicians advocate placement of resin composite and glass-ionomer materials without any tooth preparation. Although both materials have demonstrated 3-year retention rates of 80% or greater in unprepared lesions,[5,24] close to 100% retention is likely if mechanical retention is placed. Some clinicians recommend roughening the surface of sclerotic lesions with a diamond bur prior to restoration to remove the highly calcified outer layer and expose the dentinal collagen network to the adhesive.

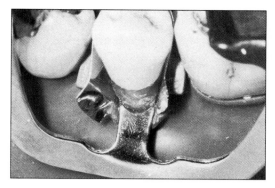

Fig 11-12 A piece of a Tofflemire band may be used without the retainer to provide lateral walls for condensation of amalgam. Wedges, compound, and/or a flat instrument may be used to support the matrix.

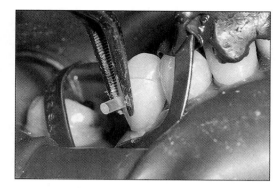

Fig 11-13 Glass-ionomer cement is injected into the cavity, and a precontoured matrix is placed.

Matrices and Insertion

Amalgam

In Class 5 preparations, the cavosurface margins should be approximately 90 degrees. This sometimes makes condensation of amalgam difficult if, because of the curvature of the tooth, the mesial and distal walls are flared so that the amalgam has no lateral walls to contain it. In this case, a custom matrix may be used.

A simple method utilizes a Tofflemire matrix band. The band is cut to a length that wraps around the lingual aspect of the tooth and extends slightly facial to the interproximal contacts (Fig 11-12). Interproximal wedges are placed to support and stabilize the band. If further support is needed, a flat hand instrument may be used to support the band during condensation, or modeling compound may be softened and pressed interproximally with the wedges. This technique provides a strong, stable matrix that will allow adequate condensation. In some situations the flat blade of a hand instrument alone will suffice to contain the amalgam for condensation.

Glass-Ionomer Restorative Materials

Because most glass-ionomer restorative materials are either autocuring or dual-curing, the restoration can be placed in one increment with an overlying matrix. The material is mixed and injected into the cavity prepara-tion until it is slightly overfilled. A precontoured matrix is then placed over the material, and the excess material is allowed to extrude out the sides. With autocured glass-ionomer cements, the edges are sealed, and the matrix is left in place until the material is set (Fig 11-13). With resin-modified (light-cured) glass-ionomer materials, a clear matrix is used, and the restoration is light polymerized through the matrix. The restoration may be contoured and polished immediately.

Resin Composite

Class 5 restorations that extend to the root surface present a special problem for resin composite, because adhesion to cementum and dentin is not as reliable as adhesion to enamel. Because of polymerization shrinkage, resin composite tends to adhere to the enamel margins but pulls away from the dentin or cementum on the gingival margin.[15,29] Improvements in dentin adhesives have decreased gap formation, and incremental placement techniques are usually recommended to further minimize effects of this phenomenon.[15,29]

Before resin composite is placed, an enamel-dentin adhesive system is applied and light polymerized. The first increment of resin composite should be placed from about the midpoint of the gingival floor to the incisal cavosurface margin and light polymerized (Fig 11-14). The second increment then fills the remainder of the preparation. Large preparations may require more than two increments. Resin composite should not be placed in increments thicker than 2 mm, to assure

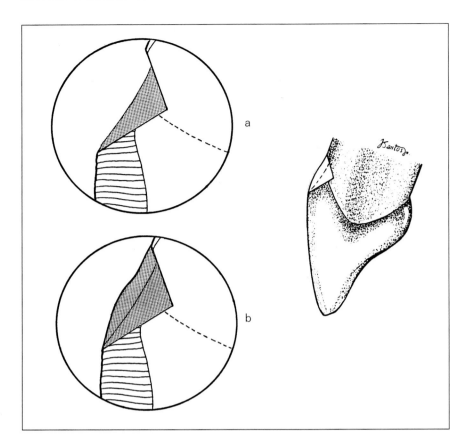

Fig 11-14 In most cases, resin composite should be placed in two increments. (a) The first should include the incisal or occlusal margin, but not the gingival margin. (b) The second increment fills the remainder of the preparation.

adequate penetration of light for polymerization.[10] Some clinicians recommend placement of glycerin over the resin composite prior to final polymerization to produce a hard external surface without an air-inhibited layer.

Finishing and Polishing

Amalgam

After the amalgam has been carved to proper contours, a slightly smoother surface may be attained with a rubber cup and a fine abrasive paste. Although polishing has been shown to have no long-term benefit,[17] a smooth surface tends to be less plaque retentive. If desired, a high shine can be obtained at a subsequent appointment with pumice, rubber polishing points or cups, polishing pastes, or a combination of these implements.

Glass-Ionomer Restorative Materials

Autocured glass-ionomer cements are inherently rough materials that do not polish well and require protection from water contamination and desiccation for 7 to 10 minutes after placement. After removal of the matrix, the restoration can be contoured with a blade, carbide or diamond burs, and disks. A No. 12 or 12b scalpel blade works well for contouring and removing flash in the interproximal areas. Fine disks work well for final polishing. These procedures should be performed with water or with the surface of the restoration coated with unfilled resin to provide lubrication and prevent desiccation. An unfilled resin glaze may be placed and polymerized after polishing is completed.

Resin-modified glass-ionomer cements can be contoured and polished immediately after polymerization. Diamond or carbide finishing burs and a No. 12 or 12b blade may be used for contouring. Polishing may be performed with disks, impregnated rubber points or cups, and polishing pastes. Some manufacturers recommend placement of an unfilled resin after polishing.

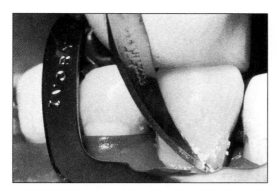

Fig 11-15a A No. 12 or 12b scalpel blade works well for removing flash with most restorative materials.

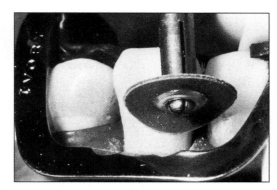

Fig 11-15b Finishing disks may be used to contour and polish Class 5 restorations

Resin Composite

Resin composite restorations should be slightly overfilled so that any air-inhibited resin is removed during finishing and polishing procedures. Diamond or carbide finishing burs may be used for contouring, along with a No. 12 or 12b scalpel blade (Fig 11-15a). Polishing may be performed with disks (Fig 11-15b), impregnated rubber points or cups, and polishing pastes. The highest luster may be achieved with microfilled materials, but most of the current composites also polish well. Rebonding, as discussed in chapters 7 and 8, is also recommended for Class 5 restorations.

Dentinal Sensitivity

Dentinal hypersensitivity is often associated with gingival recession and Class 5 lesions. It is a problem that is reported to affect about one in seven persons.[13] Sensitivity is caused by open dentinal tubules that communicate between the pulp and the oral cavity, and the degree of sensitivity is influenced by the number and size of the open tubules.[1,21] Brännström's hydrodynamic theory[2] is the most widely accepted explanation of dentinal sensitivity. According to Brännström,[2] changes in fluid movement within open dentinal tubules are perceived as pain by mechanoreceptors near the pulp. Tactile, thermal, or osmotic stimuli can induce changes in fluid flow and elicit a painful response.

Treatment or prevention of hypersensitivity is usually accomplished by use of some method to occlude the open tubules.[9,22,30] Dentin adhesives provide at least short-term relief.[3,32] Oxalate solutions, used alone or in combination with electrophoresis, are reported to be successful.[9,22] Stannous fluoride has also been used with good results.[28]

Potassium nitrate is also reported to be an effective desensitizing agent.[11,27] It is available in dentifrices or as a gel for application in the dental office. Potassium nitrate is thought to act directly on nerve membranes to reduce sensory nerve activity,[11] rather than causing occlusion of the tubules.[9]

References

1. Absi EG, Addy M, Adams D. Dentin hypersensivity. A study of the patency of dentinal tubules in sensitive and non-sensitive cervical dentin. J Clin Periodontol 1987;14:280-284.

2. Brännström M. The hydrodynamics of the dentinal tubule and of pulp fluid. A discussion of its significance in relation to dentinal sensitivity. Caries Res 1976;1:310-322.

3. Dall'Orologio GD, Malferrari S. Desensitizing effects of Gluma and Gluma 2000 on hypersensitive dentin. Am J Dent 1993;6:283-286.

4. Davis EL, Yu X, Joynt RB, Wieczkowski G Jr, Giordano L. Shear strength and microleakage of light-cured glass ionomers. Am J Dent 1993;6:127-129.

5. Duke ES, Robbins JW, Snyder DS. Clinical evaluation of a dentin adhesive system: 3 year results. Quintessence Int 1991;22:819-895.

6. Elderton RJ. Implications of recent dental health services research on the future of operative dentistry. J Public Health Dent 1985;45:101-105.

7. Gaintantzopoulou MD, Willis GP, Kafrawy AH. Pulp reactions to light-cured glass ionomer cements. Am J Dent 1994;7:39-42.

8. Heymann HO, Sturdevant JR, Bayne S, Wilder AD, Sluder TB, Brunson WD. Examining tooth flexure effects. J Am Dent Assoc 1991;122:41-47.

9. Hodosh M, Hodosh SH, Hodosh AJ. About dentinal hypersensitivity. Compend Contin Educ Dent 1994;15:658-667.

10. Jensen ME, Chan DCN. Polymerization shrinkage and microleakage. In: Vanherle G, Smith DC, eds. Posterior Composite Resin Dental Restorative Materials. The Netherlands: Szulc Utrecht, 1985:243-262.

11. Kim SA. Hypersensitive teeth: Desensitization of pulpal sensory nerves. J Endod 1986;12:482-485.

12. Knight GM. The co-cured, light-activated glass-ionomer cement–composite resin restoration. Quintessence Int 1994;25:97-100.

13. Krauser JT. Hypersensitive teeth. Part 1. Etiology. J Prosthet Dent 1986;56:153-156.

14. Lee WC, Eakle WS. Possible role of tensile stress in the etiology of cervical erosive lesions in teeth. J Prosthet Dent 1984;52:374-380.

15. Lutz F, Krejci I, Oldenburg TR. Elimination of polymerization stresses at the margins of posterior composite resin restorations: A new restorative technique. Quintessence Int 1986;17:777-784.

16. Matis BA, Carlson T, Cochran M, Phillips RW. How finishing effects glass ionomer. Results of a five-year evaluation. J Am Dent Assoc 1991;122:43-46.

17. Mayhew RB, Schmeltzer LD, Pierson WP. Effect of polishing on the marginal integrity of high-copper amalgam. Oper Dent 1986;11:8-13.

18. McLean JW, Wilson AD. The clinical development of the glass-ionomer cements. I. Formulations and properties. Aust Dent J 1977;22:31-36.

19. Mount GJ. Clinical requirements for a successful "sandwich"—Dentine to glass ionomer cement to composite resin. Aust Dent J 1989;34:259-265.

20. Mount GJ. An Atlas of Glass-ionomer Cements. London: Martin Dunitz, 1990.

21. Pashley DH. Mechanisms of dentin sensitivity. Dent Clin North Am 1990;34:449-493.

22. Pashley DH, Muzzin K. Clinical Management of Dentin Hypersensitivity. Philadelphia: Lippincott, 1990.

23. Powell LV, Gordon GE, Johnson GH. Sensitivity restored of Class V abrasion/erosion lesions. J Am Dent Assoc 1990;121:694-696.

24. Powell LV, Johnson GV, Gordon GE. Clinical evaluation of Class V abrasion/erosion restorations [abstract 1514]. J Dent Res 1992;71:705.

25. Regan SE. Periodontal access techniques for restorative dentistry. Gen Dent 1989;37:117-121.

26. Starr CB. Management of periodontal tissues for restorative dentistry. J Esthet Dent 1991;3:195-208.

27. Tarbet WJ, Silverman G, Fratarcangelo PA, Kanapka JA. Home treatment for dentinal hypersensitivity: A comparative study. J Am Dent Assoc 1982;105:227-230.

28. Thrash WJ, Dodds MWJ, Jones DL. The effect of stannous fluoride on dentinal hypersensitivity. Int Dent J 1994;44:107-118.

29. Tjan AHL, Bergh BH, Lidner C. Effect of various incremental techniques on marginal adaptation of class II composite resin restorations. J Prosthet Dent 1992;67:62-66.

30. Trowbridge HO, Silver DR. A review of current approaches to in-office management of tooth hypersensitivity. Dent Clin North Am 1990;34:561-581.

31. Tyas MJ. Cariostatic effect of glass ionomer cement: A five-year clinical study. Aust Dent J 1991;36:236-239.

32. Watanabe T, Sano M, Itoh K, Wakumoto S. The effects of primers on the sensitivity of dentin. Dent Mater 1991;7:148-150.

33. White SN, MacEntee MI, Cho G. Restorative treatment for geriatric root caries. CDA J 1994;22:55-60.

Restoration of Endodontically Treated Teeth

J. William Robbins

A great deal of research has been published regarding the restoration of endodontically treated teeth.[70] However, it is very difficult for the busy practitioner to read and synthesize this information into a logical treatment philosophy. It is the purpose of this chapter to analyze the research and present a logical approach to this subject.

When faced with the challenge of restoring an endodontically treated tooth, the dentist must decide first whether a post is required, and second, the type of restoration that is indicated. In the past, a post was thought to strengthen the root of an endodontically treated tooth. This philosophy pervaded dental education until laboratory research began to cast doubts on this assumption. It is widely held today that the primary purpose of post placement is to retain the core buildup material or to reinforce the remaining coronal tooth structure. The decision to place a post is based on several parameters, including the position of the tooth in the arch, occlusion, function of the restored tooth, amount of remaining tooth structure, and canal configuration.

Indications for Placement of Posts

Anterior Teeth

Anterior and posterior teeth function much differently; therefore, they must be evaluated separately. The anterior tooth receives predominately shear forces, which act on both the clinical crown and the root. Although some laboratory studies[36,89] have indicated that a post strengthens an intact anterior endodontically treated tooth, other studies[25,71,90] have suggested that the fracture resistance of these teeth is not affected by, or decreases with, placement of a post. Therefore, when a complete-coverage restoration is not required for esthetic or functional reasons (to serve as an abutment for a fixed or removable partial denture), a post is not indicated. However, if a complete-coverage restoration is indicated in an anterior tooth for esthetics or function, or because the remaining coronal tooth structure is inadequate, a post is commonly indicated.[95] This is especially true for maxillary lateral incisors and mandibular incisors.

With maxillary central incisors and canines, the decision to place a post should be based on the amount of remaining coronal tooth structure, as well as the occlusion and function of the tooth. If there is a significant amount of remaining coronal tooth structure, the crown preparation should be accomplished before the decision about post placement is made. Once the axial preparation is completed and the access preparation is cleaned, the dentist can make the decision as to whether the remaining coronal tooth structure needs the reinforcement of a post. If, based on the functional requirements of the tooth, the decision is made that the remaining coronal tooth structure is adequate to support the crown, resin composite can be bonded into the access preparation. However, if there is doubt regarding the adequacy of the resistance form of the coronal portion of the tooth, then a post or post and core is indicated.

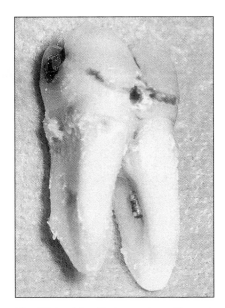

Fig 12-1 Mandibular molar with post perforation in the lingual concavity of the distal root.

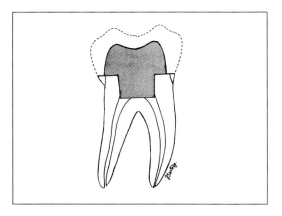

Fig 12-2a Amalcore with adequate chamber retention.

Posterior Teeth

In the posterior tooth the decisions are more clear-cut. The forces that play on posterior teeth are predominately vertical. Therefore, reinforcement of coronal tooth structure is not commonly needed, as it is in anterior teeth. Because of the morbidity associated with post placement (Fig 12-1), a post is only indicated in a posterior tooth when other more conservative retention and resistance features cannot be used for the core. These features include chamber retention, amalgam pins, and threaded pins, all of which have been shown to be exceedingly effective.[69]

In 1980, Nayyar and Walton[56] described the *amalcore*, or *coronal-radicular restoration*. Rather than placing a post, the pulp chamber and coronal 2.0 to 3.0 mm of each canal are used for retention of the buildup material (Fig 12-2a to 12-2c). Subsequently, several authors reported laboratory data on the fracture resistance of the amalcore. Kern and others[37] and Christian and others[11] reported that the placement of a post in the distal canal of a mandibular molar increases the fracture resistance of the amalcore. However, in these studies the specimens were stressed in compression at 60 degrees and 90 degrees, respectively. This angle of force does not reproduce the vertical forces that molars receive in vivo.

In a similar study, Plasmans and others[62] found no statistically significant difference between the amalcore alone and the amalcore with a post when stressed at 45 degrees. Kane and Burgess[35] reported that the placement of two horizontal threaded pins in the buccal and lingual walls of the amalcore restoration provides a significant increase in fracture resistance. In a retrospective clinical study of more than 400 coronal-radicular restorations, Nayyar and Walton[56] reported no failures that could be attributed to the core buildup.

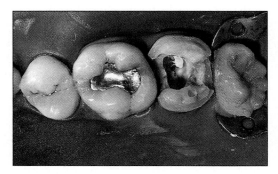

Fig 12-2b Amalcore preparation in a maxillary second molar.

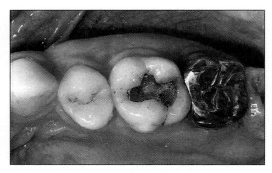

Fig 12-2c Definitive amalcore restoration in the maxillary second molar.

It has been commonly stated that threaded pins should not be placed in endodontically treated teeth because they will cause the teeth to crack. However, no clinical data are available to support this belief. In fact, current data indicate that there is very little difference between the dentin of endodontically treated teeth and vital dentin.[75] There is also a move to completely discard traditional retention and resistance features in deference to the adhesively retained buildup. Again, long-term clinical data are not available to support the efficacy of this technique. Therefore, until the efficacy of the adhesively retained buildup can be demonstrated in long-term clinical studies, it would be prudent to use adhesive materials in conjunction with traditional retention and resistance features.

Although a post is not commonly indicated in a posterior tooth, a post may be indicated when the tooth is to serve as an abutment for a removable partial denture.[79] In this circumstance, the forces that play on the tooth are not physiologic and coronal reinforcement may be necessary (Fig 12-3). In maxillary molars a post is generally placed only in the palatal canal, and in mandibular molars in the distal canal.

Maxillary premolars are a unique subset of posterior endodontically treated teeth. Because these teeth are subjected to a mixture of shear and compressive forces, the need for a post and core in maxillary premolar is not as clear-cut. If the clinical crown is tall in relation to its diameter at the point where it enters the alveolar bone, or if the tooth receives significant lateral stress, a post may be indicated (Figs 12-4a and 12-4b). In addition, if the premolar serves as an abutment for a removable partial denture, a post and core may be indicated.[79] Conversely, if the coronal portion of the tooth is relatively short, and it functions like a molar tooth, then a post is not usually indicated.

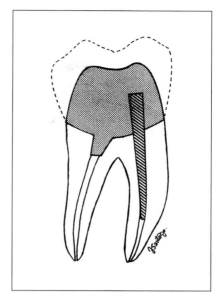

Fig 12-3 Mandibular molar that does not have a large enough pulp chamber for chamber retention of the core buildup. A post is used for retention of the core.

When the decision is made to place a post, the delicate morphologic structure of the maxillary premolar root must be considered during preparation of the post space.[93,96] Posts that necessitate minimal canal enlargement should be chosen for maxillary premolars. Ideally, after completion of the endodontic obturation, the canal should not be further enlarged. Rather, the post should be modified to fit the canal. This philosophy would commonly dictate the placement of a conservative tapered post in the maxillary premolar (Figs 12-4a and 12-4b).

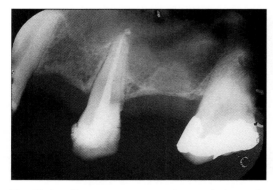

Fig 12-4a Preoperative view of an endodontically treated maxillary second premolar.

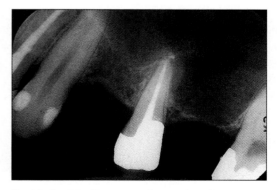

Fig 12-4b Maxillary second premolar after restoration with a tapered prefabricated post and amalgam core. The canal was not enlarged for post placement.

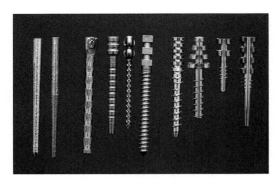

Fig 12-5 Prefabricated posts. *(left to right)* Passive tapered: Endowel (Star), Filpost (Vivadent); passive parallel: Parapost Plus (Whaledent), BCH (3M Dental), Unity (Whaledent), Boston Post (Roydent); active: Flexipost (Essential Dental Systems), V-lock (Brasseler), Radix (Caulk), Cytco (Maillefer).

Considerations in Post Design

Prior to choosing a post system, the dentist must have a clear understanding of the effect of several variables on the post-tooth combination. These variables include post design (Fig 12-5), post length, post diameter, venting, surface roughness, canal preparation, method of cementation, and luting medium.

Post Design

In general, it has been reported that the active threaded post has the greatest retention, followed by the parallel post, and the tapered post has the least retention.[14,31,83] Therefore, the post should be chosen, in part, by the amount of post retention which the clinical situation requires. If the length is adequate, usually considered to be 7.0 to 8.0 mm, and the canal configuration is normal, either the tapered or parallel post may be selected. However, if the length of post space available is minimal or the canal space is funnel shaped, an active post may be required because of the difficulty in gaining adequate axial retention of the post.

Post Length

Increased post length results in increased retention.[31,83] However, a minimum of 4.0 mm of gutta-percha should be left in the apical portion of the canal space to minimize the risk of apical leakage.[51,57] A passive post should

usually be as long as possible without encroaching on the remaining gutta-percha or causing perforation in a curved canal.[77]

Post Diameter

It is commonly stated that endodontically treated teeth are more susceptible to fracture because they exhibit increased brittleness.[8,27] However, more current research questions the validity of this assumption.[75] Regardless of the effect of endodontic therapy on the brittleness of a tooth, the dentist has no control over this variable. It is also known that the fracture resistance of a restored endodontically treated tooth decreases as the amount of dentin removed increases.[15] Increased post diameter produces minimal, if any, increase in post retention[1,82] and significantly increases internal stresses within the tooth.[49,50] Therefore, increasing the diameter of the post is not the preferred method of increasing its retention. The diameter of the post should be as small as possible, while retaining the necessary rigidity.

Venting

Because of the intraradicular hydrostatic pressure created during cementation of the post,[24] a means for cement to escape must always be provided. Because virtually all prefabricated posts have a venting mechanism incorporated in their design, this factor is most important with the custom cast post. A vent may be incorporated in the pattern before casting or cut into the post with a bur prior to cementation.

Surface Roughness

Surface roughening, such as air abrading or notching, of the post increases post retention.[12,47,68,73,87] Surface texture is usually incorporated in prefabricated posts; however, this feature must be added to the custom cast post and core.

Canal Preparation

Several methods of preparing the post space and their effect on apical seal have been investigated. These include use of rotary instruments, heated instruments, and solvents.[16,40,46,51,85] The literature is equivocal on preparation of the post space; no method has been shown to be consistently superior. When a rotary instrument is used, care must be taken to ensure that only the gutta-percha is removed. The canal space should not be routinely enlarged.

Immediate preparation (immediately after the endodontic filling) of the post space has been compared to delayed preparation (waiting at least 24 hours).[2,16,46,63,74] Again, neither method has been consistently shown to be superior.

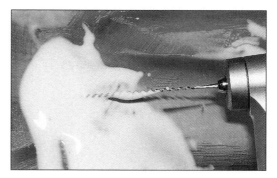

Fig 12-6 Lentulo spiral used to place cement into the canal space.

Cementation of Posts

Method of Cementation

The actual method of post cementation has been investigated,[20,22] including placement of the cement on the post, and/or placement of the cement in the canal with a lentulo spiral, a paper point, or an endodontic explorer. The lentulo spiral is the superior instrument for cement placement (Fig 12-6). The cement may also be placed in the canal with a needle tube, as long as the tip of the tube is inserted to the bottom of the canal space and the cement is extruded from the tip as it is slowly removed from the canal. After the cement is placed in the canal, the post is coated with the cement and inserted. When zinc phosphate cement is used, it has been shown that the placement of an organic solvent (Cavidry, Parkell) in the canal prior to cementation of the post increases retention.[48]

Luting Cements

Cements for posts and post-and-core restorations have been investigated extensively.[4,5,10,39,64,83,94] These include zinc phosphate, polycarboxylate, and glass ionomer, and filled and unfilled resin composites. Both zinc phosphate and glass ionomer are commonly used because of their ease of use coupled with their history of clinical success.

In recent years, interest in the use of both filled and unfilled resins as luting cements has increased. Some clinical studies have shown a significant increase in post retention with resin cements,[21,55,92] but other studies have not confirmed this finding.[59,61] There are two problems with the use of resin composite cements. First, resin cement is technique sensitive because of its short working time. Second, it is difficult to remove all of the gutta-percha and eugenol-containing cement from the prepared canal without removing excess tooth structure. This residue in the surface irregularities of the prepared canal prevents adequate conditioning of the dentin and inhibits the set of the polymer.[5]

Each cement has distinct advantages and should be chosen based on these advantages in a given situation. However, none of the cements can overcome the inadequacies of a poorly designed post.

Types of Posts

Custom Cast Post

The custom cast post and core has a long history of successful use in restorative dentistry. However, laboratory studies[45,52,58] have consistently shown that the fracture resistance of teeth restored with a custom cast post is lower than that of many different prefabricated posts. In addition, retrospective clinical studies[78,88] have shown prefabricated parallel posts to have greater clinical success than the custom cast post. This, coupled with the added expense and extra appointment required to fabricate the custom cast post, makes its routine use questionable.

There are several circumstances when the custom cast post is the post of choice.

1. When multiple post-and-core restorations are planned in the same arch, the laboratory-fabricated custom cast post is the most time- and cost-efficient method. The teeth are prepared for the posts, and the final crown preparation is completed so that all crown margins are on natural structure. It is important that the crown preparation be completed before the impression for the post and core is made

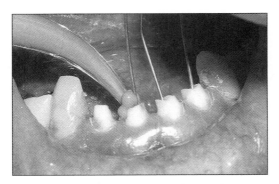

Fig 12-7a Use of 25-gauge needles to allow air to escape from canals during the impression taking to ensure a complete impression of the canal spaces.

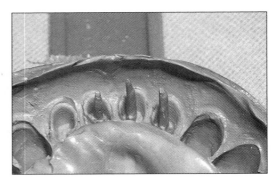

Fig 12-7b Final impression of canal spaces for laboratory fabrication of custom cast posts.

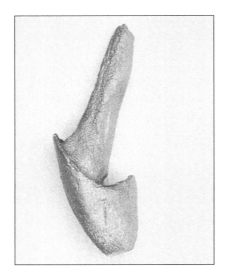

Figs 12-8a and 12-8b Custom cast post to allow a change in the angle of the core in relation to the post.

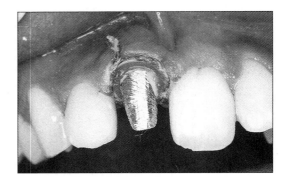

so that the axial contours of the core can be fabricated correctly.

An impression is made with an elastomeric impression material used in an injection technique, which allows the impression material to flow into the total length of the prepared canal space (Figs 12-7a and 12.7b). This can be best accomplished by placing a 25-gauge needle into the canal before the impression is made. The syringe material is then injected into the canal until it begins to flow out the top of the orifice. While the syringe material is still being injected, the needle is slowly removed from the canal. The needle serves as an escape channel for the trapped air and allows the elastomeric impression material to reproduce the entire length of the canal space.

No reinforcement of the impression material in the canal space is required with the newer impression materials. The impression is poured and the custom posts are fabricated in the laboratory. At a subsequent appointment, the posts are cemented and the final impression for the crowns is made without further tooth preparation.

2. When a small tooth, such as a mandibular incisor, requires a post and core, a prefabricated post may be difficult to use. Commonly, there is minimal space around the post for the core buildup material. In this situation, the custom cast post serves well.

3. Occasionally, the angle of the core in relation to the root must be altered. It is not advisable to bend prefabricated posts; therefore, the custom cast post and core most successfully fulfils this need (Figs 12-8a and 12-8b).

4. When an all-ceramic crown is placed, it is necessary to have a core that approximates the color of natural tooth structure. Because resin composite is not the material of choice in high-stress situations, the core of a custom cast post can have porcelain fired to the

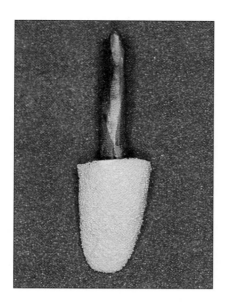

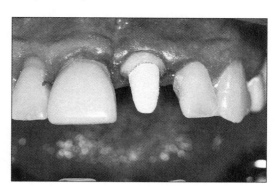

Fig 12-9a Custom cast post with porcelain fired to the core for improved esthetics.

Fig 12-9b Maxillary central incisor with a custom cast post ready to receive an all-ceramic crown.

surface to simulate natural tooth color. The porcelain on the core can be etched, and the all-ceramic crown can be adhesively bonded (Figs 12-9a and 12-9b).

Prefabricated Posts

In recent years, there has been a significant increase in the number of post systems available. Prefabricated posts may be divided into three major groups: passive tapered, passive parallel, and active.

Passive Tapered Post

A goal of all post systems should be minimal removal of tooth structure prior to post placement. Therefore, the ideal post system requires no further preparation after removal of the gutta-percha. Because the natural shape of the canal is tapered, the passive tapered post best fulfils this criterion (Fig 12-5). The major advantage of the passive tapered post is that the post can be modified to fit the tapered canal rather than the canal having to be enlarged to fit the post.

The major disadvantage is that the tapered post provides the least retention. This means that the retention must be gained through increased post length. When the root is not long enough to allow for adequate post length (7.0 to 8.0 mm), a more retentive post is indicated. A second commonly stated disadvantage of the tapered post is the alleged wedging effect, which results in increased stress and root fracture. This effect has been demonstrated in laboratory studies[9,52] with custom cast tapered post-and-core restorations. However, this theoretical wedging effect does not appear to be valid when a passive tapered post is used in conjunction with an acceptable core material and a crown.[68]

The primary indication for the passive tapered post is in teeth with small canals and thin, fragile roots, such as maxillary premolars (Figs 12-4a and 12-4b). However, it may be used routinely in teeth with normal canal configuration and sufficient canal length to provide the necessary retention.

Passive Parallel Post

The prefabricated post by which all other posts are measured has traditionally been the Parapost (Whaledent)(Fig 12-5). The success of this post style has been demonstrated clinically[78,88] as well as in the laboratory.[14,31,83] The passive parallel post has greater retention than the passive tapered post. However, a biologic price must be paid for this increased retention. The naturally tapered canal space must be enlarged to accommodate a parallel post. Enlargement of this canal space is not consistent with the ideal of maintaining as much tooth structure as possible. For this reason, use of the passive parallel post is recommended when increased retention is needed, and the parallel canal preparation will not jeopardize the integrity of the root.

Active Post

An active post is one that engages (screws into) the dentin in the canal space. There are several styles of active posts, including those requiring a tap, self-tapping posts, split-shank posts, and hybrid posts, which contain both active and passive features (Fig 12-5). It is difficult to generalize about active posts because of their design

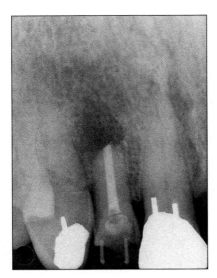

Fig 12-10a Preoperative view of a maxillary lateral incisor with a short canal space.

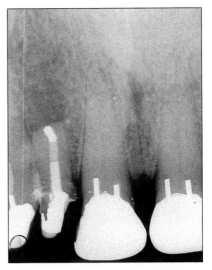

Fig 12-10b Tooth after restoration with a Brasseler V-lock active post and amalgam core.

differences. However, the V-Lock (Brasseler) and the Flexipost (Essential Dental Systems) have performed well in the laboratory,[5] and it has been the author's experience that they perform well in clinical use.

Traditionally, the major concern about active posts has been the potential for vertical fracture of the tooth during placement of the post.[6,82] However, with the newer generation of active posts, many laboratory studies support their use.[3,7,18,23,72,86] It has been shown that the active post should not be "bottomed out" when it is finally inserted.[72] After complete seating of an active post, it should be unscrewed one fourth of a turn. This results in decreased residual stress in the root. It has also been shown that, at shorter lengths, the active post produces less stress than other styles of prefabricated posts.[82] Therefore, active posts are indicated when the canal length is inadequate (eg, in a short tooth or partially occluded canal due to a broken instrument or post), to gain adequate retention with a passive post (Figs 12-10a and 12-10b).

The Retention Triad

The real difficulty in restoring an endodontically treated tooth comes when minimal coronal tooth structure remains. In this circumstance, the dentist must consider both retention of the post and core and resistance of the post-core-crown combination.

Retention is defined as the force that resists a tensile or pulling force. Retention of a post can be gained in three ways (Fig 12-11). The first method to gain retention is through adequate post *length* in the canal.[31,83] To gain this axial retention, it is imperative that the canal space has not been overenlarged iatrogenically or by caries. In an anterior tooth, adequate length is commonly considered to be in the range of 7.0 to 8.0 mm plus 4.0 mm of gutta-percha that should be left undisturbed at the apex.[57]

The design of the post may be either tapered or parallel. The tapered post requires less removal of tooth structure during preparation of the post space, but also exhibits poorer retention than does the parallel post. However, when the parallel post is employed, more tooth structure must be removed, especially at the apical end of the post space. Both of these post designs are acceptable, and the decision should be based on the canal configuration, available post space, and the amount of retention required.

The second factor affecting retention is post *style*. When the decision is made that the canal length is inadequate to retain a passive post, an active post should be selected. This can occur with short clinical roots or because of obstructions in the canal space. An active post can also serve effectively when the canal space has been overenlarged. The active post can actively engage the dentin in its terminal 2 to 3 mm to gain retention. The weakened coronal portion of the canal space is not engaged, possibly resulting in less stress.

Fig 12-11 Retention triad.

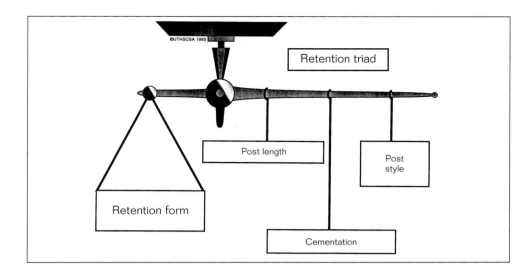

Fig 12-12 Resistance triad.

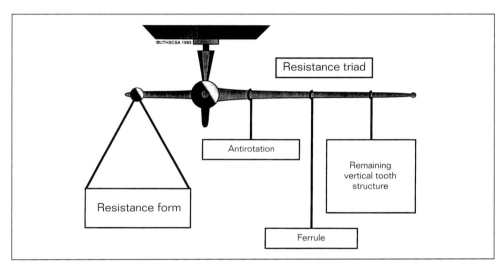

The third part of the retention triad is the *luting agent* used to cement the post. The idea of bonding a post into the canal with resin cement to increase retention is theoretically appealing. However, the gutta-percha and zinc oxide–eugenol cement smeared in the canal irregularities makes the bonded post a dream more than a reality. When technology is developed to remove the canal contaminants noninvasively, resin cement will probably be the luting agent of choice. However, until that time, no available cement can overcome the problems created by a poorly engineered post.

The Resistance Triad

The second major consideration in the design of the post restoration is the resistance of the tooth-post-crown combination. If the resistance requirements are not met,

the probability of failure is high, regardless of the retentiveness of the post. Three parameters of resistance must be considered (Fig 12-12). The resistance triad consists of the ferrule effect, vertical remaining coronal tooth structure, and antirotation. These features work in combination; therefore, if one of the features is minimal or nonexistent, one or both of the remaining features must be increased.

The first feature of the resistance triad is the *ferrule* (Fig 12-13). The ferrule is that part of the crown margin that extends past the post-and-core margin onto the natural tooth structure. To be effective, it must encircle the tooth (360 degrees) and ideally extend at least 1.5 mm onto tooth structure below the post-and-core margin.[43] It is not always possible to develop a ferrule in every crown preparation. Because all-ceramic crowns and crowns with porcelain butt-joint margins cannot be constructed with a metal collar, it is sometimes not possible to utilize a ferrule with these types of crowns. It may

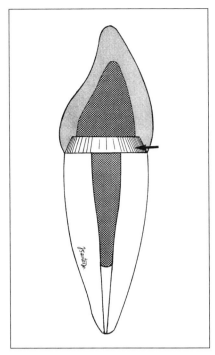

Fig 12-13 Ferrule around periphery of root surface to increase resistance form.

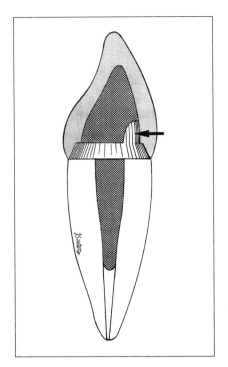

Fig 12-14 Vertical remaining tooth structure to increase resistance form.

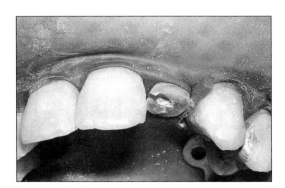

Fig 12-15 Maxillary lateral incisor that has been unnecessarily flattened prior to placement of the post and core.

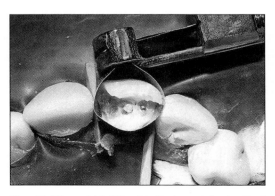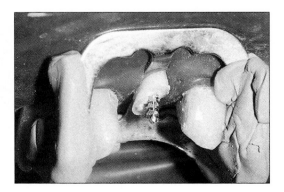

Figs 12-16a and 12-16b Vertical remaining tooth structure left in core preparations to increase resistance form.

also be difficult to prepare a ferrule when the remaining coronal tooth structure is minimal. If tooth structure has been lost to fracture or caries, it is sometimes not possible to gain the necessary ferrule because of impingement of the crown margin on the biologic width.

The second feature of the resistance triad is *vertical remaining tooth structure* (Fig 12-14). Traditionally, it was taught that the face of a root should be flattened prior to construction of the post and core (Fig 12-15). However, it has been shown that leaving as much natural vertical remaining tooth structure as possible will significantly increase the resistance of the final restoration[80] (Figs 12-16a and 12-16b). Unfortunately, because of caries, trauma, or iatrogenic removal, vertical remaining tooth structure is not always available.

The third feature of the resistance triad is *antirotation*. Every post and core must have an antirotation feature incorporated in the preparation.[58,73] An elongated or oblong canal orifice can serve as antirotation for the post and core. However, as the canal becomes more round, the need for incorporation of antirotation features becomes more important. This is especially true for anterior teeth. Auxiliary pins and keyways, which have been prepared in the face of the root prior to construction of the post are the most common antirotation devices (Fig 12-17).

The features of the resistance triad are generally easy to incorporate in the preparations of posterior teeth. If there is not enough tooth structure to allow the placement of a ferrule, a simple crown-lengthening procedure will generally expose enough tooth structure to allow for ferrule placement after healing. It is also easier to incorporate antirotation features in posterior teeth because of their larger size.

However, the features of the resistance triad are generally more difficult to incorporate in the preparations of anterior teeth. There is commonly not as much vertical tooth structure remaining and it is more difficult to incorporate antirotation features because of the smaller tooth size. If, for reasons related to the biologic width or, more commonly, for esthetic reasons, it is not possible to place a substantial metal margin, then a very important part of the resistance triad is absent. If there is also minimal vertical remaining tooth structure, the prognosis for the tooth is guarded unless more vertical tooth structure can be incorporated in the preparation. Because anterior crown lengthening generally results in an esthetically unacceptable gingival discontinuity, the treatment of choice, prior to placement of the restoration, is orthodontic eruption.[84] After forced eruption and crown-lengthening surgery, there is then sufficient remaining vertical tooth structure to significantly improve both the resistance form and the prognosis.

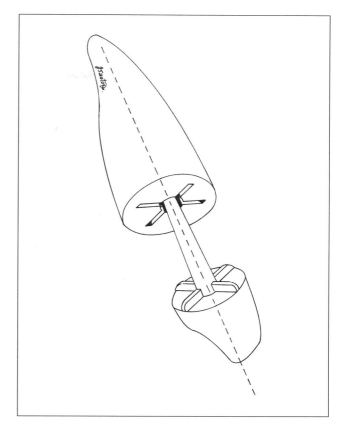

Fig 12-17 Antirotation slots.

▨ Buildup Materials

With the increased use of prefabricated posts in recent years, the choice of core material has received much interest. The ideal core material exhibits these characteristics:

- Stability in a wet environment
- Ease of manipulation
- Rapid, hard set for immediate crown preparation
- Natural tooth color
- High compressive strength
- High tensile strength
- High modulus of elasticity (rigidity)
- High fracture toughness
- Low plastic deformation
- Inert (no corrosion)
- Cariostatic properties
- Biocompatibility
- Inexpensiveness

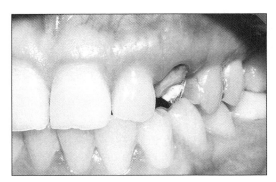

Fig 12-18a Preoperative view of an endodontically treated maxillary canine.

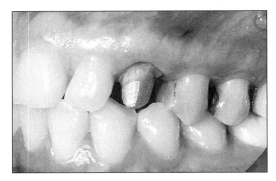

Fig 12-18b Endodontically treated maxillary canine after restoration with a prefabricated post and amalgam core.

Unfortunately, no material fulfils all of these requirements. In selecting a core buildup material, the dentist must consider both the functional requirements of the buildup as well as the amount of remaining natural tooth structure. There are currently four widely used core materials: glass ionomer, resin composite, amalgam, and cast metal.

Conventional glass-ionomer materials have the advantages of fluoride release, ease of manipulation, natural color, biocompatibility, corrosion resistance, and dimensional stability in a wet environment.[13] However, they have the major disadvantage of low fracture toughness, which indicates that the material is susceptible to propagation of cracks. Unfortunately, the fracture toughness is not improved with the addition of silver reinforcement.[44] Therefore, conventional and silver-reinforced glass ionomer can only be recommended for use in posterior teeth in which at least 50% of natural coronal tooth structure remains.

In recent years, resin-modified glass-ionomer materials have gained popularity as core materials. An initial laboratory study[42] indicated that in addition to the aforementioned advantages of glass-ionomer cement, resin-modified glass-ionomer cements have physical properties similar to those of resin composite. However, until their success can be confirmed with clinical studies, resin-modified glass-ionomer cements should be used cautiously in high-stress situations.

Resin composite is the most popular core material because it is easy to use. It is available in light-cured, dual-cured, and autocured formulations. It is provided as both a tooth-colored material to be used as a core material under anterior all-ceramic restorations and as a color-contrast material to be used under metallic restorations. Adequate compressive strength[9,52] and fracture toughness[44] have been confirmed by static load testing. However, resin composite has not performed as successfully when tested with dynamic repeated-load tests.[29,38]

This type of laboratory test is used to simulate the small, repeated loads of function and parafunction in the oral cavity. It appears that resin composite undergoes plastic deformation under a small repeated load, which may lead to core failure.

Another disadvantage of resin composite is that it is not dimensionally stable in a wet environment.[60] As it absorbs water, the buildup expands. This is clinically relevant if a provisional restoration over a resin composite core is lost after the impression has been made for the crown. At delivery, the crown will not fit accurately because of the dimensional expansion of the core.

Resin composite is an adequate buildup material when there is some remaining vertical tooth structure to help support the core buildup. However, it is not recommended for situations in which the entire coronal portion of the tooth is to be replaced with the core material.

Amalgam, as a core buildup material, has several disadvantages. Its early strength is low, necessitating a 15- to 20-minute wait, even when fast-setting spherical alloy is used, until the buildup can be prepared for the crown. It is messy to prepare and can result in irreversible staining of the marginal gingiva during preparation. However, its strength has been confirmed in laboratory studies under both static and dynamic loads.[9,29,38] Therefore, in a high-stress situation in which the entire coronal portion is replaced with the core, either amalgam or custom cast metal is the material of choice (Figs 12-18a and 12-18b).

Definitive Restorations

There are multiple materials and techniques available for the definitive restoration of the endodontically treated tooth. Because the functional requirements are significantly different for anterior and posterior teeth, they will be discussed separately.

Anterior

It has been demonstrated in the laboratory that the endodontically treated anterior tooth has a fracture resistance approximately equal to that of a vital tooth.[25,45,90] Therefore, when a significant amount of coronal tooth structure remains, there is no need to place a post, and a conventional resin composite restoration in the access preparation is the treatment of choice (Fig 12-19). When a moderate amount of coronal tooth structure is missing, but approximately 50% of the coronal enamel remains, the bonded porcelain veneer may be the restoration of choice (Figs 12-20a to 12-20d). Again, there is no need for post placement with the porcelain veneer.

When the decision is made to fabricate a crown for an anterior endodontically treated tooth, a post is commonly indicated. This is especially true for maxillary lateral incisors and mandibular incisors. The decision to place a post is based on the amount of remaining coronal tooth

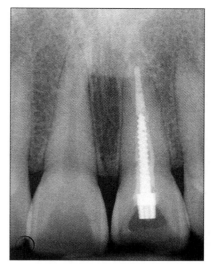

Fig 12-19 Endodontically treated maxillary central incisor that received an unnecessary post.

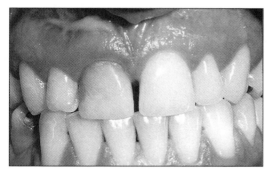

Fig 12-20a Preoperative view of an endodontically treated maxillary right central incisor. The patient did not desire correction of the gingival discontinuity or closure of the diastema. However, she wanted a long-term esthetic restoration.

Fig 12-20b Preoperative radiograph.

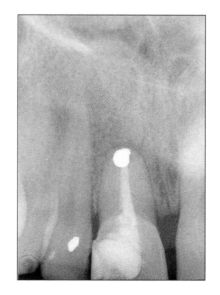

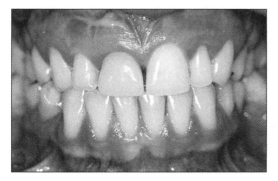

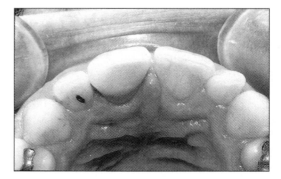

Figs 12-20c and 12-20d Endodontically treated maxillary right central incisor 6 years after restoration with a porcelain veneer.

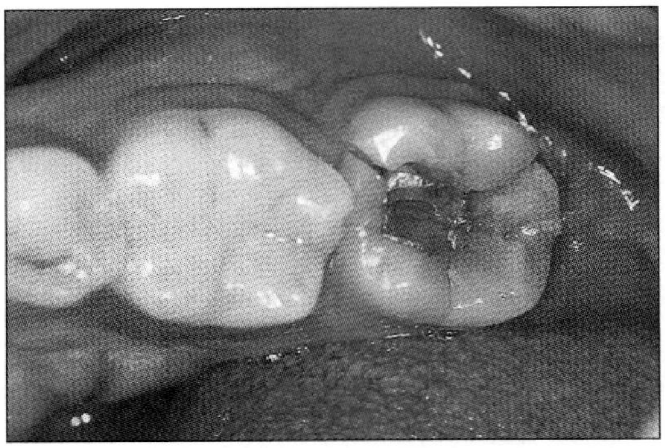

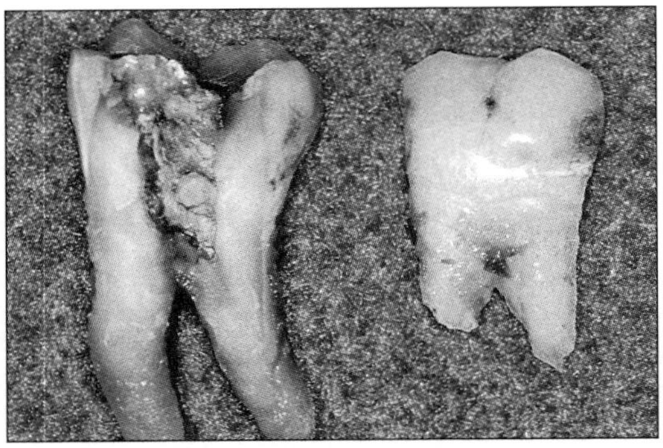

Figs 12-21a and 12-21b Unrestorable, fractured, endodontically treated mandibular second molar with an occlusal amalgam restoration.

structure after completion of the crown preparation. Therefore, the tooth should first be prepared for the crown; then the decision is made regarding the need for a post based on the strength of the remaining natural coronal tooth structure. If a post is required, the canal space is prepared, the post is cemented, and the core buildup is completed.

Posterior

In posterior teeth, the forces that play on the occlusal surfaces are more vertical. Laboratory data indicate that the access preparation has a minimal effect on the fracture resistance of posterior endodontically treated teeth.[67] Based on this data, some authors question the need for cuspal-coverage restorations in these posterior teeth. It has also been demonstrated in the laboratory that teeth with mesio-occlusodistal (MOD) preparations can be strengthened to match the values achieved by unprepared teeth if bonded restorations are placed.[30,41,53,66,76,91] In a retrospective clinical study, Kanca[34] reported a high clinical success rate in restoring endodontically treated posterior teeth with resin composite restorations.

Other laboratory studies, however, have indicated that MOD resin composite restorations in maxillary premolars have no more strengthening effect than similar MOD unbonded amalgam restorations.[32,33] In a retrospective clinical study, Hansen[26] compared the long-term efficacy of composite resin and amalgam in the restoration of endodontically treated premolars. During the first 3 years, teeth restored with amalgam had a greater incidence of cuspal fracture. However, in years 3 through 10, fractures occurred with approximately the same frequency in both groups.

In the face of confusing and contradictory data, it is difficult for the practitioner to develop a treatment philosophy with a sound scientific basis. It seems clear that in wider preparations the strengthening effect of the bonded composite restoration is real. However, it has been shown that the strengthening effect diminishes significantly with both thermal cycling[17] and functional loading[19] of the restoration. Because both of these phenomena occur in the oral environment, the long-term strengthening effect of the intracoronal bonded restoration must be questioned. It has also been proposed that a portion of the sensory feedback mechanism is lost when the neurovascular tissue has been removed from the tooth in the course of endodontic therapy. This effect has been confirmed in an in vivo study.[65] The clinical significance is that, having an impaired sensory feedback mechanism, the patient can inadvertently bite harder on an endodontically treated tooth than on a vital tooth (Figs 12-21a and 12-21b).

Both clinical[78] and laboratory studies[28] have demonstrated that the key element in the successful restoration of endodontically treated posterior teeth is the placement of a cuspal-coverage restoration. Although the intracoronal bonded restoration is appealing, based on the current data, the most prudent course of action is to place a restoration that covers all cusps. This can be one of a wide variety of restorations, including metal or ceramometal crowns and metal or ceramic onlays.

References

1. Assif D, Bliecher S. Retention of serrated endodontic posts with a composite luting agent: Effect of cement thickness. J Prosthet Dent 1986;56:689-691.

2. Bourgeois RS, Lemon RR. Dowel space preparation and apical leakage. J Endod 1981;7:66-69.

3. Boyarsky H, Davis R. Root fracture with dentin-retained posts. Am J Dent 1992;5:11-14.

4. Brown JD, Mitchem JC. Retentive properties of dowel post systems. Oper Dent 1987;12:15-19.

5. Burgess JO, Summitt JB, Robbins JW. The resistance to tensile, compression, and torsional forces provided by four post systems. J Prosthet Dent 1992;68:899-903.

6. Burns DA, Krause WR, Douglas HB, Burns DR. Stress distribution surrounding endodontic posts. J Prosthet Dent 1990;64:412-418.

7. Caputo AA, Hokama SN. Stress and retention properties of a new threaded endodontic post. Quintessence Int 1987;18:431-435.

8. Carter JM, Sorensen SE, Johnson RR, Teitelbaum RL, Levin MS. Punch shear testing of extracted vital and endodontically treated teeth. J Biomech 1983;16:841-848.

9. Chan RW, Bryant RW. Post-core foundations for endodontically treated posterior teeth. J Prosthet Dent 1982;48:401-406.

10. Chapman KKKW, Worley JL, von Fraunhofer JA. Retention of prefabricated posts by cements and resins. J Prosthet Dent 1985;54:649-652.

11. Christian GW, Button GL, Moon PC, England MC, Douglas HB. Post core restoration in endodontically treated posterior teeth. J Endod 1981;7:182-185.

12. Colley IT, Hampson EL, Lehman ML. Retention of post crowns. Br Dent J 1968;124:63-69.

13. Cooley R, Robbins J, Barnwell S. Stability of glass ionomer used as a core material. J Prosthet Dent 1990;64:651-653.

14. Cooney JP, Caputo AA, Trabert KC. Retention and stress distribution of tapered-end endodontic posts. J Prosthet Dent 1986;55:540-546.

15. Deutsch AS, Musikant BL, Cavallari J, Silverstein L, Lepley J, Ohlen K, Lesser M. Root fracture during insertion of prefabricated posts related to root size. J Prosthet Dent 1985;53:782-789.

16. Dickey DJ, Harris GZ, Lemon RR, Luebke RG. Effect of post space preparation on apical seal using solvent techniques and Peeso reamers. J Endod 1982;8:351-354.

17. Eakle WS. Effect of thermal cycling on fracture strength and microleakage in teeth restored with a bonded composite resin. Dent Mater 1986;2:114-117.

18. Felton DA, Webb EL, Kanoy BE, Dugoni J. Threaded endodontic dowels: Effects of post design on incidence of root fracture. J Prosthet Dent 1991;65:179-187.

19. Fissore B, Nicholls JI, Yuodelis RA. Load fatigue of teeth restored by a dentin bonding agent and a posterior composite resin. J Prosthet Dent 1991;65:80-85.

20. Goldman M, DeVitre R, Tenca J. Cement distribution and bond strength in cemented posts. J Dent Res 1984;63:1392-1395.

21. Goldman M, De Vitre R, White R, Nathonson D. An SEM study of posts cemented with an unfilled resin. J Dent Res 1984;63:1003-1005.

22. Goldstein GR, Hudis SI, Weintraub DE. Comparison of four techniques for cementation of posts. J Prosthet Dent 1986;55:209-211.

23. Greenfeld RS, Roydhouse RH, Marshall FJ, Schoner B. A comparison of two post systems under applied compressive shear loads. J Prosthet Dent 1989;61:17-24.

24. Gross MJ, Turner CH. Intra-radicular hydrostatic pressure changes during the cementation of post-retained crowns. J Oral Rehabil 1983;10:237-249.

25. Guzy GE, Nichols JI. In vitro comparison of intact endodontically treated teeth with and without endo-post reinforcement. J Prosthet Dent 1979;42:39-44.

26. Hansen EK. In vivo cusp fracture of endodontically treated premolars restored with MOD amalgam or MOD resin fillings. Dent Mater 1988;4:169-173.

27. Helfer AR, Melnick S, Schilder H. Determination of moisture content of vital and pulpless teeth. Oral Surg Oral Med Oral Pathol 1972;34:661-670.

28. Hoag EP, Dwyer TG. A comparative evaluation of three post and core techniques. J Prosthet Dent 1982;47:177-181.

29. Huysmans MC, Van Der Varst PG, Schafer R, Peters MC, Plasschaert AJ, Soltesz U. Fatigue behavior of direct post and core restored premolars. J Dent Res 1992;71:1145-1150.

30. Jensen ME, Redford DA, Williams BT, Gardner F. Posterior etched-porcelain restorations: An in vitro study. Compend Contin Educ Dent 1987;8:615-622.

31. Johnson JK, Sakamura JS. Dowel form and tensile force. J Prosthet Dent 1978;40:645-649.

32. Joynt RB, Wieczkowski G, Klockowoski R, Davis EL. Effects of composite restorations on resistance to cuspal fracture in posterior teeth. J Prosthet Dent 1987;57:431-435.

33. Joynt RB, Davis EL, Wieczkowski GJ, Williams DA. Fracture resistance of posterior teeth restored with glass ionomer–composite resin systems. J Prosthet Dent 1989;62:28-31.

34. Kanca J. Conservative resin restoration of endodontically treated teeth. Quintessence Int 1988;19:25-28.

35. Kane J, Burgess JO. Modification of the resistance form of amalgam coronal-radicular restorations. J Prosthet Dent 1991;65:470-474.

36. Kantor ME, Pines MS. A comparative study of restorative techniques for pulpless teeth. J Prosthet Dent 1977;38:405-412.

37. Kern SB, von Fraunhofer JA, Mueninghoff LA. An in vitro comparison of two dowel and core techniques for endodontically treated molars. J Prosthet Dent 1984;51:509-514.

38. Kovarik RE, Breeding LC, Caughman WF. Fatigue life of three core materials under simulated chewing conditions. J Prosthet Dent 1992;68:584-590.

39. Krupp JD, Caputo AA, Trabert KC, Standlee JP. Dowel retention with glass ionomer cement. J Prosthet Dent 1979;41:163-166.

40. Kwan EH, Harrington GW. The effect of immediate post preparation on apical seal. J Endod 1981;7:325-329.

41. Landy NA, Simonsen RJ. Cusp fracture strength in class 2 composite resin restorations [abstract 39]. J Dent Res 1984;63:175.

42. Lattner ML. Fracture Resistance of Five Core Materials for Cast Crowns. [thesis]. San Antonio, TX: University of Texas, 1994.

43. Libman W, Nicholls J. Load fatigue of teeth restored with cast posts and cores and complete crowns. Int J Prosthet 1995;2:155-161.

44. Lloyd CH, Adamson M. The development of fracture toughness and fracture strength in posterior restorative materials. Dent Mater 1987;3:225-231.

45. Lovdahl PE, Nicholls JO. Pin-retained amalgam cores vs. cast-gold dowel cores. J Prosthet Dent 1977;38:507-514.

46. Madison S, Zakariasen KL. Linear and volumetric analysis of apical leakage in teeth prepared for posts. J Endod 1984;10:422-427.

47. Maniatopolous C, Pilliar RM, Smith DC. Evaluation of shear strength at the cement endodontic post interface. J Prosthet Dent 1988;59:662-669.

48. Maryniuk GA, Shen C, Young HM. Effects of canal lubrication on retention of cemented posts. J Am Dent Assoc 1984;109:430-433.

49. Mattison GD. Photoelastic stress analysis of cast-gold endodontic posts. J Prosthet Dent 1982;48:407-411.

50. Mattison GD, von Fraunhofer JA. Angulation loading effects on cast-gold endodontic posts: A photoelastic stress analysis. J Prosthet Dent 1983;49:636-638.

51. Mattison GD, Delivanis PD, Thacker RW, Hassell KT. Effect of post preparation on the apical seal. J Prosthet Dent 1984;51:785-789.

52. Moll JFP, Howe DF, Svare CW. Cast gold post and core and pin-retained composite resin bases: A comparative study in strength. J Prosthet Dent 1978;40:642-644.

53. Morin D, DeLong R, Douglas WH. Cusp reinforcement by the acid-etch technique. J Dent Res 1984;63:1075-1078.

54. Nasr HH, Eskander ME, Zake AM. The luting efficacy of cements in bonding dowels of different metals. Egypt Dent J 1987;33:155-171.

55. Nathanson D. New views on restoring the endodontically treated tooth. Dental Economics 1993;August:48-50.

56. Nayyar A, Walton RE. An amalgam coronal radicular dowel and core technique for endodontically treated posterior teeth. J Prosthet Dent 1980;44:511-515.

57. Neagley RL. The effect of dowel preparation on apical seal of endodontically treated teeth. Oral Surg Oral Med Oral Pathol 1969;28:739-745.

58. Newburg RE, Pameijer CH. Retentive properties of post and core systems. J Prosthet Dent 1976;36:636-643.

59. Nourian L, Burgess JO. Tensile load to remove cemented posts cemented with different surface treatments [abstract 1788]. J Dent Res 1994;73:325.

60. Oliva RA, Lowe JA. Dimensional stability of silver amalgam and composite used as core materials. J Prosthet Dent 1987;57:554-559.

61. Paschal JE, Burgess JO. Tensile load to remove posts cemented with different cements [abstract 1362]. J Dent Res 1995;74:182.

62. Plasmans PJJM, Visseren LGH, Vrijhoef MMMA, Kayser FA. In vitro comparison of dowel and core techniques for endodontically treated molars. J Endod 1986;12:382-387.

63. Portell FR, Bernier WE, Lorton L, Peters DD. The effect of immediate versus delayed dowel space preparation on the integrity of the apical seal. J Endod 1982;8:154-160.

64. Radke RA Barkhordar RA, Podesta RE. Retention of cast endodontic posts: Comparison of cementing agents. J Prosthet Dent 1988;59:318-320.

65. Randow K, Glantz P. On cantilever loading of vital and non-vital teeth. Acta Odontol Scand 1986;44:271-277.

66. Reeh ES, Douglas WH, Messer HH. Stiffness of endodontically treated teeth related to restoration technique [abstract 1510]. J Dent Res 1988;67:301.

67. Reeh ES. Reduction in tooth stiffness as a result of endodontic restorative procedures. J Endod 1989;15:512-516.

68. Richer JB, Lautenschlager EP, Greener EH. Mechanical properties of post and core systems. Dent Mater 1986;2:63-66.

69. Robbins JW, Burgess JO, Summitt JB. Retention and resistance features for complex amalgam restorations. J Am Dent Assoc 1989;118:437-442.

70. Robbins JW. Guidelines for the restoration of endodontically treated teeth. J Am Dent Assoc 1990;120:558-566.

71. Robbins JW, Earnest L, Schumann S. Fracture resistance of endodontically treated cuspids: An in vitro study. Am J Dent 1993;6:159-161.

72. Ross RS, Nicholls JI, Harrington GW. A comparison of strains generated during placement of five endodontic posts. J Endod 1991;17:450-456.

73. Ruemping DR, Lund MR, Schnell RJ. Retention of dowels subjected to tensile and torsional forces. J Prosthet Dent 1979;41:159-162.

74. Schnell FJ. Effect of immediate dowel space preparation on the apical seal of endodontically filled teeth. Oral Surg Oral Med Oral Pathol 1978;45:470-474.

75. Sedgley CM, Messer HH. Are endodontically treated teeth more brittle? J Endod 1992;18:332-335.

76. Share J, Mishell Y, Nathanson S. Effect of restorative material on resistance to fracture of tooth structure in vitro [abstract 622]. J Dent Res 1982;61:247.

77. Sorensen JA, Martinoff JT. Clinically significant factors in dowel design. J Prosthet Dent 1984;52:28-35.

78. Sorensen JA, Martinoff JT. Intracoronal reinforcement and coronal coverage: A study of endodontically treated teeth. J Prosthet Dent 1984;51:780-784.

79. Sorensen JA, Martinoff JT. Endodontically treated teeth as abutments. J Prosthet Dent 1985;53:631-636.

80. Sorensen JA, Engelman MJ, Mito WT. Effect of ferrule design on fracture resistance of pulpless teeth [abstract 142]. J Dent Res 1988;67:130.

81. Stampalia LL, Nicholls, JI, Brudvik JS. Fracture resistance of teeth with resin-bonded restorations. J Prosthet Dent 1986;55:694-698.

82. Standlee JP, Caputo AA, Collard EW, Pollack MH. Analysis of stress distribution by endodontic posts. Oral Surg Oral Med Oral Pathol 1972;33:952-960.

83. Standlee JP, Caputo AA, Hanson EC. Retention of endodontic dowels: Effects of cement, dowel length, diameter, and design. J Prosthet Dent 1978;39:401-405.

84. Starr C. Management of periodontal tissues for restorative dentistry. J Esthet Dent 1991;3:195-208.

85. Suchina JA, Ludington JR. Dowel space preparation and the apical seal. J Endod 1985;11:11-17.

86. Thorsteinsson TS, Yaman P, Craig RG. Stress analyses of four prefabricated posts. J Prosthet Dent 1992;67:30-33.

87. Tjan AHL, Whang SB. Retentive properties of some simplified dowel-core systems to cast gold dowel and core. J Prosthet Dent 1983;50:203-206.

88. Torbjorner A, Karlsson S, Odman P. Survival rate and failure characteristics for two post designs. J Prosthet Dent 1995;73:439-444.

89. Trabert KC, Caputo AA, Abou-Rass M. Tooth fracture—a comparison of endodontic and restorative treatments. J Endod 1978;4:341-345.

90. Trope M, Maltz DO, Tronstad L. Resistance to fracture of restored endodontically treated teeth. Endod Dent Traumatol 1985;1:108-111.

91. Wendt SL, Harris BM, Hunt TE. Resistance to cusp fracture in endodontically treated teeth. Dent Mater 1987;3:232-235.

92. Wong B, Utter JD, Miller BH, Ford JP, Guo IY. Retention of prefabricated posts using three different cementing procedures [abstract 1360]. J Dent Res 1995;74:181.

93. Yaman P, Zillich R. Restoring the endodontically treated bi-rooted premolar—The effect of endodontic post preparation on width of root dentin. J Mich Dental Assoc 1986;68:79-81.

94. Young HM, Shen C, Maryniuk GA. Retention of cast posts relative to cement selection. Quintessence Int 1985;16:357-360.

95. Zakhary SY, Nasr HH. In vitro assissment of intact endodontically treated anterior teeth with different restorative procedures. Egypt Dent J 1986;32:221-239.

96. Zillich R, Yaman P. Effect of root curvature on post length in restoration of endodontically treated premolars. Endod Dent Traumatol 1985;1:135-137.

Impressions and Provisional (Temporary) Restorations

Richard S. Schwartz

Once the teeth are prepared for indirect restorations it is necessary to produce a replica of the arch that can be used in the laboratory to make the restoration. The tissue is retracted, and an impression is made and poured in an improved dental stone. Provisional or temporary restorations must be made to protect the prepared teeth and maintain their positions in the arch while the permanent restorations are fabricated.

Soft Tissue Management

Tissue management refers to the maintenance of soft tissue health during preparation, impression, and provisionalization procedures. All clinical procedures should be performed with minimal soft tissue trauma. Healthy tissue makes every clinical step easier and produces a superior end result. Every effort should be made to avoid lacerating the soft tissue during tooth preparation, and the finish lines should be kept out of the sulcus whenever possible. If this is not possible, the gingiva should be retracted for final preparation of the finish lines. Gingival damage makes impression and provisionalization procedures more difficult and may result in permanent deformities of the soft tissue (Fig 13-1).

Surgical Management

Tissue management sometimes involves periodontal surgery. If crown margins extend deep into the sulcus because of caries, fracture, or previous restorations, crown lengthening may be indicated.

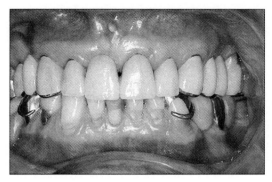

Fig 13-1 Poor tissue management may result in recession and permanent deformities of the gingiva.

If minimal crown length must be gained, gingivectomy is a simple method to uncover subgingival finish lines. For gingivectomy to be considered, there must be adequate keratinized tissue and adequate space for biologic width requirements. This means that after the gingivectomy is completed, there must be at least 3 mm from the margin of the preparation to the alveolar crest. Also, at least 1 mm of sulcus depth must remain after the gingivectomy. If the biologic width is violated during the gingivectomy procedure, chronic inflammation will result.[35] Also, if gingivectomy creates uneven gingival heights in the anterior segment, an esthetic problem may be created.

Electrosurgery is often used to perform gingivectomies at the time of tooth preparation, because it can be done quickly and provides hemostasis.[30] It is important to remove enough tissue so that the crown margins will end at the free gingival margin or slightly into the sulcus once the tissue has healed (Figs 13-2a and 13-2b). It is also important to get a good impression on the day the elec-

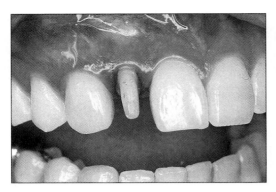

Fig 13-2a A crown preparation with subgingival finish lines is shown prior to gingivectomy.

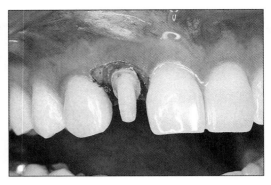

Fig 13-2b Tissue removal should be liberal when electrosurgery is used. The end result is an easy impression and crown margins located at or above the free gingival crest.

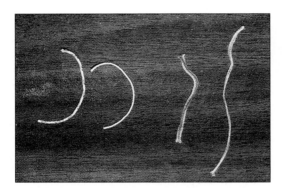

Fig 13-3 Braided and knitted cords are available to retract the gingiva.

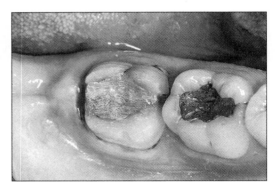

Fig 13-4 When the retraction cord is in place, all finish lines should be visible.

trosurgery is performed because the tissue will require 6 to 8 weeks of healing time. If an impression is attempted during the healing period, it will be very difficult to establish hemostasis without performing electrosurgery again.

If the clinical situation is unsuitable for gingivectomy, apically repositioned flaps may be indicated. Full-thickness flaps are reflected, bone is recontoured, if necessary, and the tissue is repositioned so that the restoration will extend only to the free gingival crest. This means positioning the bone 3 to 4 mm from the desired location for the finish lines.[35] The tissue is then allowed to heal for 3 to 6 months before final tooth preparation and impressions are completed. This is usually the preferred method of crown lengthening.

Gingival Retraction

In most cases, it is necessary to retract the gingiva before a master impression is made. The most common method of gingival retraction utilizes chemically impregnated

cord, usually braided or knitted, which contains an astringent chemical to minimize bleeding and flow of the sulcular fluid (Fig 13-3). Some cords are also impregnated with epinephrine. Epinephrine provides little or no benefit, however, and should generally be avoided, particularly in medically compromised patients.[28] Cords may be dipped in an astringent liquid such as aluminum chloride or ferric sulfate to aid in control of fluid and make placement easier.[16]

Retraction cord is pushed into the sulcus with a thin-bladed instrument, eg, a No. 1-2 plastic instrument or interproximal carver. It is left in place for several minutes to provide mechanical retraction of the gingiva in addition to its astringent effect. The cord is usually removed at the time the master impression is made. Inadequate retraction is probably the most common error that results in unsuccessful impressions. Adequate retraction means that the gingiva is clearly away from all finish lines (Fig 13-4). One useful method of retraction is to place a small cord around the tooth once, below the finish lines, and then place a larger cord on top. The larger cord is removed just before impression material is placed into the sulcus, and the smaller cord is left in the sulcus to provide retraction and hemostasis. This method is particularly helpful when bleeding is present. If the soft tissue is managed with care, little or no bleeding should be present at the time the master impression is made, and these procedures can be performed with ease.

Special care must be taken during retraction procedures if the cervical areas of prepared teeth are visible when the patient smiles. Thin, friable tissue may recede if traumatized, leaving an exposed crown margin, a situation that is esthetically unacceptable to many patients. To evaluate the risk of recession at an early appointment, the patient can be anesthetized and the bone levels can be "sounded." A thin periodontal probe is used to measure pocket depth and then is pushed through the periodontal attachment to bone. The distance from the base of the sulcus to the alveolar crest is determined. If the attachment is about 2 mm (ie, the biologic width), it is unlikely that significant recession will occur as a result of retraction procedures. If the distance is 3 mm or more, a long epithelial attachment probably exists; this is particularly susceptible to attachment loss. In this case, the finish lines should be kept supragingival, or surgical procedures should be considered to establish stable gingival levels.

Impressions

Impressions are made and cast in dental stone for a variety of purposes. The intended use for the cast usually determines the type of impression material and the type of stone that should be used.

Hydrocolloid Impression Materials

Irreversible Hydrocolloid

Irreversible hydrocolloid (alginate) is most commonly used to make impressions for diagnostic and opposing casts. Several procedures can be used to maximize the quality of casts made from alginate impressions. It is advisable to use preweighed or prepackaged alginate and measure the amount of water used to get consistent and repeatable characteristics of the mixed material. An adhesive should always be placed on the tray. This is true for all impression materials. Even with perforated or rim-lock trays the impression material will pull away from the tray in some areas if adhesive is not used.[3] Vacuum mixing will produce a smooth, thorough mix that is

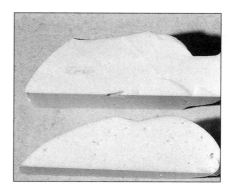

Fig 13-5 Vacuum-mixed alginate *(top)* is less porous than hand-mixed alginate *(bottom)*.

notably less porous than hand-mixed alginate (Fig 13-5). Because alginate does not flow well and traps air easily, material should be placed into critical areas with a finger or syringe before the tray is seated in the mouth.

The alginate impression should be poured as soon as possible, preferably within 10 minutes. A two-step technique should be used. The impression should be disinfected,[7,19] poured in vacuum-mixed stone, and allowed to set with the impression on the bottom (the first step). A separate mix of stone should be used to make a base after the initial set of the first pour (the second step). The cast should be separated from the impression once the exothermic setting reaction of the stone is completed, or at least within about 60 minutes. Aluminum sulfate solution, sprayed on the alginate after disinfection and prior to pouring, dramatically improves the surface quality of the stone cast. It is a recommended procedure for "important" alginate impressions.[40]

Reversible Hydrocolloid

Reversible hydrocolloid is used clinically for master impressions for fixed restorations and in the laboratory for duplicating casts. It is a firm gel at room temperature that is liquefied in a warm water bath prior to use. The warmed material is injected into the sulcus and loaded into a special stock tray, which is seated in the mouth and cooled by attached water lines.

Reversible hydrocolloid has several advantages. It is a tasteless, odorless material that sets quickly with minimal mess. It is also the least expensive impression method. The impression should be poured within minutes, however, and cannot be repoured. Reversible hydrocolloid has also been used in combination with irreversible hydrocolloid for master impressions.[25]

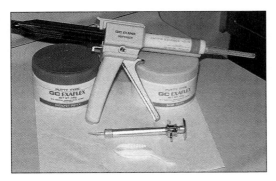

Fig 13-6 Addition silicone material is available in automix cartridges. Jars of putty materials are also shown.

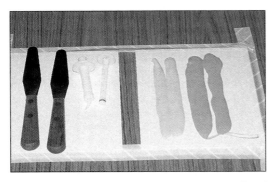

Fig 13-7a When impression materials are hand mixed, use of two pads and two spatulas is recommended. The material is mixed on the first pad with the first spatula. It is then transferred to the second pad, and mixing is completed with the second spatula. Mixing is completed when a uniform, streak-free mix is obtained.

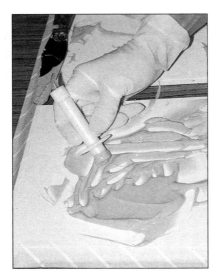

Fig 13-7b Once mixing is completed on the second pad, the material is loaded into the syringe and tray.

Elastomeric Impression Materials

Elastomeric impression materials are the materials most commonly used to make impressions for master casts. These materials are more accurate than alginate and have better detail reproduction and better tear resistance. In addition, some elastomeric materials allow delayed pouring and can be repoured several times without a significant loss of accuracy.[24] Some materials come in automix cartridges that allow injection of material directly into a tray or syringe or intraorally (Fig 13-6). Others must be hand mixed (Figs 13-7a and 13-7b).

When a master impression is made for a fixed restoration, the tissue is retracted, the impression material is mixed, retraction cord is removed from the sulcus, and light-bodied material is injected into the retracted sulcus. At this point, some clinicians gently blow a stream of air over the syringed light-bodied material to push it farther into the sulcus. In most instances, a high-viscosity material or putty is placed into an impression tray, which is seated in the mouth immediately after the light-bodied material is in place. Once the material has set, it is removed from the mouth and later poured in an improved dental stone. The clinical steps are shown in Figs 13-8a to 13-8d.

All current classes of elastomeric impression materials possess good physical properties and can be used successfully in clinical practice.[39] The most commonly used materials are discussed next.

Polysulfide Rubber

Polysulfide rubber is usually used as a dual-viscosity material. The low-viscosity (light-body) material is injected into the sulcus, and a high-viscosity (heavy-body) material is placed into the tray. A custom tray, made ahead of time, is recommended[20] to provide a uniform 2- to 3-mm thickness of material.[18] Polysulfide is an accurate material that has a long history of success. It has an extended working time, which is desirable when impressions are made of multiple tooth preparations.

Polysulfide rubber also has several undesirable characteristics. It is not available in automix cartridges and, therefore, must be hand mixed. It must be poured within about 30 minutes to minimize distortion, and should not be repoured. It also has an unpleasant taste and smell and a long setting time.

Addition Silicone

Addition silicone, or poly(vinyl siloxane), materials currently dominate the elastomeric market. They were developed in the 1970s and improved in the 1980s.[9] The initial materials were hydrophobic, making them diffi-

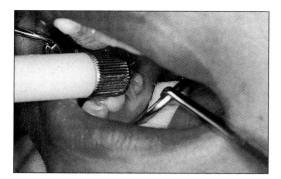

Fig 13-8a When the light-bodied material is injected, a second assistant is helpful in retracting the patient's tongue and cheeks.

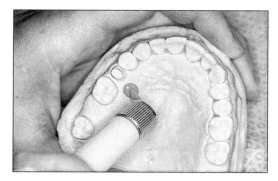

Fig 13-8b The initial injection of the light-bodied material should be directed slightly away from the sulcus.

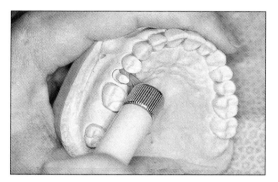

Fig 13-8c The bead of material should flow out of the sulcus ahead of the syringe tip in a smooth, continuous motion around the tooth. The syringe tip should not stop or backtrack.

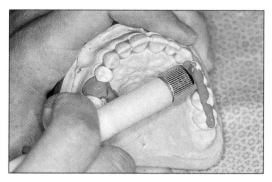

Fig 13-8d Once the preparation is completely covered with material, it is advisable to inject light-bodied material onto the other occlusal surfaces to produce sharp, bubble-free occluding surfaces in the cast.

cult to pour, and were very rigid. Current materials are more flexible and contain a surfactant that makes them easier to pour without bubbles.[38] The low-viscosity material is used as a "wash" material, to capture fine detail, such as finish lines and occlusal anatomy. The other viscosities are usually used to fill the tray, although the medium-viscosity material is sometimes used interchangeably with the low-viscosity material. Some of the addition silicone materials utilize a putty rather than a high-viscosity material.

The putty may be used in a one-step or two-step technique. In the one-step method, the freshly mixed putty is put in the tray at the time of the impression. In the two-step method, putty is used to line a stock tray ahead of time, by using a spacer on a study cast. The final impression is then made with the low-viscosity material and the putty-lined stock tray. If done correctly, both methods produce satisfactory results.[14,23,34] Care should be taken to capture areas of fine detail in the light-body material rather than the putty. If the putty shows

through when the "two-step" method is used, accuracy is compromised and the impression must be remade.

Addition silicone materials may be hand mixed but are more commonly dispensed in automix cartridges, which are easier to use and produce fewer voids.[5] The materials are tasteless and odorless and have a short setting time. Impressions should be poured within a week, and may be repoured multiple times.[24] Some of the materials release hydrogen gas for a period after initial set (Fig 13-9). For those materials, delayed pouring is necessary. Some addition silicone materials contain hydrogen-absorbing additives and may be poured immediately. Most latex gloves leave a residue on the teeth and oral surfaces that inhibits the set of addition silicone materials (Figs 13-10a and 13-10b). This is not a problem when vinyl gloves are used.[26]

Polyether

Most polyether materials are single-viscosity systems that must be hand mixed. Once manufacturer now mar-

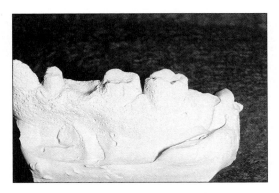

Fig 13-9 The extensive porosity in this cast was the result of hydrogen gas released from an addition silicone impression that was poured immediately.

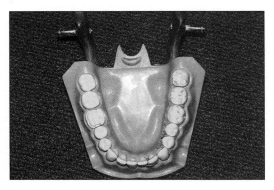

Fig 13-10a Many latex gloves leave a residue that inhibits the polymerization of addition silicone materials. This typodont was touched on the left side with latex gloves prior to a complete-arch impression.

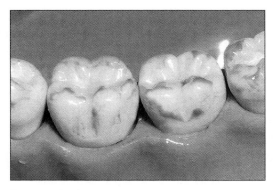

Fig 13-10b Evidence that the impression material did not completely polymerize: Unset material remains on the teeth after the impression is removed.

kets an electric-powered mixing machine (Pentamix, ESPE Premiere). Polyether material may be used with a custom or stock tray, but, because the material is quite rigid, more tray relief is necessary than with polysulfide rubber. If tray relief is insufficient, impressions are difficult to remove from the mouth and to separate from the master cast without breaking the stone, even with the less rigid polyether materials.[8] Polyether materials are accurate and stable, have a short setting time, and have the best wettability of the elastomeric materials,[36] making them the easiest to pour. The main disadvantage of polyether is the bitter, unpleasant taste.

Photoinitiated Materials

Photoinitiated elastomeric impression materials are available; they have good physical, mechanical, and clinical properties and a long working time.[10] They may be placed and light polymerized in segments.

Dual-Arch Impressions

The dual-arch technique utilizes a quadrant tray (Fig 13-11a) that records both arches in one impression and also acts as a jaw relation record (Fig 13-11b). The impression is poured on both sides and mounted in a hinge articulator (Fig 13-11c). Once mounted, the casts are separated from the impression. The mounted casts provide an accurate recording of the maximum intercuspation position of the teeth but do not accurately reproduce other jaw positions. Dual-arch impressions are recommended when there are one or two restorations that are not involved in the lateral guidance of the occlusion. Eccentric contacts, if present, must be adjusted intraorally, usually a relatively easy task if there are only one or two restorations. With more than two units, the difficulty of making intraoral adjustments greatly increases, so this technique is not recommended for more than two units.

A rigid impression material must be used with this technique, because the tray and interocclusal mesh provide little support. Polyether or rigid addition silicone materials are preferred. It is reported that dies from dual-arch impressions are as accurate as those from impressions made with a custom tray.[12,13,41]

Disinfection of Impressions

Impressions have been identified as carriers of pathogens that can be transmitted to dental personnel or other patients.[32] Because of this, recommendations have been made regarding the handling of impressions.[2,7,19]

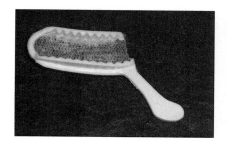

Fig 13-11a A dual-arch impression tray.

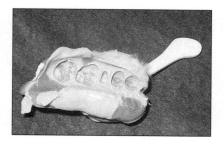

Fig 13-11b A rigid impression material, such as addition silicone or polyether, should be used for dual-arch impressions.

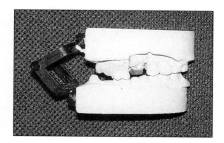

Fig 13-11c Casts from a dual-arch impression are mounted on a hinge articulator.

Impressions should be disinfected by spray or immersion in a disinfectant accepted by the American Dental Association before they are sent to the laboratory. Chlorine-based solutions are reported to be the disinfectants of choice for impressions.[22,31,33,42,46] Some alginate impression materials and some dental stones that contain disinfectants are available.[17]

Provisional (Temporary) Restorations

Provisional restorations are cemented on the teeth after tooth preparation and remain in place while the permanent restorations are fabricated. Provisional restorations serve several functions. They protect the underlying prepared tooth structure from chemical, thermal, and biologic insult that might cause pulpal damage and discomfort for the patient. In many cases, they provide temporary esthetic replacement for missing teeth or tooth structure. They should provide occlusal function and stability to both arches from solid occlusal and interproximal contacts and should maintain the health of the periodontium. They should fit well, be highly polished, and have toothlike morphology with open embrasures.[44]

Provisional restorations may also be used as aids in diagnosis and patient evaluation. They may be used to aid in the determination of width, length, and position of teeth in esthetic areas. They can be made to close or open interproximal spaces, move the midline, change the occlusal scheme, determine pontic design, or alter the vertical dimension of occlusion. If major changes are planned, the desired end result can be created in a diagnostic waxup from which the provisional restorations can be made. The patients can then "try out" provisional restorations that are similar to the planned permanent restorations.

Clinical Procedures

Provisional restorations may be made with a direct technique, on the prepared teeth,[27] or with an indirect technique, on a cast.[11] They may be made with preformed metal or resin crowns, or with a matrix and autocured resin material.[21]

Direct Techniques. Single-tooth provisional restorations are often made directly on the prepared tooth with a relined acrylic resin or metal crown form. Prefabricated soft metal or stainless steel shells are commonly used for posterior teeth. They may be trimmed and the margins crimped with a pliers so that the crown margins are well adapted to the finish lines of the preparation, and occlusal and interproximal contacts are present. The shell may be cemented with a thick mix of temporary cement or may be relined with acrylic resin to improve the marginal fit. The latter method is preferred if the provisional restorations will be in place for more than a few days. Fabrication of a soft metal shell provisional crown is shown in Figs 13-12a to 13-12c.

Pre-made resin crown forms are most commonly used for single anterior provisional restorations. The margins are trimmed with a bur made especially for acrylic resin to approximate the finish lines of the preparation. The shell is then relined with an acrylic resin or resin composite reline material directly on the tooth. The provisional restoration is removed from the mouth shortly before final set and allowed to complete polymerization. Excess material is then trimmed away from the margins, occlusion is adjusted, and the provisional restoration is polished and cemented. Fabrication of a polycarbonate provisional crown is shown in Figs 13-13a to 13-13f.

Provisional restorations may also be made of autopolymerizing acrylic with the aid of a matrix.[43] The matrix can be made on a preoperative cast, directly on the unprepared teeth, or on a stone cast of a diagnostic

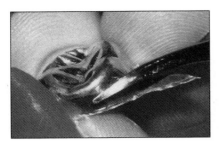

Fig 13-12a A metal shell crown may be used for single-tooth provisional restorations. The gingival margins are trimmed to the shape of the finish lines.

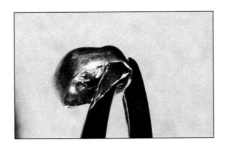

Fig 13-12b The margins are adapted with a pliers.

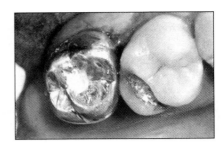

Fig 13-12c A provisional metal shell crown is shown after cementation.

waxup. The matrix can be made with wax or silicone putty, or a thin acrylic resin shell can be made in the laboratory. The matrix is filled with autopolymerizing resin, placed over the prepared teeth, and removed just before final set. Once polymerization is completed, the provisional restoration is trimmed, adjusted, polished, and cemented. Provisional restorations made with a matrix may have to be relined,[1] depending on the material used. Direct fabrication of a provisional crown from a silicone matrix is shown in Figs 13-14a to 13-14d.

Indirect Technique. Provisional restorations may also be made indirectly on a cast of the prepared teeth, through a process similar to the direct technique. The indirect process has several benefits.[11] Indirect provisional restorations reduce or eliminate the need to put unpleasant materials in the patient's mouth and minimize the possibility of hard and soft tissue damage (Fig 13-15). They can be made in the laboratory by a technician or assistant while master impressions are being made and can be polymerized under pressure, which improves their strength and hardness.[15] Indirect fabrication of the acrylic resin provisional crowns is shown in Figs 13-16a to 13-16f.

Provisional Materials

Many tooth-colored resin materials are available for provisional restorations, but only a few are commonly used.[6,45]

Poly(methyl methacrylate)

Poly(methyl methacrylate) has a long track record of successful use. It has satisfactory strength, color stability, and wear resistance for short or medium time periods,

and its properties can be improved if polymerization is allowed to occur under pressure or vacuum. It has several disadvantages, however. Fabrication of direct provisional restorations can result in tissue damage from the monomer, which is relatively caustic, or from the exothermic polymerization reaction. Poly(methyl methacrylate) resins generate the most heat of the provisional materials.[37] They exhibit the greatest amount of polymerization shrinkage, which affects marginal fit and may prevent complete seating of the restoration.[1]

Poly(ethyl methacrylate)

Poly(ethyl methacrylate) is less popular than poly(methyl methacrylate) because it is less color stable and is not as wear resistant or strong.[29] It is preferred by some clinicians, however, because it generates less heat during polymerization and shrinks less.

Bis-acryl

Bis-acryl is a combination of resin composite and acrylic resin, an attempt to take advantage of the desirable properties of both materials. It has good color stability and strength, produces little heat, exhibits little shrinkage, and may be repaired with a light-activated resin. Some bis-acryls are unesthetic, however, and are somewhat brittle and therefore subject to bulk fracture. Many of the newer provisional materials are bis-acryls.

Filled Resins

Resin composite materials with light-, auto- or dual-curing capabilities are available. Their physical properties are similar to those of the bis-acryls. Esthetics and accurate fit are the main advantages of the resin composites. They are the most esthetic of the provisional materials, but are brittle and subject to bulk fracture.

Figs 13-13a to 13-13f Preformed acrylic resin shells may be used as provisional restorations.

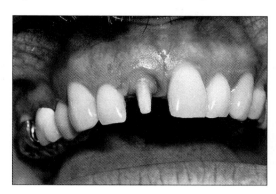

Fig 13-13a A prepared central incisor is ready for a provisional restoration.

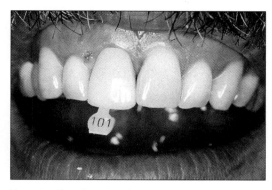

Fig 13-13b A polycarbonate shell crown of the correct mesiodistal dimension is chosen and adjusted to approximate the finish lines. It is now ready to be relined.

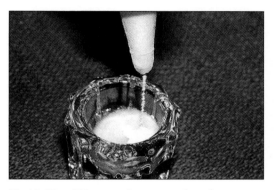

Fig 13-13c When acrylic resin is the reline material, it may be mixed in a Dappen dish. The liquid is dispensed first, and the powder is swirled into the liquid to the point of saturation.

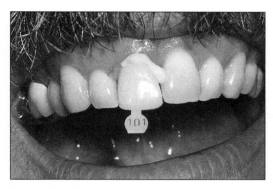

Fig 13-13d The polycarbonate crown is loaded with free-flowing acrylic resin or resin composite material and is placed on the prepared tooth.

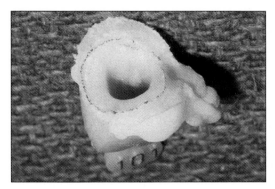

Fig 13-13e When the reline material is nearly polymerized, the restoration is removed from the tooth and polymerization is completed outside of the mouth. Once set, the margins may be marked with a pencil to aid in trimming excess reline material.

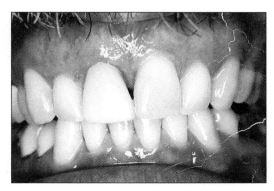

Fig 13-13f The finished provisional restoration is in place.

Figs 13-14a to 13-14d   A matrix, made from a preoperative cast, may be used to make provisional restorations.

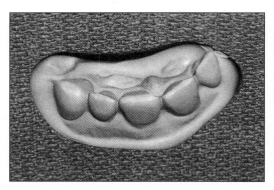

Fig 13-14a   An addition silicone matrix is made on a preoperative cast.

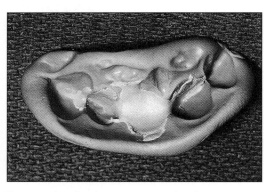

Fig 13-14b   Acrylic resin is mixed and placed in the matrix, which is placed in the mouth and removed just before final set.

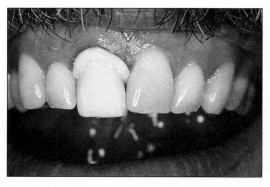

Fig 13-14c   Excess acrylic resin is trimmed away. Sometimes a provisional restoration made with this method will have to be relined.

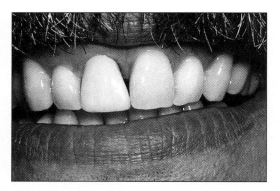

Fig 13-14d   The provisional restoration is trimmed, polished, and placed on the prepared tooth.

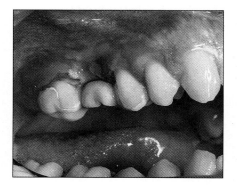

Fig 13-15   Soft tissue damage may result with the matrix technique if acrylic resin is allowed to completely polymerize in the mouth. In addition, removal of the provisional restoration may be difficult because the reline material sometimes locks into voids in the preparation or undercuts in the adjacent teeth.

Thermoplastic Materials

Thermoplastic materials flow when heated and become "rubbery" when cooled to room temperature. The material is heated and injected into a matrix, which is seated in the mouth or on a prepared cast. After cooling, the matrix is removed and the material is trimmed and contoured. The provisional restoration is then light cured to achieve its final strength and hardness. Thermoplastic materials have good physical properties but are expensive and require a special heating unit.

Figs 13-16a to 13-16f Provisional restorations may also be made indirectly, on a cast.

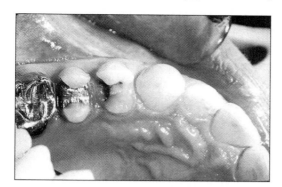

Fig 13-16a Prepared teeth are shown prior to indirect fabrication of provisional restorations.

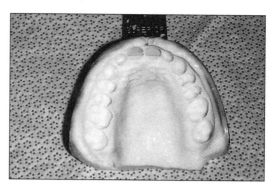

Fig 13-16b An alginate impression is made of the preparations and poured in fast-setting stone.

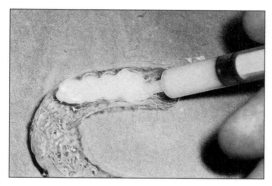

Fig 13-16c A clear matrix is made ahead of time from a preoperative cast or diagnostic waxup. The shell is loaded with provisional material.

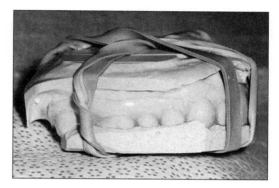

Fig 13-16d The loaded acrylic shell is then placed on the cast and may be polymerized in a pressure pot. This results in a dense, strong provisional restoration.

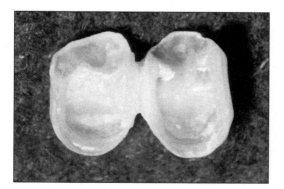

Fig 13-16e The provisional restorations are recovered, trimmed, and polished.

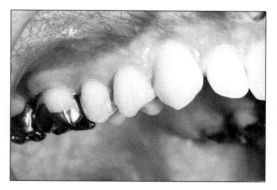

Fig 13-16f The provisional restorations are cemented in place.

References

1. Barghi N, Simmons EW. The marginal integrity of the temporary acrylic resin crown. J Prosthet Dent 1976;36:274-277.

2. Bergman B. Disinfection of prosthodontic impression materials: A Literature Review. Int J Prosthodont 1989;2:537-542.

3. Bomberg TJ, Goldfogel MH, Hoffman W. Considerations for adhesion of impression materials to impression trays. J Prosthet Dent 1988;60:681-684.

4. Chee WWL, Donovan TE. Fine detail reproduction of very high viscosity poly(vinyl siloxane) impression materials. Int J Prosthodont 1989;2:369-370.

5. Chong Y, Soh G, Wilkens JL. The effect of mixing method on void formation in elastomeric impression materials. Int J Prosthodont 1989;2:323-326.

6. Christensen GJ. Temporary restorations for fixed prosthodontics. Issue 8. Clin Res Assoc Newsletter 1988;12:1-2.

7. Council on Dental Materials, Instruments, and Equipment. Infection control recommendations for the dental office and dental laboratory. J Am Dent Assoc 1988;116:241-248.

8. Craig RG. Great impressions. Dent Advisor 1986;3:1-6.

9. Craig RG. Review of dental impression materials. Adv Dent Res 1988;2:51-64.

10. Craig RG, Hare PH. Properties of a new polyether urethane dimethacrylate photoinitiated elastomeric impression material. J Prosthet Dent 1990;63:16-20.

11. Crispin BJ, Watson JF, Caputo AA. The marginal accuracy of treatment restorations: A comparative analysis. J Prosthet Dent 1980;44:283-290.

12. Davis RD, Schwartz RS. Dual arch and custom tray impression accuracy. Am J Dent 1991;4:89-92.

13. Davis RD, Schwartz RS, Hilton TJ. Marginal adaptation of castings made with dual-arch and custom trays. Am J Dent 1992;5:253-254.

14. DeArauyo PA, Jorgenson KD. Effect of bulk and undercuts on the accuracy of impression materials. J Prosthet Dent 1985;54:791-794.

15. Donovan TE, Hurst RG, Campagni WV. Physical properties of acrylic resin polymerized by four different techniques. J Prosthet Dent 1985;54:522-524.

16. Donovan TE, Bandara BK, Nemetz H. Review and survey of medicaments used with gingival retraction cords. J Prosthet Dent 1985;53:525-531.

17. Donovan TE, Chee WWL. Preliminary investigation of a disinfected gypsum die stone. Int J Prosthodont 1989;2:245-248.

18. Eames WB, Sieweke JC, Wallace SW, Rogers CB. Elastomeric impression materials. Effect of bulk on accuracy. J Prosthet Dent 1979;41:304-307.

19. Fan PL. Council on Dental Materials, Instruments and Equipment. Disinfection of impressions. J Am Dent Assoc 1991;122:110.

20. Gordon GE, Johnson GH, Drennon DG. The effect of tray selection on the accuracy of elastomeric impression materials. J Prosthet Dent 1986;55:1-6.

21. Haddix JE. A technique for visible light-cured provisional restorations. J Prosthet Dent 1988;59:512-514.

22. Hilton TJ, Schwartz RS, Bradley DV Jr. Immersion disinfection of irreversible hydrocolloid impressions. Part II. Effects on gypsum casts. Int J Prosthodont 1994;7:424-433.

23. Hung SH, Purk JH, Tira DE, Eick JD. Accuracy of one-step versus two-step putty wash addition silicone impression technique. J Prosthet Dent 1992;67:583-589.

24. Johnson GH, Craig RG. Accuracy of four types of rubber impression materials compared with time of pour and repeat pour of models. J Prosthetic Dent 1985;53:484-490.

25. Johnson GH, Craig RG. Accuracy and bond strength of combination agar/alginate hydrocolloid materials. J Prosthet Dent 1986;55:1-6.

26. Kahn RL, Donovan TE, Chee WWL. Interaction of gloves and rubber dam with a poly(vinyl siloxane) impression material: A screening test. Int J Prosthodont 1989;2:343-346.

27. Kaiser DA, Cavazos E. Temporization techniques in fixed prosthodontics. Dent Clin North Am 1985;29:403-412.

28. Kellam SA, Smith JR, Scheffel SJ. Epinephrine absorption from commercial gingival retraction cords in clinical patients. J Prosthet Dent 1992;68:761-765.

29. Koumjian JH, Nimmo A. Evaluations of fracture resistance of resins used for provisional restorations. J Prosthet Dent 1990;64:654-657.

30. Krejci RF, Kalkwarf KL, Krause-Hohenstein U. Electrosurgery—A biological approach. J Clin Periodontol 1987;14:557-563.

31. Langenwalter EM, Aquilino SA, Turner KA. The dimensional stability of elastomeric impression materials following disinfection. J Prosthet Dent 1990;63:270-276.

32. Leung, RL, Scholfeld SE. Gypsum casts as a potential source of microbial cross-contamination. J Prosthet Dent 1983;48:210-211.

33. Look JO, Clay DJ, Gong K, Messer JJ. Preliminary results for disinfection of irreversible hydrocolloid impressions. J Prosthet Dent 1990;63:701-707.

34. Marshak B, Assif D, Pilo R. A controlled putty-wash impression technique. J Prosthet Dent 1990;64:635-636.

35. Maynard JG, Wilson RD. Physiologic dimensions of the periodontium fundamental to successful restorative dentistry. J Periodont 1979;50:170-174.

36. McCormick JT, Anthony SJ, Dial ML, Duncanson MG, Shillingburg HT. Wettability of elastomeric impression materials: Effect of selected surfactants. Int J Prosthodont 1989;2:413-420.

37. Moulding MB, Teplitsky PE. Intrapulpal temperature during direct fabrication of provisional restorations. Int J Prosthodont 1990;3:299-304.

38. Pratten DH, Craig RG. Wettability of a hydrophillic addition silicone impression material. J Prosthet Dent 1988;61:197-202.

39. Price RB, Gerrow JD, Sutow EJ, MacSween R. The dimensional accuracy of 12 impression material and die stone combinations. Int J Prosthodont 1991;4:169-174.

40. Schwartz RS, Naylor WP. Effects of aluminum sulfate on disinfected alginate impressions [abstract 2375]. J Dent Res 1991;70:563.

41. Schwartz RS, Davis RD. Accuracy of second pour casts using dual-arch impressions. Am J Dent 1992;5:192-194.

42. Schwartz RS, Bradley DV Jr, Hilton TJ, Kruse SK. Immersion disinfection of irreversible hydrocolloid impressions. Part 1. Microbiology. Int J Prosthodont 1994;7:418-423.

43. Sotera AJ. A direct technique for fabricating acrylic resin temporary crowns using the Omnivac. J Prosthet Dent 1973;29:577-580.

44. Vahidi F. The provisional restoration. Dent Clin North Am 1987;31:363-381.

45. Wang RL, Moore BK, Goodacre CJ, Swartz ML, Andres CJ. A comparison of resins for fabricating provisional fixed restorations. Int J Prosthodont 1989;2:173-184.

46. Westerholm HS, Bradley DV, Schwartz RS. Efficacy of various disinfectants on irreversible hydrocolloid impressions. Int J Prosthodont 1992;5:47-54.

Porcelain Veneers

J. William Robbins

The porcelain veneer has gained wide acceptance in recent years as a primary restoration in esthetic dentistry. Since its introduction in the early 1980s, the porcelain veneer has undergone an evolution in both techniques and materials. Although no long-term longevity data are currently available, the 2- to 5-year data suggest that porcelain veneers are meeting the profession's expectations for esthetics and durability.[3,10,14,19]

Indications and Limitations

Porcelain veneers may be used to modify a tooth's color, shape, length or alignment, to close space, and to restore fractured and endodontically treated teeth (see Fig 12-20). The patient should be informed, however, of the possible morbidity associated with a specific indication, as well as the generally accepted limitations. Informed consent should include, but not be limited to, the following information: *(1)* lack of long-term data on longevity and the possibility of *(2)* postoperative sensitivity; *(3)* marginal discoloration; *(4)* fracture; and *(5)* wear of opposing teeth.

Treatment Planning

The patient's self-image must not be overlooked during the initial patient interview.[13] A key element in the diagnostic phase is a clarification of the patient's expectations. If it can be determined initially that the patient's expectations are unrealistically high, much future grief may be avoided.

Assessment of the Face

When a treatment plan is being developed for an esthetic dentistry case, attention must be directed not only to the shape and color of the teeth, but to the shape of the face, the smile line, and the color of the skin, lips, and hair. The teeth can be used to accentuate a positive feature or deemphasize a negative feature. For example, a patient with a narrow face may desire longer and narrower teeth if he or she wants to emphasize the facial shape. However, the patient may want to soften the narrowness of the face with shorter, rounded teeth. All of these parameters must be consciously considered during the diagnostic phase if consistently excellent results are to be obtained.

Assessment of the Smile

After the facial features have been considered, attention must be directed to the smile and its components. During the initial interview, the dentist should pay close attention to the overall appearance of the patient's mouth as he or she speaks and is in repose. The dentist should note the incisal plane in relation to the lower lip and interpupillary line, the amount of gingival display during smiling and speaking, the relationship of the anterior and posterior segments, and the overall quality of the smile. In evaluating the incisal plane, it is helpful for the dentist to pull the upper lip parallel to the interpupillary line to determine if the two planes are parallel (Fig 14-1). If the incisal plane is not acceptable, this must be determined during the diagnostic phase, or the discrepancy will commonly be incorporated into the final restorations.

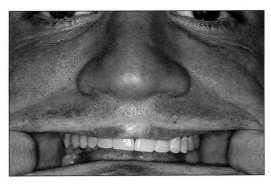

Fig 14-1 Pulling the upper lip parallel with the interpupillary line to examine the incisal plane. Note the sigmoid curve of the incisal plane.

Esthetic Guidelines

The following is a list of guidelines to assist the dentist and patient in the cocreation of a smile that is both appealing and natural. They are not rules that apply to all patients, nor must they be adhered to in all situations.

1. Natural smiles display asymmetry within symmetry. Most patients desire a smile that appears symmetric at a distance. However, closer observation should reveal small deviations from perfect symmetry, eg, notched incisal edges or slight differences in the length of the maxillary lateral incisors. Outline symmetry is essential for maxillary central incisors. As the eye moves away from the midline, outline asymmetry becomes more acceptable.

2. In a gentle smile, 3.0 to 4.0 mm of the incisal edges of the maxillary central incisors are displayed in the youthful smile, and the incisal edges of the maxillary anterior teeth are cradled by the lower lip.

3. In full smile, the upper lip should drape across the maxillary central incisors and the canines at the tooth-gingiva interface, displaying the entire clinical crown but very little marginal gingiva.

4. In full smile, the buccal corridor is almost filled with teeth. However, a minimal negative space frames the maxillary posterior teeth and is desirable.

5. The configuration of the incisal edge is dictated by personal preference. Although not supported by the literature, there is a commonly held belief that rounded edges are younger and more feminine in appearance. In contrast, square teeth and sharper angles impart a feeling of age and masculinity.

6. The long axes of maxillary anterior teeth are distally inclined. Therefore, the gingival contour of the max-

illary central and lateral incisors is not a symmetric, rounded arch form. Rather, the marginal gingiva has a parabolic shape, the high point of which is slightly distal to the midline of the tooth.

7. Interproximal contact areas move progressively more gingivally from central incisor to canine. This means that the interproximal contact between the maxillary central incisors is in the incisal third of the teeth. However, the interproximal contact between the maxillary lateral incisor and the maxillary canine is in the middle third of these teeth.

8. The incisal embrasures increase in depth from maxillary central incisor to canine. This means that the incisal embrasure between the maxillary central incisors is minimal. However, the incisal embrasure between the maxillary lateral and canine is much deeper.

9. The labial surfaces of the maxillary anterior teeth should not be highly rounded. The surfaces of the central and lateral incisors should be rather flat with resulting bold mesial and distal line angles.

10. The distoincisal line curves of the maxillary central and lateral incisors should be parallel.

11. The distal half of the maxillary canine should not be visible when viewed from the front.

12. Natural incisal edges in adults are not rounded faciolingually, but rather display a sharp incisofacial line angle as a result of wear. The incisal edges of mandibular incisors should not be flat. This imparts an aged look. If there is significant wear on the incisal edges, the mandibular incisors should be shortened enough during preparation to allow the porcelain veneer to display a natural incisal edge rather than a flat surface.

13. Normal incisal edge wear of the maxillary incisors commonly imparts a white opaque "halo effect" at the incisal edge that frames the incisal translucency.

14. The maxillary incisal plane should be parallel to the interpupillary line.

15. In an anteroposterior plane, the buccal cusp tips of the maxillary teeth should be a continuation of the anterior smile line.

16. The average length of the maxillary central incisor from gingival crest to incisal edge in the middle-aged patient is 10.7 mm for men and 9.6 mm for women. The average width of the central incisor is 9.1 mm for men and 8.2 for women. It is difficult, if not impossible, to develop optimum esthetics with short maxillary anterior teeth. The ratio of height to width in the maxillary central incisor should be approximately 1.2:1 (see Table 7-1).

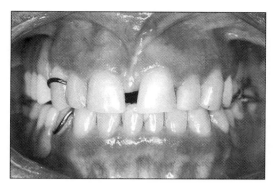

Fig 14-2a Diastema.

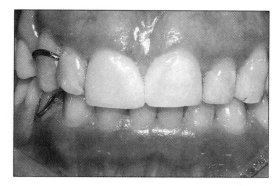

Fig 14-2b Diagnostic intraoral mock-up of diastema closure.

17. The mesiodistal proportion of the maxillary central incisor to the maxillary lateral incisor is approximately 1.5:1 (see Table 7-2).
18. Both phonetics and esthetics are used to determine the position of the maxillary incisal edges. When the patient says *F*, the maxillary incisal edges should lightly touch the lower lip at or near the wet-dry line. When the patient says *E*, approximately 50% to 70% of the space between the upper and lower lips should be occupied by maxillary anterior teeth.[11]
19. Younger teeth have more surface anatomy. With age, teeth tend to become smoother and display a higher luster.
20. Natural teeth are polychromatic, and every effort should be made to avoid monochromatic porcelain restorations.

Diagnostic Aids

Mock-ups

With a knowledge of these guidelines, the dentist can use several diagnostic methods to develop a treatment plan that will predictably result in success. Preparation and waxing on a diagnostic cast are sometimes helpful to the dentist, especially when the veneers are intended to lengthen teeth, close space, or correct malaligned teeth. However, a diagnostic waxup is not especially helpful in giving the patient a preview of the expected esthetic outcome. This can better be accomplished by one of the intraoral techniques.

A mock-up of the desired result can be accomplished with direct placement of composite in the patient's mouth to simulate the desired outcome (Figs 14-2a and 14-2b). The teeth are not acid etched prior to the intra-

oral mock-up; therefore, the composite can be easily removed from the tooth. This technique is especially helpful for simple procedures, such as diastema closure.

However, when major changes are being made, such as lengthening of several teeth, direct mock-up is time consuming. In this situation, a diagnostic waxup is done on a preoperative cast and duplicated, and a clear matrix is made. Composite material is placed in the clear matrix, which is placed over the teeth intraorally and light cured. Once the excess flash of composite is cleaned from the teeth, the patient may preview the projected outcome (Fig 14-3a to 14-3d). At this point, changes can be made, eg, shortening or lengthening of the teeth, until the patient is comfortable and satisfied. An impression can then be made of the corrected mock-up in the mouth, and the subsequent cast will serve as a "go-by" cast for the laboratory technician. Because intraoral mock-up can be time consuming, a more cost-effective method is to construct a composite shell on a diagnostic cast. The shell is placed intraorally to allow the patient to visualize the projected result. This is an especially helpful diagnostic tool for the patient with excessive gingival display. The composite shell can extend up over the gingiva to demonstrate the esthetic effect of surgically lengthening the clinical crowns (Fig 14-4a to 14-4e).

Computer Imaging

Another diagnostic method involves computer imaging of the patient's smile and making the desired esthetic changes on the screen. This provides both the patient and the dentist with a realistic preview of the expected result. However, imaging is limited because it does not allow for a dynamic evaluation in the same way that an intraoral mock-up allows the patient to experience the projected changes. Because most dentists do not have

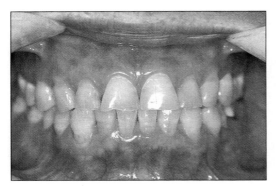

Fig 14-3a Abraded maxillary anterior teeth.

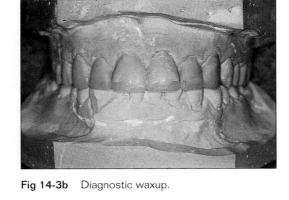

Fig 14-3b Diagnostic waxup.

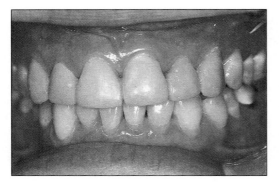

Fig 14-3c Diagnostic provisional restorations in place.

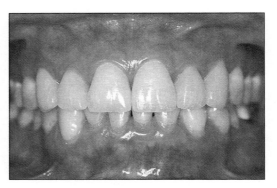

Fig 14-3d Porcelain veneers bonded on all anterior teeth.

the in-office capability to computer image, the patient or a photograph or slide of the patient may be sent to a location that offers the service.

Photographs

Another important diagnostic aid is a set of preoperative photographs. These protect the dentist, remind the patient of the preoperative condition, and most important, aid the technician in the fabrication of the veneers. The series should include a full-face smile, a retracted frontal shot of occluded maxillary and mandibular teeth, a retracted frontal view with a shade tab held directly beneath the incisal edges of the maxillary incisors, a retracted closeup view of the teeth to be veneered, with and without a shade tab, and a postpreparation view of the teeth to be veneered, with a shade tab (Fig 14-5). In addition, other photographs, such as a profile or a view of the intraoral diagnostic mock-up, should be included if they can benefit the technician.

Single Veneer

Perhaps the most difficult procedure in esthetic restorative dentistry is to perfectly match a full-coverage restoration to an adjacent natural central incisor. On occasion, the porcelain veneer is the restoration of choice in this situation. If the natural incisor is not highly characterized and the tooth to be restored is not discolored, the porcelain veneer is an excellent restorative option. However, if the adjacent incisor is highly characterized or the tooth to be restored is not the same color as the adjacent teeth, a porcelain veneer is not the restoration of choice. It is very difficult to incorporate a lot of characterization into the veneer during fabrication and also difficult to add surface stain to a veneer, although this can be done with low-fusing porcelain stains. For these reasons, the restoration of the highly characterized single anterior tooth is best attained with either a ceramometal or all-ceramic crown.

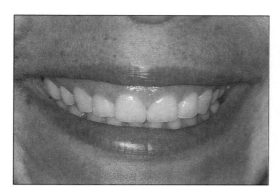

Fig 14-4a Short clinical crowns resulting from excess gingival coverage.

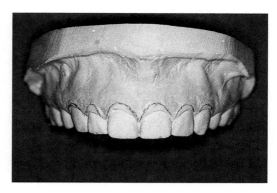

Fig 14-4b Preoperative study cast with lines drawn to aid in the fabrication of a diagnostic composite overlay.

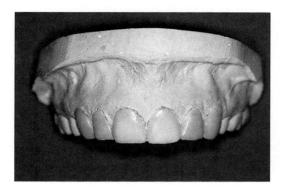

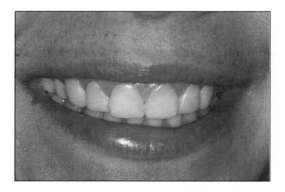

Figs 14-4c and 14-4d Diagnostic composite overlay.

Fig 14-4e Diagnostic composite overlay demonstrating the benefit of crown lengthening of the anterior teeth.

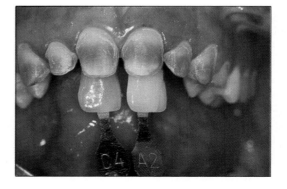

Fig 14-5 Shade tabs held under the incisal edges of the prepared teeth. Preparations on tetracycline-stained teeth are routinely extended interproximally through the contact area. In this patient, more interproximal tooth structure was removed because of existing Class 3 restorations.

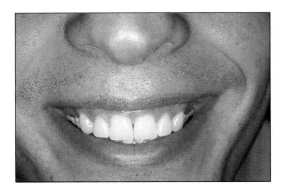

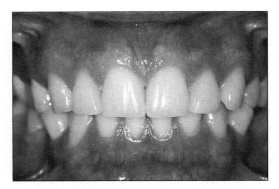

Fig 14-6 Porcelain veneers bonded on all maxillary anterior teeth. Note the apparent separation of anterior and posterior segments of the mouth because of the boldness of the porcelain veneers. (From Robbins.[18] Reprinted with permission.)

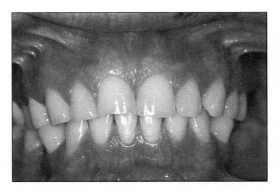

Fig 14-7a Preoperative view of maxillary central and lateral incisors.

Fig 14-7b Porcelain veneers bonded on the maxillary central and lateral incisors to blend esthetically with the maxillary canines.

Multiple Veneers

When the clinician has the option to veneer multiple anterior teeth, the problem of shade matching is minimized. It is easier to deal in even numbers when veneers are placed on anterior teeth. For example, it is much simpler to veneer two central incisors than to attempt to match a veneer to a natural tooth. Therefore, the chances of obtaining an optimally esthetic result are enhanced when either two, four, six, or eight veneers are placed versus one, three, or five veneers.

An option that is commonly chosen is the placement of six veneers from canine to canine. In this case, the anterior teeth are made brighter and bolder, while the buccal corridor appears to become darker. This accentuates the anterior teeth and commonly creates the unpleasant illusion that the anterior teeth are larger and longer as well as brighter (Fig 14-6). This does not usually occur when only the four incisors are veneered (Fig 14-7a and 14-7b). Therefore, when the incisors are treatment planned for veneers, but there is no esthetic or

functional requirement to veneer the canines, the esthetic result is enhanced when the canines are left unrestored. However, when all six anterior teeth require veneers, consideration should be given to veneering one or more posterior teeth on each side.

Tooth Preparation

The preparation of teeth for porcelain veneers is usually uncomplicated when the basic principles are understood and followed. The amount of tooth structure removed during preparation is determined by the position of the tooth in the arch and the color of the tooth. If the tooth is facioverted, more tooth structure will be removed so that the final restoration will have the correct facial contours. Conversely, if the tooth is linguoverted, very little preparation is required other than a peripheral finish line. In a routine preparation, the facial enamel is reduced approximately 0.3 to 0.5 mm (Fig 14-8). This

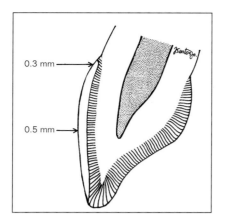

Fig 14-8 Veneer preparation that does not cover the incisal edge of the maxillary anterior tooth.

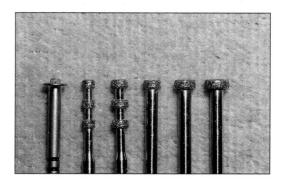

Fig 14-9 Depth cut burs of different designs and depths.

can be accomplished with depth cut burs, which are available from several manufacturers (Fig 14-9). After the depth cuts are made, the enamel is uniformly removed with a blunt, tapered diamond. However, if the underlying tooth color is dark, the preparation must be deepened to allow for increased thickness of porcelain. With darker tetracycline-stained teeth, the preparation should be approximately 0.7 mm deep.

Anterior Teeth

Gingival Finish Lines

For maxillary porcelain veneers, the gingival margin of the veneer should be routinely placed at or slightly incisal to the marginal gingiva. A primary goal of the preparation is to have all margins on sound enamel. Because the enamel is only approximately 0.3 mm thick, 0.5 mm from the cementoenamel junction,[4] it is difficult to obtain adequate preparation depth while preserving the enamel. This commonly results in a slightly overcontoured veneer, which may act as a coetiologic factor in marginal inflammation. Therefore, unless the teeth to be veneered are dark (low value), the gingival preparation should not routinely extend into the gingival sulcus.

When mandibular anterior teeth are prepared for porcelain veneers, the considerations are different from those for maxillary teeth. In most patients, the gingival half of the mandibular incisors remain covered by the lower lip at all times, resulting in no esthetic display. In addition, the marginal gingiva of the mandibular anterior teeth is commonly thin, and the gingival sulcus is narrow and shallow, making the placement of gingival retraction cord very difficult. For these reasons, the gingival mar-

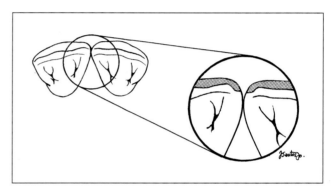

Fig 14-10 Preparation extending slightly facial to the interproximal contact area.

gin of the preparation for mandibular anterior teeth is placed at least 1.0 mm incisal to the marginal gingiva (see Fig 14-22a).

Interproximal Contact Area

For the purposes of fabrication and insertion of the veneer, it is important that the preparation not extend into the interproximal contact area. The proximal extent of the preparation should end slightly facial to the interproximal contact area in most circumstances (Fig 14-10). However, with dark teeth, eg, tetracycline-stained teeth, the preparation must extend completely through the interproximal contact area to the lingual surface (Fig 14-5). This decreases the risk of having a dark shadow around the periphery of the veneers.

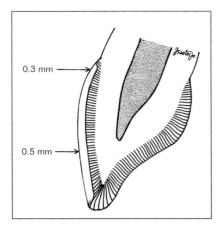

Fig 14-11 Window preparation on a maxillary anterior tooth.

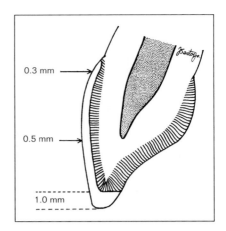

Fig 14-12 Standard veneer preparation for maxillary anterior teeth. There is 1.0 mm of incisal reduction.

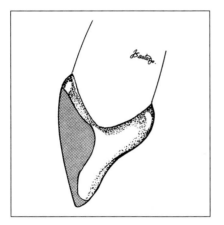

Fig 14-13 Extension of the veneer preparation into the subcontact area for improved esthetics.

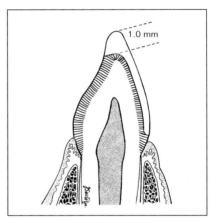

Fig 14-14 Veneer preparation on a mandibular incisor. There is a minimum of 1.0 mm of incisal reduction and the gingival margin is at least 1.0 mm incisal to the gingival crest.

Incisal Edge

There is an ongoing debate regarding the need to cover the incisal edge of a maxillary tooth with the porcelain veneer. If there is no esthetic requirement to change the incisal shape or length, and there is adequate remaining incisal tooth structure after facial reduction, the incisal margin may be terminated at the facioincisal line angle (Fig 14-8). A second alternative is the window preparation (Fig 14-11). This preparation provides the most protection for the veneer during function; however, it results in a visible composite–veneer interface at the facioincisal margin. Neither of these preparations can be used when the tooth is being lengthened incisally with the porcelain veneer. Additionally, veneers that do not cover the incisal edge are significantly more difficult to orient correctly during cementation.

Therefore, the most universally applicable preparation, which allows the technician to incorporate the natural incisal translucency into the veneer, requires incisal edge reduction. If the incisal edge is to be covered with the veneer, there must be room for at least 1.0 mm of porcelain over the incisal edge (Fig 14-12). The incisal edge should be flattened, leaving a butt margin on the lingual surface. It is then important to round the sharp incisofacial line angle of the preparation to prevent stress concentration in the cemented veneer. The proximal portion of the preparation should follow the papilla and extend slightly under the interproximal contact to

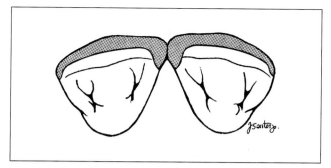

Fig 14-15a Porcelain veneer preparations for closing a small-to-moderate diastema.

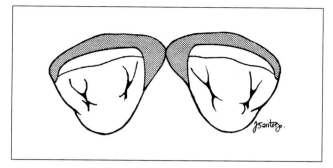

Fig 14-15b Porcelain veneer preparations for closing a large diastema. The preparations extend to the midpalatal surfaces of the central incisors to develop adequate lingual contours.

ensure coverage of the tooth in this area (Fig 14-13). If the tooth is not prepared in this manner, the unprepared triangle of natural tooth structure is darker and results in less than optimal esthetics.

The incisal edges of mandibular anterior teeth should be routinely covered with porcelain of at least 1.0 mm thickness (Fig 14-14). Incisal flattening with a resultant butt margin is recommended for mandibular anterior teeth. Again, the incisofacial line angle of the preparation must be rounded.

When multiple teeth are being prepared, incisal reduction should be symmetric, eg, both prepared lateral incisors should be the same length. This will result in more uniform esthetics in the final restorations. After completion of all veneer preparations, the dentist should stand in front of the patient, retract the patient's lips, and confirm that the preparations are symmetric and parallel to the interpupillary line.

Overlapping Teeth

When overlapping teeth are being prepared, the path of insertion of the veneer must be considered. Where there is significant malalignment of the teeth, it may not be possible to develop a path of insertion for the veneer without removing enamel from the proximal surfaces of the adjacent teeth. Also, if the path of insertion must be from the facial aspect, a chamfer preparation cannot be used on the lingual surface.

Space Closure

Preparation of teeth for space closure presents a unique situation. To obtain smooth lingual contours, the interproximal finish lines adjacent to the space must be taken farther lingually. The wider the space to be closed, the farther lingually the tooth must be prepared (Figs 14-15a and 14-15b).

Premolar Teeth

The considerations for preparing premolar teeth are similar to those for anterior teeth. The veneer preparation of the maxillary premolar may end on the facial surface of the tooth if the functional and esthetic requirements are met (Fig 14-16). Ideally, the occlusal margin should be placed so that the opposing cusp does not function across it. However, if the decision is made to cover the facial cusp, occlusal tooth reduction must be adequate to allow for a veneer of at least 2.0 mm thickness over the facial cusp (Fig 14-17). If the anterior guidance immediately disoccludes the posterior teeth, the occlusal margin can be placed anywhere on the inner incline of the buccal cusp, as long as there is no centric occlusion directly on the margin. However, when group function occlusion is present, it may be necessary to extend the occlusal margin to the central groove. In mandibular premolars, because the esthetic cusp is also the functional cusp, the tooth must generally be prepared for a porcelain onlay rather than simply for a buccal porcelain veneer (see chapter 9).

Existing Restorations

Existing composite restorations can complicate the veneer preparation. Ideally, no margins should be finished on existing composite. When feasible, the composite restoration can be removed and the missing tooth structure may be replaced as part of the porcelain veneer[2] (Fig 14-18). However, this ideal is not always possible, especially if the existing composite restoration is small, eg, a small Class 3 restoration. In this circumstance, the old composite should be replaced prior to veneer preparation, because the veneer margin will be partially on composite. If the composite restorations are large, porcelain veneers may not be indicated.

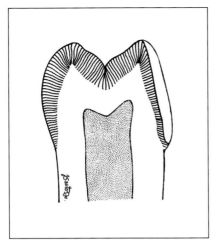

Fig 14-16 Porcelain veneer preparation that does not cover the buccal cusp of the maxillary premolar.

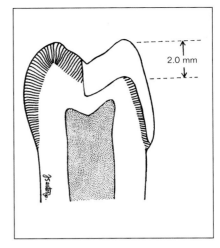

Fig 14-17 Porcelain veneer preparation that covers the buccal cusp of the maxillary premolar. The 2.0 mm of occlusal reduction on the buccal cusp.

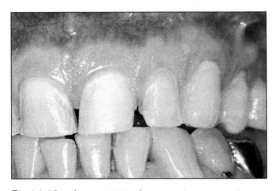

Fig 14-18 A mesioincisal composite restoration on the maxillary left lateral incisor has been removed in the veneer preparation. The porcelain veneer will replace the missing mesial surface. The gingival margin on the maxillary left canine is prepared in a glass-ionomer cement restoration.

Fractured Incisal Edge

A unique indication for the porcelain veneer is the restoration of the fractured incisal edge of an incisor tooth (Figs 14-19a to 14-19c). Although there are minimal clinical data to support this use of veneers, the laboratory data[2] are favorable. The limits for the amount of missing tooth structure that can be replaced with a porcelain veneer are not known. However, anecdotal experience seems to indicate that approximately 50% of the clinical crown can be replaced with a porcelain veneer. Because the veneer does not require endodontics for restorative reasons or the placement of a post and core, it is a highly desirable alternative to previous methods of restoring the fractured tooth. The preparation for this type of veneer extends to near the gingival crest on both the facial and lingual surfaces. Because of the wraparound design of the veneer, it must be luted with low- to moderate-viscosity composite luting resin.

Erosion/Abrasion Lesion

When erosion/abrasion lesions, caries, or restorations exist at the gingival margin, these areas are best restored with a glass-ionomer restorative material. The veneer margin may then be finished on glass-ionomer cement rather than cementum (Fig 14-18). When gingival recession has occurred without loss of tooth structure, the best alternative may be periodontal grafting procedures to cover the exposed root surface.[1] However, if the surgical option is not chosen, and the esthetic demands require that the root be covered with a veneer, then the preparation must extend onto the root surface. In this situation, a dentin bonding agent must be used in the luting process. However, when possible, it is best to finish the gingival margin on enamel. When a significant amount of tooth structure has been lost to chemical ero-

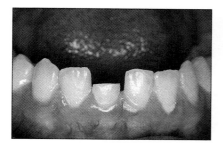

Fig 14-19a Fractured mandibular right central incisor.

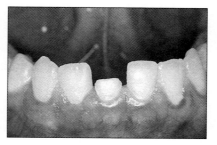

Fig 14-19b Preparation of the fractured mandibular right central incisor for a porcelain veneer.

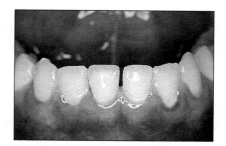

Fig 14-19c Porcelain veneer bonded on the mandibular right central incisor.

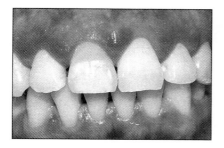

Fig 14-20a Open subcontact space between the maxillary central incisors prior to veneer preparation.

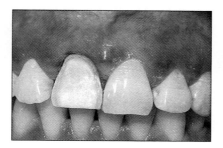

Fig 14-20b Blockout wax, placed from the palatal aspect in the subcontact space.

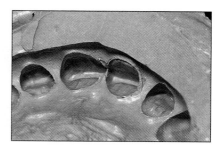

Fig 14-20c Impression of the veneer preparation, demonstrating the effectiveness of the blockout wax in keeping the impression material out of the subcontact space, which would result in a torn impression.

sion, it is sometimes difficult to determine the extent of remaining enamel. Dentin detector solutions are available for this purpose. Alternatively, a 5- to 10-second etch with phosphoric acid will disclose the remaining enamel.

Impressions

When an impression is made of the maxillary teeth, retraction cord is placed to expose all gingival margins. This step is not necessary with mandibular teeth because the preparations are at least 1.0 mm incisal to the marginal gingiva. An accurate impression material, such as poly(vinyl siloxane), polyether, or reversible hydrocolloid, is then used to make the final impression. When the interdental papilla is missing adjacent to a veneer preparation, the space must be blocked out with rope wax from the lingual aspect before the impression is made (Fig 14-20a to 14-20c). This prevents the impression material from filling the papillary space, resulting in a torn impression when it is removed from the mouth.

Provisional Restorations

Maxillary Teeth

On occasion, provisional restorations are not necessary. However, for diagnostic purposes, to meet esthetic demands, or to prevent sensitivity, provisional restorations often must be placed. This is best accomplished with direct placement of composite. A small area in the center of each tooth is etched with phosphoric acid for 15 seconds, washed, and dried. Unfilled resin is placed and light cured. A large increment of composite is then inserted, patted to place with correct contour, and light cured. There should be no overhanging composite at the margins, and the provisional restoration should require virtually no adjustment. When length has to be added to the incisal edges of the prepared teeth with the provisional restorations for esthetic or diagnostic reasons, the technique described for mandibular teeth may be used.

At the subsequent appointment, the composite over the small area of etched enamel in the center of the facial surface is lightly removed with a diamond bur, and the remaining composite is flicked off with a spoon excavator.

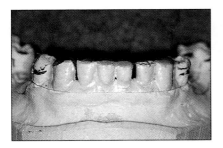

Fig 14-21a *Clear matrix on the preoperative cast.*

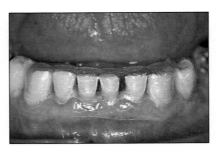

Fig 14-21b *Clear matrix placed over the teeth to verify fit and as a preparation guide to ensure adequate incisal reduction.*

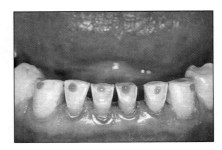

Fig 14-21c *Incisal third of each tooth spot etched with phosphoric acid.*

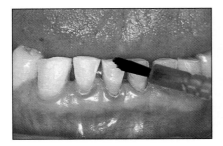

Fig 14-21d *Unfilled resin placed over etched spots on each tooth.*

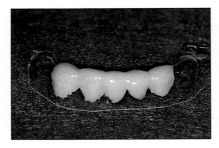

Figs 14-21e and 14-21f *Clear matrix with composite.*

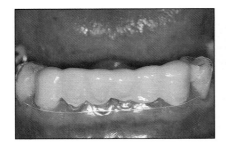

Fig 14-21g *Clear matrix and composite placed over the preparations.*

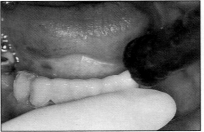
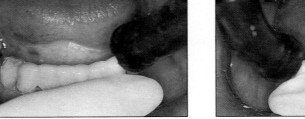

Figs 14-21h and 14-21i *Curing the incisal half of the provisional restoration on the left and right sides.*

Mandibular Teeth

Because the preparation for mandibular teeth routinely requires 1.0 mm reduction at the incisal edge, provisional restorations must be placed to avoid supereruption. The direct placement technique may be used, but is difficult because it is necessary to cover the incisal edges.

When provisional restorations are being placed on multiple mandibular teeth, it is preferable to use a clear plastic matrix made on a preoperative diagnostic cast. The teeth are spot etched, covered with unfilled resin, and light cured, as previously described. The facial and incisal areas in the matrix are filled with composite, and the matrix is placed over the prepared teeth. The gingival half of the matrix is covered by the operator and the incisal half is polymerized with the light for 10 seconds per tooth. The gingival half is then lightly cured for 1 second per tooth. The matrix is removed and the excess partially cured composite at the gingival margins is removed with a No. 12 scalpel blade. The gingival areas that have been overcarved are quickly repaired with additional composite. The light-curing process is then completed, the incisal and facial embrasures are opened with a thin separating disk, and the occlusion is adjusted (Figs 14-21a to 14-21n).

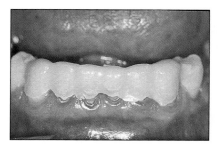

Fig 14-21j Provisional restoration immediately after removal of the clear matrix.

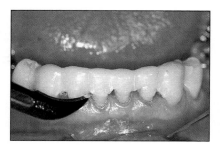

Fig 14-21k Trimming gingival margins and embrasures with No. 12 scalpel blade.

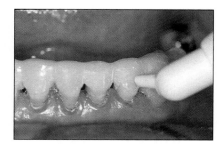

Fig 14-21l Adding composite to the gingival margins.

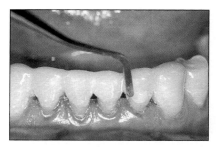

Fig 14-21m Contouring composite at the gingival margins.

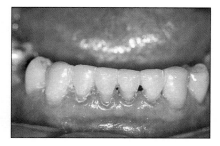

Fig 14-21n Completed provisional restoration.

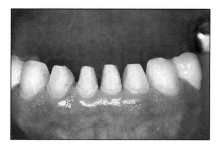

Fig 14-22a Porcelain veneer preparations on the mandibular anterior teeth. The gingival margins are located 1.0 mm above the gingival crests.

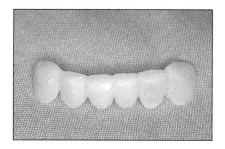

Fig 14-22b Laboratory-fabricated provisional restoration.

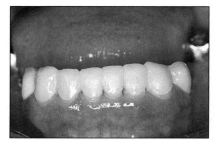

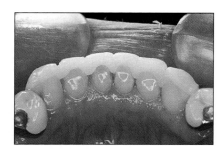

Figs 14-22c and 14-22d Provisional restoration in place.

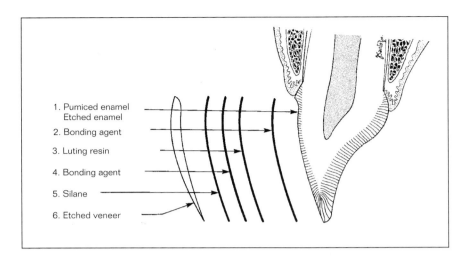

Fig 14-23 Anatomy of a porcelain veneer.

1. Pumiced enamel
   Etched enamel
2. Bonding agent
3. Luting resin
4. Bonding agent
5. Silane
6. Etched veneer

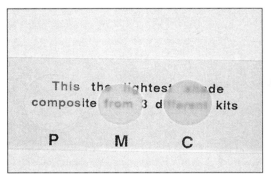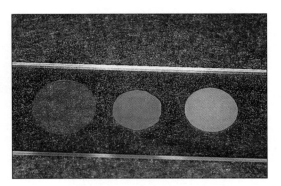

Figs 14-24a and 14-24b Lightest shade of luting composite from three different kits placed between two glass slides. The same materials are shown against two different backgrounds. Note the differences in translucency. (Fig 14-24 from Robbins.[18])

Alternatively, the provisional restoration may be made indirectly in the laboratory. After the veneer preparations are completed, an impression is made and poured in fast-setting die stone. The cast is separated from the impression in 5 minutes and covered with a separating medium, and the provisional restoration is constructed with the same matrix technique as previously described. The provisional restoration, which is constructed from either acrylic or composite, can then be cemented with polycarboxylate cement or temporarily bonded with a composite as previously described (Figs 14-22a to 14-22d).

▪ Placement

The anatomy of a porcelain veneer is illustrated in Fig 14-23. The inner surface of the veneer must be etched with hydrofluoric acid. This step is usually accomplished in the laboratory. Next, silane is painted on the etched surface of the veneer. Silane is a coupling agent that significantly increases the bond strength between porcelain and composite.[9] It is important that the silane be placed only on the etched surface of the veneer. If silane is placed on the glazed surface, removal of excess composite during finishing is much more difficult. After the silane has air dried, a thin layer of bonding agent is placed. Finally the veneer is filled with the composite luting cement and taken to the mouth.

There are many different resin luting cement kits available with differing degrees of translucency and viscosity. Figs 14-24a and 14-24b illustrate the differences in translucency offered by the lightest shade from three different kits. Translucent cements are indicated when veneers are placed on teeth that have no discoloration. The more opaque cements tend to block the natural tooth color, resulting in a less lifelike veneer. The opaque cements are more commonly used to help block

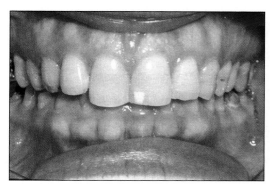

Fig 14-25a Moderately dark, tetracycline-stained teeth prior to veneer preparation.

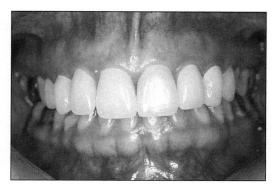

Fig 14-25b Veneers bonded on dark teeth with opaque resin cement. Note the opaque gingival margins on the right and left canines.

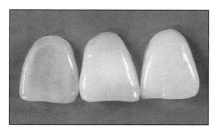

Fig 14-26 Veneers displaying different amounts of translucency. The left veneer is made from a very translucent porcelain and allows most of the underlying tooth color to show through. The center veneer has a base layer of masking dentin porcelain, which is used to block dark underlying tooth color yet maintain some degree of polychromicity. The right veneer has a layer of opaque resin cement bonded to the inner surface of the veneer. The opaque resin is very reflective and results in a displeasing, monochromatic appearance.

the darkness of discolored teeth. However, the use of these cements can result in a monochromatic appearance and an opaque line at the thin gingival margin of the veneer (Figs 14-25a and 14-25b). It is preferable to block the darkness of discolored teeth with a layer of masking dentin and/or with porcelain modifiers in the body of the veneers rather than with opaque cement (Fig 14-26).

The second major difference in veneer-luting cements is their viscosity. Initially, most resin cements had a low viscosity so that the veneers could be placed with minimal pressure, thereby decreasing the risk of fracture. However, the low-viscosity resins have some disadvantages: (1) Because of their honeylike consistency, it is more difficult to ensure correct veneer placement, especially when the veneers have no positive stop, ie, no incisal overlap; (2) cleanup of excess resin is more difficult; and (3) at least theoretically, the physical properties are compromised because of the increased percentage of resin matrix. The

major indication for the low-viscosity luting resin is the all-ceramic crown or a veneer that covers most of the tooth surfaces. As a result of friction, high-viscosity luting resins will not allow complete seating of these restorations. Recently, interest in the higher viscosity luting resins has increased because they overcome most of the disadvantages of the low-viscosity luting resins.

Friedman[6] has described a technique for using the highly filled composite from a standard restorative composite kit. The material is brought to room temperature and placed into the veneer in a thin layer through an ampule tip. The thixotropic properties of the composite allow the highly filled material to flow under moderate seating pressure. Placing the ampule of composite in a hot water bath (140°F) before use also improves the flow of the material during veneer placement. With this technique, the seating of the veneers can be more accurately controlled, and the cleanup is simplified (see box for the step-by-step technique).

Placement of Porcelain Veneers

1. Check veneers for fit on dies and transilluminate to check for fracture lines.
2. Try-in veneers individually for fit, and then all together. You may need to adjust the interproximal contact areas with a microfine diamond or disk. Do not make any other adjustments until the veneers are bonded.
3. Clean the veneers with acetone and place silane on the inner surface of each veneer and allow to air dry. If luting composite is used for the try-in, first place a thin layer of unfilled resin.
4. Choose a shade of composite or water-soluble try-in paste, place on the inside of the veneer, and try-in.
5. If water-soluble try-in paste has been used, wash the veneer with water and air dry before loading with the unfilled resin and luting composite. If the shade is correct, skip steps 6 through 13, and proceed with step 14.
6. If the shade is incorrect, remove the try-in composite and select another shade, or customize the shade by adding tint to the luting composite.
7. If characterization (eg, blue in incisal areas, yellow at gingival areas) is required, tints and opaques should be placed only on the tooth and not on the inside of the veneer. The tints and opaques are brushed on the tooth in a thin layer and light cured for 30 seconds. It is important that all try-in composite be removed from the tooth (facial, interproximal, and lingual aspects) before curing the tints and opaques. Because the tooth was not etched, the cured tints and opaques can be scraped off easily with an explorer at the end of the try-in.
8. Once you have determined a combination of composite, tint, and/or opaque, you must remember it, so that you can reproduce it exactly for final cementation.
9. Clean the try-in composite from the inside of the veneer with acetone using two different beakers. Clean the bulk of the composite with a brush dipped in the first beaker; then transfer the veneer to the second, clean beaker of acetone to remove the remaining composite.

Veneer Preparation

10. Place the veneers, etched side down, on a 2 × 2-inch gauze pad in a glass beaker of clean acetone and place in an ultrasonic cleaner for 5 minutes.
11. Remove veneers from the acetone and dry.
12. Place silane on the inner surface of the veneers and allow to air dry.
13. Place a thin layer of unfilled resin on the inner surface of all the veneers.
14. Place luting composite in the veneer, and cover to protect from light. It is helpful to write the number of each tooth to receive a veneer on a piece of paper and place each veneer on the correct tooth number to avoid placing a veneer on the wrong tooth.

Tooth Preparation

15. Place retraction cord in the sulcus of each prepared tooth (but not the mandibular incisors if the margins are more than 1.0 mm from the gingival crest).
16. Pumice both central incisors with oil-free pumice (this should be done for each tooth just before etching).
17. Place shimstock, Mylar strips, or a dead soft metal matrix between the central incisors and on the distal aspect of both central incisors.
18. Prepare the teeth to receive dentin bonding agents using an appropriate etchant. Visually inspect the etch to ensure adequacy.
19. Place primer and then a thin layer of dentin bonding agent over the entire surface. (If desired, place tints and opaques as needed in predetermined areas. Do not place tint or opaque on margins.)
20. Light cure the tint and opaque for 90 seconds. These materials are difficult to completely cure, so do not shorten the curing time. If no tints or opaques are being used, do not light cure the dentin adhesive.

Placement of Porcelain Veneers *(continued)*

Placement

21. With shimstock (0.0005-inch) between the central incisors and Mylar strips or dead soft metal matrices on the distal aspect of both central incisors, place the veneers on both central incisors and gently push to place. Make sure that excess composite appears at all margins.
22. Remove excess composite from both veneers with a small brush or explorer, depending on the viscosity of the luting composite.
23. Visually inspect to ensure that the veneers are placed correctly. Make sure that the mesial surfaces are in contact.
24. Lightly push on the facial surface of the right central veneer with an instrument; this should express a small amount of resin at all margins.
25. Light cure right central veneer at the gingival third for 5 seconds while lightly holding with an instrument.
26. Repeat steps 24 and 25 on left central veneer.
27. Light cure each veneer for 60 seconds from the lingual direction and 90 seconds from the facial direction.
28. Visually inspect for voids, and repair if possible.
29. Remove excess composite with a No. 12 scalpel blade from the proximal surfaces only to ensure that adjacent veneers will seat completely. Be careful not to start hemorrhage.
30. Repeat procedure (starting at step 16) for one veneer at a time, moving distally from the central incisors.

Finishing

31. Remove minimal gingival flash of composite with a No. 12 scalpel blade. Move the blade from the veneer gingivally so as not to chip the veneer margin. Make sure that all flash is removed from the facial and interproximal surfaces.
32. Remove excess composite from the lingual surfaces with an egg-shaped, 12-fluted carbide bur.
33. Check and adjust occlusion in maximum intercuspation and excursions.
34. Reshape incisal edges and contours, while standing in front of the patient.
35. Reshape and contour embrasures with a finishing diamond or a thin separating disk.
36. Smooth lingual surfaces with Sof-Lex disks and impregnated rubber points or disks.
37. If the gingival margins are smooth, no finishing is required. If the gingival margins are rough, smooth with a finishing diamond or 12-fluted carbide bur. Be careful not to scar the cementum.
38. Polish all roughened porcelain with a rubber porcelain-polishing point.
39. Finish interproximals with finishing and polishing strips.
40. Any visible porcelain that has been finished and smoothed with a rubber point is polished with diamond polishing paste on a wet felt wheel and prophylaxis cup at the gingival margin. Be careful not to polish the cementum.
41. With the cord still in place, re-etch and rebond all margins.
42. Remove the retraction cord.
43. Instruct the patient to return in 1 week to allow inspection for excess composite and rough areas. At this time, final esthetic reshaping can be accomplished.

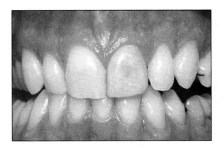

Fig 14-27a Maxillary left central incisor before veneer preparation.

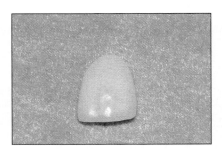

Fig 14-27b Porcelain veneer with brown characterization incorporated into the veneer.

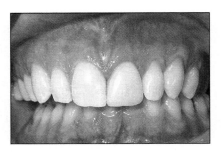

Fig 14-27c Characterized porcelain veneer bonded on maxillary left central incisor.

Color Management and Characterization

A common problem with the porcelain veneer is the lack of color differentiation between the gingival and incisal portions of the restoration. Several methods of color characterization can be used to correct the monochromism.[16-18] The best and most basic method makes the color changes in the porcelain itself. A color diagram that outlines the desired shade and color changes and any other special characterization, such as hypocalcified or hyperchromatic areas, can be given to the technician (Figs 14-27a to 14-27c). However, when characterization is incorporated in the veneer, it is there to stay. If the esthetic result is not satisfactory during the try-in, it is difficult, if not impossible, to successfully modify the veneer.

A second commonly used method involves the modification of the color with the underlying luting composite. All porcelain veneer kits have several different shades of luting composite. If an appropriate shade of luting cement is not available, resin tints can be added to the luting composite to effect virtually any desired color of luting cement.

A third and less commonly used method of characterization involves the direct placement of the resin tints on the tooth prior to placement of the veneer (Figs 14-28a to 14-28e). During the try-in, the desired resin tints are placed on the tooth and light cured. The chosen base shade of luting composite is placed in the veneer, and the veneer is placed on the tooth. A determination is then made regarding the esthetic result. The veneer can be removed, and the cured resin tint on the tooth can be easily scraped off with an explorer, because the enamel was not etched. If the esthetic result is acceptable, the

dentist can proceed with the bonding, using the same tints that were used during the try-in.

The final restoration will not always exhibit the same color it displayed at the try-in. This occurs because the luting composite becomes more translucent when it is cured, allowing more of the underlying tooth color to show through.[20] Although not usually a problem, this color-change phenomenon will occasionally result in a disappointing esthetic result, especially when the dentist is attempting to match a single veneer to an adjacent natural tooth.

Discolored Teeth

The darkly discolored tooth presents the greatest challenge for porcelain veneers. There are multiple etiologies for tooth discoloration, including extrinsic staining, fluorosis, pulpal injury, and drugs, such as tetracycline. The ideal method of dealing with stain is to remove it, when possible. Extrinsic stains are easily removed during tooth preparation. Because fluoride predominantly affects the enamel, the discoloration of fluorosis is also commonly diminished by tooth preparation.

However, the by-products of pulpal injury and tetracycline are found predominantly in the dentin, which make their removal more difficult. The restoration of the high-chroma, low-value tetracycline-stained tooth with a porcelain veneer is perhaps the most difficult treatment situation. To allow more room for thicker porcelain, more tooth structure is removed during tooth preparation. However, as more enamel is removed, the underlying color gets darker (Fig 14-29). Herein lies the major difficulty in placing porcelain veneers on tetracycline-stained teeth.

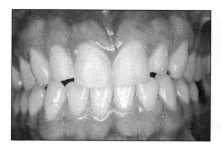

Fig 14-28a Veneer preparations on the maxillary central and lateral incisors (from Robbins[17]).

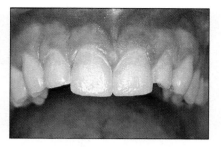

Fig 14-28b Placement of yellow resin tint in the gingival third and blue resin tint in the incisal third (from Robbins[17]).

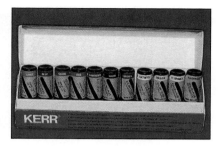

Fig 14-28c Kit of resin tints and opaques (from Robbins[17]).

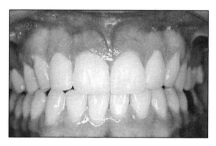

Fig 14-28d Monochromatic appearance of veneers tried in with try-in paste but without the use of resin tints (from Robbins[17]).

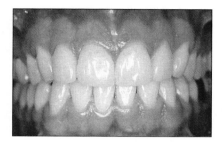

Fig 14-28e Polychromatic appearance of bonded veneers after the placement of resin tints (from Robbins[17]).

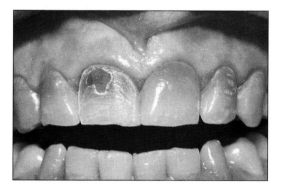

Fig 14-29 Preparation on the severely tetracycline-stained maxillary central incisor, which demonstrates increased darkness with increased depth of preparation.

Masking

It is difficult to mask out dark underlying tooth color with a natural-appearing porcelain veneer (Figs 14-30a and 14-30b). If the luting cement is opaque enough to mask the dark color, the final restoration commonly appears lifeless and monochromatic. Conversely, if the veneer and/or cement contains no opaque element, the darkness of the underlying tooth will be visible through the porcelain. It is preferable to incorporate the opaque elements into the porcelain rather than to attempt to mask the darkness with opaque composite. This requires excellent communication between the laboratory technician and the dentist. Preoperative and postpreparation photographs are very helpful to the technician when porcelain veneers are being fabricated for discolored teeth (Fig 14-5).

Several authors have discussed methods of masking dark underlying tooth color with composite resin. Friedman[6] reported successful use of a standard highly filled restorative composite resin as the luting cement. Reid[16] discussed the use of complementary colors to mask underlying dark tooth color. For example, if the tooth is predominantly yellow, a violet tint is placed and light cured. This neutralizes the high-chroma yellow to a low-value gray. Opaque resin tint is then placed over the violet tint and light cured to increase the value. The veneer is then bonded in the routine manner. Although theoretically appealing, this technique has not proven to be of practical benefit.

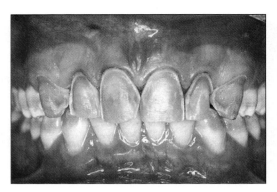

Fig 14-30a Discolored maxillary anterior teeth prepared for porcelain veneers (from Robbins[18]).

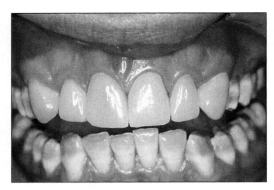

Fig 14-30b Discolored maxillary anterior teeth with bonded porcelain veneers (from Robbins[18]).

When discoloration is discrete rather than generalized, it can be mechanically removed with a bur and restored with the appropriate shade of glass ionomer or composite. This is usually done after the veneer preparation is completed but before the final impression is made; however, it can be done immediately prior to cementation of the veneer.

Composite luting resin can be used to block underlying darkness to a limited degree. However, most of the masking must be accomplished with body modifiers, which are incorporated into the porcelain veneer. Depending on the degree of darkness being masked, the technician must place 50 to 100 μm of die spacer on the refractory die prior to veneer fabrication. This allows space for additional thickness of the luting composite, which aids in the masking of the underlying darkness. Although the esthetic appearance of discolored teeth can usually be improved with porcelain veneers, the patient must understand the limitations of the restoration.

Bleaching

When a discolored tooth can be lightened prior to veneer placement, the final result is routinely improved. This can be accomplished in endodontically treated teeth with a "walking bleach" technique[5] (Figs 14-31a to 14-31c). A 2.0-mm-thick base of glass-ionomer cement or zinc phosphate cement is placed in the base of the pulp chamber to protect the cervix from the 35% hydrogen peroxide, which has been reported to cause external resorption.[8,12,15] A paste mixture of 35% hydrogen peroxide and sodium perborate is placed in the pulp chamber, which is sealed with a temporary cement for 3 to 5 days.

This can be repeated for several treatments until the desired result is attained. The mixture is ultimately removed and the access is restored with a resin composite restoration. At this point the tooth is prepared for the porcelain veneer restoration. If the darkness returns in future years, the walking bleach can be accomplished again through the lingual access without disturbing the porcelain veneer restoration.

The success of bleaching vital teeth prior to veneer placement is not as clear-cut. It is known that vital teeth that have been bleached commonly relapse to their original color with time. However, the effect that the placement of porcelain veneers will have on this relapse is not known. It is also known that bleaching teeth with 35% hydrogen peroxide[21] or carbamide peroxide[7] immediately prior to the bonding procedure has a catastrophic effect on the resultant bond strength. It is recommended that any bonding procedure be delayed at least 1 week after the completion of bleaching. It is hoped that future research will clarify the effects of bleaching on the success of porcelain veneers.

Crown and Veneer Combinations

When a combination of veneers and crowns is placed, all restorations must be tried in individually and then simultaneously. The final color of the veneers may change during the light-curing procedure.[20] For this reason, the veneers are cemented first. The porcelain crowns can then be tried in again, and if required, surface staining can be accomplished prior to final cementation.

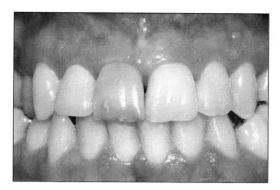

Fig 14-31a Discolored and endodontically treated maxillary right central incisor (from Robbins[18]).

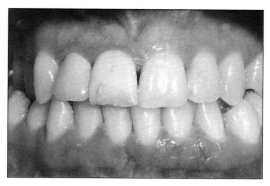

Fig 14-31b Maxillary right central incisor after completion of walking bleach procedure (from Robbins[18]).

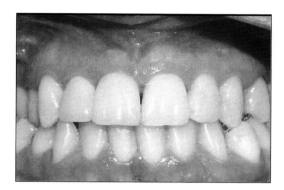

Fig 14-31c Maxillary right central incisor with a porcelain veneer bonded in place (from Robbins[18]).

Failure

On rare occasions, a porcelain veneer will debond. When this happens, it is important to determine at which bonded interface the failure occurred. If the luting composite remains on the tooth, then the failure is likely due to either inadequate etching of the veneer or the use of old silane. The shelf life of silane is approximately 1 year when it is refrigerated. If the composite remains on the inside of the veneer, then there was a problem with either the bonding materials or the placement technique.

When the composite remains on the inner surface of the veneer, it must be removed before the veneer can be rebonded. The veneer is placed in a glazing oven and the temperature is slowly increased to 600°C and held for 10 minutes to ensure burnout of the resin cement. After the veneer is removed from the oven and cooled to room temperature, it is cleaned with acetone and re-etched with 9.5% hydrofluoric acid for 4 minutes. If 9.5% hydrofluoric acid is not available, 1.23% acidulated phosphate fluoride can be used to etch the porcelain; however, this requires a 10-minute etching time. The veneer is then washed, dried, silanated, and rebonded.

A small percentage of veneers will fracture.[10] It is possible to repair fractured porcelain. First, the porcelain fracture site is etched with 9.5% hydrofluoric acid for 4 minutes. After the veneer is washed and dried, silane is placed and dried. The repair is then accomplished with conventional resin composite bonding. Because the hydrofluoric acid should not be allowed to contact natural tooth structure or soft tissue, this etching procedure should only be accomplished with rubber dam isolation. Alternatively, the porcelain can be prepared with 1.23% acidulated phosphate fluoride or by air abrasion with 50-μm aluminum oxide.

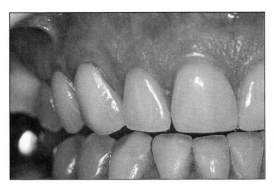

Fig 14-32 Minimally penetrating stain at the mesial margin of the maxillary right canine.

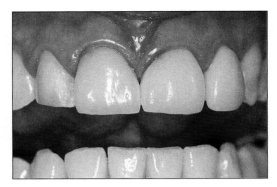

Fig 14-33 Deeply penetrating stain under the porcelain veneer on the right central incisor.

The most common cause of failure is marginal staining and leakage.[3] If the marginal stain is superficial, it can be removed by tray bleaching with 10% carbamide peroxide for several days. After the stain has been removed, the margin can be etched with 37% phosphoric acid and rebonded with unfilled resin. If the stain is slightly penetrating at the margin (Fig 14-32), it can be mechanically removed with a small bur and restored with conventional composite bonding. When there is significant penetration of stain under the veneer, the entire veneer must be removed (Fig 14-33).

Veneer Removal

Removal of porcelain veneers is not only time consuming but also difficult and technique sensitive, especially if the underlying tooth color is light. The veneer cannot be grooved with a bur and torqued in the same manner as when a gold crown is removed. The veneer must be removed with a diamond bur in the same way that enamel is removed during initial tooth preparation.

The dentist starts removing the porcelain in the midfacial area with a back-and-forth sweeping motion. This must be done without water spray so that the operator can visualize the subtle color differentiation between the veneer and the tooth as the interface is reached. Once this interface is apparent, the diamond bur is moved laterally away from the area of exposed enamel toward the periphery of the preparation. Care must be taken to remove as little enamel as possible during this step.

The procedure continues until only a small amount of porcelain remains at the margins. If there has been microleakage at the margins, the remaining marginal porcelain can be removed with a spoon excavator. However, if the marginal seal is intact, the remainder of the porcelain must be cautiously removed with the diamond bur.

It is very important that the operator not lose orientation in relation to the porcelain-tooth interface. If this occurs, it is very easy to inadvertently remove all of the enamel. For this reason, one veneer should be completely removed before starting the removal on the next tooth.

After all porcelain veneers have been removed, gingival retraction cord is packed to clearly expose all margins. As the final step of veneer removal, all margins are explored with a sharp No. 12 scalpel blade (Figs 14-34a to 14-34c). This commonly results in the removal of additional small areas of residual resin composite and porcelain.

Maintenance

The maintenance of the porcelain veneer restoration is similar to that of the porcelain crown. Devices such as an ultrasonic cleaner, air-abrasive polisher, and prophylaxis cup with pumice must be avoided. Surface stains may be removed from porcelain veneers with aluminum oxide polishing paste or diamond polishing paste on a felt wheel or rubber cup. When scaling is performed around porcelain veneers, care must be taken not to chip the margins. Acidulated phosphate fluoride should not be used intraorally because of its ability to etch porcelain.

The patient should be advised that foods and liquids with a high potential for staining, such as coffee and tea, increase the potential for marginal staining. The patient must also be made aware of the potential for the porcelain to fracture. Activities such as ice chewing and fingernail biting must be absolutely avoided. It is a good

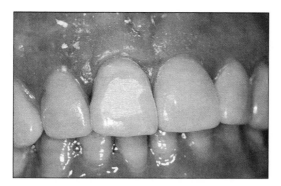

Fig 14-34a Initial removal of porcelain before tooth structure is reached.

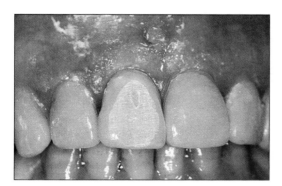

Fig 14-34b Porcelain removed until the first area of enamel is visualized.

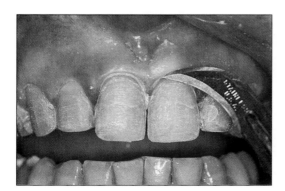

Fig 14-34c Exploring margins with a No. 12 scalpel blade to remove remaining composite and porcelain.

idea to make an occlusal guard appliance for all patients who have porcelain veneer restorations. However, when porcelain veneer restorations will oppose natural teeth or when the patient has a history of a parafunctional habit, a protective appliance should be fabricated to protect both the porcelain veneers and the opposing teeth.

References

1. Allen EP. Use of mucogingival surgical procedures to enhance esthetics. Dent Clin North Am 1988;32:307-330.

2. Andreason FM, Flugge E, Daugaard-Jensen J, Munksgaard EC. Treatment of crown fractured incisors with laminate veneer restorations. An experimental study. Endod Dent Traumatol 1992;8:30-35.

3. Calamia J. Clinical evaluation of etched porcelain veneers. Am J Dent 1989;2:9-15.

4. Crispin B. Esthetic moieties. J Esthet Dent 1993;5:37.

5. Feinman R, Goldstein R, Garber D. Bleaching Teeth. Chicago: Quintessence, 1987.

6. Friedman M. Multiple potential of etched porcelain laminate veneers. J Am Dent Assoc 1987;(special issue): 83E–87E.

7. Godwin JM, Barghi N, Berry TG, Knight GT, Hummert TW. Time duration for dissipation of bleaching effects before enamel bonding [abstract 590]. J Dent Res 1992;71:179.

8. Harrington G, Natkin E. External resorption associated with bleaching of pulpless teeth. J Endod 1979;5:344-348.

9. Hsu CS, Stangel I, Nathanson D. Shear bond strength of resin to etched porcelain [abstract 1095]. J Dent Res 1985;64:296.

10. Jordan RE, Suzuki M, Senda A. Four year recall evaluation of labial porcelain veneer restorations [abstract 544]. J Dent Res 1989;68:249.

11. Kois J. Personal communication, Austin, TX, April 1994.

12. Lado E, Stanley H, Weisman M. Cervical resorption in bleached teeth. Oral Surg Oral Med Oral Pathol 1983;55:78-80.

13. Levinson N. Psychological facets of esthetic dental health care: A developmental perspective. J Prosthet Dent 1990;64:486-491.

14. Mixson J, Pippin D, Soldan-Els A, Koh Y, Hull M. Clinical evaluation of porcelain veneers and PFM crowns [abstract 785]. J Dent Res 1995;74:110.

15. Montgomery S. External cervical resorption after bleaching a pulpless tooth. Oral Surg Oral Med Oral Pathol 1984;57:203-206.

16. Reid JS. Tooth color modification and porcelain veneers. Quintessence Int 1988;19:477-481.

17. Robbins J. Color characterization of porcelain veneers. Quintessence Int 1991;22:853-856.

18. Robbins J. Color management of the porcelain veneer. Esthetic Dent Update 1992;3:132-135.

19. Rucker L, Richter W, MacEntee M, Richardson A. Porcelain and resin veneers clinically evaluated: 2-year results. J Am Dent Assoc 1990;121:594-596.

20. Seghi R, Gritz, MD, Kim J. Colorimetric changes in composite resins due to visible light polymerization [abstract 892]. J Dent Res 1988;67:224.

21. Torneck C, Titley K, Smith D, Adibfar A. The influence of time of hydrogen peroxide exposure on the adhesion of composite resin to bleached bovine enamel. J Endod 1990;16:123-128.

Anterior Ceramic Crowns

Richard S. Schwartz

When teeth are evaluated for single-unit crowns, several things need to be considered:

1. Recent radiographs should always be reviewed before any crown preparation is initiated.
2. The existing occlusion should be analyzed, and a determination should be made whether it is necessary to develop new occlusal relationships. This may require study casts and a diagnostic mounting.
3. Caries must be identified, wear patterns determined, and the amount of useful tooth structure noted.
4. Existing restorations should be examined and, in most instances, replaced.
5. If there is any question about the health of the pulp, diagnostic pulp testing is indicated.
6. Shade selection should be made at the initial appointment and verified later. It is also important to select a shade before any dehydration of the teeth occurs because this can greatly modify the shade.
7. The depth of the gingival sulcus should be determined with a periodontal probe. The coronal margin should always be placed a minimum of 1.0 mm coronal to the epithelial attachment. Because the sulcus of the anterior teeth is often about 1.0 mm in depth, an intracrevicular margin should not be used on many anterior teeth.

Anterior ceramic crowns can be classified in several ways. For the purposes of this chapter, they will be divided into metal-ceramic and all-ceramic crowns.

Metal-Ceramic Restorations

By far the most common complete-coverage esthetic restoration today is the metal-ceramic crown. A metal-ceramic crown consists of a cast metal substructure on which several layers of porcelain are baked. The metal provides strength and the porcelain provides toothlike esthetics. Metal-ceramic restorations have a long history of success, and good to excellent esthetics can usually be attained.

Preparations

There are several key features in metal-ceramic tooth preparations that require more tooth reduction than is necessary for an all-metal crown. The combination of metal and porcelain requires approximately 1.5 mm of tooth reduction, 0.3 to 0.5 mm for the metal and 1.0 mm for the porcelain. Incisal reduction of 2.0 mm is usually necessary to allow the development of natural incisal translucency. Surfaces covered with only metal require less reduction, approximately 0.75 mm (Fig 15-1). A shoulder preparation on the facial aspect, carried into the proximal areas, is recommended, and a chamfer preparation on the lingual surface is recommended.

To ensure adequate tooth reduction, depth cuts that follow the anatomic contours of the tooth are made with a diamond bur of known dimensions. Remaining tooth structure is reduced to the same depth. The incisal edge is reduced first. This is followed by two-plane reduction of the facial surface that is carried into the interproximal areas following the contours of the soft tissue (Figs 15-2a to 15-2j). The tissue is then retracted and the fin-

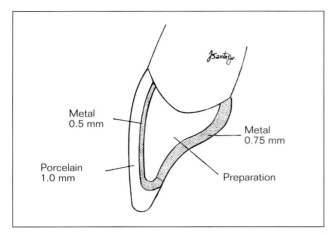

Fig 15-1 For a metal-ceramic crown, various amounts of tooth reduction are necessary for the different areas of porcelain and metal.

ish lines are refined. It is important to reduce enough tooth structure to allow the restoration to have natural contours and a flat emergence profile (ie, the vertical contours of the tooth should be nearly flat adjacent to the soft tissue), and it is important to follow the contours of the soft tissues as they rise interproximally.[40]

The type of crown margin desired will determine how the finish line is prepared.[45] A shoulder or a shoulder with a bevel are the most commonly used finish lines. If a metal facial margin is desired, a shoulder with a 45-degree bevel is usually prepared. Metal will cover the bevel and form a 90-degree butt joint with the porcelain. A metal margin is most commonly used if the margin is not visible when the patient smiles (Figs 15-3a and 15-3b). If the margin is visible, a porcelain margin is recommended, in which case a shoulder without a bevel is

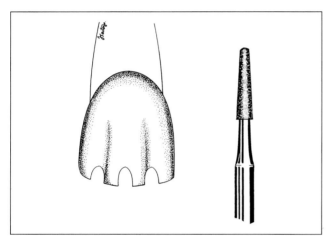

Fig 15-2a Depth cuts are made on the incisal edge with a bur of known dimensions.

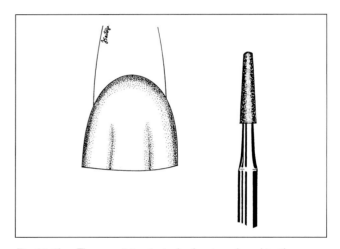

Fig 15-2b The remaining incisal edge is reduced to the same height. The incisal edge is angled slightly to the lingual.

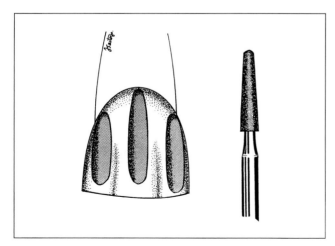

Fig 15-2c Depth cuts are made in the facial surface of the tooth, starting slightly above the projected finish line.

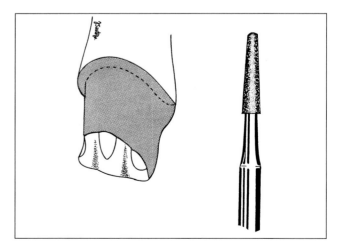

Fig 15-2d The remaining facial surface is reduced to the same depth, and the preparation is carried through the proximal contacts.

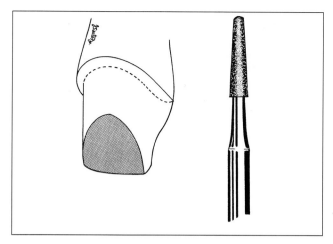

Fig 15-2e Additional tooth structure is reduced in the incisal half of the tooth at about a 30-degree angle to the long axis to allow adequate space for proper contours.

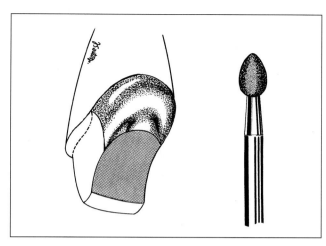

Fig 15-2f The lingual concavity is prepared with a football-shaped diamond bur.

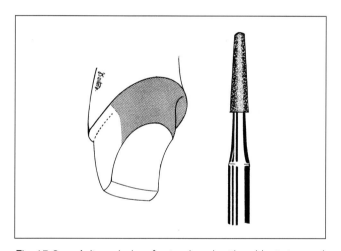

Fig 15-2g A lingual chamfer is placed with a blunt, tapered diamond bur.

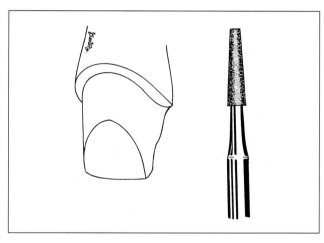

Fig 15-2h The facial and proximal shoulder is refined with a flat, cylindrical diamond bur.

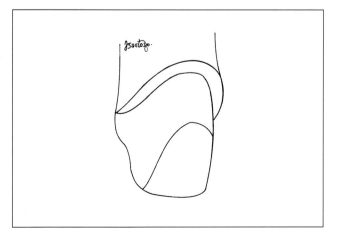

Fig 15-2i Facial view of the completed preparation.

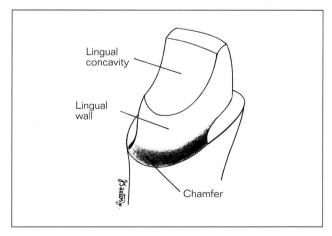

Lingual concavity

Lingual wall

Chamfer

Fig 15-2j Lingual view of the completed preparation.

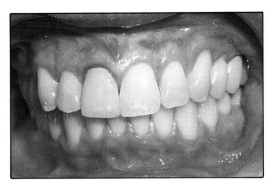

Fig 15-3a A metal margin may detract from the esthetic result if it is visible or shows through the tissue.

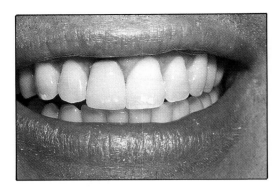

Fig 15-3b A metal margin may be the preferred design if it is not visible when the patient smiles.

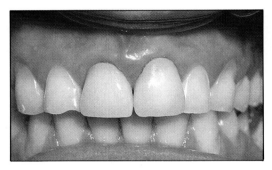

Fig 15-4 Metal-ceramic crowns on the maxillary central incisors with porcelain margins.

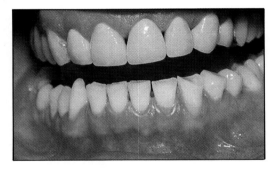

Fig 15-5 Porcelain can be highly destructive when it opposes enamel.

indicated (Fig 15-4). In either case, the finish line should be placed at the free gingival crest or slightly into the sulcus. There are few indications for placement of margins deep in the sulcus. Deep margins make the impression process difficult and cause chronic gingival inflammation.[36]

Metal-Ceramic Design

The metal substructure provides the strength and support necessary for predictable, long-term success. This is particularly true for posterior teeth. The metal substructure should be designed to support porcelain thicknesses of no more than 2.0 mm. The most common cause of metal-ceramic failure is reported to be improperly designed substructures.[54] It is desirable to keep porcelain out of occlusal contact unless it is opposed by porcelain. Porcelain is a very hard, abrasive material that can accelerate the wear of the opposing dentition and can, in some cases, be highly destructive[40,57] (Fig 15-5). Gold alloys wear at approximately the same rate as enamel.[18] With this in mind, the metal substructure should be designed so that centric contacts are in metal when possible. This is particularly true with canines (Figs 15-6a and 15-6b).

In most cases, occlusal contacts can be developed in metal in the maxillary arch. Metal can be carried to within 2.0 to 3.0 mm of the incisal edge on the lingual surface of the maxillary incisors and the centric contacts can be developed in metal (Fig 15-7a). A less desirable design is shown in Fig 15-7b. Metal occlusion can also generally be developed in the maxillary posterior teeth; a facial veneer of porcelain is carried into the interproximal surfaces and slightly onto the occlusal surface (Fig 15-8). The metal is not visible when the patient smiles, and the porcelain is kept out of occlusion because it is covering a noncentric cusp tip. In most cases, it is desirable to have the interproximal contacts in porcelain because they are easier to adjust and augment than metal and are generally more esthetic.

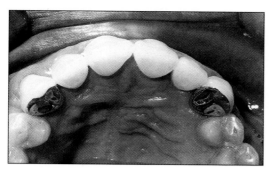

Fig 15-6a When possible, occlusal contacts should be developed in metal. In this case, metal is carried nearly to the incisal edge on the distal aspect of the canines to avoid lateral guidance on porcelain.

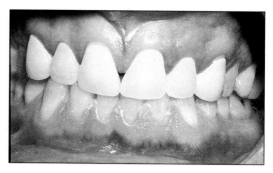

Fig 15-6b The metal protects the porcelain in lateral guidance but is not visible when viewed from the front.

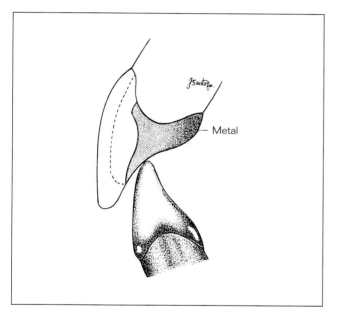

Fig 15-7a In the preferred occlusal relationship between a maxillary metal-ceramic crown and a natural mandibular incisor, the contact is in metal.

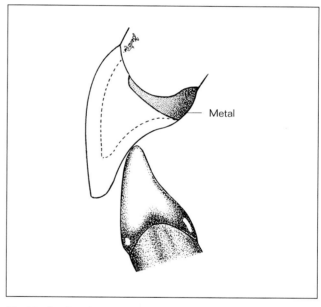

Fig 15-7b In a less desirable occlusal relationship, the opposing natural incisor contacts the restoration on porcelain. This is the recommended occlusal relationship when both maxillary and mandibular incisors are restored.

The mandibular arch can be more problematic when substructure design is planned. Porcelain is used for esthetic reasons, and therefore it is desirable to cover the metal substructure in visible areas. Because the esthetic zone for a mandibular tooth is the occlusal surface, it is not possible to cover visible areas with porcelain and place occlusal contacts in metal. Occlusal contacts are at the incisal edge of the anterior teeth and on the occlusal surfaces of the posterior teeth, both primary esthetic areas. Therefore, if esthetics is the patient's main concern, these areas must be covered with porcelain. The typical substructure design for the mandibular incisors is shown in Fig 15-9.

In the premolar area, the substructure is usually designed to allow complete porcelain coverage of the occlusal surface if esthetics are of primary importance. Porcelain coverage of only the facial surface and buccal cusp, similar to the design for maxillary posterior teeth, is not esthetic in the mandible. The facial surface is only partially visible, whereas the metal on the occlusal sur-

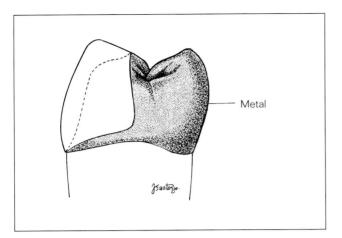

Fig 15-8 In the preferred metal-ceramic design for a maxillary premolar, the occlusion is developed in metal, yet only porcelain is visible.

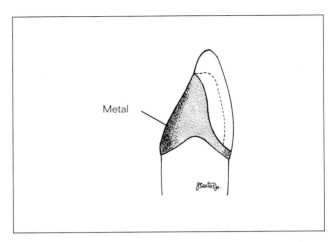

Fig 15-9 For mandibular incisors, in most cases, esthetic considerations will not allow the incisal edges to be restored in metal.

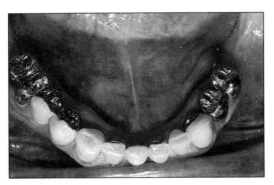

Fig 15-10a The metal-ceramic design for the mandibular right premolars is poorly conceived; these restorations are no more esthetic than the restorations on the left premolars. This metal-ceramic design combines poor esthetics with the potential for accelerated wear.

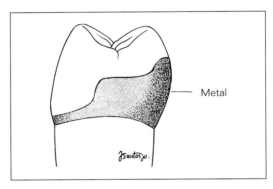

Fig 15-10b In a more esthetic metal-ceramic design, the entire occlusal surface is covered with porcelain. This is usually the preferred design for mandibular premolars, particularly if anterior guidance is present.

face is always visible (Fig 15-10a). The substructure design recommended for mandibular premolars is shown in Fig 15-10b.

The type of margin will affect the substructure design.[41] For a metal margin, the metal should cover the prepared bevel and form a butt joint with the porcelain (Fig 15-11a). For a porcelain margin, either of two metal designs may be used. The metal is usually carried down the axial wall to the shoulder, with about a 1.0-mm thickness of porcelain forming the margin (Fig 15-11b). This is the preferred design. Some technicians prefer to carry a very thin extension of the metal out to the margin (Fig 15-11c). Because the metal must be covered with opaque porcelain, this design may result in unnatural opacity at the gingival margin (Fig 15-12). This is an acceptable design, however, and can produce acceptable results.

Fig 15-11a In the preferred substructure design if a metal facial margin is desired, metal covers the bevel and forms a butt joint with the porcelain.

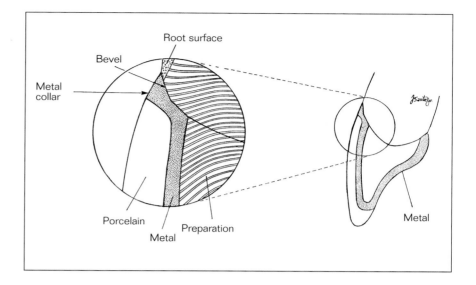

Fig 15-11b In the preferred substructure design for a porcelain facial margin, a uniform thickness of porcelain is carried to the finish line.

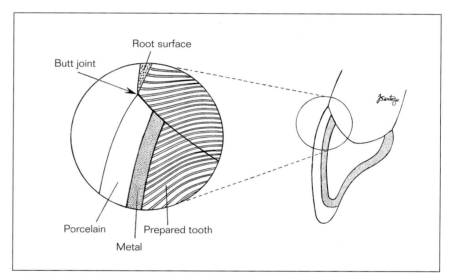

Fig 15-11c In a less desirable design for a porcelain margin, a thin extension of metal is carried out to the margin and covered with porcelain.

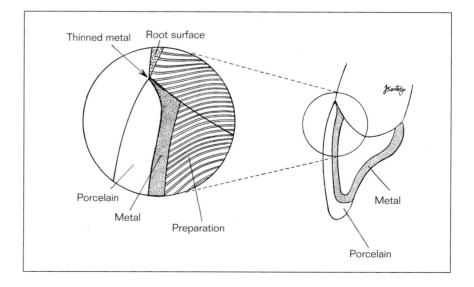

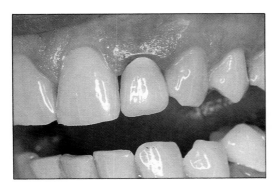

Fig 15-12 When the substructure shown in Fig 15-11c is used, the opaque porcelain may cause unnatural opacity at the gingival margin.

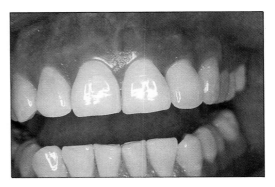

Fig 15-13 The metal substructure of the metal-ceramic crown on the maxillary left central incisor is extended only to within about 3.0 mm of the shoulder on the facial aspect, allowing light to enter the root through the cervical porcelain and provide natural illumination of the gingiva.

One other substructure design has been advocated for porcelain margins in which the metal extension on the facial surface is stopped 2.0 to 3.0 mm short of the shoulder and special porcelains that have more translucency than traditional shoulder porcelains are used. This design allows light to enter the root and "illuminates" the soft tissue covering the root, avoiding the shadowing that is sometimes present in the tissue adjacent to metal-ceramic restorations (Fig 15-13).

Matching Natural Teeth

In attempts to match natural teeth with porcelain crowns, the most important factors are shape, characterization, and shade. Restorations that are shaped correctly can be esthetic despite an imperfect color match. The shape of a porcelain crown should generally mirror that of the same tooth on the opposite side of the arch and should blend in with the shapes of the adjacent teeth (Fig 15-14).

Characterization refers to both the surface texture and the nonuniform aspects of color. It is important to become proficient at identifying the subtle characteristics present in teeth. Characterization of the teeth, once identified, can usually be incorporated into the porcelain. An example of characterization is shown in Fig 15-15.

The natural color of teeth is yellow-orange, but there are more than 700 visibly different shades.[15] Shades are usually described in three terms: *hue, value,* and *chroma. Hue* refers to the actual color, such as red or yellow. All teeth fall within the yellow range, but most range toward yellow-red and some slightly toward yellow-green.[52] *Value* refers to the brightness of the shade and is considered by many to be the most important aspect of shade selection.

The value describes where the shade falls in the gray range, from white to black. *Chroma* describes the concentration of color from faint to intense. The cervical areas of teeth are usually high and the incisal areas are usually low in chroma. These descriptive terms can be used to aid in shade selection and characterization and in describing errors in shade matching. For example, when a shade is not right, it can be analyzed: Is the value too high? Is the chroma too low? If the shape and characterization are correct, the shade usually only needs to be close.

Shades are selected with the aid of a shade guide, which consists of shade tabs arranged in some fashion to represent different combinations of opaque, body, and incisal porcelains (Fig 15-16). When the shade guides are utilized, it is advisable to attempt to match the color in the gingival and middle thirds of the tooth. The incisal porcelains are gray and translucent and nearly identical on all of the shade guide tabs. Often the incisal portion will have localized areas of high chroma or translucency that are not present on the shade guide and must be specified on the laboratory prescription. Body porcelain or modifiers are sometimes used in the incisal third when less translucency or more color is needed. It is important to select shades at the beginning of an appointment, because the teeth often become dehydrated during clinical procedures (Fig 15-17). Once the basic shade is determined, color characterization can be added internally with colored porcelains or externally with surface stains.

Materials Considerations

Many different alloys are used for metal-ceramic restorations. The American Dental Association classifies

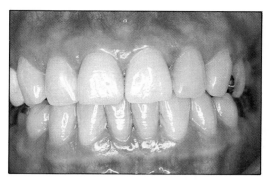

Fig 15-14 The shape and characterization of the metal-ceramic crown should mirror that of the same tooth on the opposite side of the arch. Despite being slightly high in value, the result is acceptable in the all-ceramic crown on the maxillary left central incisor.

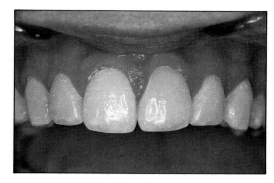

Fig 15-15 The metal-ceramic crowns on the maxillary central incisors are highly characterized.

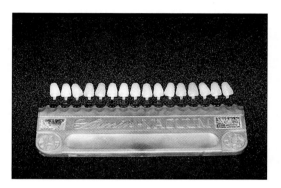

Fig 15-16 Ceramic shade guide.

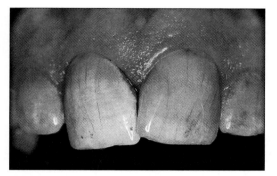

Fig 15-17 Shades should be chosen before the teeth have a chance to dehydrate. Significant dehydration can occur within a few minutes, as it did in the maxillary right central incisor shown here after removal of the rubber dam. The right central incisor is lighter and chalkier than is the left central incisor. Cotton roll isolation has the same effect. If the shade is selected after dehydration occurs, it will almost always be too light (high in value).

them as *high noble* (60% or greater noble metals and at least 40% gold, palladium, or platinum), *noble* (greater than 40% noble metals), or primarily *base* (less than 25% noble metals).[16] Recently, titanium-based metal-ceramic alloys have been developed.[31,55]

Any metal selected must have certain characteristics. It must form an oxide layer that allows bonding with porcelain. It must have a coefficient of thermal expansion that is compatible with that of the porcelain used and have a melting temperature sufficiently high that it will not melt or sag when the porcelain is fired. It must cast accurately and polish well.

Many porcelain systems are available for metal-ceramic applications, but all have certain characteristics in common. They are feldspathic porcelains that have similar compositions. They utilize an opaque porcelain that is applied in a thin layer on the metal substructure to mask the underlying color and provide the basic shade for the porcelain. The bulk of the ceramic is provided by body porcelain, which is more translucent and has lower chroma. This is supplemented with incisal or enamel porcelain, which forms the incisal edge and thins to blend with the body porcelain (Fig 15-18).

Precementation Procedures

Precementation procedures for metal-ceramic crowns are similar to those for cast restorations. They are discussed in detail in chapter 16.

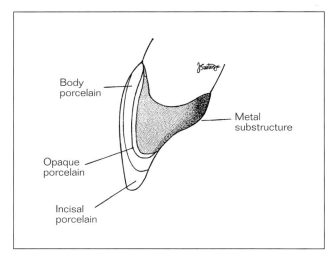

Fig 15-18 Porcelain is layered over the metal substructure.

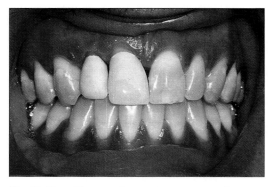

Fig 15-19a The metal-ceramic crowns on the maxillary right central and lateral incisors appear to be a poor match with the other teeth.

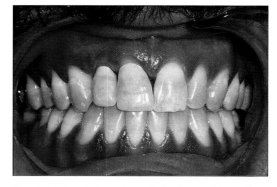

Fig 15-19b After characterization with surface stains, the restorations are better matched to the natural teeth. If the basic shade is close, surface stains can improve the match.

Surface Stains and Glazing Procedures

Once the porcelain has been shaped and the occlusion has been adjusted, characterization will usually improve the esthetic result. Surface smoothness should be increased or decreased, as necessary, by polishing or roughening the surface. Subtle surface color can be added with metal oxide stains. Surface stains are not very effective in changing the basic color of the porcelain. They increase metamerism (the tooth looks different under different types of light) and decrease translucency. Surface stains are very effective in adding subtle characterization, however. For example, they are effective at mimicking decalcified areas (Figs 15-3b and 15-15), adding brown or orange to the cervical or proximal areas, or adding to the translucent look at the incisal edge. If the basic shade is close, surface stains can greatly enhance the esthetic result (Figs 15-19a and 15-19b). The surface gloss can be duplicated with a high or low glaze (Fig 15-14). The level of the glaze (shiny or dull) is determined by the temperature and duration of the final firing of the porcelain.

If minor areas of adjustment are necessary on a previously glazed surface, a high shine can be obtained with rubber points, followed by diamond paste applied with a ragwheel.

Cementation

All of the efforts that have gone into fabrication of a fixed restoration can be nullified during cementation. Problems such as contamination of the cement or incomplete seating can prevent the successful completion of a restoration. To avoid these pitfalls, a rigid protocol for cementation is recommended. The casting and preparation should be thoroughly cleaned so that the cement is placed between clean, dry surfaces. The preparation can be cleaned with pumice or a mild solvent, and the casting can be cleaned with a detergent or solvent. Some clinicians clean their preparations with antimicrobial solutions, such as chlorhexidine. If the soft tissue interferes with seating or sulcular fluid is a problem, retraction cord should be placed.

The cement should be mixed according to the manufacturer's instructions; the crown is then loaded with cement and seated. The patient should be instructed to bite on an orangewood stick or another device, which should be moved up and down and back and forth for a few seconds. This technique, called *dynamic seating*, results in more complete seating of the crown.[42] The physical properties of most cements deteriorate if the cement gets wet during their initial setting phase, so every effort should be made to keep the cement dry for 5 minutes after cementation. The excess cement at the margin will protect the cement under the casting from contamination.[17] The final step is removal of the excess set cement. If the operator does not pay attention to detail, cement can easily be left in the sulcus. A discussion of cements is included in chapter 16.

All-Ceramic Restorations

Prior to the development of metal ceramics, porcelain jacket (all-ceramic) crowns were commonly used for single-unit anterior crowns. Porcelain fused-to-metal technology was developed in the 1960s and soon dominated the market. Metal-ceramic crowns had some esthetic shortcomings, but generally provided acceptable esthetics, increased strength, and improved fit. In recent years, the demand for superior esthetics has resulted in renewed interest in porcelain jacket crowns.

Prior to the development of metal-ceramic technology, porcelain jackets were made by adapting platinum foil to the master die. The foil acted as the matrix on which the porcelain was built. Once completed, the foil was peeled out, leaving an all-ceramic crown. By the 1980s, however, most of the laboratory skills needed to work with platinum foil had been lost. New techniques were developed that utilized refractory die materials and were considered more user-friendly by most laboratory technicians.

All-ceramic crowns may be used on any tooth, but are indicated primarily in the anterior segment when esthetics is of primary importance. They may be used on posterior teeth, but most all-ceramic porcelain systems have only about one fourth to one third the strength of metal-ceramic restorations.[20,24] Because a great amount of force can be generated between the posterior teeth, and acceptable esthetics can be attained with metal-ceramic crowns, all-ceramic crowns should be limited to the anterior teeth in most instances.[29] Despite manufacturers' claims, most of the all-ceramic systems have similar strength.[19,44,47] Generally speaking, ceramic materials do not have sufficient strength to be used alone for fixed partial dentures except, perhaps, in areas that are not in function. A high-alumina ceramic core material, InCeram (Vident), is stronger than other available dental ceramics[44] and has been recommended by some researchers for posterior use.[49,50] Further research and clinical experience will determine if InCeram is appropriate for these applications.

Most all-ceramic crowns provide superior esthetics because they allow transmission of light through the body of the tooth, like natural teeth, and because they allow some of the underlying tooth color to come through the crown. Lack of translucency is a major shortcoming of metal-ceramic restorations (Figs 15-20a and 15-20b). All-ceramic crowns represent a trade-off: improved esthetics for decreased strength. They are thought to have adequate strength for most anterior applications, however.

Preparations

A minimum of 1.2 mm of tooth reduction is necessary in all dimensions or strength is compromised[24]; reduction of 1.5 mm is preferred. The preparation for an all-ceramic crown requires more tooth reduction on the lingual surface than does the preparation for a metal-ceramic crown (Fig 15-21). For this reason, these preparations are not possible on some teeth. A smooth, 360-degree shoulder is recommended, with a sharp axiogingival line angle and no cavosurface bevel.[20] The shoulder is usually carried to the free gingival crest, and a taper of about 10 degrees is recommended.[24]

Porcelain Systems

Several methods are used to fabricate all-ceramic crowns,[59] and these methods may be used to classify different systems. For the purposes of this chapter, the materials will be classified as single-composition ceramics made on refractory die materials, crowns made with a distinct ceramic substructure, and castable glass ceramics.

Ceramic Crowns Made on Refractory Dies
The term *refractory* refers to materials that are stable at high temperatures.[38] In the fabrication of an all-ceramic restoration, the master impression is poured in die stone. A second (refractory) die is made, either by duplication of the master die or repouring of the impression in a refractory material. Porcelain is built on the refractory die and fired in a porcelain oven. One or more porcelain additions may be necessary. Once the desired contours are attained, the refractory material is carefully removed from the porcelain with burs, air abrasives, and/or acids. The restoration is then fit to the master (stone) die, preferably with the aid of magnification.

Many different porcelain systems that utilize refractory materials are available. Some utilize feldspathic

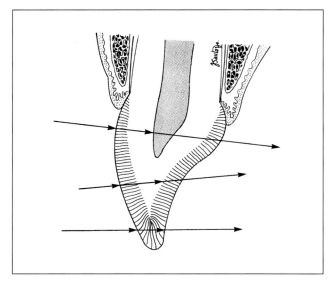

Fig 15-20a The translucent nature of a natural tooth allows some light to be transmitted through the body of the tooth.

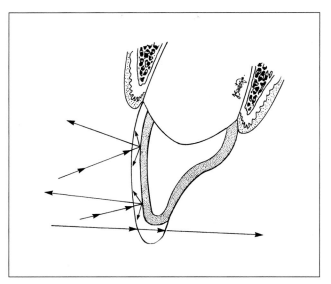

Fig 15-20b A metal-ceramic crown will not allow any light to transmit through the body of the tooth. The opaque layer masks the metal and reflects much of the incident light. For this reason, metal-ceramic crowns tend to lack natural translucency and often look more opaque than the surrounding natural teeth.

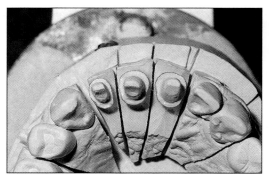

Fig 15-21 An all-ceramic crown requires more lingual tooth reduction than does a metal-ceramic crown. If enamel can be maintained on the lingual surface, however, reduction of only 0.5 mm is necessary with most ceramic materials.

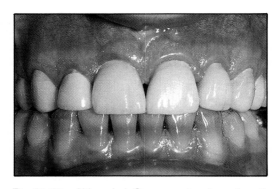

Fig 15-22 Although InCeram restorations (maxillary anterior teeth and first premolars) tend to be opaque, they are effective in masking dark underlying tooth structure, such as occurs from tetracycline staining.

porcelain, some utilize aluminous porcelain, and some incorporate a core material with a veneer of feldspathic or aluminous porcelain. Some laboratory technicians can manipulate the refractory materials well and produce excellent results, but many technicians have difficulty producing restorations with an accurate marginal fit.

In addition to laboratory difficulties, chairside surface staining can be a problem. Once the crown is recovered from the refractory die, an additional firing can cause rounding or distortion of the margins because the glazing temperature for traditional stains is only slightly less

than the fusing temperature of the porcelain. Special low-fusing surface stains that can be used with all-ceramic crowns are available.

Crowns with Ceramic Cores

Some all-ceramic systems incorporate a ceramic core material that is veneered with traditional dental porcelains. The core material usually adds strength and is stable at the sintering temperature of the veneering porcelain, allowing the margins to be fabricated in the core material. Current ceramic technology is such that, for

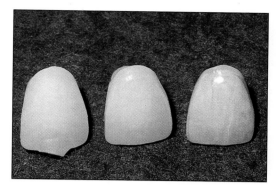

Fig 15-23 Cerammed, shaded, and characterized Dicor crowns.

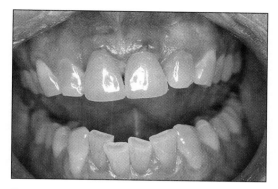

Fig 15-24 Dicor restorations (maxillary central incisors) are best suited to match teeth that are translucent and low in value.

the desired physical properties to be incorporated in the core materials, they tend to be rather opaque and unesthetic. Compatible veneering porcelains are used to cover the core materials in visible areas.

InCeram is a reinforced-alumina core material made on a refractory die. A lengthy, two-step process involves fabrication of a high-alumina porcelain framework followed by infiltration with a clear glass. This results in a coping that is considerably stronger than other ceramic materials.[13,44,51] Aluminous porcelain is built up and fired on the InCeram core to complete the restoration. The strength of this material is such that it has been advocated for use in the posterior segments, although its primary use is for single-unit anterior crowns.

The InCeram system overcomes some of the shortcomings of other all-ceramic systems. The coping is high strength, fits accurately, and is easily recovered from the refractory die. The margins may be fabricated in the InCeram material, which has a high fusing temperature so that repeated firings have little effect on marginal adaptation. The main drawbacks to the material are the lack of translucency in the core material (Fig 15-22), which limits its use in some cases, and additional cost.

The Empress System (Ivoclar) utilizes a compression-molded, high-leucite core material.[59] While not as strong as InCeram, Empress has excellent marginal adaptation and is more translucent. The core material comes in several shades and utilizes a proprietary veneering porcelain.

Spark-erosion technology is being adapted for use with dental ceramics. In this process, a die replica is eroded into a block of high-alumina ceramic material. The ceramic is then contoured to the desired substructure configuration and thickness. The high alumina content of the core material imparts strength, and the material has some translucency.

Castable Glass-Ceramic Crowns

Castable ceramics (Dicor, Dentsply) were introduced in the 1980s after modification of the process used to make cookware. A wax pattern is made on a stone die, invested, and cast into a clear glassy material. This is then heat treated, a process called *ceramming*, which strengthens the restoration and changes it from clear to frosty and colorless. Shading porcelain is applied to the surface to produce the desired color; three or four layers are usually required. Additional color can be imparted with surface stains and colored luting cements. Cerammed, shaded, and characterized Dicor crowns are shown in Fig 15-23.

Cast ceramic has a thin, crystalline layer on the surface that is referred to as the *skin*. It is thought to result from a reaction of the ceramic with the investment. The skin imparts some opacity and may be removed to add translucency to the restoration. It should not be partially removed in visible areas, however, because this will result in uneven color after shading porcelain is added. Any adjustment to a shaded surface results in show-through of the underlying translucent parent material. The parent material has about the same hardness[35] and rate of wear[18,28,37] as enamel. The skin is much harder than enamel, however; harder, in fact, than traditional porcelain. Shaded Dicor has hardness comparable to that of most porcelains. When possible, areas that are in occlusion, such as the lingual aspect of maxillary incisors, should be left unshaded and the skin should be removed.[11]

Castable ceramics have been shown to fit well[1] and to have strengths comparable to those of most other dental ceramic materials.[19,44] They are less plaque retentive than natural tooth structure, although that is true of ceramic materials in general.[2,14] They are the most translucent of the ceramic materials[43] and are particular-

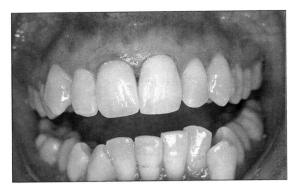

Fig 15-25 The Willi's Glass crown (maxillary right central incisor) combines the advantages of Dicor in the substructure and traditional ceramics in the visible areas.

ly well suited to matching teeth that are gray and translucent (Fig 15-24). They are not well suited to matching teeth that are opaque and highly characterized. Surface stains may be added without risk to the margins, because the melting temperature of castable ceramics is about 400°C higher than the firing temperature of the stains.

Combination Porcelain and Castable Ceramic

Willi Geller, a Swiss laboratory technician, developed the technique of veneering a castable ceramic substructure with aluminous porcelain. Crowns of this type are often referred to as the Willi's Glass crowns.[25] The system is marketed as Dicor Plus (Dentsply). The bond between the two ceramic materials is strong and uniform,[12] and the Willi's Glass crown is as strong as castable ceramic by itself.[5,12,23]

Willi's Glass incorporates the advantages of both materials and eliminates some of the disadvantages. It can usually be designed to take advantage of the desirable wear characteristics and high melting temperature of the castable ceramic and the ability to incorporate in-depth color and surface texture in the aluminous porcelain. The substructure is usually designed to incorporate occlusal contacts and margins in the castable ceramic, similar to the metal substructure design used for a crown with a metal margin, but without bevels. Visible areas are then veneered with the aluminous porcelain. The optical properties of the materials are such that excellent results are possible with Willi's Glass crowns (Figs 15-14 and 15-25), particularly when teeth with low values are being matched.

There are two drawbacks to Willi's Glass crowns. The tendency toward low value makes it difficult to match

teeth that are opaque or high in value. In addition, the extra procedures involved in fabrication usually result in extra charges from the laboratory.

Cementation

The cementation process is critical to the success of all-ceramic restorations, because the cement affects the final strength and color of the restoration. The common luting agents, such as zinc phosphate or glass-ionomer cement, should not be used. Resin composite cements offer several distinct advantages for most all-ceramic systems. Resin cements have been shown to increase the strength of all-ceramic restorations[6,22,26,30,33,34] and exhibit less microleakage than other cements.[8,46,51,56] This is particularly true when enamel that may be etched is present.[21] Resin composite cements tend to have a greater film thickness than the other cements, however.[32,53] Because all-ceramic crowns are weaker than other types of crowns, a cement that will improve the strength of the restoration is highly desirable.

The goal of cementation is to seal the margins of the crown and bond it to the prepared tooth. It is thought that forces are transmitted through the ceramic and distributed to and absorbed by the underlying tooth structure. The stronger the ceramic-tooth bond, the more efficient the distribution of force.[27,34] Resin composite cement best meets these criteria because it can be mechanically bonded to both tooth structure and ceramic materials.

A very durable bond can be formed between most ceramic materials and resin composite. The ceramic material is etched with hydrofluoric acid or a similar etchant to create micromechanical areas of retention. A thin layer of silane, a coupling agent, is then painted over the etched surface to provide better wetting by the resin cement and a chemical bond to supplement the mechanical bond.[3,48] The resin cement will form a strong, leak-resistant bond to the ceramic material[4] that is, in fact, stronger than the cohesive strength of the ceramic material itself.[39] The ceramic material is usually etched at the laboratory before the restoration is returned for cementation. Silane should be applied shortly before cementation.

Bonding to the tooth is not as reliable as bonding to the ceramic. At the cement-tooth interface, a strong bond is possible if enamel that can be etched is present.[9,21] In most cases, however, only dentin and cementum are present after tooth preparation. Several materials are recommended for the cementation process to maximize bond strength. A dentin adhesive system should be applied to the dentin surface to prepare it for

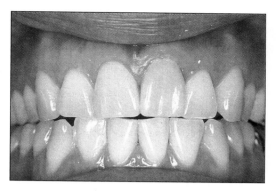

Fig 15-26 Unlike metal-ceramic crowns, cemented all-ceramic restorations are significantly influenced by the underlying color. In this case, an amalgam buildup shows through an all-ceramic crown on the maxillary left central incisor, making it too gray.

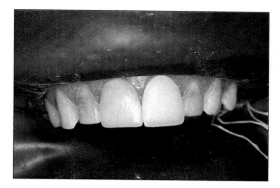

Fig 15-27 The cement draws the underlying tooth color through the ceramic. At try-in, the restoration on the left central incisor is significantly lighter than the cemented restoration on the right central incisor, although they were made at the same time with the same porcelain.

cementation. Use of dual-cured resin cement is recommended to bond the crown to the prepared dentinal surface. Dual-cured resins have a slow, autocured component and a light-cured component. The light will quickly polymerize most of the resin, but light polymerization decreases with increased thickness of porcelain.[7,10] In those areas that the light does not penetrate, a slow chemical reaction will complete the polymerization process. This is the preferred cementation process for most currently available ceramic materials.

The cementation process also affects the esthetic result of all-ceramic restorations. Unlike the color of metal-ceramic crowns, the color of an all-ceramic restoration may be greatly affected by the cement. If a translucent cement is used, it tends to draw the color of the underlying tooth or buildup material through the crown. This is desirable in many instances, but may be undesirable if, for example, an underlying amalgam restoration causes graying (Fig 15-26). Most of the resin cements are translucent, but opaque cements are also available. One consideration in cement selection is the need to cover up or draw out the underlying color.

The color of an all-ceramic restoration tried in without cement is significantly different from the color after cementation (Fig 15-27). To estimate the postcementation color, it is advisable to experiment with different cements prior to cementation. The colored component of a resin cement may be used for try-in but must be cleaned out of the restoration with a solvent such as acetone prior to final cementation. Some resin cements come with water-soluble try-in pastes that attempt to mimic the optical effects of the cements and rinse away after try-in.

The clinical steps involved in cementing an all-ceramic crown are outlined in the box.

Cementation of All-Ceramic Crowns with Resin Cements

1. Apply a thin layer of silane to the clean, etched inner surface of the crown and allow to dry.
2. Clean the preparation with pumice or a solvent or detergent.
3. Apply a dentin adhesive system to the preparation, according to the manufacturer's instructions. In most cases, this includes an etchant, a primer, and an adhesive. Thin the adhesive as much as possible with a brush and avoid pooling. Light cure.
4. Partially fill the crown with a light- or dual-cured cement. Cover all of the margins.
5. Gently push the crown to place with finger pressure.
6. Remove excess cement with a clean brush.
7. Gently tap the incisal edge of the crown with a mirror handle or another instrument to extrude excess cement. A bead of cement should form around the margins.
8. Light cure from the facial and lingual aspects for 1 minute each.
9. Remove excess cement with a spoon excavator or scaler. Break off the cement bead by sliding the instrument from the ceramic to the tooth.
10. Carefully examine all margins with an explorer and air stream for any remaining cement.

References

1. Abbate MF, Tjan AH, Fox WM. Comparison of the marginal fit of various ceramic crown systems. J Prosthet Dent 1989;61:527-531.

2. Adamcyk E, Spiechowicz E. Plaque accumulation on crowns made of various materials. Int J Prosthodont 1990;3:285-291.

3. Bailey L, Bennett R. Dicor surface treatments for enhanced bonding. J Dent Res 1988;67:925-931.

4. Bailey L, Bennett R. Two year bond results of Dicor ceramic/LA cement system [abstract 1734]. J Dent Res 1989;68:398.

5. Bales DJ, Duffin JL, Johnson GH. Evaluation of the fracture resistance of two ceramic crown techniques [abstract 538]. J Dent Res 1990;69:176.

6. Bernal G, Jones RM, Brown DT, Munoz CA, Goodacre CJ. The effect of finish line form and luting agent on the breaking strength of Dicor crowns. Int J Prosthodont 1993;6:286-290.

7. Blackman R, Barghi N, Duke ES. Influence of ceramic thickness on the polymerization of light-cured resin cement. J Prosthet Dent 1990;63:295-300.

8. Blair KF, Koeppen RG, Schwartz RS, Davis RD. Microleakage associated with resin composite–cemented, cast glass ceramic restoration. Int J Prosthodont 1993;6:579-584.

9. Bowen RL, Cobb EN. A method for bonding to dentin and enamel. J Am Dent Assoc 1983;107:734-736.

10. Boyer DB, Chan KC. Curing light-activated composite cement through porcelain [abstract 1289]. J Dent Res 1989;68:476.

11. Campbell SD, Kelly JR. The influence of surface preparation on the strength and surface microstructure of a cast dental ceramic. Int J Prosthodont 1989;2:459-468.

12. Campbell SD. Esthetic modification of cast dental-ceramic restorations. Int J Prosthodont 1990;3:123-130.

13. Castellani D, Baccetti T, Giovannoni A, Bernardini UD. Resistance to fracture of metal ceramic and all-ceramic crowns. Int J Prosthodont 1994;7:149-154.

14. Chan C, Webber H. Plaque retention on teeth restored with full ceramic crowns: A comparative study. J Prosthet Dent 1986;6:666-671.

15. Clark EB. The color problem in dentistry. Dent Digest 1931;37:499-509.

16. Council on Dental Materials, Instruments and Equipment. Classification system for cast alloys. J Am Dent Assoc 1984;109:766.

17. Curtis SR, Richards MW, Meiers JC. Early erosion of glass-ionomer cement at crown margins. Int J Prosthodont 1993;6:553-557.

18. Delong R, Pintado MR, Douglas WH. The wear of enamel opposing shaded ceramic restorative materials: An in vitro study. J Prosthet Dent 1992;68:42-48.

19. Dickinson AJG, Moore BK, Harris RK, Dykema RW. A comparative study of the strength of aluminous porcelain and all-ceramic crowns. J Prosthet Dent 1989;61:297-304.

20. Doyle MG, Munoz CA, Goodacre CJ, Friedlander LD, Moore BK. The effect of tooth preparation design on the breaking strength of Dicor crowns. Part 2. Int J Prosthodont 1990;3:241-245.

21. Duffin JL, Bales DJ, Johnson GH. Fracture resistance of castable ceramic crowns [abstract 429]. J Dent Res 1989;68:235.

22. Eden GT, Kacicz JM. Dicor crown strength improvement due to bonding [abstract 801]. J Dent Res 1987;66:207.

23. Ferro KJ, Myers ML, Graser GN. Fracture strength of full-contoured ceramic crowns and porcelain-veneered crowns of ceramic copings. J Prosthet Dent 1994;71:462-467.

24. Friedlander LD, Munoz CA, Goodacre CJ, Friedlander LD, Moore BK. The effect of tooth preparation design on the breaking strength of Dicor crowns. Part 1. Int Prosthodont 1990;3:159-166.

25. Geller WG, Kwialkowski SJ. The Willi's glass crown: A new solution in the dark and shadowed zones of esthetic porcelain restorations. Quintessence Dent Technol 1987;11:233-242.

26. Grossman DG, Nelson JW. The bonded Dicor crown [abstract 800]. J Dent Res 1987;66:206.

27. Grossman DG. Photoelastic examination of bonded crown interfaces [abstract 719]. J Dent Res 1989;68:271.

28. Hankinson JA, Cappeta EG. Five years' clinical experience with a leucite-reinforced porcelain crown system. Int J Periodont Rest Dent 1994;14:139-153.

29. Jacob R, Shillingburg H, Duncanson M. Abrasiveness of gold and eight ceramic surfaces against tooth structure [abstract 1701]. J Dent Res 1989;68:394.

30. Jensen ME, Sheth JJ, Toliver D. Etched porcelain resin-bonded full-veneer crowns: In vitro fracture resistance. Compend Contin Educ Dent 1989;10:336-342.

31. Leong D, Chai J, Lautenschlager E, Gilbert J. Marginal fit of machine-milled titanium and cast titanium single crowns. Int J Prosthodont 1994;7:440-447.

32. Levine WA. An evaluation of the film thickness of resin luting agents. J Prosthet Dent 1989;62:175-178.

33. McInnes-Ledoux PM, Ledoux WR, Weinberg R. A bond strength study of luted castable ceramic restorations. J Dent Res 1989;68:823-825.

34. Meseros AJ, Evans DB, Schwartz RS. Influence of a dentin bonding agent on the fracture load of Dicor. Am J Dent 1994;7:137-140.

35. Naylor WP, Munoz CA, Goodacre CJ, Swartz ML, Moore BK. The effect of surface treatment on the Knoop hardness of Dicor. Int J Prosthodont 1991;4:147-151.

36. Newcombe GM. The relationship between the location of subgingival crown margins and gingival inflammation. J Periodontal 1974;45:151-159.

37. Palmer DS, Barco MT, Pelleu GB. Wear of human enamel against a commercial castable ceramic restorative material. J Prosthet Dent 1991;65:192-195.

38. Phillips RW. Skinners Science of Dental Materials, ed 8. Philadephia: Saunders, 1982.

39. Pratt RC, Burgess JO, Schwartz RS, Smith JD. Evaluation of bond strength of six porcelain repair systems. J Prosthet Dent 1989;62:11-13.

40. Preston J. Rational approach to tooth preparation for ceramo-metal procedures. Dent Clin North Am 1977;21:683-703.

41. Rhodes SK. The porcelain butt margin with hydrocolloid impression technique. J Prosthet Dent 1988;59:418-420.

42. Rosenstiel SF, Gegauff AF. Improving cementation of complete cast crowns: A comparison of static and dynamic seating methods. J Am Dent Assoc 1988;117:845-848.

43. Seghi RR, Sorensen J, Brown J. Relative translucency of esthetic restorative materials [abstract 821]. J Dent Res 1990;69:211.

44. Seghi RR, Sorensen JA, Engelman MJ, Rouranas E, Torres TJ. Flexural strength of new ceramic materials [abstract 1521]. J Dent Res 1990;69:299.

45. Shillingburg HT, Hobo S, Fisher DW. Preparation design and margin distortion in porcelain-fused-to-metal restorations. J Prosthet Dent 1973;29:276-284.

46. Shortall AC, Fayyad MA, Williams JD. Marginal seal of injection-molded ceramic crowns cemented with three adhesive systems. J Prosthet Dent 1989;61:24-27.

47. Sobanski DB, Pameijer CH. Resistance to fracture of Optec porcelain vs. conventional porcelain [abstract 178]. J Dent Res 1989;68:204.

48. Sorensen JA, Kang SK, Avera SA. Porcelain-composite interface microleakage with various porcelain surface treatments. Dent Mater 1991;7:118-121.

49. Sorensen JA, Kang SK, Roumanas E, Avera SP. Effect of preparation design on flexural strength of all-ceramic bridges [abstract 1642]. J Dent Res 1991;70:471.

50. Sorensen JA, Kang SK, Kyomen SM, Avera SP, Faulkner R. Marginal fidelity of all-ceramic bridges [abstract 2192]. J Dent Res 1991;70:540.

51. Sorensen JA. Marginal fidelity and microleakage of porcelain veneers made by two techniques. J Prosthet Dent 1992;67:16-22.

52. Sproull RC. Color matching in dentistry. Part II. Practical applications of the organization of color. J Prosthet Dent 1973;29:556-566.

53. Staninec M, Giles WS Saiku JM, Hattori M. Caries penetration and cement thickness of three luting agents. Int J Prosthodont 1988;1:259.

54. Stein RS, Kuwata M. A dentist and a dental technologist analyze ceramo-metal procedures. Dent Clin North Am 1977;21:729-749.

55. Valderrama S, Van Roekel N, Andersson M, Goodacre CJ, Munoz CA. A comparison of the marginal and internal adaptation of titanium and gold-platinum-palladium metal ceramic crowns. Int J Prosthodont 1995;8:29-37.

56. White SN, Sorensen JA, Kang SK, Caputo AA. Microleakage of new luting agents [abstract 514]. J Dent Res 1990;69:173.

57. Wiley MG. Effects of porcelain on occluding surfaces of restored teeth. J Prosthet Dent 1989;61:133-137.

58. Wohlwend A, Strub JR, Schärer P. Metal ceramic and all-porcelain restorations: Current considerations. Int J Prosthodont 1989;40:13.

59. Wohlwend A, Schärer P. The Empress Technique. Quintessenz Zahntech 1990;16:966-978.

Cast-Gold Restorations

Thomas G. Berry / David A. Kaiser / Richard S. Schwartz

The cast-gold restoration has lessened in popularity over the past 20 years because of the increased emphasis on esthetics, but it remains an excellent restoration with a long history of success. If used with care, gold is considered to have the greatest longevity of any restorative material used in dentistry. This opinion is generally supported by longitudinal studies,[2,38,40] although it is disputed by other studies.[39,41,66] Cast gold may be used for intracoronal (inlays) or extracoronal (complete coverage crowns) restorations, or for restorations that are a combination of both (onlays or partial-coverage crowns) (Fig 16-1).

Gold castings present several advantages over direct restorative materials, such as silver amalgam or resin composite. Because castings are fabricated with an indirect technique, it is possible to achieve nearly ideal contours and occlusion.[59] Gold is a strong material that rarely fractures and, when used as an extracoronal restoration, can provide protection to the tooth.[55,62] Gold wears at a rate similar to that of enamel, so it does not cause accelerated wear of the opposing teeth.[10] It casts easily and accurately, and, if a type II or type III gold is used, marginal adaptation can usually be improved after the restoration is cast.

The primary drawback to use of cast-gold rather than direct restorations is higher cost, because castings require at least two appointments for the patient and have associated laboratory costs. For esthetic reasons, gold castings are usually used to restore posterior teeth, where they are not as visible. For the more anterior teeth, preparations are usually designed so that the gold is hidden from direct observation (Figs 16-2a and 16-2b).

This chapter will address the indications, materials, and clinical steps for the fabrication of cast-gold restorations.

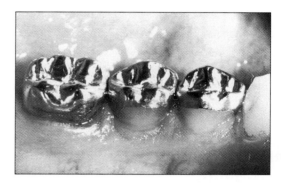

Fig 16-1 Partial and complete-coverage cast restorations.

Indications

The indications for a cast-gold restoration range from a relatively small carious lesion, restored with an inlay, to a severely weakened and/or malfunctioning tooth, restored with a complete-coverage crown. Cast-gold restorations may be used to restore teeth with carious lesions or to replace existing restorations. They are generally indicated for situations in which other, less expensive materials are not suitable for establishing proper proximal and/or occlusal contacts, creating appropriate axial contours, or protecting the remaining tooth structure. A cast-gold restoration may also be indicated when gold has been used to restore adjacent and/or opposing teeth so that problems arising from use of dissimilar metals do not occur.[8,52]

The morphology of posterior teeth, the number of carious surfaces, the number of restored surfaces, the width and depth of existing restorations,[34] and the occlusal

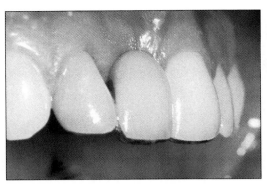
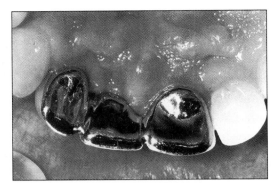

Figs 16-2a and 16-2b These anterior restorations are designed to display very little of the gold from the facial aspect. The incisal gold is angled so that light is not reflected directly back at the viewer.

relationships must be considered when the need for a cast restoration is determined. Non–working-side contacts can be especially important. Hiatt[21] has shown a significant increase in the number of vertical fractures in teeth with non–working-side contacts.

Basic Principles of Cast Restorations

There are many acceptable techniques and designs for cast restorations that enable them to be adapted to many situations. Certain principles always apply, however.

Conservation of Tooth Structure

It is desirable to make preparations as conservative as possible. This maximizes the strength of the remaining tooth structure, lessens the likelihood of postoperative sensitivity and pulpal pathosis, and decreases the likelihood of tooth fracture.

Tooth preservation involves more than simply minimizing the removal of tooth structure. Preparations must be designed to protect remaining tooth structure. This may necessitate additional reduction to remove weak tooth structure or it may necessitate cuspal coverage. Studies have shown that, as a cavity preparation gets wider[35,65] and deeper,[4] progressive weakening of the tooth occurs. When an inlay preparation exceeds one third the intercuspal width, an onlay or another extracoronal restoration should be considered to protect the cusps of the tooth. Because an extracoronal restoration covers both facial and lingual surfaces, it protects the remaining tooth structure to reduce the incidence of tooth fracture.[55]

Retention and Resistance Form

Retention and resistance form are two separate but related features of a preparation. Correctly incorporated, they resist unseating forces that are placed on the restoration during function or parafunction. *Retention form* resists forces attempting to remove a restoration along the path of insertion. *Resistance form* resists forces attempting to dislodge a restoration obliquely to the path of insertion. Although retention and resistance are two separate features of the preparation, they are usually closely interrelated and may be difficult to distinguish clinically as separate features.

Retention is gained when two or more walls oppose each other. These walls may be intracoronal, extracoronal, or a combination of the two (Figs 16-3a and 16-3b). The amount of retention created by these opposing walls is determined by several factors. The degree of convergence toward the occlusal (extracoronal walls) or divergence toward the occlusal (intracoronal walls) and the length of the walls are the most important factors. The longer[18] and more nearly parallel the walls, the greater the retention.[27] One long wall opposed by a short wall provides retention equivalent only to the short wall. Additionally, the greater the circumference, the greater the retention. Retention and resistance form may also be gained by adding intracoronal walls. Twisting or rotational forces are countered by the presence of grooves, boxes, or other features, such as pins or potholes[19] (Figs 16-4a and 16-4b).

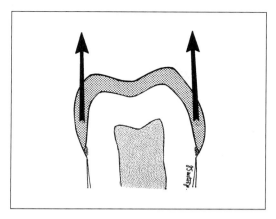

Fig 16-3a Complete-coverage crowns rely on the opposing external walls to provide retention for the restoration. A slight taper of the walls in the occlusal direction provides a path of insertion.

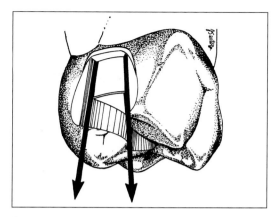

Fig 16-3b Inlays (pictured) and onlays rely on tapering opposing internal walls for retention.

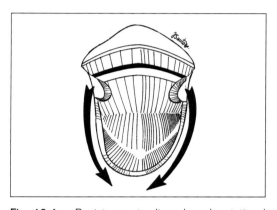

Fig 16-4a Resistance to lingual and rotational forces may be provided by proximal grooves.

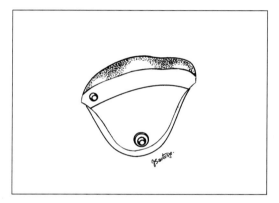

Fig 16-4b Pinholes also provide resistance to lingual displacement.

All the preparation types must allow the cast restoration to seat in and/or on the tooth. To allow this seating, the walls of the preparation must taper to some degree. A taper of 3 to 6 degrees of each wall toward the occlusal is considered ideal,[14,39] and a convergence angle of 2.5 to 6.5 degrees has been shown to minimize concentration of stresses.[14] In reality, however, preparations with this degree of parallelism rarely occur. Although a rapid loss of retention occurs as the taper progresses from 5 to 10 degrees for each wall,[11] a total convergence up to 16 degrees still provides adequate retention.[19,69] Insufficient retention is a major cause of failure of fixed prostheses.[66]

Recent developments in luting agents and techniques of metal conditioning allow the cast restoration to be bonded to the tooth, adding to the resistance to displacement from the preparation. To take advantage of this bonding, the metal may be treated by tin plating and luted with a resin luting cement. The long-term effectiveness of bonded castings in not yet known.

Pulpal Considerations

Tooth preparation for any cast restoration involves dentin, and therefore affects the pulp. Often, in situations in which a restoration is indicated, the pulp has already been traumatized by caries and/or previous restorations. Prior to tooth preparation, the pulp should be tested for vitality and radiographs should be made. The additional trauma created by tooth preparation can be enough to cause necrosis of an unhealthy pulp. If the vitality of the pulp is in doubt, endodontic therapy should be performed prior to preparation.

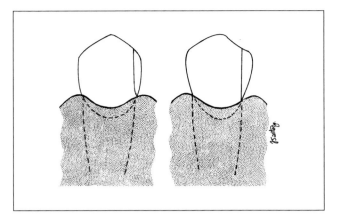

Fig 16-5 Flat proximal surfaces *(left)* allow the easy formation of a chamfered finish line, while bell-shaped anatomy *(right)* makes it difficult to create such a finish line without severe reduction of the proximal surface.

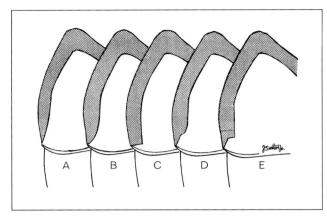

Fig 16-6 Forms of finish line: (A) knife-edged; (B) chamfer; (C) shoulder; (D) beveled chamfer; (E) beveled shoulder.

Pulpal considerations for cast restorations are the same as those for direct restorations. The best pulpal protection is a thick layer of sound dentin. A thorough discussion of the subject can be found in chapter 3.

Certain anatomic considerations are critical to the planning of the preparation, especially in younger patients. The pulp horns may be large enough to be exposed during tooth preparation. Examination of preoperative radiographs is imperative to identify such potential problems. Because the pulp is narrower in the cervical region of the tooth, pulpal exposures are less likely to occur in this area.

Postcementation thermal sensitivity is sometimes a problem. Several methods to prevent or minimize this problem have been recommended. Some clinicians scrub the preparations with antimicrobial solutions to remove bacterial contamination. Bacterial contamination under restorations is thought to be the major cause of postoperative sensitivity.[5,7] Some clinicians apply a varnish or dentin adhesive to seal the dentinal surface prior to cementation to prevent migration of bacteria into the tubules. Techniques vary depending on the cement used, and these are discussed later in the chapter.

Finish Lines

The term *finish line* refers to the border of the preparation where the prepared tooth structure meets the unprepared surface of the tooth. The type of finish line depends on the clinical situation. A smooth, well-defined finish line is beneficial, regardless of the design used, to facilitate laboratory procedures and finishing of the restoration. Selection of the type of finish line may be dictated by the shape of the tooth (bell shaped versus flat) (Fig 16-5), the desired location of the finish line, or operator preference. The most common types of finish lines for cast restorations are knife-edged, chamfer, and shoulder. Both the chamfer and the shoulder may be beveled or unbeveled (Fig 16-6).

Knife-edged

A knife-edged finish line requires the least amount of tooth reduction. It is sometimes used when the tooth is bell shaped, because creation of a heavier margin would require excessive removal of tooth structure. Generally, a knife-edged finish line is not desirable because it is more difficult to discern on a die than other finish lines, and it tends to result in overcontoured restorations.

Chamfer

A chamfer is often the preferred finish line for extracoronal restorations. It creates a sharp, easily identified margin that provides room for adequate thickness of gold without overcontouring the restoration.

Shoulder

The shoulder finish line is chosen primarily in situations where a bulk of material is needed to strengthen the restoration in the marginal areas, as for all porcelain or metal-ceramic restorations. It is the least conservative of the finish line types for cast gold and causes the most difficulty in fitting the margin of the restoration.

Chamfer or Shoulder with a Bevel

This design is preferred by some clinicians who believe that a beveled margin is easier to detect in an impression and that it makes the margins of the casting more burnishable. A bevel is recommended for proximal boxes.

Gingival Considerations

Gargiulo et al[15] described the dentogingival junction as consisting of the junctional epithelium and the gingival fiber attachment to cementum, coronal to the alveolar crest. In healthy tissue, the average length of each of these zones is approximately 1.0 mm in an apicocoronal direction (Fig 16-7). The combined zones of the junctional epithelium and the supracrestal fibers are often referred to as the *biologic width.*[24] If restorative margins violate the biologic width and impinge on the supracrestal fibers, gingival inflammation results and may lead to loss of periodontal attachment.[12,24,44,75] If possible, finish lines should not be prepared further than 0.5 to 1.0 mm into the sulcus,[13,43] or closer than 1.0 mm to the base of the sulcus.[76] A more complete discussion of this subject may be found in chapter 1.

Because gingival health may be adversely affected by subgingival finish lines,[25,45,60,61,68] the finish lines should be placed supragingivally if the situation permits. When it is necessary to place finish lines within the gingival crevice because of caries, existing restorations, fractures, root sensitivity, or short clinical crowns,[31,44] care must be exercised to minimize the damage to gingival tissues. The fragile soft tissue may be reflected by careful placement of retraction cord prior to final preparation of the finish line to avoid damaging these soft tissues.

Contours

The establishment of proper contours of the restoration is dependent on proper tooth preparation. An overcontoured casting is often the result of an underprepared tooth. If removal of tooth structure is insufficient, the crown has to be overcontoured to obtain sufficient thickness of metal.

Overcontoured crowns have been reported to encourage plaque retention, resulting in gingival inflammation[42,51,77] (Fig 16-8). Even with overcontoured crowns, however, the gingival health can be maintained if the patient practices excellent oral hygiene.

Wheeler[70] proposed that convexities be created in the gingival third of artificial crowns to deflect food away from the free gingiva. Herlands et al[20] however, showed

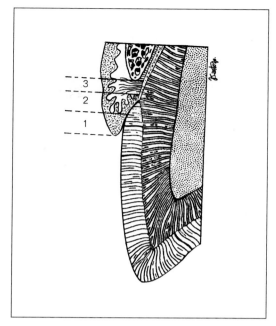

Fig 16-7 Anatomy of the periodontium: (1) gingival sulcus; (2) junctional epithelium; (3) connective tissue attachment.

that the maximum bulge in the natural crown at its greatest diameter is no more than 0.5 mm greater than at the cementoenamel junction and that the impaction mechanism of gingival injury does not occur. The biologic acceptability of undercontouring is often observed when a provisional crown is lost from a prepared tooth for an extended time without adverse effects on the surrounding gingiva. A natural contour (ie, the exact replacement of the axial and proximal morphology) is the desired form for cast-gold restorations when the gingival crest is at a normal level.

When the free gingival margin is at a more apical position because of recession or surgery, a flattened contour best reproduces the contour of the root surface.[77] Flat contours are recommended occlusal to furcations to allow access for cleaning.

Stein[64] described the contours of restorations adjacent to the gingiva as the *emergence profile.* He stated that the proximal emergence profiles of all natural teeth are either flat or concave. This natural contour provides an open gingival embrasure that promotes good oral hygiene (Fig 16-9).

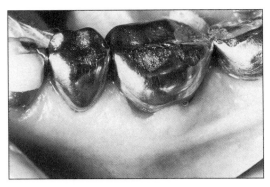

Fig 16-8 Overcontoured restorations lead to problems. Note the loss of normal gingival contours and the edematous appearance of the tissue.

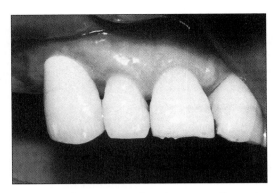

Fig 16-9 Open proximal embrasures allow adequate space for healthy tissues and access for good oral hygiene.

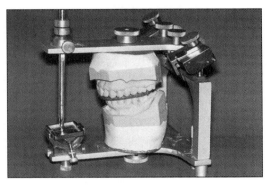

Fig 16-10 The semiadjustable articulator, shown with a jaw relation record in place, simulates mandibular movements more closely than the simple articulators.

Occlusion

No restoration, no matter how well crafted, will be successful if it does not function correctly. Satisfactory occlusion is a necessity if the restoration is to achieve adequate function and patient comfort.

Establishing biologically acceptable occlusion starts with careful planning. The teeth opposing the one to be restored (whether in a natural or restored state) should be properly aligned and in the desired occlusal plane. Occlusal surfaces should be well formed. If these conditions do not exist, the opposing dentition should be recontoured or restored, if possible. Failure to do so may seriously compromise the occlusal relationships and, in turn, the future health and function of the involved teeth[33] as well as the patient's comfort.[1]

Acceptable occlusion has several characteristics. Multiple contact points exist between opposing teeth that come into contact simultaneously during closure. The maximum closure position is referred to as *maximum intercuspation.* Ideally, the facial cusps of the mandibular teeth and the lingual cusps of the maxillary teeth contact the opposing teeth in a fossa or on a marginal ridge so that the occlusal contacts stabilize the teeth in both arches. In most cases, contact on the anterior teeth separates the posterior teeth during any eccentric movement of the jaw. This occlusal relationship is referred to as *anterior guidance* or *mutually protected occlusion.* Another occlusal relationship, referred to as *group function,* sometimes exists or is created. In this relationship, teeth on the functional side share equally in the contact during lateral movements of the mandible.

A major benefit of indirect fabrication of a restoration is the ability to form the wax pattern to fit the desired occlusal relationships. The wax pattern (and ultimately the restoration) must contact its antagonist in the prescribed contact areas at precisely the instant the other teeth contact. A premature contact or a noncentric interference may be uncomfortable, produce loosening or accelerated wear of the restoration or its antagonist, and/or damage the health of the tooth and its supporting structures.

Occlusion should be developed with mounted casts on an articulator. For single-unit castings, a simple hinge articulator may be adequate, although it allows accurate reproduction of maximum intercuspation only. Lateral or protrusive interferences must be adjusted in the mouth. In more complicated situations, as for multiple units, use of a more sophisticated semiadjustable articulator may be indicated (Fig 16-10). When casts are mounted on a semiadjustable articulator with a facebow, the lateral and protrusive movements of the mandible may be simulated with reasonable accuracy.[17]

To verify the accuracy of the relationship of the mounted casts, the patient's occlusal contacts should be checked intraorally with shimstock. If a small discrepancy exists between the patient's occlusal contacts and those on the the mounted casts, the casts can be corrected with shimstock, thin articulating paper, and a carving instrument. If the discrepancy is great, it will be necessary to remount the casts. If the casts are mounted accurately and the casting is correctly fabricated, minimal adjustments will be necessary at the insertion appointment.

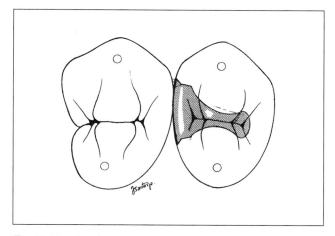

Fig 16-11   An inlay is an intracoronal restoration.

Types of Cast Restorations

The variety of cast restorations ranges from inlays (small intracoronal restorations) to complete-coverage castings (restorations that cover the entire coronal surface of the tooth). Onlays and partial-coverage castings are hybrids that possess both intracoronal and extracoronal features. The design chosen should be the one that removes the least sound tooth structure while it restores the missing tooth structure and allows the tooth to withstand functional and parafunctional forces.

Inlay

The gold inlay is a treatment option for conservative Class 2 lesions. Although used less frequently than in the past, the inlay has a long history of success. It is not uncommon to see a patient who has multiple inlays that are 30 years old and still clinically serviceable.

Inlays are entirely intracoronal restorations, most commonly with occlusal and proximal extensions (Fig 16-11). The preparation should be as conservative as possible to maintain tooth strength. If the occlusal width of the preparation exceeds one third to one half the buccolingual intercuspal distance, a restoration offering more protection for the cusps, such as an onlay, should be planned.[65] The occlusal contacts should be entirely on gold or enamel, not on a margin of the restoration.

Occlusal Preparation

Initial entry is made in the central fossa with a tapered fissure bur to establish the pulpal floor (Fig 16-12). The depth is determined by the extent of existing caries or restorations or the need for additional retention. The occlusal outline is extended mesiodistally along the central groove and stopped just short of the marginal ridge. The bur is kept in the vertical position in the long axis of

the tooth throughout the preparation so that its taper provides the 3- to 5-degree divergence toward the occlusal to the facial and lingual walls (total divergence of 6 to 10 degrees) (Fig 16-13).

Proximal Boxes

The tapered fissure bur is used to create proximal boxes mesially and/or distally. A thin layer of proximal enamel is left to protect the adjacent tooth while the proximal box is formed (Fig 16-14). The faciolingual dimension is determined by any existing restoration, caries, and the relationship of the proximal surface to the adjacent tooth. The gingival floor of the box should have an axial depth of approximately 1.5 mm. Ideally, the gingival extension should be established occlusal to the height of the papilla (Fig 16-15). However, the presence of caries or an existing restoration or the need for a longer wall to assure adequate retention may require extension to a subgingival location. The contour of the axial wall of the box should follow the faciolingual contour of the external surface of the tooth (Fig 16-16). The box should extend to the facial and lingual borders of the contact area, and the bevels should extend the preparation slightly beyond the box. This extension allows access to the gold margins facially and lingually for finishing with a disk.

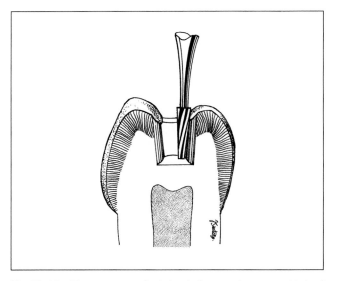

Fig 16-12 The correct pulpal depth for an inlay is established with a tapered fissure bur. It can be used to create the flat floors and well-defined internal angles.

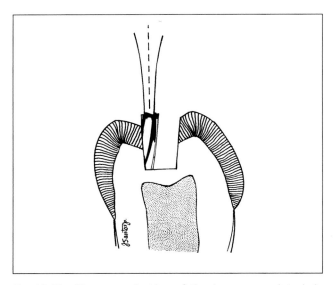

Fig 16-13 The tapered sides of the bur are used to help establish the desired divergence of the walls

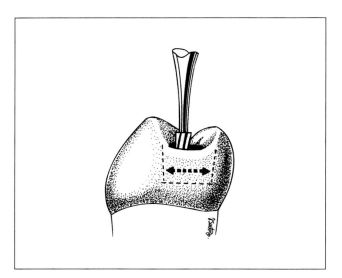

Fig 16-14 A thin layer of enamel is left on the proximal surface to protect the adjacent tooth while the proximal box is being prepared.

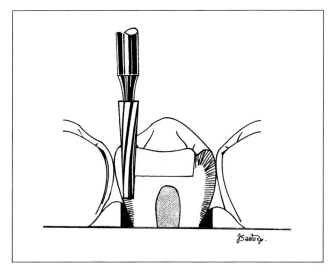

Fig 16-15 A flat gingival floor with a slightly converging axial wall is created. The gingival floor is established occlusal to the gingival tissue, unless otherwise dictated.

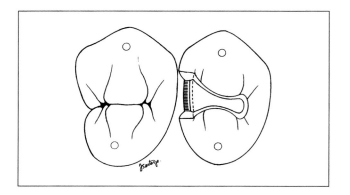

Fig 16-16 The axial wall is made an even depth into the tooth from the facial to the lingual wall.

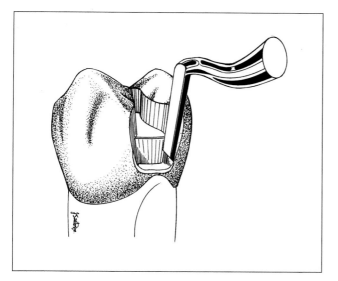

Fig 16-17 A hand instrument, such as an enamel hatchet, is helpful in smoothing the walls of the preparation.

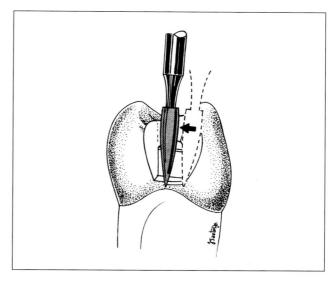

Fig 16-18 The proximal bevel or flare should be established slightly beyond the contact area and is blended with the gingival bevel.

Refinement

The operator should make certain that all the floors and walls are smooth, that all walls *except* the axial walls are divergent, that the axial walls are convergent occlusally, and that the internal angles are well defined (Fig 16-12). It is critical that no undercut area exists that could interfere with insertion and withdrawal. All cavosurface margins must be sharply defined (Fig 16-17).

Proximal Bevel

The proximal bevel or flare is established on the facial and lingual walls of the box with a garnet disk, a No. 7901 bur, or a thin diamond bur (Figs 16-18 and 16-19). A finishing bur or diamond bur must be used carefully to avoid developing an undercut in the facial and lingual walls at the faciogingival or linguogingival line angles. An undercut is less likely to be a problem when a disk is used (Fig 16-19). The walls of the preparation should diverge from the gingival floor in the occlusal direction. The proximal bevel should blend smoothly with the gingival and occlusal bevels.

Horizontal Bevels

A No. 7901 finishing bur or a thin tapered diamond is used to place 0.5-mm-wide occlusal and gingival bevels along the entire cavosurface finish line (Figs 16-18 and 16-20). A gingival margin trimmer may also be used to place the gingival bevels if access is too limited to use a bur. The bevels should be at an angle of approximately 45 degrees to the external surface of the tooth.

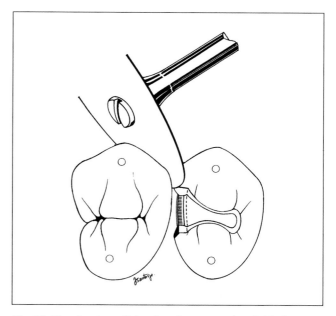

Fig 16-19 A rotary disk, placed at an angle of 45 degrees, can provide a smooth, flat bevel without undercuts.

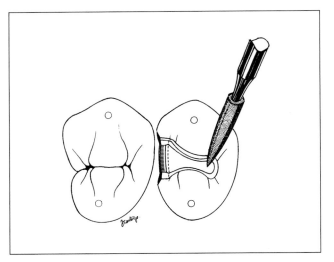

Fig 16-20a A tapered diamond or bur is used to create a short but distinct bevel at the occlusal finish lines.

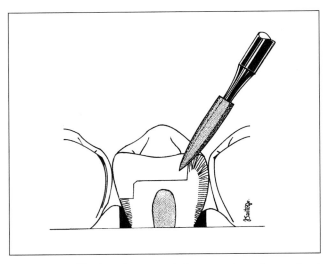

Fig 16-20b The bevel is extended across the entire occlusal margin and blended with the other bevels.

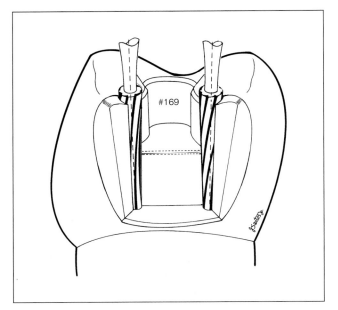

Fig 16-21 The tapered fissure bur is positioned at an angle to give an occlusal divergence for the retentive grooves. The grooves should be at a depth of half the diameter of the bur.

Retention Grooves

A No. 169 bur is used to place retention grooves that bisect the facioaxial and linguoaxial line angles (Fig 16-21). The grooves must diverge toward the occlusal aspect in a facial and lingual direction, and the axial walls should converge occlusally.

Onlay

The onlay is essentially an inlay that covers one or more cusps. It incorporates the principles of both extracoronal and intracoronal restorations. Although it is generally more conservative than a partial- or complete-coverage crown, it provides the same protection of the remaining tooth structure (Fig 16-22).

There are several important features of the preparation. All finish lines are beveled. A bevel or flare creates a second plane designed to allow close adaptation of the gold to the tooth. A beveled shoulder is used for the centric cusp and a long bevel or chamfer is used for the noncentric cusp. The gingival margin and the facial and lingual walls of the proximal boxes are designed like those for the inlay with their well-defined bevel or flare. These finish lines are blended to form an uninterrupted finish line around the entire preparation. The gingival floor is essentially a beveled shoulder.

The width and depth of the occlusal portion of the preparation and of the proximal boxes are often dictated by the presence of an old restoration and/or caries. If additional resistance and retention form are needed, retention grooves may be placed at the axiofacial and axiolingual line angles.

A tapered fissure bur is recommended for preparing the outline form because its taper helps to establish the desired occlusal divergence of 6 to 10 degrees for the internal walls.

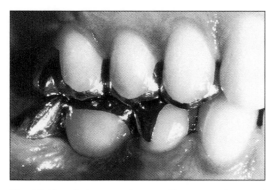

Fig 16-22 Onlays on the maxillary premolars and first molar provide protection to the facial cusps.

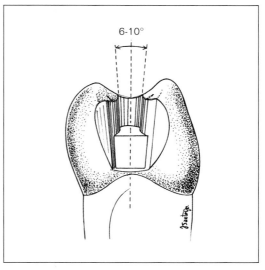

Fig 16-23 Ideally, opposing walls diverge 6 to 10 degrees for the inlay preparation.

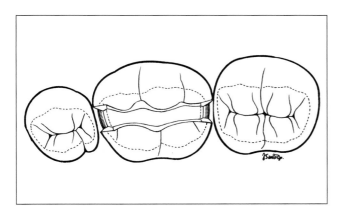

Fig 16-24 The proximal box is extended to or slightly beyond the contact area. Bevels will provide the desired proximal clearance.

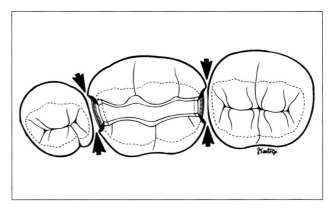

Fig 16-25 After the bevels are placed, there is access for completing the preparation's finish lines and the margins of the restoration.

Occlusal Preparation

The initial entry is made in the central fossa to a depth of approximately 1.0 mm into dentin (total depth of approximately 2.5 mm in the tooth). In some cases, it may be necessary to extend some portions of the preparation to a greater depth because of caries or a previous restoration or for additional retention. The occlusal outline form is extended by moving the bur laterally, cutting with the side of the bur. The occlusal outline form should be as conservative as the carious lesion or old restoration permits. The bur is kept in the long axis of the intended path of insertion so that the taper of the bur provides the desired 3- to 5-degree divergence for each internal cavity wall.

Proximal Boxes

The boxes are created on the proximal surfaces. The facial and lingual walls should exhibit a combined divergence of 6 to 10 degrees from each other as was provided in the occlusal area of the preparation (Fig 16-23). The faciolingual dimension is likely to be determined by the presence of a restoration, caries, and/or the relationship of the proximal surface to the adjacent tooth (Fig 16-24). The bevels will extend the preparations slightly beyond the proximal contact area so that the margins of the restoration will be accessible for finishing with a disk (Fig 16-25).

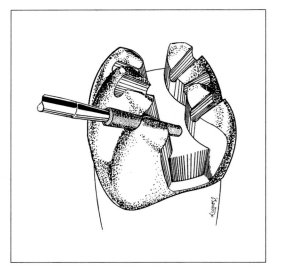

Fig 16-26 A bur of known diameter is used to establish the correct reduction of the cusps.

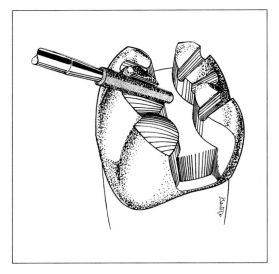

Fig 16-27 The cusps are reduced in accordance with the occlusal anatomy of the tooth.

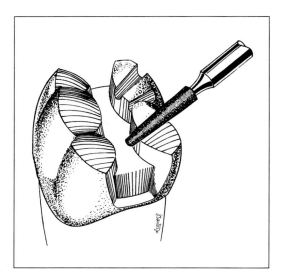

Fig 16-28 The lingual cusps of the mandibular teeth require less reduction because they are not holding cusps.

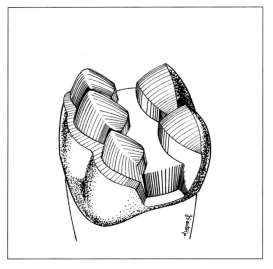

Fig 16-29 The shoulder should have precise line angles.

Cuspal Reduction

A carbide or diamond bur is used to reduce the cusps. Depth cuts of 1.5 to 2.0 mm are made for the centric (vertical holding) cusp(s) and of 1.0 to 1.5 mm are made for the noncentric cusp(s) (Fig 16-26). A bur with a measured diameter is used to gauge the depth of the cuts. The side of the bur is angled at the same angle as the cuspal inclines to make the depth cuts. After the depth cuts are placed, a uniform reduction of the cusps that parallels the general anatomic contours of the occlusal surface is made. The cuspal heights are reduced to the full extent of the depth cuts (Fig 16-27). The non-

centric cusp(s) is reduced in the same fashion, but only to a depth of 1.0 to 1.5 mm (Fig 16-28). Reduction for the centric cusps generally needs to be greater than that for the noncentric cusps because less occlusal force tends to be exerted against a noncentric cusp.

Shoulder Preparation

A shoulder is prepared on the external surface of the centric cusp to provide a band of metal (ferrule) to protect the tooth. The bur is held parallel to the external surface of the tooth, and a shoulder about 1.0 mm in height and 1.0 mm in axial depth is cut. The finish line

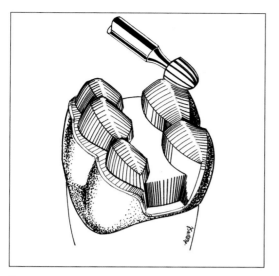

Fig 16-30 A barrel-shaped bur can be used to create the chamfer on the noncentric cusp.

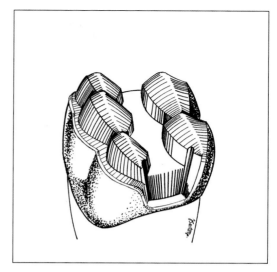

Fig 16-31 Finished onlay. Internal angles are precise, occlusal line angles are rounded, the walls have the correct taper, the grooves are correctly positioned, and all the finish lines are smooth and continuous.

should extend gingivally at least 1.0 mm beyond any occlusal contacts. The occlusoaxial line angles are rounded (Fig 16-29). There must be adequate (1.0- to 1.5-mm) clearance in all lateral movements.

Noncentric Cusp

A chamfer or long bevel may be used instead of a shoulder on the noncentric cusp(s). The bur is positioned at an angle of approximately 45 degrees to the axial surface (Fig 16-30). This provides a ferrule effect for additional protection of the cusp.

Gingival Bevel

A smooth and distinct bevel is established on the gingival margins with a No. 7901 finishing bur, a thin tapered diamond, or a gingival margin trimmer. This bevel should be approximately 0.5 mm in width and at an angle of approximately 45 degrees to the external surface of the tooth.

Shoulder Bevel

A 1.0-mm bevel is placed on the shoulder with a No. 7901 or fine diamond bur. This bevel is blended with the proximal bevels. Any corners or sharp angles at the junction of the various bevels and across the occlusoaxial line angle are eliminated (Fig 16-31).

Proximal Bevels

The proximal bevel or flare is established with a garnet disk, fine tapered diamond, or a No. 7901 bur. Creation of an undercut at the faciogingival or linguogingival line

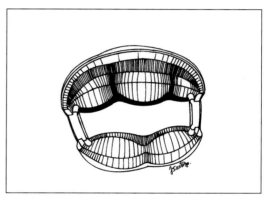

Fig 16-32 The retention grooves are placed at the linguoaxial and facioaxial line angles but do not undermine the facial and lingual enamel.

angles must be avoided. Divergence is established from the gingival floor occlusally. The proximal bevel should blend smoothly with the gingival bevel and the buccal and lingual bevels.

Retention Grooves

If retention grooves are needed, grooves are placed in both proximal boxes. A No. 169 bur is used to bisect the facioaxial and linguoaxial line angles. The grooves must diverge toward the occlusal aspect faciolingually and be aligned with the internal path of insertion (Fig 16-32).

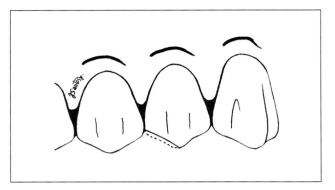

Fig 16-33 Limited reduction of the mesiofacial incline of the facial cusp and greater reduction of the distofacial incline of a maxillary tooth provide some protection to the cusp while limiting the display of gold in a partial-coverage restoration.

Partial-Coverage Crown

The partial-coverage crown covers only a portion of the outer circumference of the tooth. Leaving part of the external surface of the tooth uncovered offers several potential benefits. It conserves tooth structure and avoids potential insult to the periodontium on the unrestored tooth surface.[60] Cementation is generally easier and seating is more complete than for a complete-coverage crown because escape of the excess cement is facilitated. The uncovered tooth surface allows pulp testing.[28] Preservation of the facial surface eliminates the need to match the shade of the adjacent teeth. Because it is not necessary to veneer the casting with a tooth-colored material, the laboratory procedures are simplified.[57]

Retention and resistance of the partial veneer crown are provided by a combination of extracoronal and intracoronal features. The extracoronal retention is created by opposing axial walls on the mesial and distal surfaces that have a combined convergence toward the occlusal of approximately 6 to 10 degrees. This is supplemented with grooves or boxes in the proximal walls that provide not only added retention but also resistance to lingual displacement. A slight overlay of the facial cusp protects it from fracture and provides some resistance form.

The extensions of the proximal and facial portions of the preparation can vary in design according to the specific needs. If the tooth is located so that the facial cusps are readily visible, esthetic concerns may dictate a modification of the standard design to conceal the margin. In such cases, the mesial proximal wall is extended toward the facial surface only far enough to barely break contact. The mesial incline of the mesiofacial cusp of molars

and the mesial incline of the facial cusp of premolars are left unreduced. The distal incline is reduced to provide protection and the ferrule effect. This more esthetic design is shown in Fig 16-33.

Because partial-coverage crowns are infrequently placed on anterior teeth, this section will concentrate on the posterior teeth.

Occlusal Reduction

Depth cuts are made by laying the side of the bur (of measured diameter) against the cuspal inclines (Fig 16-34) and reducing them to the desired depth (Fig 16-35). The total reduction of the centric cusp should be 1.5 to 2.0 mm and that of the noncentric cusp should be 1.0 to 1.5 mm. The remaining occlusal surface is reduced, but the general anatomic contours are maintained (Fig 16-36). As previously mentioned, less reduction may be desirable in some areas for esthetic reasons. The placement of an occlusal channel and the facial bevel will be discussed later.

Lingual Reduction

The axial wall of the lingual surface is reduced with a blunt tapered diamond. Close attention must be paid to the desired path of insertion to maintain parallelism. A two-plane reduction of the tooth is needed to maintain natural contours. Because of the anatomic differences in the lingual contours of the maxillary and the mandibular teeth, the second plane on the lingual surface of maxillary teeth will be more pronounced. The gingival portion of the lingual surface should have a 3- to 5-degree convergence occlusally to the path of insertion (Fig 16-37), and the second plane should be offset about 30 degrees.

Proximal Reduction

The proximal surfaces are reduced in one plane. A 3- to 5-degree taper is established from the finish line to the occlusoaxial line angle. Space limitations may require use of a thin tapered diamond initially until enough space has been created to use a blunt tapered diamond bur. The blunt diamond bur has a more appropriate shape to create a chamfer finish line (Fig 16-38).

Finish Lines

The junction of each proximal wall and the lingual wall is blended so that there is a smooth transition. This procedure is especially important at the finish line. The gingival finish lines are placed slightly coronal to the gingival tissue if possible. The presence of caries or existing restorations may alter the level of finish line placement but, no matter where the finish line is located, the transition should be smooth and well defined.

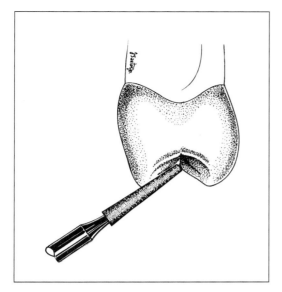

Fig 16-34 The diamond bur is held at the same angle as the natural slope of the cusp to create an even reduction for the partial-coverage crowns.

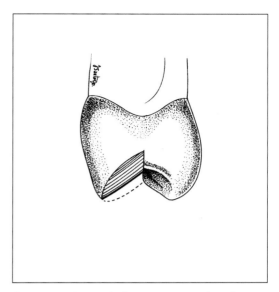

Fig 16-35 Removal of 1.0 to 1.5 mm of tooth structure from the noncentric cusp serves as a guide to reducing the rest of the occlusal surface.

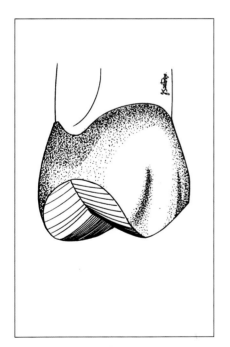

Fig 16-36 The occlusal reduction has followed the original contours of the tooth.

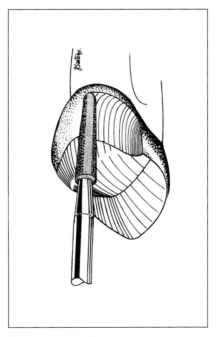

Fig 16-37 The blunt tapered diamond is very effective in creating the proper taper and in creating a chamfer finish line.

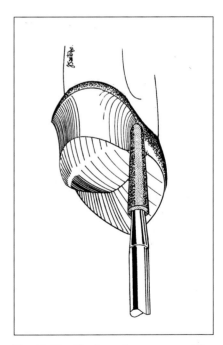

Fig 16-38 The lingual contours and finish line should be carried into the proximal surfaces. Lack of access may require use of a thinner diamond initially.

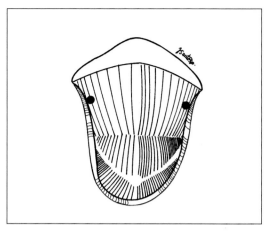

Fig 16-39a Before the proximal grooves are prepared, their desired location is marked with a pencil or an indentation made by a bur. This aids in obtaining the correct faciolingual location.

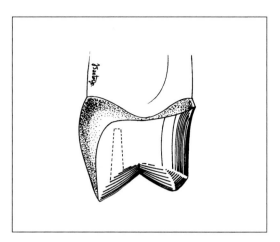

Fig 16-39b The angulation of the proximal groove is equally important, so visualization is critical.

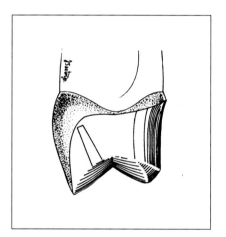

Fig 16-40a This proximal groove is angulated too much toward the lingual surface and will not provide resistance to lingual rotation.

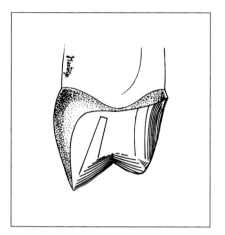

Fig 16-40b This proximal groove is angulated too much toward the facial surface, creating an undercut in relation to the lingual surface of the preparation.

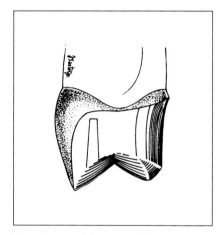

Fig 16-40c Alignment of the proximal groove with the long axis of the tooth provides the best compatibility with the rest of the preparation design.

Proximal Grooves

The groove is initiated in the proximal areas with a No. 170 bur (or a No. 169 for a small tooth). The grooves are located as far facially as possible without undermining the facial enamel. It may be helpful to mark the proposed location of the grooves before they are prepared (Figs 16-39a and 16-39b). Because the grooves must have a path of draw compatible with each other and with the axial walls, their angulation is carefully planned before they are begun. As a general rule, the grooves should be parallel to the long axis of the tooth in posterior teeth. The axial walls of the two grooves should converge occlusally. Failure to align the grooves correctly will result in a preparation that does not have an acceptable path of insertion (Figs 16-40a and 16-40b).

The axial depth of the groove is made equal to or slightly greater than the diameter of the No. 170 bur (Fig 16-41). The groove on the opposing wall is then prepared in the same fashion so that it aligns with the first groove and the axial walls. The grooves may be enlarged, and the internal walls may be left rounded or more acutely refined to form boxes. In many cases, boxes are present after the removal of existing restorations. These may be modified and incorporated in the preparation in lieu of grooves (Fig 16-42).

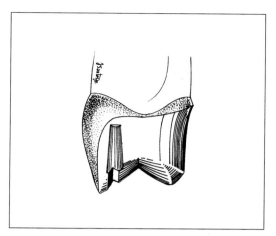

Fig 16-41 Properly designed and placed proximal groove.

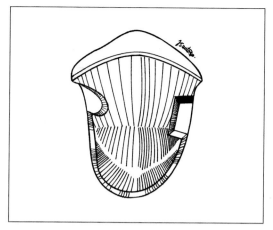

Fig 16-42 A groove is located on one proximal surface and a box of the other. Both meet the requirements for divergence on the facial and lingual walls and convergence on the axial wall toward the opposite proximal wall. The groove has a lingual "lip" to provide resistance to lingual displacement.

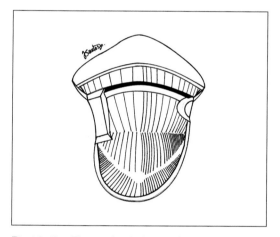

Fig 16-43 The occlusal channel follows the general contours of the facial surface rather than cutting straight across the tooth to the opposite wall. Note the inadequate proximal groove, which provides little resistance to lingual displacement.

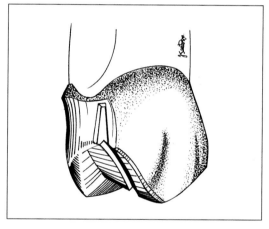

Fig 16-44 The preparation in Fig 16-43 is shown from another view. Note the shape of the occlusal channel as it comes across the occlusal surface to connect to the proximal groove and the small facial bevel.

Occlusal Channel

The resistance form and strength of the restoration can be enhanced by preparation of an occlusal channel. A channel may already exist if an occlusal restoration has been removed. If not, it may be prepared. A tapered carbide or diamond bur is used to cut the channel or to remove undercuts in an existing channel. The channel allows the space for a "staple" of thicker metal in the restoration that resists lingual displacement and that strengthens the restoration against deformation under pressure (Fig 16-43).

Facial Bevel

Placement of the facial finish line differs in the maxillary teeth and the mandibular teeth. Because the maxillary facial cusp is usually the noncentric cusp, only a 1.0-mm layer of metal and a short bevel are required to protect the cusp (Fig 16-44). Placement of a shoulder and a bevel are recommended for the facial cusp of mandibular teeth, to help restorations withstand the forces directed on a centric cusp. A shoulder that is 1.0 mm long occlusogingivally and 1.0 mm deep is placed into the facial surface across the facial cusp with a straight

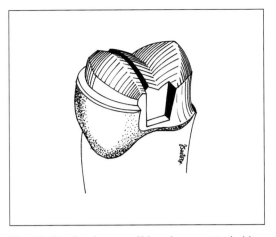

Fig 16-45 In the mandible, the centric holding cusp requires a facial design similar to that of the onlay preparation.

fissure bur held parallel to the external surface of the tooth (Fig 16-45). A 0.5- to 1.0-mm wide bevel is placed with a fine diamond or a finishing bur. The finish line should be placed gingival to any occlusal contacts.

Final Refinement

All the sharp external angles of the preparation are rounded. Sharp angles make it more difficult to pour the stone into the impression without bubbles. Even if the die is poured without bubbles, it has fragile edges that

are easily abraded during laboratory procedures. After all the angles of the preparation are rounded, the surfaces are smoothed with a fine-grit diamond bur (Figs 16-46a and 16-46b).

Complete-Coverage Gold Castings

The complete-coverage casting, as the name implies, includes coverage of the entire coronal portion of the tooth. Extensive loss of tooth structure is the most common indication for complete coverage. This restoration tends to be limited to molars for esthetic reasons. Because the restoration involves the entire circumference of the tooth, control of occlusal and proximal relationships allows improvements in occlusion and proximal contacts. Correction of malpositioning of the tooth is sometimes possible.

Retention is provided primarily or entirely by the extracoronal walls. A complete-coverage crown is the most retentive of the casting designs.[37,53] One or more grooves or boxes can be added to the preparation if additional retention and resistance form are needed.

Proximal Reduction

A thin tapered diamond bur is placed at either the facial or lingual embrasure and used to cut proximal tooth structure toward the opposite embrasure (Figs 16-47a and 16-47b). The bur should be extended cervically to the desired location of the gingival finish line. Unless caries or an old restoration dictates otherwise, the gingival finish line should be established at least 0.5 mm

Figs 16-46a and 16-46b Preparations for partial-coverage crowns require the same refinement of walls, floors, and bevels as are needed for inlay and onlay preparations.

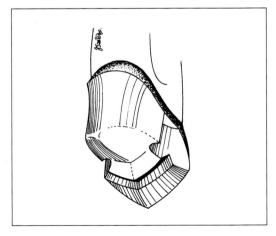

Fig 16-46a Maxillary preparation.

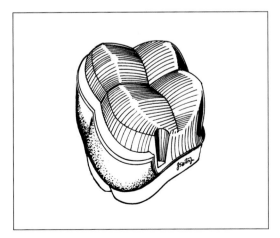

Fig 16-46b Mandibular preparation.

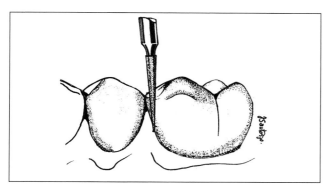

Fig 16-47a Use of a thin tapered diamond is recommended to initiate the proximal reduction of the preparation for a complete-coverage restoration.

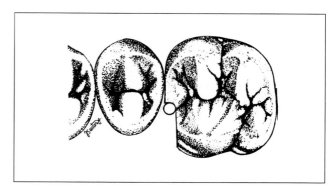

Fig 16-47b The reduction is kept within the original contours of the tooth so that abrasion of the adjacent tooth is avoided.

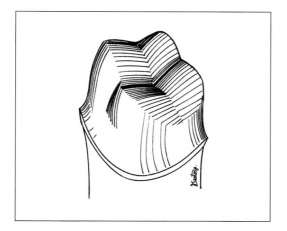

Fig 16-48 Reduction of the axial walls for a complete-coverage restoration is identical to that for the partial-coverage crowns, except the facial wall is also included. At this stage, the facial and lingual walls are each in one plane.

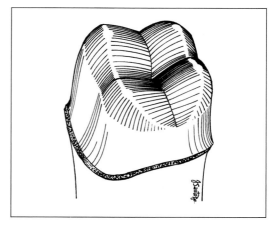

Fig 16-49 The second plane is added to the facial and lingual walls. The second plane should be at a 30- to 45-degree angle to the long axis and involves the occlusal third of the centric holding cusp and the occlusal fourth of the noncentric cusp.

supragingivally. The reduction must be at the expense of the tooth being prepared to avoid damage to the enamel of the adjacent tooth. The reduction, when completed, should taper occlusally 3 to 5 degrees toward the opposing proximal wall. The opposing wall is prepared in the same manner. Once enough space has been created to permit access, a blunt tapered diamond is used to complete the proximal reduction and place a gingival chamfer.

Occlusal Reduction

A series of depth cuts is made on the occlusal surface with a diamond or tapered fissure bur. Both the facial and lingual cuspal inclines are cut to a depth of at least 1.5 mm. The 1.5-mm reduction allows an adequate thickness of metal for strength and wear. An even reduc-

tion that follows the original anatomic contours allows the development of the appropriate occlusal anatomy in the restoration. The corrugated form of the preparation adds strength to the crown.

Facial and Lingual Reduction

The facial and lingual surfaces are each reduced in two planes. The first plane, extending occlusally from the gingival finish line, should have a 3- to 5-degree taper to the path of insertion (Fig 16-48). The second plane should be angled at 30 to 45 degrees to the first plane to allow natural facial and lingual contours to be reestablished (Fig 16-49). This second plane should begin at the occlusal third of the wall for the centric cusp and the occlusal fourth of the noncentric cusp. A blunt tapered diamond is used to make these reductions.

Refinement

The parts of the preparation are blended to eliminate indefinite areas of the finish line, irregularities in the walls, and sharp corners. A finish line that is distinct around the whole preparation is established. The areas at the facioproximal and linguoproximal line angles often need to be rounded and distinctly defined. All of the sharp corners of the preparation, such as the occlusoaxial line angles, are rounded. The surfaces of the preparation should be relatively smooth. A fine-grit diamond or a rubber polishing cup may be used. The preparation is carefully viewed from more than one angle to ensure there are no undercuts within any wall, between the walls, or in relationship to an adjacent tooth.

Impressions and provisional restorations are covered in detail in chapter 13 and will not be discussed in this chapter.

◼ Try-In

Before the casting is fitted to the patient's tooth, it should be adjusted to fit the master die. The casting is inspected under magnification for bubbles or other imperfections,[16,49] which can be removed with a small round bur. The die is checked for defects or abraded areas. The casting should not be forced onto the die. If the casting does not seat easily, the die should be sprayed with a disclosing medium and the crown should then be gently reseated. The disclosing medium should mark areas that are binding on the inside of the casting. These areas can be relieved with a bur (No. 2 or No. 4 round bur). This process is repeated until the casting is fully seated.

Once the casting is fully seated on the die, the interproximal contacts are checked, and needed adjustments are made. This is best accomplished on a solid cast, especially if there are multiple castings. The occlusion is adjusted until the restoration holds a shim equally with the adjacent natural teeth. The location and size of the occlusal contacts are marked with articulating paper. A stone is used to make any modifications needed. If these steps are done with precision before the patient arrives, minimal chair time should be required for adjustments.

The internal surface of the casting is carefully air abraded with aluminum oxide, avoiding the margins, in preparation for the clinical try-in. Air abrasion provides a dull, matte finish. Any area that binds during intraoral seating of the casting will create a bright, burnished mark.

Once adjustments have been made on the cast, the casting is tried on the tooth to determine the fit. Adjustments to the proximal contacts are made if needed. The internal surface is inspected for shiny spots. The shiny spots are adjusted. and the casting is reseated. The casting is removed and reinspected for new shiny spots. This process may need to be repeated several times until the casting is fully seated.

Any alternative method to seat castings uses disclosing media. Disclosing media include chloroform and rouge, disclosing pastes or waxes,[29] and impression materials.[16] Whatever the choice, the medium is placed on the internal surface of the casting, which is then seated. The casting is removed and inspected for abrasion of the disclosing medium that allows the gold to show through. These areas are adjusted as needed, more disclosing medium is placed, and the casting is reseated. This process is continued until the casting is fully seated.

The fitting process is completed when the margins are flush against the finish lines of the preparation and there is no binding when the restoration is seated. The casting should go passively to place. A tight fit usually means the casting is not fully seated.

◼ Marginal Finishing

Marginal finishing is done prior to cementation to thin and/or smooth margins already determined to be satisfactory. The goal is to develop a margin that is adapted to the tooth, extends to, but not beyond, the finish line, and blends with the contours of the tooth.[30] The casting must be fully seated before an attempt can be made to adapt and finish the margins.

Marginal location determines whether any finishing can be done on the tooth. Subgingival and/or interproximal margins are very difficult to reach without damaging the soft tissue, bone, or the tooth itself. In such cases, all finishing must be done on the die. Easily accessible margins can be finished while the casting is seated on the tooth (Fig 16-50). If the margin is tightly adapted but slightly overcontoured or undercontoured, a white stone or abrasive disk can be used in a low-speed handpiece to reduce the protruding surface, whether it is gold or enamel. When finished, the gold margin should be flush with the tooth structure, and adjacent contours of the restoration should be continuous with natural tooth contours. The stone or disk should be rotated from the metal to the tooth or parallel to the margin, but never from tooth to gold. Rubber points or sandpaper disks may be used to produce a high luster if access permits. Care must be exercised to

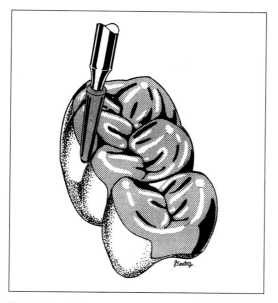

Fig 16-50 A fine diamond bur or finishing stone is held perpendicular to the margin and moved parallel to the margin to reduce small discrepancies in the marginal area.

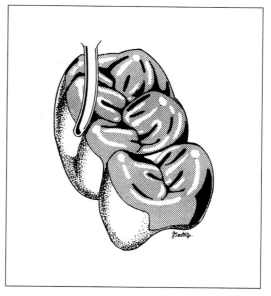

Fig 16-51 Pressure is applied with the side or tip of the burnisher parallel to the marginal area to adapt it more tightly to the tooth.

avoid damage to the soft tissue or abrasion of the tooth surface.

Marginal adaptation can sometimes be improved by hand burnishing, both on the die and on the tooth prior to cementation of the crown. Well-controlled pressure is applied with a beavertail or ball burnisher held adjacent and moved parallel to the gold margin (Fig 16-51). The burnisher should not be placed directly on the margin. Pressure should be applied with a back-and-forth motion that moves slowly closer to the margin. Because a small area of the burnisher is contacting the gold, a great deal of pressure (force per unit area) is applied. The casting is stabilized during the burnishing process to ensure that it does not change position. It is also critical to have good finger rests to assure that the burnisher does not slip off the tooth and injure the soft tissue or the tooth itself if the burnishing is done in the mouth. Some additional benefit may be achieved by burnishing the margins of the casting on the tooth during the cementing procedure, before the cement sets.

Cementation

The final step in the process is luting or cementation of the casting. A thin layer of the luting agent (cement) is placed in the casting and on the walls of the preparation, and the casting is then seated on or in the tooth. The

cement hardens within a few minutes, and the excess is removed. The luting agent fills the gap between the casting and tooth to provide retention and to minimize leakage at the margin. Some luting agents, such as zinc phosphate cement, provide retention entirely from frictional resistance to displacement. Others, such as the adhesive resin cements, bond to the casting and/or the tooth to provide both frictional resistance to displacement and adhesion.

Selection of a Luting Agent

Many different types of luting agents are available, each with inherent advantages and disadvantages. The primary luting agents in use today are zinc phosphate, glass ionomer, polycarboxylate, and resin cements.[20] A survey of 10,000 dentists conducted in 1990 revealed that glass-ionomer cements were used most frequently for cementation of crowns (42%), followed by polycarboxylate (33%), zinc phosphate (22%), resin cement (2%), and zinc oxide–eugenol (1%) cements.[6] Since that time, resin cements have gained in popularity, and much of the current research in the area of cements is aimed at improving resin cements. Because the indications and procedures for the use of each luting agent are different, they will be discussed separately.

Zinc Phosphate Cement

Among the many luting agents available, zinc phosphate has the longest record of successful use. It has good compressive strength, low film thickness, and is easy to manipulate. The excess cement is easily removed after it has set. It has a coefficient of thermal expansion similar to that of tooth structure, and its setting shrinkage is minimal. Relatively high compressive and tensile strengths make zinc phosphate a good choice for long-span fixed partial dentures.[58]

Zinc phosphate cement is slightly soluble in oral fluids, allows relatively high levels of microleakage,[74] and is sometimes associated with postoperative sensitivity.[46,71] Despite these drawbacks, it is not unusual to see patients with gold castings that were cemented more than 30 years ago with zinc phosphate cement.

Zinc phosphate cement is usually mixed on a chilled glass slab. The powder is mixed into the liquid in small increments over a large area of the glass slab. This method dissipates the heat released during the exothermic setting reaction and provides a longer working time. The slower the mix and cooler the glass slab, the longer the working time. Powder is added until the mixed material strings out after the spatula for 1 inch or so when the spatula is lifted. The mixing should be completed within 90 seconds after initiation. If the mixing is prolonged beyond approximately 90 seconds, the hardening of the cement caused by the setting reaction may be confused with having achieved the proper powder-liquid ratio.[48] Its relatively long working time makes zinc phosphate cement a good choice when multiple castings are luted at the same time.

Glass-Ionomer Cement

Glass-ionomer luting cement is a modification of the glass-ionomer restorative material. It bonds to tooth structure (as discussed in chapter 6) and has the potential to prevent caries because of fluoride release. It has a low film thickness (20 to 25 μm) and relatively good physical properties. It may be hand mixed or is available in preweighed capsules that allow mixing in an amalgamator. Despite persistent reports of excessive postoperative sensitivity associated with glass-ionomer luting agents, this was not borne out in a multicenter clinical study.[26]

Glass-ionomer cement is very sensitive to early moisture contamination. If exposed to moisture during the setting reaction (usually 5 minutes), the reaction is interrupted, resulting in a cement with high solubility and poor physical properties. Therefore, glass-ionomer cement should not be used when bleeding is present or isolation is a problem. Excess cement should not be removed from the margins for at least 5 minutes after the crown is seated. Leaving a bead of excess cement in place protects the underlying layers of cement from moisture contamination.[9] Glass-ionomer cement bonds to the tooth surface so it is somewhat difficult to remove once set, particularly in the interproximal areas. The resin-modified glass-ionomer cements have also been adapted for use as luting agents and have made the luting process less technique sensitive because they are slightly less affected by moisture.

When glass-ionomer cement is mixed by hand, the powder is incorporated into the liquid in bulk as quickly as possible with a premeasured amount of powder and liquid. The ratio is usually one level scoop of powder to two drops of liquid. Most manufacturers now offer the encapsulated form, which results in a correctly proportioned cement thoroughly mixed in a few seconds. Glass-ionomer cement has a relatively short working time, so a single mix should be limited to luting no more than two or three units. If additional units have to be luted, a new mix of cement should be used.

Resin Luting Agents

The resin cements are especially designed for use with bonded porcelain restorations, but they may also be used with cast restorations. They differ from resin composite restorative materials primarily in their reduced filler content. This results in better flow and reduced film thickness, which are necessary for a luting agent.

Resin cements have the best physical properties of all of the cements. They are virtually insoluble in oral fluids and have the highest compressive and tensile strengths of all the cements. They also exhibit less microleakage[3] than other luting agents. If used in combination with a dentin adhesive system, they bond to tooth structure and some types of metals,[20,71,73] and they are often recommended for less retentive preparations.[32,50]

There are, however, several potential problems associated with resin cements. There is great variation in the physical properties and handling characteristics among resin cements.[72] Their film thickness tends to be greater than that of other cements,[36,63,72] so incomplete seating of the casting can be a problem. This is especially true when a dentin adhesive is used if it is allowed to pool in the internal angles of the preparation. Resin cements are relatively new, so there are no long-term clinical studies to determine if the high retention values and low microleakage are long lasting. Although a bond between the casting and the tooth is generally considered advantageous, it can be a problem if it becomes necessary to remove the restoration.

Polycarboxylate and Zinc Oxide–Eugenol Cements

Polycarboxylate and zinc oxide–eugenol cements are no longer widely used with cast restorations. Their properties are generally inferior to those of the cements previously discussed. Historically, some clinicians have used them if a tooth has had a history of sensitivity. They have also been used as temporary luting agents and with stainless steel crowns.

Preparing the Tooth for Cementation

Although some materials are more strongly affected by the presence of contaminants than are others, no material fares well if used in the presence of oils, debris, saliva, blood, or other significant contamination. It is important to assure that the area is cleaned, free of excess moisture, and well isolated. Bleeding and other significant moisture must be well controlled. Temporary cements leave a layer of debris on the dentinal surface[56] that should be removed prior to cementation. This may be accomplished with pumice, detergents, or cleaning agents.

Some clinicians recommend the additional step of disinfecting the preparation with chlorhexidine or other disinfectants. The rationale is that because bacteria are a primary cause of postoperative sensitivity,[5,7] disinfection of the dentinal surface will lower the number of microbes and thus lessen the sensitivity. Whether the disinfection has any significant effect is not yet known.

In addition to cleaning and isolating the preparation, specific additional steps are recommended to prepare the tooth to receive certain cements.

Zinc Phosphate Cement

Because zinc phosphate cement exhibits the most microleakage of any cement[72] and has been associated with postcementation sensitivity, several methods have been recommended to prevent sensitivity by "sealing" the dentin prior to cementation. Copal varnish has a long history of use for this purpose with anecdotal reports of success. More recently, use of dentin primers and adhesives to seal the dentin before cementation have resulted in reports of decreased sensitivity. Neither method has been tested in a controlled clinical study, however.

Glass-Ionomer Cements

For glass-ionomer cements, the tooth should be clean and dry, but it should not be dehydrated. No cavity varnish or other coating agent should be placed because this would prevent bonding of this luting agent to the tooth. The area should be well isolated to prevent moisture contamination during the luting process and for several minutes following the seating of the restoration.

Resin Composite Cements

Most resin composite cements have corresponding dentin adhesive systems that are applied immediately prior to cementation. In most cases, the preparation is etched and then a primer and adhesive are placed. Each adhesive system has specific instructions for its use that must be followed precisely to obtain the best results. Failure to follow the specific directions for both the adhesive and the luting agent can mean the difference between success and failure of the luting process.

A small amount of the cement should be mixed and observed before cementation procedures are started to confirm that the cement will set. Some autocuring resin cements have short shelf lives and lose their ability to polymerize.

Preparing the Casting for Cementation

After adjustments have been made and the external surface of the casting has been polished, the internal surface of the casting should be air abraded with aluminum oxide to produce a uniform, slightly roughened finish. The casting should then be cleaned to remove any contaminants, such as polishing compounds. Ammonia, detergents or various other cleaning solutions may be used in an ultrasonic bath, or the casting can be cleaned with a steam cleaner.

If an adhesive resin cement is used, additional retention can be obtained by tin plating the inside of the casting.[23,47] A number of inexpensive tin-plating systems that can be used to deposit a thin layer of tin on the surface of gold are commercially available. This simple process can be done in the laboratory or operatory in a few minutes.[23]

Seating the Casting

The luting agent is mixed and placed in the casting. Some clinicians also like to place a layer of the luting agent on the walls of the preparation for intracoronal restorations. The casting should be half filled and all the margins should be covered. Once the casting is seated with finger pressure, the patient is instructed to bite on an orangewood stick or other seating instrument. The instrument is moved up and down, and then side to side. This technique, called *dynamic seating*, results in more complete seating of the casting.[54] The margins are checked with an explorer to determine if complete seating has been accomplished. Once complete seating has been assured, the patient is told to maintain steady pressure until cement has completely set.

The excess cement must be removed with proper timing and care. If removal is attempted before the cement is set, thin strands of cement may be dragged from under the margins, thus creating voids. The bead of extruded cement has been shown to protect the cement at the margin from moisture contamination.[9] Therefore, it is important to check the cement to assure that it has set before the excess is removed. Excess cement may be removed with an explorer or curette and floss or yarn. The gingival crevice should be flushed with water frequently to remove any loose particles. As a final step, an assistant should blow a continuous stream of air on each margin while the clinician reflects the gingiva gently with an explorer to check for any remaining cement. Cement left subgingivally can initiate tissue inflammation. A knot is tied in the floss and then the floss is pulled back and forth through the gingival embrasure to remove loose pieces from the interproximal areas.

The occlusion is reevaluated and final adjustments are made, if necessary. The patient is informed of the possibility of postcementation sensitivity and that a minor additional adjustment of the occlusion may be necessary. The patient is instructed in the proper oral hygiene measures to assure prevention of caries and periodontal problems.

References

1. Bell WE. Tempromandibular Disorders: Classification/Diagnosis/Management, ed 2. Chicago: Year Book, 1986:219.

2. Bentley C, Drake EW. Longevity of restorations in dental school clinic J Dent Educ 1986;50:594-600.

3. Blair KF, Koeppen RG, Schwartz RS, Davis RD. Microleakage associated with resin composite–cemented, cast glass ceramic restoration. Int J Prosthodont 1993;6:579-584.

4. Blazer PK, Land MR, Cochran RA. Effects of designs of class 2 preparations on resistance of teeth to fracture. Oper Dent 1983;8:6-10.

5. Brännström M, Vojinovic O. Response of the dental pulp to invasion of bacteria around three filling materials. J Dent Child 1976;43:83-89.

6. Christensen GJ, Christensen R. Use Survey—1990. Clin Res Assoc Newsletter 1990;14: 1-3.

7. Cox CF, Suzuki S. Re-evaluating pulp protection: Calcium hydroxide liners vs. cohesive hybridization. J Am Dent Assoc 1994;125:823-831.

8. Craig RG. Restorative Dental Materials, ed 6. St Louis: Mosby, 1980:57.

9. Curtis SR, Richards MW, Dhuru VB, Meiers JC. Early erosion of glass-ionomer cement at crown margins. Int J Prosthdont 1993; 6:553-557.

10. Delong R, Pintado MR, Douglas WH. The wear of enamel opposing shaded ceramic restorative materials: An in vitro study. J Prosthet Dent 1992;68:42-48.

11. Dodge WR, Weed RM, Baez RJ, Buchanan RN. The effect of convergence angle on retention and resistance form. Quintessence Int 1985;16:191-197.

12. Donnenfeld OW. Therapeutic end-points in periodontal therapy. Int J Periodont Rest Dent 1981;1(4):51-59.

13. Dragoo JR, Williams GB. Periodontal tissue reactions to restorative procedures. Int J Periodont Rest Dent 1981;1(1):9-23.

14. El-Ebrashi MK, Craig RG, Payton FA. Experimental stress analysis of dental restorations IV. Concept of parallelism of axial walls. J Prosthet Dent 1969;22:346-356.

15. Gargiulo AW, Wentz FM, Orban BJ. Dimensions and relations of the dentogingival junction in humans. J Periodont 1961;32:261-267.

16. Gerhardt DE. Seating the cast gold restoration. Gen Dent 1987; 35:479-480.

17. Gibbs CH, Lundeen HL. Advances in Occlusion. Littleton, MA: PSG, 1982:2-32.

18. Gilbar DB, Teteruck WR. Fundamental of extracoronal tooth preparation. Retention and resistance form. J Prosthet Dent 1974; 32:651-656.

19. Guyer SE. Multiple preparations for fixed prosthodontics. J Prosthet Dent 1970;32:529-553.

20. Herlands RE, Lucca JJ, Morris HL. Forms, contours, and extensions of full coverage restorations in occlusal reconstruction. Dent Clin North Am 1962;6:147-162.

21. Hiatt WH. Incomplete crown–root fracture in pulpal periodontal disease. J Periodontol 1973;44:369-379.

22. Hunsaker JK, Christensen GJ, Christensen RP, Coo D, Lewis RG. Retentive characteristics of dental cementation materials. Gen Dent 1993;44:464-467.

23. Imbery TA, Davis RD. Evaluation of tin plating systems for a high-noble alloy. Int J Prosthodont 1993;6:55-59.

24. Ingber JS, Rose LF, Coslet JG. The "biologic width"—A concept in periodontics and restorative dentistry. Alpha Omegan 1977;70: 62-65.

25. Jameson LM. Comparison of the volume of crevicular fluid from restored and nonrestored teeth. J Prosthet Dent 1979;41:209-214.

26. Johnson GH, Powell LV, DeRouen TA. Evaluation and control of post-cementation pulpal sensitivity: Zinc phosphate and glass ionomer cements. J Am Dent Assoc 1993;124:38-46.

27. Jorgensen KD. The relationship between retention and convergence angle in cemented veneer crowns. Acta Odontol Scand 1955;13:35-40.

28. Kahn AE. Partial versus full coverage. J Prosthet Dent 1960;10:167-172.

29. Kaiser DA, Wise HB. Fitting cast gold restorations with the aid of disclosing wax. J Prosthet Dent 1980;43:227-228.

30. Kaiser DA. Anatomy of the cast gold margin. J Prosthet Dent 1983;50:437-440.

31. Kay HB. Esthetic considerations in the definitive periodontal prosthetic management of the maxillary anterior segment. Int J Periodont Rest Dent 1982;2(3):45-59.

32. Krabbendam CA, Ten Harkel HC, Duijesters PPE, Davidson CL. Shear bond strength determinations on various kinds of luting cements with tooth structure and cast alloys using a new testing device. J Dent 1987;15:77-81.

33. Krough-Paulsen WG, Olsson A. Occlusal disharmonies and dysfunction of the stomatognathic system. Dent Clin North Am 1966;10:627-635.

34. Lagouvardos P, Sourai P, Douvitsas G. Coronal fractures in posterior teeth. Oper Dent 1989;14:28-32.

35. Larson TD, Douglas WH, Geistfeld RE. Effects of prepared cavities on the strength of teeth. Oper Dent 1981;6:2-5.

36. Levine WA. An evaluation of the film thickness of resin luting agents. J Prosthet Dent 1989;62:175-181.

37. Lorey RE, Myers GE. The retentive qualities of bridge retainers. J Am Dent Assoc 1968;76:568-572.

38. Marynuik GA. In search of treatment longevity—A 30 year perspective. J Am Dent Assoc 1984; 109:7932-44.

39. Minker JS. Simplified full coverage preparations. Dent Clin North Am 1965;9:355-372.

40. Mjör IA. Placement and replacement of restorations. Oper Dent 1981;6:49-54.

41. Mjör IA, Jokstad A, Qvist V. Longevity of posterior restorations Int Dent J 1990:40;11-17.

42. Morris ML. Artificial crown contours and gingival health. J Prosthet Dent 1962;12:1146-1156.

43. Mount GJ. Crown and the gingival tissues. Aust Dent J 1970;15:253-258.

44. Nevins M, Skurow HM. The intracrevicular restorative margin, the biologic width, and the maintenance of the gingival margin. Int J Periodont Rest Dent 1984;4(3):31-49.

45. Newcomb GM. The relationship between the location of subgingival crown margins and gingival inflammation. J Periodontol 1974;5:151-154.

46. Norman RD, Swartz ML, Phillips RW, Vermani RV. A comparison of the intraoral disintegration of three dental cements. J Am Dent Assoc 1969;78:777-782.

47. Olin PS, Hill EME. Tensile strength of air abraded vs tin plated metals luted with three cements [abstract 188]. J Dent Res 1991;70:387.

48. Osborne JW, Wolff MS, Berry JC. Variance in powder-liquid ratio in zinc phosphate cement for luting castings [abstract 468]. J Dent Res 1986;65:778.

49. Ostlund LE. Improving the marginal fit of the cast restorations. J Am Acad Gold Foil Oper 1974;17:56-60.

50. O'Sullivan BP, Johnson PF, Blosser RL, Rupp NW, Li SH. Bond strength of a luting composite to dentin with different bonding systems. J Prosthet Dent 1987;58:171-175.

51. Parkinson CF. Excessive crown contours facilitate endemic plaque niches. J Prosthet Dent 1976;35:424-429.

52. Phillips RW. Skinner's Science of Dental Materials, ed 9. Philadelphia: Saunders, 1991:296.

53. Potts RG, Shillingburg HT, Duncanson MG. Retention and resistance of preparations for cast restorations. J Prosthet Dent 1980;43:303-308.

54. Rosenstiel SF, Gegauff AF. Improving cementation of complete cast crowns: A comparison of static and dynamic seating methods. J Am Dent Assoc 1988;117:845-848.

55. Salis SG, Good J, Stokes A, Kirk E. Patterns of indirect fracture in intact and restored human premolar teeth. Endod Dent Traumatol 1987;3:10-14.

56. Schwartz RS, Davis RD, Hilton TJ. Effect of temporary cements on the bond strength of a resin cement. Am J Dent 1992;5:147-150.

57. Shillingburg HT. Cast gold restorations. In: Clark JW (ed). Clinical Dentistry. New York: Harper & Row, 1976.

58. Shillingburg HT, Hobo S, Whitsett LD. (1981) Fundamentals of Fixed Prosthodontics. Chicago: Quintessence, 1981:376-377.

59. Shillingburg HT, Jacobi R, Brackett SE. Fundamentals of Tooth Preparation. Chicago: Quintessence, 1987:112.

60. Silness J. Periodontal conditions in patients treated with dental bridges. II. The influence of full and partial crowns on plaque accumulation, development of gingivitis and pocket formation. J Periodont Res 1970;5:219-230.

61. Silness J. Periodontal conditions in patients treated with dental bridges. Part III. The relationship between the location of the crown and margin and the periodontal condition. J Periodont Res 1970;5:225-229.

62. Sorensen JA, Martinoff JT. Intracoronal reinforcement and coronal coverage: A study of endodontically treated teeth. J Prosthet Dent 1984;51:780-784.

63. Staninec M, Giles WS, Saiku JM, Hattori M. Caries penetration and cement thickness of three luting agents. Int J Prosthodont 1988;1:259-265.

64. Stein RS. Periodontal dictates for esthetic ceramomental crowns. J Am Dent Assoc 1987;(special issue):63E-75E.

65. Vale WA. Cavity preparation. Ir Dent Rev 1956;2:33-41.

66. Vanderhaug J. A 15-year clinical evaluation of fixed prosthodontics. Acta Odontol Scand 1991;49:35-40.

67. Van Nortwick WG, Gettlemen L. Effect of internal relief, vibration and venting on the vertical seating of cemented crowns. J Prosthet Dent 1981;45:395-399.

68. Waerhaug J. Histologic consideration which govern where the margins of restorations should be located in relation to the gingiva. Dent Clin North Am 1960;4:161-176.

69. Weed RM. Determining adequate crown convergence. Tex Dent J 1980;98:14-16.

70. Wheeler RC. Complete crown form and the periodontium. J Prosthet Dent 1961;11:722-734.

71. White SN, Sorensen JA, Kang SK, Caputo AA. Microleakage of new crown and fixed partial denture luting agents. J Prosthet Dent 1992;67:156-161.

72. White SN, Yu Z. Film thickness of new adhesive luting agents. J Prosthet Dent 1992;67:782-785.

73. White SN, Yu Z. Physical properties of fixed prosthodontic resin composite luting agents. Int J Prosthodont 1993;6:384-389.

74. White SN, Yu Z, Tom JFMD, Sangsurasak S. In vivo microleakage of luting cements for cast crowns. J Prosthet Dent 1994;71:333-338.

75. Wilson AD, Prosser JK, Powis DM. Mechanism of adhesion of polyelectrolyte cements to hydroxyapatite J Dent Res 1983;62:590-592.

76. Wilson RD, Maynard G. Intracrevicular restorative dentistry. Int J Periodont Rest Dent 1981;1(4):35-49.

77. Youdelis RA, Weaver JD, Sapkos S. Facial and lingual contours of artificial complete crown restorations and their effect on periodontium. J Prosthet Dent 1973;29:61-66.

Index

B

Bases
  categories of, 61–62
  placement guidelines for, 61
  uses of, 58, 58f
Bevels, blade, 75, 75f
Biocompatibility, of dentin adhesives and
    pulp, 153, 155
Biologic width, 18, 20f
  periodontal health and, 34, 34f
Bis-acryl, for provisional restorations, 344
Bite blocks, 130, 130f
Bitine ring
  in matrix application, 219f, 219–220
  in Palodent matrix system, 288, 289f
Black, G.V.
  cavity preparation and, 74
  classification of carious lesions and tooth
      preparations, 72–74, 73f
  instrument kit recommendation of, 83, 106
  instrumentation nomenclature of, 77
  numeric formulas of, 80, 81f, 83
    centigrade scale in, 80, 82f
Bleaching, of discoloration, 368f, 369
Boley gauge, 269f
Bonding
  amalgam, 174, 174f
  ceramic, 174f, 174–175, 175f, 176f
  to composite restorations, 231
  substrate for, 13
Box cavity preparation, 7, 7f
Buccal pit preparation, 7, 7f
Buildup material(s)
  amalgam, 332, 332f
    effect on ceramic restoration, 387
  composite, 332
  glass-ionomer, 332
    resin-modified, 332
  ideal characteristics for, 332
Bur head, measurement for length, 266, 269,
    269f
Burnishers, 85–86, 86f
Burnishing
  of amalgam restoration
    postcarve, 296–297
    precarve, 292–293
Bur(s)
  carbide
    12-bladed for finishing, 102t–103t, 103
    for tooth preparation, 100t–101t
  components of, 98, 98f
  diamond, 103
    versus carbide, 202, 202f
  shapes of, 98, 99f
  standards for, 98f, 99

C

Calcium hydroxide, as base or liner, 61, 218
Caps. See Pulp cap(s)
Caries
  abbreviations of, 74
  antimicrobial management and, 56–57

around existing restorations, 35f, 35–36, 36f
Black's classification of, 72–74, 73f
Classes 1–6, 70–72, 70f–73f
dentinal anterior, 189, 190f, 191
development and progression of, 53, 53f,
    54f, 55f
diagnosis of, 31, 53
enamel, incipient anterior, 189, 190f
identification and removal of, 54, 55f
initiation of, 51f, 51–52
interproximal, 32f
occlusal, 31f
  amalgam restoration of, 253–257, 301f
  sealing of, 252, 253f, 253–254
pit and fissure, 31f, 31–32
prevention of
  fluoride in, 55–56
  sealants in, 56, 57f
risk for, 30–31
root, 32, 32f, 55f
secondary
  from posterior composite restorations,
      210, 212, 212f
smooth surface, 32, 32f, 54f
Caries detectors, 54, 55f
Carver(s), 85, 85f, 86f
  cleoid-discoid, 85, 85f, 86f, 293, 294f
  interproximal, 294–295, 295f
  No. 14L sickle-shaped, 297f, 299f
  sharpening of, 88, 91f
Carving, of occlusal amalgam, 293, 294f,
    294–295, 295f
Cast-gold restorations. See Gold restoration(s)
Casts, evaluation of, 41–42
Cavity preparation
  anatomic and clinical crown in, 70, 72, 72f
  Black's steps in, 74
  Class 2, 70f
  Class 3, 71f
  Class 5, 70f
  nomenclature for, 70–72
  steps in, 74
  walls and margins in, 70, 71f
Cavity sealers, 58, 281–282
Cavity wall preparation, 7, 7f
Cement spatulas, 87f, 87–88
Cement(s), 61
  composite
    technique for, 363, 364–365
    dual-cured versus light-cured, 231–232
  glass-ionomer, 176–179, 412. See also
      Glass-ionomer cement(s)
  polycarboxylate, 413
  for porcelain veneers
    translucency of, 362f, 362–363
    viscosity of, 363
  for posts and post-and-core, 325
  resin, 412, 413
    for gold castings, 230, 412, 413
    for indirect posterior bonded restora-
        tions, 230–231, 232
  resin luting, 230
  zinc oxide–eugenol, 413
  zinc phosphate, 412

Ceramic restoration(s)
  anterior crowns, 373–389. See also All-
      ceramic restorations; Metal-ceramic
      restorations
    all-ceramic, 383–387
    metal-ceramic, 373–383
  inlays
    computer-assisted design of, 243, 245f
    computer-assisted manufacture of, 243,
        246, 246f
    preparation for, 243, 244f
    try-in and cementation of, 246–247, 247f
  onlays
    computer-assisted design of, 248
    computer-assisted manufacture of, 248,
        248f
    preparation for, 247–248, 248
Ceramic surface
  bonding to, 174, 174f, 175f, 176f
  silanization of, 175, 175f
Charting, pictorial, 47f, 48f
Chisel, 77, 78f, 79f
  versus hoe, 83
  sharpening of, 88, 90f
Chlorhexidine rinses, for caries management,
    57
Circumferential slots, 277f, 277–278
Clamp forceps, 114, 115f
Clamp(s), 114–119, 116t, 117f, 118f. See also
    Rubber dam
  butterfly, 118f, 118–119
  design of, 114, 115f
  floss ligatures with, 119
  modeling compound and, 119–120, 121f
  No. 212, 313, 313f, 314
  No. W8A, 116, 117f, 118
  placement of, 114, 116f, 133
  recommended, 114, 116f
  supplemental, 116, 117f
  tooth contact and, 119, 119f
  use of multiple, 133
  winged, 126, 127f
  wingless, 127f, 126–127
Class 1 preparation
  for amalgam restoration
    resistance and retention form in, 255–256
  of defective restorations and recurrent
      caries, 255, 256f
  indications for, 252–255
  of occlusal caries, 252–255
  outline form of, 255–256, 257f
    for fissure caries, 256, 257f
    for occlusal caries, 255, 257f
  posterior, 71f
Class 2 preparation
  for amalgam restoration, 258–266
    of fissures, 258
    mechanical retention, 264, 264f. See also
        Pin(s)
    of occlusal caries, 258
    outline form of, 258, 259f, 260
    of proximal caries, 258
    replacement with occlusal extensions,
        265, 266f

of esthetic inlay/onlay, 231f, 233
of incisal edge
    anterior porcelain veneer restoration of, 358, 359f
of veneer
    in crown-veneer restorations, 369–370
Frame holders
    Nygard-Ostby, 113f, 114
    strap- or harness-type, 113f
    Young-type, 112, 113f, 114

G

Gingiva
    healthy, 18, 19f
    relaxation incisions in, 133, 134f
Gingival margin trimmer, 77, 79f, 80f
Gingivectomy, 337
    electrosurgical, 337–338, 338f
Glass-ceramic crowns, castable, 385, 386f
Glass-ionomer cement(s), 61–62
    for Class 5 restorations, 311, 313
    for composite/ceramic inlays and onlays, 229
    conventional, 176, 176f
    Dyract, 178f, 179
    for gold castings, 412, 413
    resin-modified, 177–179, 311, 312f, 313
        versus conventional, 178–179
        grouping by setting mechanism, 177t
        mechanism of, 178, 179f
        Photac Bond, 178f
        structure of, 177f
    Vitremer, 178f
Glass-ionomer materials, 189
    in Class 5 restorations, 315, 317, 317f, 318
        finishing and polishing of, 318
        matrix and insertion of, 317, 317f
        preparation for, 315
    in core buildup, 332
    in liners and bases, 218
    resin-modified
        for tunnel preparation, 224–225
Glazing. See Rebonding (glazing)
Gold foil restoration, 313
Gold inlay, 397–400
    cementation of, 411–414
    for Class 5 restorations, 313
    description of, 397, 397f
    marginal finishing of, 410–411
    preparation for
        bevels in, 399, 399f, 400f
        occlusal, 397, 398f
        proximal boxes in, 397, 398f
        refinement of, 399, 399f
        retention grooves in, 400, 401f
    try-in of, 410
Gold onlay, 400–403
    cementation of, 411–414
    description of, 400, 401f
    marginal finishing of, 410–411
    preparation of
        bevels in, 403, 403f
        cuspal reduction in, 402, 402f

noncentric cusp in, 403, 403f
occlusal, 401
proximal boxes, 401, 401f
retention grooves in, 403, 403f
shoulder in, 402f, 402–403
try-in of, 410
Gold restoration(s), 391–414. See also specific, eg, Gold inlay
    advantages of, 391
    in anterior teeth, 391, 392f
    applications for, 391
    basic principles of
        conservation of tooth structure, 392
        finish lines in, 394f, 394–395
        pulpal considerations, 383
        resistance form in, 392, 393, 393f
        retention form in, 392, 393, 393f
    biologic width and, 395
    bonded, 393
    cementation of, 411–414
        casting preparation for, 413
        selection of luting agent for, 411–413
        tooth preparation for, 413
    contours in, 395–396, 396f
    crowns
        complete-coverage, 391f, 408–410
        partial-coverage, 391f, 404–408
    finish lines for
        types and selection of, 394f, 394–395
    gingival considerations in, 395, 395f
    indications for, 391–392
    inlay, 397–400
    marginal finishing of, 410–411
    occlusion and, 396f, 396–397
    onlay, 400–403
    seating of, 413–414
    thermal sensitivity from, 394
    try-in of, 410
Grasps, 94f, 95, 95f, 96f
Groove
    definition of, 252

H

Hand instrument(s)
    cutting, 74–83
        centigrade scale and, 80, 82f
        classification of, 76f, 77
        components of, 75, 75f
        design of, 75, 75f, 76f, 77
        metals for, 75
        nomenclature for, 76f, 77
        numeric formulas for, 80, 81f, 82f
        usage of, 77, 80, 81f
    grasps for, 94f, 95, 95f, 96f
    motions of, 96
    noncutting, 83–88
    rotating, 97–103
    sharpening of, 88–93
Handpiece(s), 97–98
    contra-angle, 97f, 98f
    low-speed and high-speed, 97–98
    straight, 97f
Hatchet, 76f, 77, 78f

off-angle, 77
Hoe, 77, 79f
    sharpening of, 88, 90f
Hydrocolloid impression material(s)
    irreversible, 339, 339f
        vacuum mixing versus hand mixing of, 339, 339f
    reversible, 339
Hydrodynamics
    dentin sensitivity and, 12, 13f
    pulpal and thermal sensitivity, 60, 60f, 319
Hydrolytic breakdown, of composite restorations, 214

I

Impressions, 339–343
    disinfection of, 342–343
    dual-arch, 342, 343f
    materials for, 339–342
        elastomeric, 340–342
        hydrocolloid, 339, 339f
        photoinitiated, 342
        polyether, 341–342
    for porcelain veneer, 359, 359f
InCeram system all-ceramic restorations, 384f, 385
Incisor, restoration for fracture of incisal edge, 358, 359f
Inlay(s)
    ceramic, 243–247. See also under Ceramic restoration(s)
    esthetic, 229–250. See also Esthetic inlay(s)/onlay(s)
    gold, 397–403. See also Gold onlay
Instrument kit, 106
    bur block in, 105f
Instrumentation
    hand, 74–97. See also Hand instrument(s)
    rotating, 97–104. See also Rotating instruments
Interproximal carver, 294–295, 295f

L

Latex allergies, rubber dam and, 136, 136f
Latex gloves, effect on addition silicone materials, 341, 342f
Lentulo spiral, for cement placement, 325, 325f
Light-curing units, 201
Liners, 58, 58f
    adhesive, 62
    categories of, 61–62
Loupes, 104, 105f
Lubricant
    lip, 122, 123f
    rubber dam, 122–123, 123f
Luting agents, 412–413. See also Cement(s)

M

Magnifiers, 104, 105f
Margins
  gap formation at, 152
  leakage from, 370
Marginal opening, of restorations, 33, 35f
Masking, for porcelain veneer placement, 367, 368f, 369
Matrices
  in anterior restorations, 187
    Class 3, 198, 199f
    Class 4, 199, 199f
  for Class 5 restorations
    amalgam, 317, 317f
    composite, 317–318, 318f
    glass-ionomer, 317, 317f
  clear, 219, 219f, 220, 221f
  in composite restorations, 187
    posterior, 219f, 219–220
    metal, 219, 219f, 220, 221f
    Mylar, 198, 199
  in provisional restorations
    of mandibular teeth, 360
    techniques for, 344, 346f
  reinforcement with modeling compound, 288, 290f, 291
Matrix system(s)
  AutoMatrix, 288, 289f
  Denovo, 288, 289f
  Omni-Matrix, 288, 289f
  Palodent, 288, 289f
  Tofflemire. See Tofflemire matrix system
Metal-ceramic restorations, 373–383
  alloys for, 380–381
  cementation of, 382–383
  design of, 376–380
  dynamic seating of, 382
  glazing procedures for, 382
  margins
    metal facial, 379, 379f, 380f
    porcelain facial, 379, 379f, 380f
  matching natural teeth in
    color and characterization of, 380, 381f
    shade guide for, 380, 381f
    shape and, 380, 381f
  occlusal contacts in
    mandibular arch, 377
    maxillary arch, 376, 377f, 378f
  porcelain systems for, 381, 382f
  precementation procedures for, 381
  preparation for, 373–374, 374f–375f
    crown margin in, 376f
    finish line in, 374, 376, 376f
  substructure of, 376, 376f
    margins and, 378, 379f
    premolar area, 377, 378f
  surface stains and, 382, 382f
Microleakage
  adhesive techniques and, 141
  in restored teeth, 11, 12f
Miniflap procedure, in Class 5 restorations, 314, 314f
Mirrors, 92f, 93

Mock-up(s)
  composite shell on diagnostic cast, 351, 353f
  intraoral of diastema closure, 351f
  wax-up, 351, 352f
Modeling compound
  in application of clamp, 119–120, 120f
  in support of metal matrix, 288, 290f, 291

N

Nerves, 17

O

Occlusion
  acceptable, 396
  adjustment of
    in amalgam restorations, 295–296
    articulating paper in, 296f
    shimstock in, 296f
  development of with casts and articulator, 396f, 396–397
Off-angle hatchet, 77
O'Leary index of plaque, 30
Onlay(s)
  esthetic, 229–250. See also under Ceramic restoration(s)
  gold, 400–403. See also Gold onlay
  porcelain, 240, 241
Oral mucosa, external appearance of, 19, 19f
Oxalate solutions, for dentin hypersensitivity, 319

P

Palm grasp, 95, 95f, 96f
Palm-thumb grasp, 95, 95f, 96f
Paper, absorbent, 138, 138f
Partial-coverage gold crowns
  advantages of, 404
  cementation of, 411–414
  description of, 404, 404f
  marginal finishing of, 410–411
  preparation for
    facial bevel in, 407f, 407–408, 408f
    final refinement in, 408, 409f
    finish lines in, 404
    lingual, 404, 405f
    mandibular, 409f
    maxillary, 409f
    occlusal, 404, 405f
    occlusal channel in, 407, 407f
    proximal, 404, 405f
    proximal grooves in, 406, 406f, 407f
  try-in of, 410
Patient evaluation. See also Problem-oriented treatment planning; Treatment Plan
  clinical examination in, 29–42
    elements of, 30
  dental history and chief complaint in, 29
  dentition in, 30–40

diagnostic casts in, 41–42
  periodontium in, 40
  radiographs in, 40–41, 41f
Pen grasp, 94f, 95, 95f
Perikymata, 3, 4f
Periodontal disease, 18, 19
Periodontal probes, 93, 93f
Periodontium
  anatomy of, 395, 395f
  evaluation of, 40
Phosphoric acid
  effect on dentin, 163f
  for enamel etching, 155, 156f
Photographs, preoperative for porcelain veneer, 352, 353f
Pin bender, 275f, 2754
Pin channel drills, 271, 272f, 273, 273f
Pin(s)
  channel preparation for, 271–274
    cavity varnish and bonding agents in, 274
    location of, 271, 272f, 273, 274f
    perforation during, 277
    size of, 274
    twist drills for, 271, 272f, 273
  in Class 4 restorations, 193, 194f
  in failed complex amalgam restoration, 279, 280f–281f
  horizontal, 276f, 277, 277f
    channel preparation for, 277
  insertion of
    bending in, 274, 275f
    by hand, 274, 275f
    with low-speed handpiece, 274, 275f
    shortening of, 276, 276f
  number to use, 271
  pin channel drills and pins, 271, 271f
  and pin drivers, 275f
  risks with, 279
  self-threading, 270
  vertical, 270–276
Pit, definition of, 70, 252
Plaque
  bacterial etiology of, 52
  O'Leary index of, 30
  pH of, 51
Plastic instruments, 87, 87f
Polishing. See Finishing and polishing
Polycarboxylate cement, for gold castings, 413
Poly(ethyl methacrylate), for provisional restorations, 344
Polymerization
  initiation at resin-tooth interface, 149f, 152
  of visible light–cured composites, 214
Polymerization shrinkage
  of composite restorations, 149, 149f, 188, 234
  with composites
    autocured and light-cured, 210, 211f
Poly(methyl methacrylate), for provisional restorations, 344
Porcelain jacket crowns, 383. See also All-ceramic restorations